T0344708

Neurobiological Basis of Migraine

Neurobiological Basis of Migraine

Edited by

Turgay Dalkara, MD, PhD
Hacettepe University
Ankara
Turkey

Michael A. Moskowitz, MD
Harvard Medical School
Massachusetts General Hospital
Boston
Massachusetts
USA

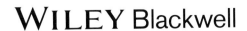

Registered Offices
John Wiley & Sons, Inc., 111 River Street, Hoboken, NJ 07030, USA

Editorial Office
111 River Street, Hoboken, NJ 07030, USA

For details of our global editorial offices, customer services, and more information about Wiley products visit us at www.wiley.com.

Wiley also publishes its books in a variety of electronic formats and by print-on-demand. Some content that appears in standard print versions of this book may not be available in other formats.

Library of Congress Cataloguing-in-Publication Data applied for.

ISBN: 9781118967195

Cover Design: Wiley
Cover Images: Courtesy of Rami Burstein; (Background) © Tetra Images/Gettyimages

Set in 10/12pt WarnockPro by SPi Global, Chennai, India
Printed and bound in Malaysia by Vivar Printing Sdn Bhd
10 9 8 7 6 5 4 3 2 1

We dedicate this book to our wives, Sevim and Mary as well as to our children and grandchildren, Deniz Dalkara-Mourot, Defne Dalkara, Jenna Moskowitz, Ozan and Esin Dalkara-Mourot, Mattia and Talia Farmer. Their unconditional support and encouragement continue as our inspiration

Contents

List of Contributors

Isamu Aiba
Developmental Neurogenetics
Laboratory
Department of Neurology
Baylor College of Medicine
Houston
Texas
USA

Messoud Ashina
Danish Headache Center, Department of
Neurology
Rigshospitalet, Glostrup
Faculty of Health and Medical Sciences
University of Copenhagen
Copenhagen
Denmark

Christopher W. Atcherley
Department of Collaborative Research
and Neurology
Mayo Clinic
Scottsdale
Arizona
USA

Cenk Ayata
Stroke Service and Neuroscience
Intensive Care Unit
Department of Neurology
Massachusetts General Hospital
Harvard Medical School
Boston
Massachusetts
USA

David A. Boas
Martinos Center for Biomedical Imaging
MGH
Harvard Medical School
Charlestown
Massachusetts
USA

David Borsook
P.A.I.N. Group
Department of Anesthesiology
Perioperative & Pain Medicine
Boston Children's Hospital, Harvard
Medical School
Boston
Massachusetts
USA

K.C. Brennan
Headache Physiology Laboratory
Departments of Neurology
University of Utah
Utah
USA

Rami Burstein
Department of Anesthesia
Critical Care and Pain Medicine
Beth Israel Deaconess Medical Center
Harvard Medical School
Boston
Massachusetts
USA

Shih-Pin Chen
Department of Neurology
Taipei Veterans General Hospital
Taipei
Taiwan

F. Michael Cutrer
Department of Neurology
Mayo Clinic
Rochester
Minnesota
USA

Markus A. Dahlem
Department of Physics
Humboldt University of Berlin
Berlin
Germany

Turgay Dalkara
Department of Neurology
Faculty of Medicine and Institute of
Neurological Sciences and Psychiatry
Hacettepe University
Ankara
Turkey

Milena De Felice
School of Clinical Dentistry
University of Sheffield
South Yorkshire
United Kingdom

Anna Devor
Departments of Neurosciences and
Radiology
UCSD
La Jolla
California
USA

David W. Dodick
Mayo Clinic Hospital
Phoenix
Arizona
USA

Gregory Dussor
Behavioral and Brain Sciences
BSB-14, The University of Texas at Dallas
Richardson
Texas
USA

Mária Dux
Department of Physiology
University of Szeged
Szeged
Hungary

Else Eising
Department of Human Genetics
Leiden University Medical Center
Leiden
The Netherlands

Michel D. Ferrari
Department of Neurology
Leiden University Medical Center
Leiden
The Netherlands

G.F. Gebhart
Center for Pain Research
Department of Anesthesiology
School of Medicine
University of Pittsburgh
Pittsburgh
Pennsylvania
USA

Peter J. Goadsby
Headache Group – NIHR-Wellcome
Trust
King's Clinical Research Facility
King's College London
London
UK

Michael S. Gold
Center for Pain Research
Department of Neurobiology
School of Medicine
University of Pittsburgh
Pittsburgh
Pennsylvania
USA

Jakob Møller Hansen
Danish Headache Center
Department of Neurology
Rigshospitalet
Glostrup
Faculty of Health and Medical Sciences
University of Copenhagen
Copenhagen
Denmark

Richard J. Hargreaves
Biogen
Cambridge
Massachusetts
USA

Duncan J. Hodkinson
P.A.I.N. Group
Department of Anesthesiology
Perioperative & Pain Medicine
Boston Children's Hospital, Harvard
Medical School
Boston
Massachusetts
USA

Kıvılcım Kılıç
Department of Neurosciences
UCSD
La Jolla
California
USA

Jonghwan Lee
Martinos Center for Biomedical Imaging
MGH
Harvard Medical School
Charlestown
Massachusetts
USA

Dan Levy
Department of Anesthesia
Critical Care and Pain Medicine
Beth Israel Deaconess Medical Center
Harvard Medical School
Boston
Massachusetts
USA

Agustin Melo-Carrillo
Department of Anesthesia
Critical Care and Pain Medicine
Beth Israel Deaconess Medical Center
Harvard Medical School
Boston
Massachusetts
USA

Karl Messlinger
Institute of Physiology and
Pathophysiology
Friedrich-Alexander University
Erlangen-Nürnberg
Erlangen
Germany

Michael A. Moskowitz
Departments of Radiology and Neurology
Massachusetts General Hospital
Harvard Medical School
Boston
Massachusetts
USA

Kelsey Nation
Department of Pharmacology
University of Arizona
Tucson
Arizona
USA

Jeffrey Noebels
Developmental Neurogenetics
Laboratory
Department of Neurology
Baylor College of Medicine
Houston
Texas
USA

Rodrigo Noseda
Department of Anesthesia
Critical Care and Pain Medicine
Beth Israel Deaconess Medical Center
Harvard Medical School
Boston
Massachusetts
USA

Michael H. Ossipov
Department of Pharmacology
University of Arizona
Tucson
Arizona
USA

Daniela Pietrobon
Department of Biomedical Sciences
University of Padova

and

CNR Institute of Neuroscience
Padova
Italy

Frank Porreca
Department of Collaborative Research
and Neurology
Mayo Clinic
Scottsdale
Arizona
USA

and

Department of Pharmacology
University of Arizona
Tucson
Arizona
USA

Andrew F. Russo
Neuroscience Program
Department of Molecular Physiology and
Biophysics
VA Center for the Prevention and
Treatment of Visual Loss
University of Iowa
Iowa City
Iowa
USA

Payam A. Saisan
Department of Neurosciences
UCSD
La Jolla
California
USA

Sava Sakadžić
Martinos Center for Biomedical Imaging
MGH
Harvard Medical School
Charlestown
Massachusetts
USA

Aaron Schain
Department of Anesthesia
Critical Care and Pain Medicine
Beth Israel Deaconess Medical Center,
Harvard Medical School
Boston
Massachusetts
USA

Ryan Smith
Department of Molecular Physiology and
Biophysics
VA Center for the Prevention and
Treatment of Visual Loss
Iowa City
Iowa
USA

Levi P. Sowers
Department of Molecular Physiology and
Biophysics
VA Center for the Prevention and
Treatment of Visual Loss
University of Iowa
Iowa City
Iowa
USA

Andrew M. Strassman
Department of Anesthesia
Critical Care and Pain Medicine
Beth Israel Deaconess Medical Center
Harvard Medical School
Boston
Massachusetts
USA

Gisela M. Terwindt
Department of Neurology
Leiden University Medical Center
Leiden
The Netherlands

Jeremy Theriot
Headache Physiology Laboratory
Department of Neurology
University of Utah
Salt Lake City
Utah
USA

Peifang Tian
Department of Physics
John Carroll University
University Heights
Ohio
USA

Else A. Tolner
Department of Neurology
Leiden University Medical Center
Leiden
The Netherlands

Annie E. Tye
Neuroscience Program
University of Iowa
Iowa City
Iowa
USA

Hana Uhlirova
Department of Radiology
UCSD
La Jolla
California
USA

Arn M.J.M. van den Maagdenberg
Department of Human Genetics
Leiden University Medical Center
Leiden
The Netherlands

Michele Viana
Headache Science Center
C. Mondino National Neurological
Institute
Pavia
Italy

Luis Villanueva
Institut National de la Santé et de la
Recherche Médicale/Université Paris
Descartes
Centre de Psychiatrie et Neurosciences
Paris
France

Sergei A. Vinogradov
Departments of Biochemistry and
Biophysics and Chemistry
University of Pennsylvania
Philadelphia
Pennsylvania
USA

Sophie L. Wilcox
P.A.I.N. Group
Department of Anesthesiology
Perioperative & Pain Medicine
Boston Children's Hospital
Harvard Medical School
Boston
Massachusetts
USA

Jennifer Y. Xie
Department of Pharmacology
University of Arizona
Tucson
Arizona
USA

Mohammad Abbas Yaseen
Martinos Center for Biomedical Imaging
MGH
Harvard Medical School
Charlestown
Massachusetts
USA

Foreword

When I studied psychology between 1969 and 1975, I took a course on psychosomatic diseases. The professor presented migraine as a typical example of disease which was clearly a psychological problem without a biological basis. There were compelling arguments, like migraine attacks triggered by stress and a strong co-morbidity with anxiety disorders. How much has changed since these times?

When I started to see migraine patients as a young neurology resident, it became immediately clear to me that migraine was clearly more than a psychological problem. Why had the psychologists neglected the results from twin studies? The phenotype of migraine attacks was extremely homogeneous across patients.

Now is the time to summarize the progress in the neurobiological basis of migraine we have made in the last 40 years. The editors have recruited the best scientists and clinicians in the field of migraine research for a display of amazing research results. We are now able to assign all phases of a migraine attack, from prodromes, aura, headache, autonomic symptoms, photo- and phonophobia and postdromes, to anatomical structures, modifications in the pain transmission and modulation system and higher cortical functions.

A major challenge is still the treatment of acute migraine attacks and migraine prevention. Triptans were developed as attack treatment, under the assumption that they would constrict dilated vessels in the dura and the base of the brain. Later, it turned out that they have major effects on pain transmission in the trigemino-thalamic pathways. We desperately need more effective and better tolerated drugs for migraine prevention. The migraine-preventive properties of available medications like beta-blockers, flunarizine, valproic acid, topiramate, amitriptyline and onabotulinum-toxin A were detected "by chance" when these drugs were used for other indications in patients with migraine. CGRP was identified as a major player in the pathophysiology of migraine. At present, four antibodies against CGRP or the CGRP receptor are under development for migraine prevention. This is a good example of translational research, where observations from pathophysiological studies have resulted in new treatment approaches.

Who should read this book? Anyone who is interested in migraine as a disease and in migraine patients. I hope that many young researchers and clinicians will become motivated to move into the very promising field of headache research.

Hans-Christoph Diener
Senior Professor of Clinical Neurosciences
Department of Neurology
University Duisburg-Essen
Essen Germany
E-Mail: hans.diener@uk-essen.de

Part I

Anatomy and physiology

1

Functional anatomy of trigeminovascular pain

Karl Messlinger[1] and Mária Dux[2]

[1] *Institute of Physiology and Pathophysiology, Friedrich-Alexander University Erlangen-Nürnberg, Erlangen, Germany*
[2] *Department of Physiology, University of Szeged, Szeged, Hungary*

1.1   Anatomy of the trigeminovascular system

The trigeminal system, consisting of afferent nerve fibers mostly arising from the trigeminal ganglion, conveys sensory information from extra- and intracranial structures to the central nervous system via the fifth cranial nerve. The term "trigeminovascular system" has been formed to describe the close morpho-functional relationship of trigeminal afferents with intracranial blood vessels, originally in the context of vascular headaches (Moskowitz, 1984). Nowadays, the term may be extended to extracranial tissues, as well as to the central projections of trigeminal afferents into the trigeminal nuclear brainstem complex, as specified below.

1.1.1   Vascularization and innervation of the dura mater encephali

Large arteries run in the outer (periosteal) layer of the dura mater, accompanied by one or two venous vessels. In the human dura, arterial branches form arterio-venous shunts and supply a rich capillary network of the inner (arachnoid-near) layer (Kerber and Newton, 1973; Roland *et al.*, 1987). The remarkable dense vascularization of the dura mater is in contrast to the light red color of meningeal veins, suggesting very low oxygen consumption that leaves other functional interpretations, such as thermoregulation, open (Zenker and Kubik, 1996; Cabanac and Brinnel, 1985).

The meningeal innervation has been studied extensively in rodents, but there is general agreement that the findings conform, in principle, with the human meningeal system. The dura mater is innervated by bundles consisting of unmyelinated and myelinated nerve fibers (Andres *et al.*, 1987), with diameters ranging from 0.1–0.4 μm (unmyelinated) and from 1–6 μm (myelinated including myelin sheath) in rat (Schueler *et al.*, 2014).

Immunohistochemical observations indicate that most of the nerve bundles consist of mixed afferent and autonomic fibers, which split up into smaller branches and, finally, into single fibers. Trigeminal fibers, which originate in the ipsilateral trigeminal ganglion, and sympathetic fibers, predominantly arising from the ipsilateral superior cervical ganglion, form dense plexus around the middle, anterior and posterior meningeal

Neurobiological Basis of Migraine, First Edition. Edited by Turgay Dalkara and Michael A. Moskowitz.
© 2017 John Wiley & Sons, Inc. Published 2017 by John Wiley & Sons, Inc.

artery, suggesting a vasomotor function (Keller and Marfurt, 1991; Mayberg *et al.*, 1984; Uddman *et al.*, 1989). An especially dense network of nerve fibers is found around dural sinuses (Andres *et al.*, 1987). In addition, a prominent system of cholinergic nerve fibers originating from the otic and sphenopalatine ganglia surrounds mainly large meningeal blood vessels (Amenta *et al.*, 1980; Edvinsson and Uddman, 1981; Artico and Cavallotti, 2001).

Ultrastructural analyses of trigeminal fibers reveal the typical details of non-corpuscular sensory endings, which can be extensively ramified, forming short bud-like extensions or longer branches at the vessel wall, but also within the connective tissue between blood vessels (Messlinger *et al.*, 1993). In addition, at sites where the cerebral (bridging) veins enter the sagittal superior sinus, non-encapsulated Ruffini-like receptor endings have been described (Andres *et al.*, 1987). Particular features of the sensory endings (von Düring *et al.*, 1990) are the free areas not covered by Schwann cells, and the equipment with vesicles and a specific fibrous plasma ("receptor matrix") accumulating adjacent to the cell membrane of the free areas (Andres *et al.*, 1987).

Functionally, the trigeminal and the parasympathetic fibers mediate arterial vasodilatation, and the postganglionic sympathetic nerve fibers mediate vasoconstriction (Jansen *et al.*, 1992; Faraci *et al.*, 1989). The vasodilatation of meningeal arteries induced by cortical spreading depression in rat was abolished after sphenopalatine ganglionectomy (Bolay *et al.*, 2002). There are multiple functional measurements of the meningeal vasoregulation, employing video microscopy and laser Doppler flowmetry, which all indicate regulation of meningeal arteries but obviously no venous vasoregulation (Gupta *et al.*, 2006; Kurosawa *et al.*, 1995; Fischer *et al.*, 2010; Williamson *et al.*, 1997).

The arterial vessels are accompanied by mast cells, arranged in a street-like manner frequently close to nerve fiber bundles, suggesting signaling functions (Dimlich *et al.*, 1991; Dimitriadou *et al.*, 1997; Keller *et al.*, 1991). In addition, extensive networks of dendritic cells with access to the cerebrospinal fluid and resident macrophages exist in all meningeal layers, suggesting competent immune functions within these tissue (McMenamin, 1999; McMenamin *et al.*, 2003).

1.1.2 Extracranial extensions of the meningeal innervation

Postmortem tracings with DiI show two systems of trigeminal fibers transversing the rat dura mater of the middle cranial fossa in a roughly orthogonal direction, one accompanying the middle meningeal artery (MMA), and the other running from the transverse sinus across the artery in a rostromedial direction (Strassman *et al.*, 2004). Recent neuronal tracing (Schueler *et al.*, 2014) has revealed that the MMA accompanying fiber plexus is formed by the spinosus nerve originating in the mandibular division (V3) of the trigeminal ganglion, while the MMA crossing plexus arises from the tentorius nerve originating in the ophthalmic division (V1). This innervation pattern conforms to the historical observations on the human meningeal system described by Luschka and Wolff's group (Luschka, 1856; Ray and Wolff, 1940).

Previous retrograde tracing studies in cat and monkey aimed at the question of whether intracranial structures may be innervated by divergent axon collaterals that also supply facial skin to explain pain referred to the surface of the head (Borges and

Moskowitz, 1983; McMahon *et al.*, 1985), but these studies brought no evidence for this hypothesis. Recently, however, it became clear that the rodent meningeal nerve fibers may traverse the cranium, and may communicate with extracranial structures such as the galea aponeurotica (Kosaras *et al.*, 2009). Postmortem anterogradely traced meningeal nerve fibers in rat and human preparations were found to split up in several branches, some of which pass through sutures and along emissary veins and innervate the periosteum and deep layers of pericranial muscles (Schueler *et al.*, 2014). *In vivo* retrograde tracing has confirmed this, and functional measurements have showed that at least some of the nerve fibers innervating pericranial muscles are collaterals of meningeal afferents innervating the dura mater (Schueler *et al.*, 2013; Zhao and Levy, 2014).

1.1.3 Neuropeptides and their receptors in meningeal tissues

Immunohistochemical studies have identified various neuropeptides in nerve fibers innervating the dura mater (O'Connor and van der Kooy, 1986; von Düring *et al.*, 1990; Keller and Marfurt, 1991; Messlinger *et al.*, 1993) and blood vessels of the pia mater in different species, including humans (Edvinsson *et al.*, 1988; You *et al.*, 1995). The peptidergic nerve fibers form a dense network around blood vessels, but can also be found in non-vascular regions of the dura mater (Messlinger *et al.*, 1993; Strassman *et al.*, 2004). Meningeal nerve fibers immunoreactive for calcitonin gene-related peptide (CGRP), substance P (SP) or neurokinin A (NKA) are considered to be afferents of the trigeminal sensory system. A few nerve fibers immunopositive for pituitary adenylate cyclase-activating polypeptide (PACAP) have been found in rat dura mater, some of them colocalized with CGRP, indicating two likely sources of PACAP-containing fibers: a minor sensory and a larger putatively parasympathetic one (Edvinsson *et al.*, 2001). SP-like immunoreactivity is found coexpressed with CGRP in a small proportion of thin unmyelinated nerve fibers. However, the CGRP-immunoreactive nerve fibers outnumber the SP-positive ones and, consequently, many CGRP-containing fibers display no SP-immunoreactivity. The majority of the CGRP-immunoreactive fibers are distributed to branches of the anterior and middle meningeal arteries, and to the superior sagittal and transverse sinuses (Keller and Marfurt, 1991; Messlinger *et al.*, 1993).

Nerve fibers immunoreactive for neuropeptide Y (NPY), which are most likely of sympathetic origin, are also found located around cerebral and dural blood vessels of human and rodents (Edvinsson and Uddman, 1981; Edvinsson *et al.*, 1998). These nerve fibers are similarly numerous in the cranial dura mater (Keller *et al.*, 1989). They form generally more intimate contact with the blood vessel wall than sensory peptidergic fibers (von Düring *et al.*, 1990; Keller and Marfurt, 1991; Edvinsson *et al.*, 1987). NPY potentiates the vasoconstrictor action of noradrenaline (Jansen *et al.*, 1992). In addition, a sparse innervation of nerve fibers immunoreactive for vasoactive intestinal polypeptide (VIP), most likely of parasympathetic origin, has been identified around dural and pial blood vessels in different species (Keller and Marfurt, 1991; Edvinsson *et al.*, 1998).

Release of VIP from the parasympathetic endings induces vasodilatation in meningeal tissues (Jansen *et al.*, 1992). Nitric oxide synthase (NOS) immunoreactivity has been identified in some trigeminal sensory neurons, and in parasympathetic postganglionic fibers innervating pial arteries and proximal parts of the anterior and middle cerebral arteries. In some of these neurons, NOS is colocalized with VIP, implying a modulatory role of nitric oxide (NO) on VIP-induced vasorelaxation (Nozaki *et al.*, 1993).

Antibodies raised against two components of the CGRP receptor, the calcitonin receptor-like receptor (CLR) and the receptor activity-modifying protein 1 (RAMP1), mark smooth muscle of dural arterial blood vessels, as well as mononuclear and Schwann cells (Lennerz *et al.*, 2008). Also, some thicker CGRP-negative A-fibers of rodent and human dura may express CLR and RAMP1 (Eftekhari *et al.*, 2013). Binding of CGRP to the vascular CGRP receptors in dural and pial tissues causes vasodilatation and increased meningeal blood flow (Edvinsson *et al.*, 1987; Kurosawa *et al.*, 1995). Endothelial cells of blood vessels in the dura mater and in cerebral blood vessels express the neurokinin-1 (NK-1) receptor. SP acting at the NK-1 receptor appears to be mainly responsible for plasma extravasation (Stubbs *et al.*, 1992; O'Shaughnessy and Connor, 1993), but intravascular SP may also cause dilatation of cerebral microvessels (Kobari *et al.*, 1996).

Blockade of NK-1 receptors effectively reduces the plasma protein extravasation in the rodent dura, acting most likely on postcapillary venules (Shepheard *et al.*, 1993; Lee *et al.*, 1994). Both CGRP and NK-1 receptors are also expressed on the surface of mononuclear cells, most of which may be mast cells (Ottosson and Edvinsson, 1997; Lennerz *et al.*, 2008). Release of CGRP and SP from peripheral terminals of meningeal afferents may thus degranulate dural mast cells and release their vasoactive mediator content, such as histamine (Schwenger *et al.*, 2007). In addition, application of the neuropeptide PACAP can degranulate mast cells, but the receptor type mediating this effect is not yet clear (Baun *et al.*, 2012). Mast cell degranulation is considered as a peripheral component of headache pathophysiology (Levy, 2009), but vasodilatation and neurogenic plasma extravasation induced by SP release seems to be negligible in the generation or maintenance of headaches (Dux *et al.*, 2012; see Figure 1.1).

Figure 1.1 Peripheral trigeminovascular structures of nociceptive transduction. Thin myelinated and unmyelinated afferent fibers (Aδ/C, yellow) of all trigeminal partitions and autonomic fibers, mostly postsynaptic sympathetic (Sy) and few parasympathetic fibers (Pa) innervate the cranial dura mater and cerebral arteries, which run on the cortical surface through the subarachnoidal space. Collaterals of meningeal Aδ/C fibers transverse the cranium and innervate also periosteum and deep layers of pericranial muscles. The inset shows multiple G-protein coupled receptors and ion channels involved in sensory transduction and efferent functions of Aδ and C fibers: Voltage-gated sodium and calcium channels (Na_v, Ca_v) cause excitation and release of neuropeptides like CGRP and substance P (SP), which can also be induced by opening of calcium conducting transient potential receptor channels (TRPV1, TRPA1) activated by thermal and chemical stimuli. TRPV1 and acid sensing ion channels (ASIC3) respond to low pH, purinergic receptor channels ($P2X_3$) and receptors (P2Y) to purines like ATP. CGRP activates CGRP receptors on arterial smooth muscle cells causing vasodilatation, which is supported by vasodilatory substances like VIP released from parasympathetic fibers (Pa), whereas vasoconstriction is caused by monoamines like norepinephrine (NE) released from sympathtic efferents (Sy). SP induces mainly plasma extravasation through endothelial NK-1 receptors. CGRP and SP can also degranulate mast cells (MC), thereby releasing tryptase (Try) that activates afferent PAR-2 receptors and histamine (HA) that causes arterial vasodilatation through H2 receptors. Vascular serotonin ($5\text{-}HT_{1B}$) and afferent $5\text{-}HT_{1D/1F}$ as well as cannabinoid (CB1) receptors are inhibitory, acting against vasodilatation and neuropeptide release.

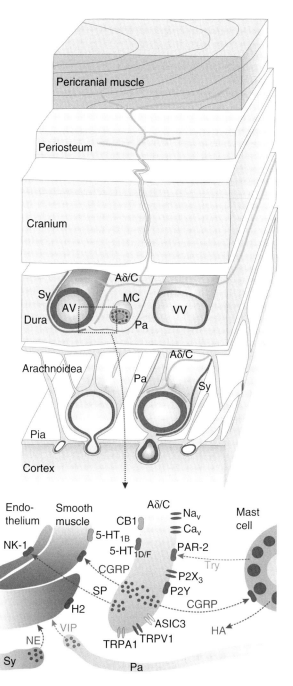

1.1.4 Transduction channels and receptors in the trigeminovascular system

Chemosensitive meningeal afferents express different members of the transient receptor potential (TRP) cation channel family. In rats, a dense network of TRP vanilloid 1 (TRPV1) channel expressing fibers has been identified (Huang *et al.*, 2012). TRPV1 immunoreactivity is colocalized with CGRP in most of the afferents (Hou *et al.*, 2002; Dux *et al.*, 2003), which has proved to be sensitive to capsaicin (Dux *et al.*, 2007). TRPV1 cannot only be activated by exogenous substances like capsaicin or resiniferatoxin, but also by noxious heat, acidic pH (pH < 5.3) and different endogenous compounds such as some membrane lipid metabolites (anandamide, N-arachidonoyl-dopamine; Price *et al.*, 2004).

The TRP ankyrin 1 (TRPA1) ion channel is another member of the TRP receptor family that is highly colocalized with TRPV1 receptors on trigeminal neurons innervating the dura mater and activated by substances like mustard oil and cannabinoids (Salas *et al.*, 2009; Jordt *et al.*, 2004). Recent observations indicate the activation of trigeminal TRPA1 receptors as a link between the two major vasodilator mechanisms. Vasodilatation induced by the production of NO in the vascular endothelium and by release of CGRP from trigeminal afferents (Eberhardt *et al.*, 2014) – that is, nitroxyl (HNO), the one-electron-reduced sibling of NO, modifies cysteine residues of the receptor, leading to activation of the ion channel and consequent release of CGRP. TRPA1 receptors can also be activated by environmental irritants or a volatile constituent of the "headache tree" – the umbellulone (Nassini *et al.*, 2012). Given that TRPA1 receptors are expressed not only on intracranial axons but also on their extracranial collaterals innervating (e.g., nasal mucosa, periosteum and pericranial muscles) (Schueler *et al.*, 2014), nociceptive stimulation of extracranial tissues may activate intracranial collaterals by an axon reflex mechanism, release vasoactive neuropeptides in meningeal tissue, increase intracranial blood flow, and contribute to the pathomechanisms of headaches (Schueler *et al.*, 2013).

Sensitization of meningeal nociceptors by a variety of blood- and tissue-borne agents may be an important peripheral mechanism in the initiation of headaches (Burstein *et al.*, 1998a). The proteinase activated receptor 2 (PAR-2), activated through cleavage by the serine protease tryptase released from stimulated mast cells, amplifies the vasodilatation caused by sensory neuropeptides (Bhatt *et al.*, 2010) and possibly also the central transmission of nociceptive signals (Zhang and Levy, 2008). The effect of PAR-2 activation is at least partly mediated by TRPV1 and TRPA1 receptor sensitization (Dux *et al.*, 2009).

Acid-sensing ion channels (ASICs), predominantly the ASIC3 subtype responding to low meningeal pH, has been identified on meningeal afferents (Yan *et al.*, 2011). ASICs are members of the ENaC/DEG (epithelial amiloride-sensitive Na^+ channel and degenerin) family of ion channels (Wemmie *et al.*, 2006). Acidic metabolites may be released by activated mast cells, or during ischemia developing as a consequence of cortical spreading depression linked to the aura phase of migraine.

Purinergic P2Y receptors and P2X receptor channels activated by ATP are richly expressed in trigeminal afferents, partly colocalized with TRPV1 receptors (Ichikawa and Sugimoto, 2004; Ruan and Burnstock, 2003).The majority (52%) of retrogradely labeled trigeminal ganglion neurons innervating the dura mater expresses either $P2X_2$ or $P2X_3$ or both receptors (Staikopoulos *et al.*, 2007). ATP enhances the proton-induced

CGRP release through P2Y receptors from the isolated rat dura mater (Zimmermann *et al.*, 2002). Conversely, CGRP caused delayed upregulation of purinergic P2X receptors in cultivated trigeminal ganglion neurons (Fabbretti *et al.*, 2006).

G-protein-coupled 5-HT$_{1D/1F}$ receptors are located on peripheral and central terminals of meningeal afferents (Amrutkar *et al.*, 2012; Buzzi and Moskowitz, 1991). Their activation inhibits the release of neuropeptides and transmitters from the trigeminal afferents, leading to attenuation of the central transmission of nociceptive signals. Recent findings indicate the presence of 5-HT$_7$ receptors on trigeminal terminals. Vasodilatation induced by the activation of trigeminal 5-HT$_7$ receptors seems to be the result of CGRP release from nerve terminals (Wang *et al.*, 2014).

In the trigeminal system, cannabinoid CB1 receptor immunoreactive neurons are found mainly in the maxillary and mandibular divisions of the trigeminal nerve (Price *et al.*, 2003). Activation of trigeminal CB1 receptors inhibits arterial blood vessel dilatation induced by electrical stimulation of the dura mater (Akerman *et al.*, 2004) and CGRP release induced by thermal stimulation in an *in vitro* dura mater preparation (Fischer and Messlinger, 2007). Activation of CB1 receptors may have a particular role in the regulation of CGRP release from TRPV1 expressing neurons, since both receptors can be activated by the same endogenous lipid metabolites as anandamide and N-arachidonoyl-dopamine, acting on both TRPV1 and CB1 receptors with different efficacies (Price *et al.*, 2004; Figure 1.1).

1.2   Trigeminal ganglion

The trigeminal ganglion is located extracranially in the Meckel's space and wrapped with a duplicature of the cranial dura mater. It is subdivided into the ophthalmic (V1), maxillary (V2) and mandibular (V3) division, and contains the cell bodies of the respective sensory trigeminal nerves. Furthermore, transition of nerve fibers of mesencephalic trigeminal neurons has been found in all three partitions within the trigeminal nerve (Byers *et al.*, 1986).

1.2.1   Types of trigeminal ganglion cells

The number of trigeminal ganglion cells varies considerably. In human trigeminal ganglia, 20–35 thousand neurons and about 100 times more non-neuronal cells have been counted (LaGuardia *et al.*, 2000). Each cell body is surrounded by satellite glial cells, other cell types are resident microglia-like macrophages (Glenn *et al.*, 1993) and fibroblasts. A functional crosstalk between neurons and macrophages and/or satellite glial cells is assumed, at least in pathological states (Franceschini *et al.*, 2012, 2013; Villa *et al.*, 2010).

1.2.2   Neuropeptides and their receptors in the trigeminal ganglion

The largest peptidergic neuron population in the trigeminal ganglion expresses CGRP. In different species, including human, immunoreactivity for CGRP is found in 29–49% of trigeminal ganglion neurons (Alvarez *et al.*, 1991; Eftekhari *et al.*, 2010; Lennerz *et al.*, 2008), predominantly in small and medium-sized cells. Accordingly,

CGRP immunoreactivity is preferably found in unmyelinated fibers of the trigeminal nerve (Bae *et al.*, 2015). In a minor group of neurons, CGRP is coexpressed with SP immunoreactivity (Lee *et al.*, 1985), which has been found in up to 33% of neurons (Del Fiacco *et al.*, 1990; Prins *et al.*, 1993; Prośba-Mackiewicz *et al.*, 2000). The isolectin IB4 from *Griffonia simplicifolia*, which binds to a subpopulation of small trigeminal ganglion neurons, stains less than 25% of CGRP or SP immunoreactive neurons (Ambalavanar and Morris, 1992). Immunoreactivity for PACAP is present in 29% of neurons, of which CGRP is coexpressed in 23% (Eftekhari *et al.*, 2015).

Immunoreactivity for the CLR and RAMP1 components of the CGRP receptor has been found in Schwann and satellite cells, and in a large proportion of neurons, but colocalization with CGRP is extremely rare (Alvarez *et al.*, 1991; Eftekhari *et al.*, 2010; Lennerz *et al.*, 2008). *In vitro* studies have provided evidence that CGRP release from neurons can stimulate surrounding satellite cells to increase intracellular calcium, which leads to an enhancement of purinergic (P2Y) receptors (Ceruti *et al.*, 2011), expression of different cytokines (Vause and Durham, 2010) and release of NO (Li *et al.*, 2008). In this way, CGRP could function as a paracrine factor to stimulate nearby glial cells and neurons (Figure 1.2).

Human trigeminal ganglia express all three receptor subtypes of the VIP/PACAP receptor family VPAC1, VPAC2 and PAC1 (Knutsson and Edvinsson, 2002). Provided that trigeminal ganglion neurons can release PACAP, the presence of PAC1 receptors on neuron somata suggests the possible existence of a signaling pathway for PACAP-mediated communication between neighboring trigeminal sensory neurons (Chaudhary and Baumann, 2002).

Figure 1.2 Trigeminal ganglion (TG) and structures in the trigeminal nuclear brainstem complex (TBNC) subserving nociceptive transmission. While the central processes of most mechanoreceptive Aβ fibers of the trigeminal ganglion (TG) project to the pontine subnucleus principalis (Vp), Aδ and C fibers run down the spinal trigeminal tract terminating in the spinal trigeminal nucleus (Vsp). Intracranial afferents terminate mainly in the trigemino-cervical complex (TCC), which is composed of subnucleus caudalis (Vc) and the dorsal horn of the first cervical segments (C1-3), and some also in the subnucleus interpolaris (Vi). The upper inset shows two trigeminal afferents with C fibers, wrapped by Schwann cells (SC), and somata, surrounded by satellite glial cells (SGC). The neuropeptides CGRP and PACAP are expressed by major proportions of TG neurons and may be released within the TG. VPAC and PAC receptors are present on neurons. CGRP receptors are present on neurons not producing CGRP, on SGC and SC, possibly enabling crosstalk between neurons and glia, which may include nitric oxide (NO) release from SGC. The lower inset shows important neuronal elements of transmission. Voltage-dependent conduction channels (Na_v, Ca_v) subserve depolarisation and neurotransmitter release. Glutamate (Glu), as the main transmitter, activates NMDA and non-NMDA receptor channels and metabotropic glutamate receptors (mGluR) on second-order neurons, among them projection neurons (PN) projecting to the thalamus and other nuclei involved in nociceptive processing. Glutamate receptors are also found presynaptically, possibly modulating neurotransmitter and neuropeptide release. The same function may apply to activating CGRP and purinergic ($P2X_3$) receptors and inhibiting $5-HT_1$ receptors, while SP may preferably act through postsynaptic NK-1 receptors. Inhibitory interneurons (IN) release GABA and other inhibitory neurotransmitters acting pre- and postsynaptically through $GABA_A$ receptor channels and $GABA_B$ receptors.

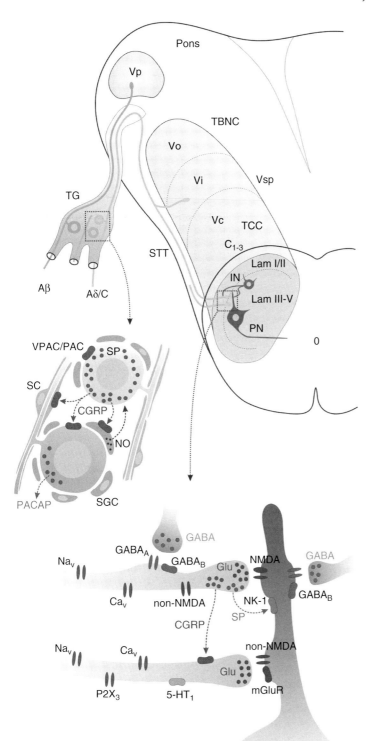

1.2.3   Representation of intracranial structures in the trigeminal ganglion

According to old anatomic observations in primates, all three divisions of the trigeminal nerve contribute to the innervation of the meninges (McNaughton, 1938), though not equally. Tracing experiments using application of horseradish peroxidase (HRP) to dural structures in the cat has confirmed this view (Steiger and Meakin, 1984). Afferents around the middle meningeal artery are found projecting predominantly to the ophthalmic division (V1) of the ipsilateral trigeminal ganglion, but to a minor extent also to the maxillary (V2) and mandibular (V3) divisions (Mayberg *et al.*, 1984). The medial anterior cranial fossa and the tentorium cerebelli are represented mainly in V1, the orbital region of the anterior cranial fossa in V2 (Steiger and Meakin, 1984). In the rat, retrograde labeling with DiI of the dural spinosus nerve stains neuronal cell bodies, preferably in the V3 and, to a lesser extent, in the V2 division (Schueler *et al.*, 2014). True blue application to the middle meningeal artery labels not only ipsilateral trigeminal ganglion cells, but also some neurons in the contralateral trigeminal ganglion and in the dorsal root ganglion at the C2 level (Uddman *et al.*, 1989).

HRP labeled cell bodies innervating the intracranial carotid and the middle cerebral artery in the cat are located in the ophthalmic division of the trigeminal ganglion (Steiger and Meakin, 1984). Using Wallerian degeneration in monkey, the vessels of the circle of Willis are also found to be innervated by the V1 division, with a small maxillary contribution (Simons and Ruskell, 1988). In the rat, retrograde HRP labeling around basal intracranial arteries (Arbab *et al.*, 1986) and true blue labeling of the middle cerebral artery (Edvinsson *et al.*, 1989) is found not only in the trigeminal ganglion, but also in the first and preferably the second cervical spinal ganglion.

1.3   Trigeminal brainstem nuclear complex

1.3.1   Organization of the trigeminal brainstem nuclear complex

The trigeminal nerve enters the brain stem at the pontine level and projects to the trigeminal brain stem nuclear complex (TBNC), which is composed of the principal sensory nucleus (Vp) and the spinal trigeminal nucleus (Vsp). The bulk of myelinated mechanoreceptive afferents projects to the Vp, while both large diameter and small diameter fibers descend in the spinal trigeminal tract and project into the Vsp, which is subdivided into the rostral subnucleus oralis (Vo), the middle subnucleus interpolaris (Vi), and the caudal subnucleus caudalis (Vc) (Olszewski, 1950). The Vc is often referred to as the medullary dorsal horn (MDH), and some researchers emphasize its anatomic and functional transition to the cervical dorsal horn, terming the Vc, including the dorsal horn of the C1-C3 segments, trigeminocervical nucleus (TCN) (Goadsby *et al.*, 2001; Hoskin *et al.*, 1999). Using transganglionic tracing, central trigeminal terminals have been found throughout the TBNC and sparsely in the upper cervical dorsal horn, even contralaterally (Marfurt, 1981; Figure 1.2).

Gobel *et al.* (1977) proposed a laminar subdivision of the MDH similar to Rexed's nomenclature of the spinal dorsal horn (Rexed, 1952), in which lamina I corresponds to the marginal layer, lamina II to the substantia gelatinosa, and laminae III and IV to the magnocellular region. The most ventral lamina V merges with the medullary reticular formation without clear boundary (Nord and Kyler, 1968). Within the spinal trigeminal tract, some groups of neurons are termed interstitial islands of Cajal, or paratrigeminal or interstitial nucleus (Phelan and Falls, 1989). These cells may be homologues to laminae I and II neurons of the Vc, according to their nociceptive specific character and small receptive fields (Davis and Dostrovsky, 1988). Anatomical and electrophysiological studies have demonstrated that the Vp and the subnuclei of the Vsp are topographically organized in a largely ventrodorsal direction (Hayashi *et al.*, 1984; Shigenaga *et al.*, 1986; Strassman and Vos, 1993). Mandibular afferents terminate preferentially in the dorsal region, ophthalmic afferents terminate ventrally, and maxillary afferents terminate in between.

Early anatomical and neurophysiological studies suggest that each subnucleus receives information from all parts of the head (Kruger *et al.*, 1961; Torvik, 1956). The rostrocaudal axis of the face is represented from rostral to caudal in the TBNC in an "onion-leaf-like" fashion (Yokota and Nishikawa, 1980; Jacquin *et al.*, 1986). Labeling of various mandibular nerves in the rat with HRP has revealed that the oral afferents tend to terminate most heavily in the rostral TBNC, whereas the posterior perioral-auricular afferents terminate preferentially in the caudal aspect of the complex (Jacquin *et al.*, 1988).

It is not entirely clear if a similar somatotopic distribution in ventrodorsal and rostrocaudal directions exists for intracranial trigeminal structures.

1.3.2 Nociceptive afferent projections to the spinal trigeminal nucleus

The Vc is primarily responsible for processing nociceptive and temperature information, whereas the Vp is involved in processing tactile information. Trigeminal tractotomy (i.e., transection of the spinal trigeminal tract at the level of the obex) has been found to relieve facial pain (Sjoqvist, 1938). Isolated lesions of the Vc cause complete or partial loss of pain and temperature sensation on the ipsilateral side, whereas tactile sensations remain nearly intact (Lisney, 1983). These clinical data have been supplemented with a large body of neurophysiological evidence showing that the Vc is essential for the perception of pain in trigeminal tissues. Since the loss of facial pain sensation after trigeminal tractotomy is not complete, but frequently spares peri- and intraoral areas, rostral parts of the TNBC may contribute to trigeminal nociception in the oral region (Young, 1982). Similarly, behavioral responses to noxious orofacial stimuli may persist following tractotomy or Vc lesions in animals (Vyklický *et al.*, 1977) while, conversely, nociceptive responsiveness and intraoral pain may be diminished by more rostral lesions of the trigeminal complex (Broton and Rosenfeld, 1986; Graham *et al.*, 1988).

The projection of nociceptive facial afferents to the spinal trigeminal nucleus has been studied by a series of elegant experiments combining intraaxonal recordings in the Vsp and HRP injections to examine the central terminations of labeled axons. Hayashi (1985) found high-threshold mechanoreceptive Aδ afferents in the cat forming extensive terminal arbors in superficial layers of the Vi as well as in lamina I and, to a lesser extent, in outer lamina II of the Vc. Jacquin *et al.* (1986, 1988) confirmed these findings in the rat, and localized a second termination area in laminae III to V of the Vc. In line with the above findings, the sensory projection from the cornea, which is thought to be mainly nociceptive, has been shown to be focused in the outer laminae of Vc (Panneton and Burton, 1981).

The projection of intracranial trigeminal afferents to the TNBC has not been studied in detail by axonal tracing, but functional data suggest a similar distribution as for the facial nociceptive afferents.

1.3.3 Functional representation of meningeal structures in the spinal trigeminal nucleus

Electrophysiological studies in the cat have shown that the cranial meninges are mainly represented in Vc, but also in Vi and Vo (Davis and Dostrovsky, 1988). The neurons in Vc are preferentially located in the ventrolateral (ophthalmic) portion of the nucleus. Nearly all Vc neurons with meningeal afferent input evoked from the middle meningeal artery and the superior sagittal sinus (SSS) have facial receptive fields located in the ophthalmic division, whereas a considerable proportion of neurons in Vo and Vi have facial receptive fields in maxillary and mandibular areas. These neurons are typically nociceptive, responding either exclusively (nociceptive-specific) or at a higher rate of action potentials (wide-dynamic range) to noxious mechanical stimuli.

Another cluster of neurons with input from the SSS has been found to be located in the dorsal horn of the upper cervical spinal cord, particularly in C2 (Lambert *et al.*, 1991; Storer and Goadsby, 1997). This meningeal representation is largely confirmed by measuring regional blood flow and metabolism, using the 2-deoxyglucose method, and by c-fos expression following electrical and mechanical stimulation of dural structures (Goadsby and Zagami, 1991; Hoskin *et al.*, 1999; Kaube *et al.*, 1993). Remarkably, two-thirds of the neurons in the upper cervical cord of the cat have convergent input from the superior sagittal sinus and the occipital nerve (Angus-Leppan *et al.*, 1997), and a similar convergent input has been found in the rat (Bartsch and Goadsby, 2003).

In the rat, the number of neurons activated by electrical stimulation of dural sites (sinus transversus or parietal dura mater) peaks in the caudal Vc, but there is another cluster around the obex level corresponding to the Vi/Vc region (Burstein *et al.*, 1998b; Schepelmann *et al.*, 1999). Intracellular labeling has shown that such neurons give rise to an extensive axonal projection system that arborizes at multiple levels of the Vc and the caudal part of the Vi (Strassman *et al.*, 1994a). The widespread meningeal representation extending from upper cervical to medullary levels has also been confirmed by immunocytochemical labeling for c-fos (Strassman *et al.*, 1994b). As in the cat, most of these neurons have convergent cutaneous input, and their facial receptive fields are located in periorbital, frontal or parietal areas – that is, the same areas in which the patients of the early investigators like Ray and Wolff (1940) felt head pain elicited by stimulation of supratentorial dural structures. It appears possible that neurons in the Vc/C1-2 region are most important in signaling nociceptive information to higher centers of the CNS, whereas the Vi/Vc region may be more involved in autonomic and motor reflexes, as has been suggested for neurons with corneal afferent input (Meng *et al.*, 1997).

1.3.4 Efferent projections from the spinal trigeminal nucleus

There have been numerous reports about efferent projections from the spinal trigeminal nucleus to higher centers of the CNS in various species (Stewart and King, 1963; Tiwari and King, 1973; Ring and Ganchrow, 1983; Van Ham and Yeo, 1992). Old data in the cat used reversible block of nuclei and antidromic stimulation to show that neurons in the Vc are mainly relayed in the contralateral ventroposteromedial nucleus (VPM) to neurons projecting into the somatosensory cortex (Rowe and Sessle, 1968), which has recently been confirmed (Lambert *et al.*, 2014). In addition, projections from the Vc to the contra- and ipsilateral nucleus submedius and the intralaminar nuclei centralis medialis and lateralis have been identified by HRP tracing in the rat (Peschanski, 1984).

Using tracing techniques, projections to the nucleus of the solitary tract (Menétrey and Basbaum, 1987), facial nucleus (Hinrichsen and Watson, 1983), the contralateral inferior olivar complex (Huerta *et al.*, 1983), the parabrachial and the Kölliker-Fuse nucleus (Cechetto *et al.*, 1985; Panneton *et al.*, 1994), the tectum and the cerebellar cortex (Steindler, 1985; Yatim *et al.*, 1996) and even the ventral cochlear nucleus (Haenggeli *et al.*, 2005) have been identified. Neurons with intracranial afferent input in the Vc and the cervical dorsal horn at the level of C1 have been found projecting to the hypothalamus, which may be of significance regarding endocrine and rhythmic disorders in migraine (Malick and Burstein, 1998; Malick *et al.*, 2000).

In addition to the ascending projections, spinal trigeminal neurons have been seen projecting ipsilaterally to all levels of the spinal cord and forming an extensive network of efferent connections, which may be important for motor reflexes associated with cranial pain (Ruggiero *et al.*, 1981; Hayashi *et al.*, 1984).

1.3.5 Neuropeptides and their receptors in the trigeminal nucleus

Corresponding to the distribution of nociceptive afferent terminals visualized by neuronal tracing, SP and CGRP immunoreactive nerve fibers are localized in different species, including humans, preferentially in Vc and in the caudal part of Vi, but less in Vo and Vp (Boissonade *et al.*, 1993; Helme and Fletcher, 1983; Pearson and Jennes, 1988; Tashiro *et al.*, 1991). The nerve fibers are mainly located in outer laminae I and II (substantia gelatinosa) of the Vsp, where CGRP immunoreactivity appears most dense (Lennerz *et al.*, 2008; Tashiro *et al.*, 1991). SP immunoreactivity is also found in deeper layers (IV/V; Salt *et al.*, 1983). Also in the human trigeminal tract, the proportion of nerve fibers immunoreactive for CGRP is higher than that immunoreactive for SP (Smith *et al.*, 2002).

In contrast, another study revealed a rich supply of SP and a moderate supply of CGRP- and PACAP-immunoreactive nerve fibers in the human Vc and dorsal horn at the C1-2 level (Uddman *et al.*, 2002). After trigeminal rhizotomy in the cat, most of the CGRP immunoreactive fibers disappeared throughout the TBNC, whereas a certain number of SP immunoreactive fibers remained intact (Henry *et al.*, 1996; Tashiro *et al.*, 1991), suggesting that these are of central origin. SP immunoreactive fibers originating from neurons in lamina I of the MDH have been found projecting into the hypothalamus (Li *et al.*, 1997) and to the solitary tract (Guan *et al.*, 1998).

Morphological and functional data suggest that neuropeptides are implicated in the trigeminal nociceptive processing within the Vsp. Following electrical stimulation of the trigeminal ganglion in the rat, depletion of CGRP, SP and NKA immunoreactivity have been observed in the ipsilateral medullary brainstem (Samsam *et al.*, 2000). Noxious stimulation causes CGRP release from medullary brainstem slices (Jenkins *et al.*, 2004; Kageneck *et al.*, 2014). Microiontophoretic injections of CGRP into the cat trigeminocervical complex at C1/2 level increases the firing of second order neurons to electrical stimulation of the dura mater or glutamate injection, reversed by CGRP receptor blockade (Storer *et al.*, 2004a).

Electron microscopy in the cat Vsp has revealed CGRP immunoreactivity within the substantia gelatinosa in axon terminals presynaptic to dendritic profiles (Henry *et al.*, 1996). Immunoreactivity for CLR and RAMP1, components of the CGRP receptor, has been observed associated with terminals of trigeminal afferents in the rat trigeminal tract entering Vsp (Lennerz *et al.*, 2008). Neither CGRP nor its receptor components have been identified in cell bodies of the Vsp. The functional interpretation of these findings is that CGRP-releasing terminals of primary afferents synapse at CGRP receptor-expressing central axons of trigeminal neurons. The action of CGRP within the trigeminal nucleus is most likely a presynaptic effect, whereby distinct terminals of primary afferents control the neurotransmitter release in other populations of primary afferents (Messlinger *et al.*, 2011; Figure 1.2).

Stimulation of the rat dura mater with acidic solution provokes release of immunoreactive SP in the rat medullary trigeminal brain stem measured with the microprobe technique (Schaible *et al.*, 1997). Henry *et al.* (1980) found that iontophoretical administration of SP in the cat Vc selectively activates nociceptive neurons. In the rat, iontophoretically applied SP has predominantly excitatory actions on both nociceptive and non-nociceptive nucleus caudalis neurons (Salt *et al.*, 1983). Selective blockade of the receptors for SP (NK-1) or NKA (NK-2), as well as NMDA and non-NMDA receptors (see below) reduced the expression of c-fos protein following corneal stimulation in the rat Vc (Bereiter and Bereiter, 1996; Bereiter *et al.*, 1998).

1.3.6 Channels and receptors involved in synaptic transmission in the trigeminal nucleus

Trigeminal afferents projecting to the spinal trigeminal nucleus release glutamate as primary excitatory neurotransmitter, binding to glutamate receptors of various types expressed pre- and postsynaptically. Activation of NMDA and non-NMDA receptors of second order neurons seems to play a dominant role in the transmission of nociceptive information (Leong *et al.*, 2000). Blockade of NMDA receptors reduces c-fos expression in the Vsp following stimulation of the superior sagittal sinus in the cat (Classey *et al.*, 2001). Ultrastructural data suggest that kainate receptors mediate nociceptive transmission postsynaptic to SP-containing afferents, but may also modulate the presynaptic release of neuropeptides and glutamate in the trigeminal nucleus (Hegarty *et al.*, 2007). Metabotropic glutamate receptors seem to be involved in the mechanisms of long-term potentiation in the Vsp (Youn, 2014). Recent expression studies show that glutamatergic neurons in the Vsp projecting to the thalamus differ from projecting neurons in the Vp by their exclusive equipment with vesicular glutamate transporter VGLUT2 (Ge *et al.*, 2014).

Agonists of the 5-HT$_{1B/1D/1F}$ receptors, which act on central terminals of meningeal afferents, modulate glutamate release (Choi *et al.*, 2012) that may play a central role in trigeminovascular activation, central sensitization and cortical spreading depression (Amrutkar *et al.*, 2012). Glutamatergic kainate receptors may also be targets of the migraine prophylactics topiramate (Andreou and Goadsby, 2011).

Immunohistochemical observations indicate that GABA receptors are involved in both pre- and postsynaptic inhibitory mechanisms of synaptic transmission in the

Vc (Basbaum *et al.*, 1986). GABA receptor activation has been shown to decrease c-fos expression in the Vc following intracisternal application of capsaicin (Cutrer *et al.*, 1995), and to attenuate the activity of neurons in the TNC, following electrical stimulation of cat sinus sagittalis (Storer *et al.*, 2004b).

Purinergic receptors have long been assumed to be involved in nociceptive transduction but also transmission in the spinal trigeminal system (Burnstock, 2009). Throughout the whole TBNC, thin nerve fibers immunoreactive for $P2X_3$ receptors are seen, mostly colocalized with the nonpeptidergic marker IB4, and sometimes with SP immunoreactivity (Kim *et al.*, 2008). The distribution is most dense in the superficial laminae of Vc, especially in the inner lamina II, and appears in electron microscopic sections presynaptic to dendrites or postsynaptic to axonal endings, suggesting different modes of nociceptive transmission (Figure 1.2).

A direct descending orexinergic projection, terminating in the spinal and trigeminal dorsal horn (Hervieu *et al.*, 2001; Marcus *et al.*, 2001), is considered to play a role in central pain modulation. Orexin is believed to have a major role in modulating the release of glutamate and other amino acid transmitters dependent on the wake-sleep rhythm (Siegel, 2004). In an animal model of trigeminovascular nociception, systemically administered orexin A was found to significantly inhibit nociceptive responses of neurons in the TNC to electrical stimulation of the dura mater surrounding the middle meningeal artery (Holland *et al.*, 2006).

References

Akerman, S., Kaube, H., Goadsby, P.J. (2004). Anandamide acts as a vasodilator of dural blood vessels *in vivo* by activating TRPV1 receptors. *British Journal of Pharmacology* **142**: 1354–1360.

Alvarez, F.J., Morris, H.R., Priestley, J.V. (1991). Sub-populations of smaller diameter trigeminal primary afferent neurons defined by expression of calcitonin gene-related peptide and the cell surface oligosaccharide recognized by monoclonal antibody LA4. *Journal of Neurocytology* **20**: 716–731.

Ambalavanar, R., Morris, R. (1992). The distribution of binding by isolectin I-B4 from Griffonia simplicifolia in the trigeminal ganglion and brainstem trigeminal nuclei in the rat. *Neuroscience* **47**: 421–429.

Amenta, F., Sancesario, G., Ferrante, F., Cavallotti, C. (1980). Acetylcholinesterase-containing nerve fibers in the dura mater of guinea pig, mouse, and rat. *Journal of Neural Transmission* **47**: 237–242.

Amrutkar, D.V., Ploug, K.B., Hay-Schmidt, A., Porreca, F., Olesen, J., Jansen-Olesen, I. (2012). mRNA expression of 5-hydroxytryptamine 1B, 1D, and 1F receptors and their role in controlling the release of calcitonin gene-related peptide in the rat trigeminovascular system. *Pain* **153**: 830–838.

Andreou, A.P., Goadsby, P.J. (2011). Topiramate in the treatment of migraine: a kainate (glutamate) receptor antagonist within the trigeminothalamic pathway. *Cephalalgia* **31**: 1343–1358.

Andres, K.H., von Düring, M., Muszynski, K., Schmidt, R.F. (1987). Nerve fibres and their terminals of the dura mater encephali of the rat. *Anatomy and Embryology (Berlin)* **175**: 289–301.

Angus-Leppan, H., Lambert, G.A., Michalicek, J. (1997). Convergence of occipital nerve and superior sagittal sinus input in the cervical spinal cord of the cat. *Cephalalgia* **17**: 625–630; discussion 623.

Arbab, M.A., Wiklund, L., Svendgaard, N.A. (1986). Origin and distribution of cerebral vascular innervation from superior cervical, trigeminal and spinal ganglia investigated with retrograde and anterograde WGA-HRP tracing in the rat. *Neuroscience* **19**: 695–708.

Artico, M., Cavallotti, C. (2001). Catecholaminergic and acetylcholine esterase containing nerves of cranial and spinal dura mater in humans and rodents. *Microscopy Research and Technique* **53**: 212–220.

Bae, J.Y., Kim, J.H., Cho, Y.S., Mah, W., Bae, Y.C. (2015). Quantitative analysis of afferents expressing substance P, calcitonin gene-related peptide, isolectin B4, neurofilament 200, and Peripherin in the sensory root of the rat trigeminal ganglion. *Journal of Comparative Neurology* **523**: 126–138.

Bartsch, T., Goadsby, P.J. (2003). Increased responses in trigeminocervical nociceptive neurons to cervical input after stimulation of the dura mater. *Brain – A Journal of Neurology* **126**: 1801–1813.

Basbaum, A.I., Glazer, E.J., Oertel, W. (1986). Immunoreactive glutamic acid decarboxylase in the trigeminal nucleus caudalis of the cat: a light- and electron-microscopic analysis. *Somatosensory & Motor Research* **4**: 77–94.

Baun, M., Pedersen, M.H.F., Olesen, J., Jansen-Olesen, I. (2012). Dural mast cell degranulation is a putative mechanism for headache induced by PACAP-38. *Cephalalgia* **32**: 337–345.

Bereiter, D.A. and Bereiter, D.F. (1996). N-methyl-D-aspartate and non-N-methyl-D-aspartate receptor antagonism reduces Fos-like immunoreactivity in central trigeminal neurons after corneal stimulation in the rat. *Neuroscience* **73**: 249–258.

Bereiter, D.A., Bereiter, D.F., Tonnessen, B.H., Maclean, D.B. (1998). Selective blockade of substance P or neurokinin A receptors reduces the expression of c-fos in trigeminal subnucleus caudalis after corneal stimulation in the rat. *Neuroscience* **83**: 525–534.

Bhatt, D.K., Ploug, K.B., Ramachandran, R., Olesen, J., Gupta, S. (2010). Activation of PAR-2 elicits NO-dependent and CGRP-independent dilation of the dural artery. *Headache* **50**: 1017–1030.

Boissonade, F.M., Sharkey, K.A., Lucier, G.E. (1993). Trigeminal nuclear complex of the ferret: anatomical and immunohistochemical studies. *Journal of Comparative Neurology* **329**: 291–312.

Bolay, H., Reuter, U., Dunn, A.K., Huang, Z., Boas, D.A., Moskowitz, M.A. (2002). Intrinsic brain activity triggers trigeminal meningeal afferents in a migraine model. *Nature Medicine* **8**: 136–142.

Borges, L.F., Moskowitz, M.A. (1983). Do intracranial and extracranial trigeminal afferents represent divergent axon collaterals? *Neuroscience Letters* **35**: 265–270.

Broton, J.G., Rosenfeld, J.P. (1986). Cutting rostral trigeminal nuclear complex projections preferentially affects perioral nociception in the rat. *Brain Research* **397**: 1–8.

Burnstock, G. (2009). Purines and sensory nerves. *Handbook of Experimental Pharmacology*, pp. 333–392. Springer.

Burstein, R., Yamamura, H., Malick, A., Strassman, A.M. (1998a). Chemical stimulation of the intracranial dura induces enhanced responses to facial stimulation in brain stem trigeminal neurons. *Journal of Neurophysiology* **79**: 964–982.

Burstein, R., Yamamura, H., Malick, A., Strassman, A.M. (1998b). Chemical stimulation of the intracranial dura induces enhanced responses to facial stimulation in brain stem trigeminal neurons. *Journal of Neurophysiology* **79**: 964–982.

Buzzi, M.G., Moskowitz, M.A. (1991). Evidence for 5-HT1B/1D receptors mediating the antimigraine effect of sumatriptan and dihydroergotamine. *Cephalalgia* **11**: 165–168.

Byers, M.R., O'Connor, T.A., Martin, R.F., Dong, W.K. (1986). Mesencephalic trigeminal sensory neurons of cat: axon pathways and structure of mechanoreceptive endings in periodontal ligament. *Journal of Comparative Neurology* **250**: 181–191.

Cabanac, M., Brinnel, H. (1985). Blood flow in the emissary veins of the human head during hyperthermia. *European Journal of Applied Physiology* **54**: 172–176.

Cechetto, D.F., Standaert, D.G., Saper, C.B. (1985). Spinal and trigeminal dorsal horn projections to the parabrachial nucleus in the rat. *Journal of Comparative Neurology* **240**: 153–160.

Ceruti, S., Villa, G., Fumagalli, M., Colombo, L., Magni, G., Zanardelli, M., Fabbretti, E., Verderio, C., van den Maagdenberg, A.M.J.M., Nistri, A., *et al.* (2011). Calcitonin gene-related peptide-mediated enhancement of purinergic neuron/glia communication by the algogenic factor bradykinin in mouse trigeminal ganglia from wild-type and R192Q Cav2.1 Knock-in mice: implications for basic mechanisms of migraine pain. *Journal of Neuroscience* **31**: 3638–3649.

Chaudhary, P., Baumann, T.K. (2002). Expression of VPAC2 receptor and PAC1 receptor splice variants in the trigeminal ganglion of the adult rat. *Molecular Brain Research* **104**: 137–142.

Choi, I.-S., Cho, J.-H., An, C.-H., Jung, J.-K., Hur, Y.-K., Choi, J.-K., Jang, I.-S. (2012). 5-HT(1B) receptors inhibit glutamate release from primary afferent terminals in rat medullary dorsal horn neurons. *British Journal of Pharmacology* **167**: 356–367.

Classey, J.D., Knight, Y.E., Goadsby, P.J. (2001). The NMDA receptor antagonist MK-801 reduces Fos-like immunoreactivity within the trigeminocervical complex following superior sagittal sinus stimulation in the cat. *Brain Research* **907**: 117–124.

Cutrer, F.M., Limmroth, V., Ayata, G., Moskowitz, M.A. (1995). Attenuation by valproate of c-fos immunoreactivity in trigeminal nucleus caudalis induced by intracisternal capsaicin. *British Journal of Pharmacology* **116**: 3199–3204.

Davis, K.D., Dostrovsky, J.O. (1988). Responses of feline trigeminal spinal tract nucleus neurons to stimulation of the middle meningeal artery and sagittal sinus. *Journal of Neurophysiology* **59**: 648–666.

Del Fiacco, M., Quartu, M., Floris, A., Diaz, G. (1990). Substance P-like immunoreactivity in the human trigeminal ganglion. *Neuroscience Letters* **110**: 16–21.

Dimitriadou, V., Rouleau, A., Trung Tuong, M.D., Newlands, G.J., Miller, H.R., Luffau, G., Schwartz, J.C., Garbag, M. (1997). Functional relationships between sensory nerve fibers and mast cells of dura mater in normal and inflammatory conditions. *Neuroscience* **77**: 829–839.

Dimlich, R.V., Keller, J.T., Strauss, T.A., Fritts, M.J. (1991). Linear arrays of homogeneous mast cells in the dura mater of the rat. *Journal of Neurocytology* **20**: 485–503..

Dux, M., Sántha, P., Jancsó, G. (2003). Capsaicin-sensitive neurogenic sensory vasodilatation in the dura mater of the rat. *Journal of Physiology* **552**: 859–867.

Dux, M., Rosta, J., Pintér, S., Sántha, P., Jancsó, G. (2007). Loss of capsaicin-induced meningeal neurogenic sensory vasodilatation in diabetic rats. *Neuroscience* **150**: 194–201.

Dux, M., Rosta, J., Sántha, P., Jancsó, G. (2009). Involvement of capsaicin-sensitive afferent nerves in the proteinase-activated receptor 2-mediated vasodilatation in the rat dura mater. *Neuroscience* **161**: 887–894.

Dux, M., Sántha, P., Jancsó, G. (2012). The role of chemosensitive afferent nerves and TRP ion channels in the pathomechanism of headaches. *Pflügers Archiv European Journal of Physiology* **464**: 239–248.

Eberhardt, M., Dux, M., Namer, B., Miljkovic, J., Cordasic, N., Will, C., Kichko, T.I., de la Roche, J., Fischer, M., Suárez, S.A., *et al.* (2014). H2S and NO cooperatively regulate vascular tone by activating a neuroendocrine HNO-TRPA1-CGRP signalling pathway. *Nature Communications* **5**: 4381.

Edvinsson, L., Uddman, R. (1981). Adrenergic, cholinergic and peptidergic nerve fibres in dura mater – involvement in headache? *Cephalalgia* **1**: 175–179.

Edvinsson, L., Ekman, R., Jansen, I., McCulloch, J., Uddman, R. (1987). Calcitonin gene-related peptide and cerebral blood vessels: distribution and vasomotor effects. *Journal of Cerebral Blood Flow & Metabolism* **7**: 720–728.

Edvinsson, L., Brodin, E., Jansen, I., Uddman, R. (1988). Neurokinin A in cerebral vessels: characterization, localization and effects *in vitro*. *Regulatory Peptides* **20**: 181–197.

Edvinsson, L., Hara, H., Uddman, R. (1989). Retrograde tracing of nerve fibers to the rat middle cerebral artery with true blue: colocalization with different peptides. *Journal of Cerebral Blood Flow & Metabolism* **9**: 212–218.

Edvinsson, L., Gulbenkian, S., Barroso, C.P., Cunha e Sá, M., Polak, J.M., Mortensen, A., Jørgensen, L., Jansen-Olesen, I. (1998). Innervation of the human middle meningeal artery: immunohistochemistry, ultrastructure, and role of endothelium for vasomotility. *Peptides* **19**: 1213–1225.

Edvinsson, L., Elsås, T., Suzuki, N., Shimizu, T., Lee, T.J. (2001). Origin and Co-localization of nitric oxide synthase, CGRP, PACAP, and VIP in the cerebral circulation of the rat. *Microscopy Research and Technique* **53**: 221–228.

Eftekhari, S., Salvatore, C.A., Calamari, A., Kane, S.A., Tajti, J., Edvinsson, L. (2010). Differential distribution of calcitonin gene-related peptide and its receptor components in the human trigeminal ganglion. *Neuroscience* **169**: 683–696.

Eftekhari, S., Warfvinge, K., Blixt, F.W., Edvinsson, L. (2013). Differentiation of nerve fibers storing CGRP and CGRP receptors in the peripheral trigeminovascular system. *Journal of Pain* **14**: 1289–1303.

Eftekhari, S., Salvatore, C.A., Johansson, S., Chen, T.-B., Zeng, Z., Edvinsson, L. (2015). Localization of CGRP, CGRP receptor, PACAP and glutamate in trigeminal ganglion. Relation to the blood-brain barrier. *Brain Research* **1600**: 93–109.

Fabbretti, E., D'Arco, M., Fabbro, A., Simonetti, M., Nistri, A., Giniatullin, R. (2006). Delayed upregulation of ATP P2X3 receptors of trigeminal sensory neurons by calcitonin gene-related peptide. *Journal of Neuroscience* **26**: 6163–6171.

Faraci, F.M., Kadel, K.A., Heistad, D.D. (1989). Vascular responses of dura mater. *American Journal of Physiology* **257**: H157–H161.

Fischer, M.J.M., Messlinger, K. (2007). Cannabinoid and vanilloid effects of R(+)-methanandamide in the hemisected meningeal preparation. *Cephalalgia* **27**: 422–428.

Fischer, M.J.M., Uchida, S., Messlinger, K. (2010). Measurement of meningeal blood vessel diameter *in vivo* with a plug-in for ImageJ. *Microvascular Research* **80**: 258–266.

Franceschini, A., Nair, A., Bele, T., van den Maagdenberg, A.M., Nistri, A., Fabbretti, E. (2012). Functional crosstalk in culture between macrophages and trigeminal sensory neurons of a mouse genetic model of migraine. *BMC Neuroscience* **13**: 143.

Franceschini, A., Vilotti, S., Ferrari, M.D., van den Maagdenberg, A.M.J.M., Nistri, A., Fabbretti, E. (2013). TNFα levels and macrophages expression reflect an inflammatory potential of trigeminal ganglia in a mouse model of familial hemiplegic migraine. *PloS One* **8**: e52394.

Ge, S.-N., Li, Z.-H., Tang, J., Ma, Y., Hioki, H., Zhang, T., Lu, Y.-C., Zhang, F.-X., Mizuno, N., Kaneko, T., *et al*. (2014). Differential expression of VGLUT1 or VGLUT2 in the trigeminothalamic or trigeminocerebellar projection neurons in the rat. *Brain Structure and Function* **219**: 211–229.

Glenn, J.A., Sonceau, J.B., Wynder, H.J., Thomas, W.E. (1993). Histochemical evidence for microglia-like macrophages in the rat trigeminal ganglion. *Journal of Anatomy* **183**(Pt. 3): 475–481.

Goadsby, P.J., Zagami, A.S. (1991). Stimulation of the superior sagittal sinus increases metabolic activity and blood flow in certain regions of the brainstem and upper cervical spinal cord of the cat. *Brain – A Journal of Neurology* **114**(Pt. 2): 1001–1011.

Goadsby, P.J., Akerman, S., Storer, R.J. (2001). Evidence for postjunctional serotonin (5-HT1) receptors in the trigeminocervical complex. *Annals of Neurology* **50**: 804–807.

Gobel, S., W. M. Falls, Hockfield, S. (1977). The division of the dorsal and ventral horns of the mammalian caudal medulla into eight layers using anatomical criteria. In: *Pain in the Trigeminal Region*, pp. 443–453. Elsevier/North-Holland Biomedical Press.

Graham, S.H., Sharp, F.R., Dillon, W. (1988). Intraoral sensation in patients with brainstem lesions: role of the rostral spinal trigeminal nuclei in pons. *Neurology* **38**: 1529–1533.

Guan, Z.L., Ding, Y.Q., Li, J.L., Lü, B.Z. (1998). Substance P receptor-expressing neurons in the medullary and spinal dorsal horns projecting to the nucleus of the solitary tract in the rat. *Neuroscience Research* **30**: 213–218.

Gupta, S., Akerman, S., van den Maagdenberg, A.M.J.M., Saxena, P.R., Goadsby, P.J., van den Brink, A.M. (2006). Intravital microscopy on a closed cranial window in mice: a model to study trigeminovascular mechanisms involved in migraine. *Cephalalgia* **26**: 1294–1303.

Haenggeli, C.-A., Pongstaporn, T., Doucet, J.R., Ryugo, D.K. (2005). Projections from the spinal trigeminal nucleus to the cochlear nucleus in the rat. *Journal of Comparative Neurology* **484**: 191–205.

Hayashi, H. (1985). Morphology of terminations of small and large myelinated trigeminal primary afferent fibers in the cat. *Journal of Comparative Neurology* **240**: 71–89.

Hayashi, H., Sumino, R., Sessle, B.J. (1984). Functional organization of trigeminal subnucleus interpolaris: nociceptive and innocuous afferent inputs, projections to thalamus, cerebellum, and spinal cord, and descending modulation from periaqueductal gray. *Journal of Neurophysiology* **51**: 890–905.

Hegarty, D.M., Mitchell, J.L., Swanson, K.C., Aicher, S.A. (2007). Kainate receptors are primarily postsynaptic to SP-containing axon terminals in the trigeminal dorsal horn. *Brain Research* **1184**: 149–159.

Helme, R.D., Fletcher, J.L. (1983). Substance P in the trigeminal system at postmortem: evidence for a role in pain pathways in man. *Clinical and Experimental Neurology* **19**: 37–44.

Henry, J.L., Sessle, B.J., Lucier, G.E., Hu, J.W. (1980). Effects of substance P on nociceptive and non-nociceptive trigeminal brain stem neurons. *Pain* **8**: 33–45.

Henry, M.A., Johnson, L.R., Nousek-Goebl, N., Westrum, L.E. (1996). Light microscopic localization of calcitonin gene-related peptide in the normal feline trigeminal system and following retrogasserian rhizotomy. *Journal of Comparative Neurology* **365**: 526–540.

Hervieu, G.J., Cluderay, J.E., Harrison, D.C., Roberts, J.C., Leslie, R.A. (2001). Gene expression and protein distribution of the orexin-1 receptor in the rat brain and spinal cord. *Neuroscience* **103**: 777–797.

Hinrichsen, C.F., Watson, C.D. (1983). Brain stem projections to the facial nucleus of the rat. *Brain, Behavior and Evolution* **22**: 153–163.

Holland, P.R., Akerman, S., Goadsby, P.J. (2006). Modulation of nociceptive dural input to the trigeminal nucleus caudalis via activation of the orexin 1 receptor in the rat. *European Journal of Neuroscience* **24**: 2825–2833.

Hoskin, K.L., Zagami, A.S., Goadsby, P.J. (1999). Stimulation of the middle meningeal artery leads to Fos expression in the trigeminocervical nucleus: a comparative study of monkey and cat. *Journal of Anatomy* **194** (Pt. 4): 579–588.

Hou, M., Uddman, R., Tajti, J., Kanje, M., Edvinsson, L. (2002). Capsaicin receptor immunoreactivity in the human trigeminal ganglion. *Neuroscience Letters* **330**: 223–226.

Huang, D., Li, S., Dhaka, A., Story, G.M., Cao, Y.-Q. (2012). Expression of the transient receptor potential channels TRPV1, TRPA1 and TRPM8 in mouse trigeminal primary afferent neurons innervating the dura. *Molecular Pain* **8**: 66.

Huerta, M.F., Frankfurter, A., Harting, J.K. (1983). Studies of the principal sensory and spinal trigeminal nuclei of the rat: projections to the superior colliculus, inferior olive, and cerebellum. *Journal of Comparative Neurology* **220**: 147–167.

Ichikawa, H., Sugimoto, T. (2004). The co-expression of P2X3 receptor with VR1 and VRL-1 in the rat trigeminal ganglion. *Brain Research* **998**: 130–135.

Jacquin, M.F., Renehan, W.E., Mooney, R.D., Rhoades, R.W. (1986). Structure-function relationships in rat medullary and cervical dorsal horns. I. Trigeminal primary afferents. *Journal of Neurophysiology* **55**: 1153–1186.

Jacquin, M.F., Stennett, R.A., Renehan, W.E., Rhoades, R.W. (1988). Structure-function relationships in the rat brainstem subnucleus interpolaris: II. Low and high threshold trigeminal primary afferents. *Journal of Comparative Neurology* **267**: 107–130.

Jansen, I., Uddman, R., Ekman, R., Olesen, J., Ottosson, A., Edvinsson, L. (1992). Distribution and effects of neuropeptide Y, vasoactive intestinal peptide, substance P, and calcitonin gene-related peptide in human middle meningeal arteries: comparison with cerebral and temporal arteries. *Peptides* **13**: 527–536.

Jenkins, D.W., Langmead, C.J., Parsons, A.A., Strijbos, P.J. (2004). Regulation of calcitonin gene-related peptide release from rat trigeminal nucleus caudalis slices *in vitro*. *Neuroscience Letters* **366**: 241–244.

Jordt, S.-E., Bautista, D.M., Chuang, H.-H., McKemy, D.D., Zygmunt, P.M., Högestätt, E.D., Meng, I.D., Julius, D. (2004). Mustard oils and cannabinoids excite sensory nerve fibres through the TRP channel ANKTM1. *Nature* **427**: 260–265.

Kageneck, C., Nixdorf-Bergweiler, B.E., Messlinger, K., Fischer, M.J. (2014). Release of CGRP from mouse brainstem slices indicates central inhibitory effect of triptans and kynurenate. *Journal of Headache and Pain* **15**: 7.

Kaube, H., Keay, K.A., Hoskin, K.L., Bandler, R., Goadsby, P.J. (1993). Expression of c-Fos-like immunoreactivity in the caudal medulla and upper cervical spinal cord following stimulation of the superior sagittal sinus in the cat. *Brain Research* **629**: 95–102.

Keller, J.T., Marfurt, C.F. (1991). Peptidergic and serotoninergic innervation of the rat dura mater. *Journal of Comparative Neurology* **309**: 515–534.

Keller, J.T., Marfurt, C.F., Dimlich, R.V., Tierney, B.E. (1989). Sympathetic innervation of the supratentorial dura mater of the rat. *Journal of Comparative Neurology* **290**: 310–321.

Keller, J.T., Dimlich, R.V., Zuccarello, M., Lanker, L., Strauss, T.A., Fritts, M.J. (1991). Influence of the sympathetic nervous system as well as trigeminal sensory fibres on rat dural mast cells. *Cephalalgia* **11**: 215–221.

Kerber, C.W., Newton, T.H. (1973). The macro and microvasculature of the dura mater. *Neuroradiology* **6**: 175–179.

Kim, Y.S., Paik, S.K., Cho, Y.S., Shin, H.S., Bae, J.Y., Moritani, M., Yoshida, A., Ahn, D.K., Valtschanoff, J., Hwang, S.J., *et al.* (2008). Expression of P2X3 receptor in the trigeminal sensory nuclei of the rat. *Journal of Comparative Neurology* **506**: 627–639.

Knutsson, M., Edvinsson, L. (2002). Distribution of mRNA for VIP and PACAP receptors in human cerebral arteries and cranial ganglia. *Neuroreport* **13**: 507–509.

Kobari, M., Tomita, M., Tanahashi, N., Yokoyama, M., Takao, M., Fukuuchi, Y. (1996). Intravascular substance P dilates cerebral parenchymal vessels through a specific tachykinin NK1 receptor in cats. *European Journal of Pharmacology* **317**: 269–274.

Kosaras, B., Jakubowski, M., Kainz, V., Burstein, R. (2009). Sensory innervation of the calvarial bones of the mouse. *Journal of Comparative Neurology* **515**: 331–348.

Kruger, L., Siminoff, R., Witkovsky, P. (1961). Single neuron analysis of dorsal column nuclei and spinal nucleus of trigeminal in cat. *Journal of Neurophysiology* **24**: 333–349.

Kurosawa, M., Messlinger, K., Pawlak, M., Schmidt, R.F. (1995). Increase of meningeal blood flow after electrical stimulation of rat dura mater encephali: mediation by calcitonin gene-related peptide. *British Journal of Pharmacology* **114**: 1397–1402.

LaGuardia, J.J., Cohrs, R.J., Gilden, D.H. (2000). Numbers of neurons and non-neuronal cells in human trigeminal ganglia. *Neurological Research* **22**: 565–566.

Lambert, G.A., Zagami, A.S., Bogduk, N., Lance, J.W. (1991). Cervical spinal cord neurons receiving sensory input from the cranial vasculature. *Cephalalgia* **11**: 75–85.

Lambert, G.A., Hoskin, K.L., Michalicek, J., Panahi, S.E., Truong, L., Zagami, A.S. (2014). Stimulation of dural vessels excites the SI somatosensory cortex of the cat via a relay in the thalamus. *Cephalalgia* **34**: 243–257.

Lee, W.S., Moussaoui, S.M., Moskowitz, M.A. (1994). Blockade by oral or parenteral RPR 100893 (a non-peptide NK1 receptor antagonist) of neurogenic plasma protein extravasation within guinea-pig dura mater and conjunctiva. *British Journal of Pharmacology* **112**: 920–924.

Lee, Y., Kawai, Y., Shiosaka, S., Takami, K., Kiyama, H., Hillyard, C.J., Girgis, S., MacIntyre, I., Emson, P.C., Tohyama, M. (1985). Coexistence of calcitonin gene-related peptide and substance P-like peptide in single cells of the trigeminal ganglion of the rat: immunohistochemical analysis. *Brain Research* **330**: 194–196.

Lennerz, J.K., Rühle, V., Ceppa, E.P., Neuhuber, W.L., Bunnett, N.W., Grady, E.F., Messlinger, K. (2008). Calcitonin receptor-like receptor (CLR), receptor activity-modifying protein 1 (RAMP1), and calcitonin gene-related peptide (CGRP) immunoreactivity in the rat trigeminovascular system: differences between peripheral and central CGRP receptor distribution. *Journal of Comparative Neurology* **507**: 1277–1299.

Leong, S., Liu, H., Yeo, J. (2000). Nitric oxide synthase and glutamate receptor immunoreactivity in the rat spinal trigeminal neurons expressing Fos protein after formalin injection. *Brain Research* **855**: 107–115.

Levy, D. (2009). Migraine pain, meningeal inflammation, and mast cells. *Current Pain and Headache Reports* **13**: 237–240.

Li, J., Vause, C.V., Durham, P.L. (2008). Calcitonin gene-related peptide stimulation of nitric oxide synthesis and release from trigeminal ganglion glial cells. *Brain Research* **1196**: 22–32.

Li, J.L., Kaneko, T., Shigemoto, R., Mizuno, N. (1997). Distribution of trigeminohypothalamic and spinohypothalamic tract neurons displaying substance P receptor-like immunoreactivity in the rat. *Journal of Comparative Neurology* **378**: 508–521.

Lisney, S.J. (1983). Some current topics of interest in the physiology of trigeminal pain: a review. *Journal of the Royal Society of Medicine* **76**: 292–296.

Luschka, H. (1856). *Die Nerven der harten Hirnhaut*. Tübingen: H. Laupp.

Malick, A., Burstein, R. (1998). Cells of origin of the trigeminohypothalamic tract in the rat. *Journal of Comparative Neurology* **400**: 125–144.

Malick, A., Strassman, R.M., Burstein, R. (2000). Trigeminohypothalamic and reticulohypothalamic tract neurons in the upper cervical spinal cord and caudal medulla of the rat. *Journal of Neurophysiology* **84**: 2078–2112.

Marcus, J.N., Aschkenasi, C.J., Lee, C.E., Chemelli, R.M., Saper, C.B., Yanagisawa, M., Elmquist, J.K. (2001). Differential expression of orexin receptors 1 and 2 in the rat brain. *Journal of Comparative Neurology* **435**: 6–25.

Marfurt, C.F. (1981). The central projections of trigeminal primary afferent neurons in the cat as determined by the tranganglionic transport of horseradish peroxidase. *Journal of Comparative Neurology* **203**: 785–798.

Mayberg, M.R., Zervas, N.T., Moskowitz, M.A. (1984). Trigeminal projections to supratentorial pial and dural blood vessels in cats demonstrated by horseradish peroxidase histochemistry. *Journal of Comparative Neurology* **223**: 46–56.

McMahon, M.S., Norregaard, T.V., Beyerl, B.D., Borges, L.F., Moskowitz, M.A. (1985). Trigeminal afferents to cerebral arteries and forehead are not divergent axon collaterals in cat. *Neuroscience Letters* **60**: 63–68.

McMenamin, P.G. (1999). Distribution and phenotype of dendritic cells and resident tissue macrophages in the dura mater, leptomeninges, and choroid plexus of the rat brain as demonstrated in wholemount preparations. *Journal of Comparative Neurology* **405**: 553–562.

McMenamin, P.G., Wealthall, R.J., Deverall, M., Cooper, S.J., Griffin, B. (2003). Macrophages and dendritic cells in the rat meninges and choroid plexus: three-dimensional localisation by environmental scanning electron microscopy and confocal microscopy. *Cell and Tissue Research* **313**: 259–269.

McNaughton, M. (1938). The innervation of the intracranial blood vessels and dural sinuses. *Association for Research in Nervous and Mental Disease* **18**: 178–200.

Ménétrey, D., Basbaum, A.I. (1987). Spinal and trigeminal projections to the nucleus of the solitary tract: a possible substrate for somatovisceral and viscerovisceral reflex activation. *Journal of Comparative Neurology* **255**: 439–450.

Meng, I.D., Hu, J.W., Benetti, A.P., Bereiter, D.A. (1997). Encoding of corneal input in two distinct regions of the spinal trigeminal nucleus in the rat: cutaneous receptive field properties, responses to thermal and chemical stimulation, modulation by diffuse noxious inhibitory controls, and projections to the parabrachial area. *Journal of Neurophysiology* **77**: 43–56.

Messlinger, K., Hanesch, U., Baumgärtel, M., Trost, B., Schmidt, R.F. (1993). Innervation of the dura mater encephali of cat and rat: ultrastructure and calcitonin gene-related peptide-like and substance P-like immunoreactivity. *Anatomy and Embryology (Berlin)* **188**: 219–237.

Messlinger, K., Fischer, M.J.M., Lennerz, J.K. (2011). Neuropeptide effects in the trigeminal system: pathophysiology and clinical relevance in migraine. *Keio Journal of Medicine* **60**: 82–89.

Moskowitz, M.A. (1984). The neurobiology of vascular head pain. *Annals of Neurology* **16**: 157–168.

Nassini, R., Materazzi, S., Vriens, J., Prenen, J., Benemei, S., De Siena, G., la Marca, G., Andrè, E., Preti, D., Avonto, C., *et al.* (2012). The "headache tree" via umbellulone and TRPA1 activates the trigeminovascular system. *Brain – A Journal of Neurology* **135**: 376–390.

Nord, S.G., Kyler, H.J. (1968). A single unit analysis of trigeminal projections to bulbar reticular nuclei of the rat. *Journal of Comparative Neurology* **134**: 485–494.

Nozaki, K., Moskowitz, M.A., Maynard, K.I., Koketsu, N., Dawson, T.M., Bredt, D.S., Snyder, S.H. (1993). Possible origins and distribution of immunoreactive nitric oxide synthase-containing nerve fibers in cerebral arteries. *Journal of Cerebral Blood Flow & Metabolism* **13**: 70–79.

O'Connor, T.P., van der Kooy, D. (1986). Pattern of intracranial and extracranial projections of trigeminal ganglion cells. *Journal of Neuroscience* **6**: 2200–2207.

Olszewski, J. (1950). On the anatomical and functional organization of the spinal trigeminal nucleus. *Journal of Comparative Neurology* **92**: 401–413.

O'Shaughnessy, C.T., Connor, H.E. (1993). Neurokinin NK1 receptors mediate plasma protein extravasation in guinea-pig dura. *European Journal of Pharmacology* **236**: 319–321.

Ottosson, A., Edvinsson, L. (1997). Release of histamine from dural mast cells by substance P and calcitonin gene-related peptide. *Cephalalgia* **17**: 166–174.

Panneton, W.M., Burton, H. (1981). Corneal and periocular representation within the trigeminal sensory complex in the cat studied with transganglionic transport of horseradish peroxidase. *Journal of Comparative Neurology* **199**: 327–344.

Panneton, W.M., Johnson, S.N., Christensen, N.D. (1994). Trigeminal projections to the peribrachial region in the muskrat. *Neuroscience* **58**: 605–625.

Pearson, J.C., Jennes, L. (1988). Localization of serotonin- and substance P-like immunofluorescence in the caudal spinal trigeminal nucleus of the rat. *Neuroscience Letters* **88**: 151–156.

Peschanski, M. (1984). Trigeminal afferents to the diencephalon in the rat. *Neuroscience* **12**: 465–487.

Phelan, K.D., Falls, W.M. (1989). The interstitial system of the spinal trigeminal tract in the rat: anatomical evidence for morphological and functional heterogeneity. *Somatosensory & Motor Research* **6**: 367–399.

Price, T.J., Helesic, G., Parghi, D., Hargreaves, K.M., Flores, C.M. (2003). The neuronal distribution of cannabinoid receptor type 1 in the trigeminal ganglion of the rat. *Neuroscience* **120**: 155–162.

Price, T.J., Patwardhan, A., Akopian, A.N., Hargreaves, K.M., Flores, C.M. (2004). Modulation of trigeminal sensory neuron activity by the dual cannabinoid-vanilloid agonists anandamide, N-arachidonoyl-dopamine and arachidonyl-2-chloroethylamide. *British Journal of Pharmacology* **141**: 1118–1130.

Prins, M., van der Werf, F., Baljet, B., Otto, J.A. (1993). Calcitonin gene-related peptide and substance P immunoreactivity in the monkey trigeminal ganglion, an electron microscopic study. *Brain Research* **629**: 315–318.

Prośba-Mackiewicz, M., Zółtowska, A., Dziewiatkowski, J. (2000). Substance-P of neural cells in human trigeminal ganglion. *Folia Morphologica* **59**: 327–331.

Ray, B.S., Wolff, H.G. (1940). Experimental studies on headache: pain sensitive structures of the head and their significance in headache. *Archives of Surgery* **1**: 813–856.

Rexed, B. (1952). The cytoarchitectonic organization of the spinal cord in the cat. *Journal of Comparative Neurology* **96**: 414–495.

Ring, G., Ganchrow, D. (1983). Projections of nucleus caudalis and spinal cord to brainstem and diencephalon in the hedgehog (Erinaceus europaeus and Paraechinus aethiopicus): a degeneration study. *Journal of Comparative Neurology* **216**: 132–151.

Roland, J., Bernard, C., Bracard, S., Czorny, A., Floquet, J., Race, J.M., Forlodou, P., Picard, L. (1987). Microvascularization of the intracranial dura mater. *Surgical and Radiologic Anatomy* **9**: 43–49.

Rowe, M.J., Sessle, B.J. (1968). Somatic afferent input to posterior thalamic neurones and their axon projection to the cerebral cortex in the cat. *Journal of Physiology* **196**: 19–35.

Ruan, H.Z., Burnstock, G. (2003). Localisation of P2Y1 and P2Y4 receptors in dorsal root, nodose and trigeminal ganglia of the rat. *Histochemistry and Cell Biology* **120**: 415–426.

Ruggiero, D.A., Ross, C.A., Reis, D.J. (1981). Projections from the spinal trigeminal nucleus to the entire length of the spinal cord in the rat. *Brain Research* **225**: 225–233.

Salas, M.M., Hargreaves, K.M., Akopian, A.N. (2009). TRPA1-mediated responses in trigeminal sensory neurons: interaction between TRPA1 and TRPV1. *European Journal of Neuroscience* **29**: 1568–1578.

Salt, T.E., Morris, R., Hill, R.G. (1983). Distribution of substance P-responsive and nociceptive neurones in relation to substance P-immunoreactivity within the caudal trigeminal nucleus of the rat. *Brain Research* **273**: 217–228.

Samsam, M., Coveñas, R., Ahangari, R., Yajeya, J., Narváez, J.A., Tramu, G. (2000). Simultaneous depletion of neurokinin A, substance P and calcitonin gene-related peptide from the caudal trigeminal nucleus of the rat during electrical stimulation of the trigeminal ganglion. *Pain* **84**: 389–395.

Schaible, H.G., Ebersberger, A., Peppel, P., Beck, U., Messlinger, K. (1997). Release of immunoreactive substance P in the trigeminal brain stem nuclear complex evoked by chemical stimulation of the nasal mucosa and the dura mater encephali--a study with antibody microprobes. *Neuroscience* **76**: 273–284.

Schepelmann, K., Ebersberger, A., Pawlak, M., Oppmann, M., Messlinger, K. (1999). Response properties of trigeminal brain stem neurons with input from dura mater encephali in the rat. *Neuroscience* **90**: 543–554.

Schueler, M., Messlinger, K., Dux, M., Neuhuber, W.L., De Col, R. (2013). Extracranial projections of meningeal afferents and their impact on meningeal nociception and headache. *Pain* **154**: 1622–1631.

Schueler, M., Neuhuber, W.L., De Col, R., Messlinger, K. (2014). Innervation of rat and human dura mater and pericranial tissues in the parieto-temporal region by meningeal afferents. *Headache* **54**: 996–1009.

Schwenger, N., Dux, M., de Col, R., Carr, R., Messlinger, K. (2007). Interaction of calcitonin gene-related peptide, nitric oxide and histamine release in neurogenic blood flow and afferent activation in the rat cranial dura mater. *Cephalalgia* **27**: 481–491.

Shepheard, S.L., Williamson, D.J., Hill, R.G., Hargreaves, R.J. (1993). The non-peptide neurokinin1 receptor antagonist, RP 67580, blocks neurogenic plasma extravasation in the dura mater of rats. *British Journal of Pharmacology* **108**: 11–12.

Shigenaga, Y., Okamoto, T., Nishimori, T., Suemune, S., Nasution, I.D., Chen, I.C., Tsuru, K., Yoshida, A., Tabuchi, K., Hosoi, M. (1986). Oral and facial representation in the trigeminal principal and rostral spinal nuclei of the cat. *Journal of Comparative Neurology* **244**: 1–18.

Siegel, J.M. (2004). Hypocretin (orexin): role in normal behavior and neuropathology. *Annual Review of Psychology* **55**: 125–148.

Simons, T., Ruskell, G.L. (1988). Distribution and termination of trigeminal nerves to the cerebral arteries in monkeys. *Journal of Anatomy* **159**: 57–71.

Sjoqvist, O. (1938). Studies on pain conduction in the trigeminal nerve. A contribution to the surgical treatment of facial pain. *Acta Psychiatrica Scandinavica* **17**(Suppl): 1–139.

Smith, D., Hill, R.G., Edvinsson, L., Longmore, J. (2002). An immunocytochemical investigation of human trigeminal nucleus caudalis: CGRP, substance P and 5-HT1D-receptor immunoreactivities are expressed by trigeminal sensory fibres. *Cephalalgia* **22**: 424–431.

Staikopoulos, V., Sessle, B.J., Furness, J.B., Jennings, E.A. (2007). Localization of P2X2 and P2X3 receptors in rat trigeminal ganglion neurons. *Neuroscience* **144**: 208–216.

Steiger, H.J., Meakin, C.J. (1984). The meningeal representation in the trigeminal ganglion--an experimental study in the cat. *Headache* **24**: 305–309.

Steindler, D.A. (1985). Trigeminocerebellar, trigeminotectal, and trigeminothalamic projections: a double retrograde axonal tracing study in the mouse. *Journal of Comparative Neurology* **237**: 155–175.

Stewart, W.A., King, R.B. (1963). Fiber projections from the nucleus caudalis of the spinal trigeminal nucleus. *Journal of Comparative Neurology* **121**: 271–286.

Storer, R.J., Goadsby, P.J. (1997). Microiontophoretic application of serotonin (5HT)1B/1D agonists inhibits trigeminal cell firing in the cat. *Brain – A Journal of Neurology* **120** (Pt. 12): 2171–2177.

Storer, R.J., Akerman, S., Goadsby, P.J. (2004a). Calcitonin gene-related peptide (CGRP) modulates nociceptive trigeminovascular transmission in the cat. *British Journal of Pharmacology* **142**: 1171–1181.

Storer, R.J., Akerman, S., Shields, K.G., Goadsby, P.J. (2004b). GABAA receptor modulation of trigeminovascular nociceptive neurotransmission by midazolam is antagonized by flumazenil. *Brain Research* **1013**: 188–193.

Strassman, A.M., Vos, B.P. (1993). Somatotopic and laminar organization of fos-like immunoreactivity in the medullary and upper cervical dorsal horn induced by noxious facial stimulation in the rat. *Journal of Comparative Neurology* **331**: 495–516.

Strassman, A.M., Potrebic, S., Maciewicz, R.J. (1994a). Anatomical properties of brainstem trigeminal neurons that respond to electrical stimulation of dural blood vessels. *Journal of Comparative Neurology* **346**: 349–365.

Strassman, A.M., Mineta, Y., Vos, B.P. (1994b). Distribution of fos-like immunoreactivity in the medullary and upper cervical dorsal horn produced by stimulation of dural blood vessels in the rat. *Journal of Neuroscience* **14**: 3725–3735.

Strassman, A.M., Weissner, W., Williams, M., Ali, S., Levy, D. (2004). Axon diameters and intradural trajectories of the dural innervation in the rat. *Journal of Comparative Neurology* **473**; 364–376.

Stubbs, C.M., Waldron, G.J., Connor, H.E., Feniuk, W. (1992). Characterization of the receptor mediating relaxation to substance P in canine middle cerebral artery: no evidence for involvement of substance P in neurogenically mediated relaxation. *British Journal of Pharmacology* **105**: 875–880.

Tashiro, T., Takahashi, O., Satoda, T., Matsushima, R., Uemura-Sumi, M., Mizuno, N. (1991). Distribution of axons showing calcitonin gene-related peptide- and/or substance P-like immunoreactivity in the sensory trigeminal nuclei of the cat. *Neuroscience Research* **11**: 119–133.

Tiwari, R.K., King, R.B. (1973). Trigeminothalamic projections from nucleus caudalis in primates. *Surgical Forum* **24**: 444–446.

Torvik, A. (1956). Afferent connections to the sensory trigeminal nuclei, the nucleus of the solitary tract and adjacent structures; an experimental study in the rat. *Journal of Comparative Neurology* **106**: 51–141.

Uddman, R., Hara, H., Edvinsson, L. (1989). Neuronal pathways to the rat middle meningeal artery revealed by retrograde tracing and immunocytochemistry. *Journal of the Autonomic Nervous System* **26**: 69–75.

Uddman, R., Tajti, J., Hou, M., Sundler, F., Edvinsson, L. (2002). Neuropeptide expression in the human trigeminal nucleus caudalis and in the cervical spinal cord C1 and C2. *Cephalalgia* **22**: 112–116.

Van Ham, J.J., Yeo, C.H. (1992). Somatosensory Trigeminal Projections to the Inferior Olive, Cerebellum and other Precerebellar Nuclei in Rabbits. *European Journal of Neuroscience* **4**: 302–317.

Vause, C.V., Durham, P.L. (2010). Calcitonin gene-related peptide differentially regulates gene and protein expression in trigeminal glia cells: findings from array analysis. *Neuroscience Letters* **473**: 163–167.

Villa, G., Ceruti, S., Zanardelli, M., Magni, G., Jasmin, L., Ohara, P.T., Abbracchio, M.P. (2010). Temporomandibular joint inflammation activates glial and immune cells in both the trigeminal ganglia and in the spinal trigeminal nucleus. *Molecular Pain* **6**: 89.

von Düring, M., Bauersachs, M., Böhmer, B., Veh, R.W., Andres, K.H. (1990). Neuropeptide Y- and substance P-like immunoreactive nerve fibers in the rat dura mater encephali. *Anatomy and Embryology (Berlin)* **182**: 363–373

Vyklický, L., Keller, O., Jastreboff, P., Vyklický, L., Butkhuzi, S.M. (1977). Spinal trigeminal tractotomy and nociceptive reactions evoked by tooth pulp stimulation in the cat. *Journal of Physiology (Paris)* **73**: 379–386.

Wang, X., Fang, Y., Liang, J., Yan, M., Hu, R., Pan, X. (2014). 5-HT7 Receptors Are Involved in Neurogenic Dural Vasodilatation in an Experimental Model of Migraine. *Journal of Molecular Neuroscience* **54**(2): 164–70.

Wemmie, J.A., Price, M.P., Welsh, M.J. (2006). Acid-sensing ion channels: advances, questions and therapeutic opportunities. *Trends in Neurosciences* **29**: 578–586.

Williamson, D.J., Hargreaves, R.J., Hill, R.G., Shepheard, S.L. (1997). Intravital microscope studies on the effects of neurokinin agonists and calcitonin gene-related peptide on dural vessel diameter in the anaesthetized rat. *Cephalalgia* **17**: 518–524.

Yan, J., Edelmayer, R.M., Wei, X., De Felice, M., Porreca, F., Dussor, G. (2011). Dural afferents express acid-sensing ion channels: a role for decreased meningeal pH in migraine headache. *Pain* **152**: 106–113.

Yatim, N., Billig, I., Compoint, C., Buisseret, P., Buisseret-Delmas, C. (1996). Trigeminocerebellar and trigemino-olivary projections in rats. *Neuroscience Research* **25**: 267–283.

Yokota, T., Nishikawa, N. (1980). Reappraisal of somatotopic tactile representation within trigeminal subnucleus caudalis. *Journal of Neurophysiology* **43**: 700–712.

You, J., Gulbenkian, S., Jansen Olesen, I., Marron, K., Wharton, J., Barroso, C.P., Polak, J.M., Edvinsson, L. (1995). Peptidergic innervation of guinea-pig brain vessels: comparison with immunohistochemistry and in vitro pharmacology in rostrally and caudally located arteries. *Journal of the Autonomic Nervous System* **55**: 179–188.

Youn, D.-H. (2014). Long-term potentiation by activation of group I metabotropic glutamate receptors at excitatory synapses in the spinal trigeminal subnucleus oralis. *Neuroscience Letters* **560**: 36–40.

Young, R.F. (1982). Effect of trigeminal tractotomy on dental sensation in humans. *Journal of Neurosurgery* **56**: 812–818.

Zenker, W., Kubik, S. (1996). Brain cooling in humans – anatomical considerations. *Anatomy and Embryology (Berlin)* **193**: 1–13.

Zhang, X.-C., Levy, D. (2008). Modulation of meningeal nociceptors mechanosensitivity by peripheral proteinase-activated receptor-2: the role of mast cells. *Cephalalgia* **28**: 276–284.

Zhao, J., Levy, D. (2014). The sensory innervation of the calvarial periosteum is nociceptive and contributes to headache-like behavior. *Pain* **155**: 1392–1400.

Zimmermann, K., Reeh, P.W., Averbeck, B. (2002). ATP can enhance the proton-induced CGRP release through P2Y receptors and secondary PGE(2) release in isolated rat dura mater. *Pain* **97**: 259–265.

2

Physiology of the meningeal sensory pathway

Andrew M. Strassman and Agustin Melo-Carrillo

Department of Anesthesia, Critical Care and Pain Medicine, Beth Israel Deaconess Medical Center,
Harvard Medical School, Boston, Massachusetts, USA

2.1   Role of the meningeal sensory pathway in headache

Anatomical studies in man and animals have shown that the intracranial meninges (dura and pia) receive a sensory innervation that originates from cells in the trigeminal, as well as the upper cervical dorsal root ganglia (see Chapter 1). This innervation supplies both the major branches of the Circle of Willis, which carry the blood supply to the brain, as well as the major dural venous sinuses which carry a large portion of the venous outflow from the brain. A very large body of evidence now strongly supports the view that this sensory innervation is critically involved in mediating the headache of migraine (see Chapter 1 and Chapter 7).

One seminal piece of evidence was the finding that direct stimulation of the meninges can evoke painful headache-like sensations in awake human neurosurgical patients (Fay, 1935; Ray and Wolff, 1940). The meninges were the only intracranial tissue from which pain could be evoked in these studies, and pain was the only sensation that could be evoked, regardless of whether the stimulus was electrical, mechanical, or thermal. The pain was typically referred to a region within the trigeminal or, in some cases, the upper cervical dermatomes, depending on the stimulus site. In these respects, the sensory properties of the meningeal innervation are similar to those of certain visceral organs, in that the sensations that can be evoked are primarily painful, and the pain can be referred to a somatic region that is spatially separate from the stimulus site.

Although extracranial tissues of the head and face can also give rise to pain, the meninges seem to stand apart in consistently evoking headache-like, referred pain. These properties prompted Moskowitz to propose the meninges as the trigeminal analog of the visceral organs of the body (Moskowitz, 1991). Beginning especially with Moskowitz's reformulation of its potential role in headache within the framework of modern neurobiology (Moskowitz, 1984), the meningeal sensory innervation has become the focus of intensive research into its basic anatomical and physiological properties. This chapter will give an overview of the major findings from research on the physiology of the meningeal sensory pathway, as well as some of the current unresolved questions and controversies.

Neurobiological Basis of Migraine, First Edition. Edited by Turgay Dalkara and Michael A. Moskowitz.
© 2017 John Wiley & Sons, Inc. Published 2017 by John Wiley & Sons, Inc.

2.2 Nociceptive response properties of peripheral and central neurons in the meningeal sensory pathway

Electrophysiological studies of the meningeal sensory pathway have, so far, focused on the innervation of the dura rather than the pia (i.e., proximal branches of the Circle of Willis), probably owing to the greater accessibility and ease of delivering controlled, localized stimuli. Such studies have shown that the primary afferent neurons that innervate the dura display response properties broadly similar to those of nociceptive neurons that innervate other tissues of the body, and this sensory information is conveyed centrally to neurons in the medullary and upper cervical dorsal horn that also receive convergent sensory input from facial receptive fields.

2.2.1 Primary afferent neurons

Electrophysiological studies of primary afferent neurons that innervate the dura have recorded discharge activity, either from the neurons' axons in the nasociliary nerve (Bove and Moskowitz, 1997) or, in most studies, from the neurons' cell bodies in the trigeminal ganglion (Dostrovsky *et al.*, 1991; Strassman *et al.*, 1996; Strassman and Raymond, 1999; Levy and Strassman, 2002b; Levy *et al.*, 2004; Zhang *et al.*, 2013; Zhao and Levy, 2015; see Strassman and Levy (2006) for a more detailed review). These studies have identified neurons with axons that conduct in the A-delta and C-fiber range that display sensory response properties consistent with a nociceptive function and, thus, have been termed meningeal nociceptors (Levy and Strassman, 2002a). Such neurons can be activated by mechanical, thermal, or chemical stimulation of the dura, and individual neurons have been shown to respond to all three modalities (Bove and Moskowitz, 1997), as is found for polymodal nociceptors in other tissues.

Neurons display one or more spot-like mechanical receptive fields to punctate (von Frey) stimuli that can be distributed at vascular sites on the dura (transverse sinus, middle meningeal artery), as well as dural sites away from any major blood vessels (Strassman *et al.*, 1996; Bove and Moskowitz, 1997; Strassman and Raymond, 1999; Zhao and Levy, 2015). Neurons could also be activated by traction (Dostrovsky *et al.*, 1991), whereas intraluminal distention produced by rapid infusion of normal saline is ineffective. Mechanical and thermal response thresholds are much lower than those of cutaneous nociceptors, but are consistent with a nociceptive function for a deep tissue. Thus, the neurons' response thresholds to temperatures of less than 42°C (Bove and Moskowitz, 1997) are lower than those of cutaneous nociceptors. However, they are consistent with a nociceptive function for intracranial tissues, since they might potentially allow the neurons to detect conditions such as fever or heat stroke, which can be associated with headache. Mechanical response thresholds to punctate stimuli are also much lower than those of cutaneous nociceptors, with the lowest thresholds being just above the normal range of intracranial pressures (Levy and Strassman, 2002b; Strassman and Levy, 2006).

In addition to thermal and mechanical stimuli, meningeal nociceptors can also be activated by a variety of chemical stimuli, in common with nociceptors innervating other tissues. These chemicals, applied topically to the dura, include hypertonic saline, KCl, capsaicin, acidic buffer, pH-neutral buffer solutions of low or high osmolarity, serotonin, PGI_2, ATP, and a mixture of inflammatory mediators given in combination

Table 2.1 Stimuli or agents that activate cranial meningeal nociceptors.

Mechanical	
Traction on superior sagittal sinus	Dostrovsky *et al*, 1991
Stroking with blunt probe or indenting with punctate probe within dural receptive fields away from or overlying dural blood vessels (superior sagittal or transverse sinus, or middle meningeal artery)	Bove and Moskowitz, 1997; Strassman *et al.*, 1996; Levy and Strassman, 2002a, 2002b
NOTE: no response to intravascular distention produced by rapid infusion of normal saline into the superior sagittal sinus (Strassman *et al.*, 1996)	
Thermal	
Heating to 39°C or higher; cooling to 25–32°C	Bove and Moskowitz, 1997
Chemical	
Infusion into superior sagittal sinus of 400 mM hypertonic saline	Strassman *et al.*, 1996
Topical application to the dura of:	
Potassium chloride, hypertonic saline (>500 mOsm), high osmolarity sucrose solution (>600 mOsm), low osmolarity buffer (<200 mOsm), capsaicin, acidic buffer(pH 5), mixture of inflammatory mediators (bradykinin, serotonin, histamine, PGE_2), ATP	Strassman *et al.*, 1996; Bove and Moskowitz, 1997; Levy and Strassman, 2002a; Zhao and Levy, 2015
Mast cell mediators: serotonin, PGI_2, histamine, agonist for proteinase-activated receptor 2; no response to PGD2 and leukotriene C_4	Zhang *et al.*, 2007; Zhang and Levy, 2008
TNF-alpha: mechanical sensitization, but not activation, via dural endothelial vascular cyclooxygenase and p38 MAP kinase	Zhang *et al.*, 2011
Systemic administration of mast cell degranulating agent	Levy *et al.*, 2007
Sumatriptan, i.v. or topical application to the dura (transient activation)	Strassman and Levy, 2004; Burstein *et al.*, 2005
NOTE: no response to vasodilatation induced by dural application or systemic administration of CGRP (Levy *et al.*, 2005)	
Headache-related stimuli	
Cortical spreading depression: delayed activation	Zhang *et al.*, 2010
Intravenous nitroglycerin: delayed mechanical sensitization, but not activation, via dural arterial ERK phosphorylation	Zhang *et al.*, 2013

(histamine, bradykinin, serotonin, and prostaglandin E_2) (Strassman *et al.*, 1996; Bove and Moskowitz, 1997; Zhang *et al.*, 2007; Zhao and Levy, 2015). Hypertonic saline also activates neurons when infused into the dural venous sinuses, showing that the dural nerve endings could be accessed by chemicals on either the intra- or extraluminal side of the dural venous sinuses.

One additional, crucial property of meningeal nociceptors, in common with nociceptors in other tissues, is chemically induced sensitization, expressed as an enhanced sensitivity to mechanical stimuli (Chapter 7, Figure 7.2). Activation and mechanical sensitization may occur together or independently in meningeal nociceptors, depending

Table 2.2 Meningeal vs cutaneous vs corneal nociceptor response thresholds.

Meningeal nociceptors	Cutaneous nociceptors	Corneal nociceptors
Mechanical (punctate indenting stimulation)		
25 kPa, C fibers, guinea pig (Bove and Moskowitz, 1997) 16 kPa, C fibers; 10 kPa, slow A fibers, rat (Levy and Strassman, 2002b)	approximately 60 kPa, C fibers, rat (Schlegel *et al.*, 2004)	39 kPa, A-delta fibers, cat (Belmonte and Giraldez, 1981)
Note: 1 kPa = 1 mN/sq.mm. = approx. 0.1 g/sq.mm.		
Heat		
39°C, C fibers, guinea pig (Bove and Moskowitz, 1997)	45–46.5°C, C fibers, rat (Martin *et al.*, 1988; Rau *et al.*, 2007; Cuellar *et al.*, 2010)	41.5°C, A-delta fibers, cat (Belmonte and Giraldez, 1981) 41.2°C, A-delta fibers, rabbit (MacIver and Tanelian, 1993)
Cold		
25–32°C, C fibers, guinea pig (Bove and Moskowitz, 1997)	4.6°C, A-delta fibers, rat (Simone and Kajander, 1997)	32°C, C-fibers, cat (Gallar *et al.*, 1993) <2°C decrease from baseline, thermosensitive C-fibers, rabbit (MacIver and Tanelian, 1993); rat (Hirata and Meng, 2010)

on the neuron and the sensitizing agent. Mechanical sensitization may consist of either an increase in suprathreshold responses, an increase in threshold responses, or both (Levy and Strassman, 2002a, 2004; Levy *et al.*, 2008; Zhang *et al.*, 2011b, 2012; Burstein *et al.*, 2014).

One study found evidence that the pattern of mechanical sensitization differed for different subpopulations of meningeal nociceptors (Levy and Strassman, 2002a). That study used a cAMP analog, rather than inflammatory mediators, as the sensitizing agent, in order to selectively activate only one of the intracellular signaling pathways implicated in primary afferent sensitization – the cAMP/PKA cascade. Unlike the actions of inflammatory mediators, the cAMP analog produced selective sensitizing effects that were subpopulation-specific, in that individual neurons exhibited an increase in either threshold responses or suprathreshold responses, but not both. The two subpopulations so defined by these two patterns of sensitization also differed in their baseline mechanosensitivity and conduction velocity; the neurons that exhibited an increase in threshold responses had higher baseline thresholds and lower conduction velocities. These differences between the two subpopulations show parallels with the differences found between two subpopulations of presumed nociceptive dorsal root ganglion cells that are distinguished by their voltage gated membrane currents (Scroggs *et al.*, 1994; Petruska *et al.*, 2000), and are suggestive of different subpopulation-specific mechanisms of sensitization (Strassman and Levy, 2006; see further discussion below).

The property of mechanical sensitization is of great relevance for understanding the clinical symptoms of migraine (see Chapter 7), in particular, those symptoms that indicate the presence of an exaggerated intracranial mechanosensitivity. In migraine, as well in certain headaches that accompany intracranial pathologies such as meningitis, the headache is worsened by coughing, straining, or sudden head movement (Blau and Dexter, 1981). Such activities would be expected to increase intracranial pressure, or otherwise change the distribution of mechanical forces within the intracranial space (Williams, 1976). The throbbing quality of migraine headache has been attributed to arterial pulsations, which produce a pressure pulse that propagates throughout the intracranial space (Daley *et al.*, 1995). Post-dural puncture headache has a positional dependence that suggests the involvement of a gravity-induced displacement of intracranial tissue (Wolff, 1963). Each of these symptoms is evidence of an intracranial mechanosensitive sensory system that, during clinically occurring headaches, can develop abnormally elevated sensitivity that results in activation and generation of pain by normally innocuous intracranial mechanical forces.

2.2.2 Central neurons (dorsal horn and thalamus)

Sensory inputs from the head and face are transmitted centrally to neurons in the medullary and upper cervical dorsal horn (see Chapter 1). Sensory inputs from the dura converge centrally on a subpopulation of dorsal horn neurons that also receive inputs from a facial receptive field, which is commonly in the periorbital region, and is usually nociceptive, either wide-dynamic-range or nociceptive specific (Strassman *et al.*, 1986; Davis and Dostrovsky, 1986, 1988d; Angus-Leppan *et al.*, 1994; Burstein *et al.*, 1998). Such convergence of peripheral sensory inputs from separate deep and superficial tissues onto individual dorsal horn neurons is also found in neurons of the spinal dorsal horn (Blair *et al.*, 1981), and is regarded as the neural basis for the phenomenon of referred pain originating from deep or visceral tissues.

   The facial receptive fields of dorsal horn neurons that respond to dural stimulation are consistent with a role for these neurons in mediating the pain evoked by dural stimulation, in that their distribution strongly overlaps with the area of dural-evoked pain referral in humans, and the receptive fields are primarily nociceptive. In addition, sensitization of such central neurons, which can be induced by sustained nociceptive input such as from dural application of inflammatory mediators, results in a state of prolonged neuronal hypersensitivity, with marked enhancement of the responses to stimulation of both the facial and the dural receptive fields. This phenomenon of central sensitization of dorsal horn neurons with convergent inputs from deep tissues is thought to be the basis for the phenomenon of referred visceral hyperalgesia and, in the meningeal sensory pathway, provides a mechanism to explain the facial cutaneous allodynia that can occur in migraine (Chapter 7, Figure 7.3).

   Dorsal horn neurons that receive dural inputs can be activated by potentially noxious forms of mechanical and chemical meningeal stimulation, including traction or distension of dural blood vessels (Davis and Dostrovsky, 1988c, 1988d; Lambert *et al.*, 1991, 1992; Kaube *et al.*, 1992) and dural or subarachnoid application of bradykinin and other algesic or inflammatory agents (Davis and Dostrovsky, 1988a; Ebersberger *et al.*, 1997; Burstein *et al.*, 1998). In addition to the dorsal horn, neurons that respond to dural stimulation are also found in more rostral parts of the spinal trigeminal nucleus, nucleus interpolaris and oralis (Davis and Dostrovsky, 1988d). The responses of neurons in these more rostral regions are reduced by cold block applied to the medullary dorsal horn, indicating that inputs reach these neurons in part via a relay in the dorsal horn (Davis and Dostrovsky, 1988b).

Neurons that respond to dural stimulation are present in both superficial and deep laminae of the dorsal horn. Studies that used expression of c-*fos* as an anatomical marker for neuronal activation found neuronal labeling following dural stimulation in a relatively restricted laminar distribution – primarily in dorsal horn laminae I and V – but in a widespread rostrocaudal distribution that extended from medullary to upper cervical levels (Kaube *et al.*, 1993; Strassman *et al.*, 1994). Intracellular labeling of dorsal horn lamina V neurons that are activated by dural stimulation revealed a subpopulation with an extensive system of axonal projections to multiple levels of the dorsal horn and the caudal part of trigeminal nucleus interpolaris (Strassman *et al.*, 1994). These extensive intratrigeminal projections might contribute to the rostrocaudally widespread distribution of neuronal activation found in the c-*fos* studies.

Electrophysiology studies have also examined neurons that are activated by dural stimulation in the thalamus, where they have been found within or at the periphery of the ventroposteromedial nucleus, the posterior nucleus, and the intralaminar nuclei (Davis and Dostrovsky, 1988c; Zagami and Lambert, 1990; Angus-Leppan *et al.*, 1995; Burstein *et al.*, 2010; Noseda *et al.*, 2010a). As in the dorsal horn, most of the neurons had receptive fields on the face that often included the ophthalmic region. Thus, the convergent dural and facial inputs that are present in dorsal horn neurons are also found in thalamic neurons, as expected, since the dorsal horn is a major source of inputs to the thalamus. However, the thalamic neurons with dural and facial receptive fields are also activated by light, indicating an additional, unexpected convergent input to these somatosensory neurons from visual pathways (Noseda *et al.*, 2010b). This visual input is of great clinical significance for understanding the mechanism of photophobia, or exacerbation of headache by light – one of the defining characteristics of migraine (see Chapter 7).

As is found for other nociceptive dorsal horn neurons, dorsal horn neurons in the meningeal sensory pathway are subject to multiple descending modulatory influences from higher levels of the neuraxis, including the periaqueductal gray, acting through CGRP, cannabinoids, and the 5HT 1B/D receptor (Strassman *et al.*, 1986; Knight and Goadsby, 2001; Knight *et al.*, 2003; Bartsch *et al.*, 2004; Akerman *et al.*, 2013; Pozo-Rosich *et al.*, 2015), and the hypothalamus, acting through somatostatin, dopamine (D(2) receptor) and orexin A(OX(1) receptor) (Bartsch *et al.*, 2004, 2005; Holland *et al.*, 2006; Bergerot *et al.*, 2007; Charbit *et al.*, 2009).

A critical question is to what degree these modulatory systems differentially target the meningeal sensory pathway. Such specificity would presumably be required for theories of migraine that propose a central modulatory mechanism as the initiator of the attack, in order to be able to explain why the pain of migraine is specifically a headache, rather than a pain in other parts of the body. Such specificity would also be important for possible therapeutic strategies that make use of these neurochemical modulatory systems.

2.3 Activity of neurons in the meningeal sensory pathway under conditions associated with headache: CSD and nitroglycerin

The studies described above examined activity of neurons in the meningeal sensory pathway in response to direct stimulation of their receptive fields in the dura or the facial skin, using stimuli that are generally known to be effective for activating nociceptive neurons, but are not specifically related to conditions associated with the generation of headache. Such studies have investigated the consequences of activating the nociceptive pathway that is believed to mediate the pain of migraine, but they do not, themselves, directly shed light on the question of how this pathway might become activated during a clinically occurring headache in humans.

More recently, activity in this sensory pathway has been studied during experimental manipulations that are potentially more relevant to conditions associated with the generation of a headache. A key difference in these studies is that the experimental manipulation does not, itself, directly activate the meningeal nerve endings but, instead, serves to initiate an endogenous process that somehow generates the eventual excitatory neural stimulus. One such finding, of critical importance to current theories of migraine, was the recent demonstration of a delayed activation of both primary afferent nociceptors and dorsal horn neurons, following the induction of cortical spreading depression (CSD) (Chapter 7, Figure 7.1) (Zhang *et al.*, 2010, 2011a; Zhao and Levy, 2015); an earlier study by Bolay *et al.* (2002) had provided indirect evidence for such activation based on a delayed increase in dural blood flow). The spreading depression theory of migraine, originally proposed more than 70 years ago, hypothesized that CSD, a slowly propagating wave of altered activity in the cerebral cortex, was the basis for the migraine aura (see Chapter 16). It was further hypothesized that CSD produced the headache of migraine by activating meningeal sensory nerve fibers, but a major obstacle in further understanding was the difficulty in finding direct neurophysiological evidence that such activation occurred (Lambert *et al.*, 1999; Ebersberger *et al.*, 2001), as well as conflicting evidence from c-fos studies (Moskowitz *et al.*, 1993; Ingvardsen *et al.*, 1997).

One striking aspect of the CSD-induced activation of neurons in the meningeal sensory pathway is that it occurs at a characteristic delay that is comparable to the typical delay between the migraine aura and onset of headache, as proposed in the CSD theory of migraine. A major remaining question is how to account for such a long delay in activation, since the delay is much longer than the time required for propagation of the CSD wave across the cortex. If the trigeminal activation were, in fact, produced by the release of excitatory chemicals (e.g., potassium, glutamate) that accompanies the CSD wave, as has been hypothesized, then no such delay would be expected.

A recent study supports the idea that the delayed trigeminal activation, as reflected in dural blood flow levels, results from a cascade in which the initial brief CSD-induced depolarization of cortical neurons induces the activation of pannexin 1 megachannels and the release of the pro-inflammatory molecule high-mobility group box 1 which, in turn, triggers activation and sustained release of inflammatory mediators from cortical astrocytes (Karatas *et al.*, 2013). One further question is whether the CSD-induced activation of neurons in the dorsal horn might occur through a purely central mechanism, such as via descending cortical projections, rather than through the activation of meningeal nerve endings (Lambert *et al.*, 2011). An ongoing technical problem that must be considered in the interpretation of all such studies of CSD-induced neuronal activation of the meningeal sensory pathway is the possibility of a false positive finding resulting from an artifactual direct excitatory action of the CSD-initiating stimulus (e.g., potassium chloride) on the meningeal sensory nerve endings, independent of the CSD wave.

Another headache-associated condition which has been used as a test stimulus for activation of the meningeal sensory pathway is intravenous infusion of nitroglycerin or related nitric oxide donor molecules. This treatment induces in migraineurs a delayed headache that reproduces the features of the subject's spontaneously occurring migraine attacks (Iversen *et al.*, 1989; Thomsen *et al.*, 1994), including relief by triptans (Iversen and Olesen, 1996), and elevation of blood levels of CGRP (calcitonin gene-related peptide) (Juhasz *et al.*, 2003). Neurophysiological studies have shown that such infusion induces a sensitization of primary afferent neurons (Zhang *et al.*, 2013) and activation of dorsal horn neurons (Koulchitsky *et al.*, 2004, 2009) in the meningeal sensory pathway. These findings are of great significance as the first direct neurophysiological demonstration that the meningeal sensory pathway is activated or sensitized by a treatment that causes headache in humans, and with a similar time course, thereby strengthening the evidence in support of the role of this pathway in headache.

As with the CSD findings described above, a key open question is: how do the nitric oxide donor molecules cause these delayed excitatory effects? The delay means that the nitric oxide is not acting as a direct excitatory agent on the neurons, because it has a short half-life, and so is no longer present in the body at the time the effects start to appear. Therefore, these agents must instead be serving as a trigger for an endogenous process that results in the neuronal effects. There is evidence that nitroglycerin infusion is followed by a delayed meningeal inflammation (Reuter *et al.*, 2001, 2002), and that the sensitizing effects on meningeal nociceptors are dependent specifically on activation within meningeal arterial cells of a signaling cascade that involves phosphorylation of extracellular signal-related kinase (ERK) (Zhang *et al.*, 2013).

2.4 Role of blood vessels in activation of the meningeal sensory pathway

The original idea of Wolff (1963) – that the pain of migraine results from dilatation of intra- or extracranial blood vessels and consequent mechanically evoked excitation of perivascular sensory nerve fibers – ultimately suffered from a failure of supporting evidence, and has largely been replaced by new concepts about the role of vascular mechanisms in migraine (Strassman and Levy, 2006; Dodick, 2008; Brennan and Charles, 2010). Neurophysiology studies have demonstrated that dural vasodilatation induced by local or systemic administration of CGRP has no detectable effect on activity or mechanosensitivity of dural nociceptors (Levy *et al.*, 2005). More generally, there appears to be no evidence that physiological vasodilatation is capable of activating sensory neurons, or producing pain, in any body tissue. Instead, current evidence on the role of blood vessels in migraine has focused on other factors, such as the generation of inflammatory mediators (Zhang *et al.*, 2013).

However, it should be noted that neurophysiological studies of the meningeal sensory pathway have focused on the dural innervation, and the sensory properties of the pial innervation are unexplored. Although the dural sensory innervation is referred to as the trigeminovascular system, it is not specifically vascular in its anatomical distribution, in that it supplies both vascular and nonvascular dural territories (Strassman *et al.*, 2004) and, in fact, the number of sensory nerve endings in the dura is greater at non-vascular sites (Messlinger *et al.*, 1993). Unlike the dural innervation, the pial sensory innervation has a specifically vascular distribution, along the proximal branches of the major cerebral arteries, and so might potentially have different properties than the dural innervation, with respect to the effects of vasodilatation.

2.5   Unique neuronal properties of the meningeal sensory pathway

One ongoing question is whether the neurons of the meningeal sensory pathway display any properties that distinguish them from nociceptive neurons in sensory pathways from other tissues. As outlined above, the neurons of the meningeal sensory pathway display sensory response properties in common with nociceptive neurons of sensory pathways from other body tissues, such as: sensitivity to noxious forms of stimulation, including algesic chemicals and inflammatory mediators; central convergence of nociceptive somatic input; and peripheral and central sensitization. Also, in common with nociceptors in other tissues, dural primary afferent neurons exhibit resistance to tetrodotoxin (Strassman and Raymond, 1999), a property which is conferred by a type of voltage-gated sodium channel that is, remarkably, expressed only by nociceptors, and not any other population of peripheral or central neuron.

In general, the neuropeptides and receptors that have been identified in the meningeal primary afferent neurons are common to other sensory innervations, including the neuropeptide CGRP, and the receptor for triptans, 5-HT1D. Furthermore, the percentage of neurons that express the 5-HT1D receptor is no greater in trigeminal ganglion than in dorsal root ganglia (Potrebic *et al.*, 2003). However there is some recent evidence that the axonal density of 5HT1D receptors (in distinction from the number of expressing neurons) does differ between tissues, and may be greater in the meninges than in extracranial tissues (Harriott and Gold, 2008). There is also an enrichment of CGRP in meningeal sensory neurons, compared with trigeminal ganglion neurons that innervate extracranial tissues (O'Connor and van der Kooy, 1988).

Although meningeal primary afferent neurons display sensory signaling properties that are typical of nociceptive neurons in other tissues, there is recent evidence that the ionic mechanisms underlying these properties can differ for nociceptor populations, and that meningeal nociceptors, in particular, display distinctive membrane properties (Harriott and Gold, 2009). Compared with afferent neurons that innervate extracranial tissue (temporalis muscle), dural primary afferents exhibit higher baseline conductance, indicative of larger number of open ion channels, and greater excitability in response to intracellular current injection (Harriott and Gold, 2009).

Most strikingly, dural primary afferent neurons display a mechanism of inflammatory mediator-induced sensitization that is unique among primary afferent populations that have been examined thus far (Vaughn and Gold, 2010). This mechanism of sensitization is dependent on a type of chloride channel that is apparently unique to dural nociceptors, insofar as it has not been described in previous studies of nociceptors or any other neuronal population. A phenomenon that is common among other nociceptor populations, enhancement of tetrodotoxin-resistant sodium current (NaV1.8), is also present, but apparently does not make a significant contribution to sensitization in dural nociceptors. This dual finding, of a type of ion channel, and a mechanism of sensitization that is apparently unique to dural nociceptors, is potentially of great therapeutic significance, since it offers a possible target for selective pharmacological blockade of sensitization of the dural afferent pathway. It should be noted that these findings are from *in vitro* studies of dissociated cells, and it would be of great interest to investigate this mechanism further *in vivo*.

Aside from such differences in intrinsic neuronal properties, the signaling properties of the meningeal sensory pathway are bound to the distinctive properties of the tissue that it innervates. The intracranial tissues are unusual, in being enclosed within a rigid structure and, thus, subject to compressive forces that do not routinely occur in other tissues. The close proximity to the central nervous system endows the meningeal nerve endings with the capacity to detect central disturbances such as those caused by CSD, as well as epileptic seizure, which can be associated with the occurrence of a migraine-like headache (Ekstein and Schachter, 2010).

The dura is well endowed with inflammatory cells such as mast cells and, as noted above, develops an inflammatory reaction with a distinctive delayed time course, following administration of headache-causing agents such as nitroglycerin. As discussed by Levy (see Chapter 6), meningeal nociceptors are strongly activated by mast cell degranulation (Levy *et al.*, 2007) and mast cell mediators (Zhang *et al.*, 2007). Systemic administration of mast cell degranulators produces a regionally selective distribution of dorsal horn activation, restricted to two distinct peaks at the medullary and sacral level, indicating a selective nociceptive action on afferents in a specific subset of tissues (Levy *et al.*, 2012). The activation in medullary dorsal horn was attenuated by prior depletion of dural mast cells, indicating that dural afferents were the primary source of the medullary activation. It is not yet known whether this selectivity results from tissue-specific differences in the properties of the mast cells (e.g., density, type of mediators) or the nociceptors.

2.6 Intracranial vs extracranial mechanisms of migraine: new findings

While this review has focused on the sensory pathway from intracranial tissues, the question of intra- versus extracranial contributions to migraine has been discussed, since the original studies of Wolff (Ray and Wolff, 1940) up to the present time. Recently, a reformulation of this question has been prompted by novel anatomical evidence that the peripheral axons of dural primary afferent neurons can give rise to axonal branches that, after coursing distally through the dura, exit the cranium through calvarial sutures to innervate extracranial tissues, particularly the sutures themselves and the overlying periosteum (Kosaras *et al.*, 2009; Schueler *et al.*, 2013; Burstein *et al.*, 2014; Zhao and Levy, 2014).

A detailed electrophysiological analysis showed that the majority of the periosteal innervation is supplied by extracranial nerves, as previously believed, but about 30% of the periosteal afferent axons instead originate from axonal branches that enter the sutures via an intracranial trajectory through the underlying dura and, in these neurons, the periosteal receptive field is always restricted to the region immediately overlying a suture (Zhao and Levy, 2014). The presence of a population with such dual intra- and extracranial receptive fields in the dura and the sutures means that extracranial stimuli that reach the area of the sutures could activate a subset of the neurons that constitute the meningeal sensory pathway and, thus, potentially produce sensory effects and symptoms at least partly in common with those produced by intracranial stimuli.

There is also some evidence that intracranial afferents can innervate other extracranial tissues beyond the immediate vicinity of the sutures (Kosaras *et al.*, 2009; Schueler *et al.*, 2013), but the degree of such innervation that has been documented thus far is extremely sparse. It may be noted that a much larger population of primary afferent neurons with divergent intracranial and extracranial (e.g., facial) branches is present at early stages of development, but is eliminated by selective cell death prior to adulthood (O'Connor and van der Kooy, 1986).

References

Akerman, S., P. R. Holland, M. P. Lasalandra and P. J. Goadsby (2013). Endocannabinoids in the brainstem modulate dural trigeminovascular nociceptive traffic via CB1 and "triptan" receptors: implications in migraine. *Journal of Neuroscience* **33**(37): 14869–14877.

Angus-Leppan, H., B. Olausson, P. Boers and G. A. Lambert (1994). Convergence of afferents from superior sagittal sinus and tooth pulp on cells in the upper cervical spinal cord of the cat. *Neuroscience Letters* **182**(2): 275–278.

Angus-Leppan, H., B. Olausson, P. Boers and G. A. Lambert (1995). Convergence of afferents from superior sagittal sinus and tooth pulp on cells in the thalamus of the cat. *Cephalalgia* **15**(3): 191–199.

Bartsch, T., M. J. Levy, Y. E. Knight and P. J. Goadsby (2004). Differential modulation of nociceptive dural input to [hypocretin] orexin A and B receptor activation in the posterior hypothalamic area. *Pain* **109**(3): 367–378.

Bartsch, T., M. J. Levy, Y. E. Knight and P. J. Goadsby (2005). Inhibition of nociceptive dural input in the trigeminal nucleus caudalis by somatostatin receptor blockade in the posterior hypothalamus. *Pain* **117**(1–2): 30–39.

Belmonte, C. and F. Giraldez (1981). Responses of cat corneal sensory receptors to mechanical and thermal stimulation. *Journal of Physiology (London)* **321**: 355–368.

Bergerot, A., R. J. Storer and P. J. Goadsby (2007). Dopamine inhibits trigeminovascular transmission in the rat. *Annals of Neurology* **61**(3): 251–262.

Blair, R. W., R. N. Weber and R. D. Foreman (1981). Characteristics of primate spinothalamic tract neurons receiving viscerosomatic convergent inputs in T3-T5 segments. *Journal of Neurophysiology* **46**(4): 797–811.

Blau, J. N. and S. L. Dexter (1981). The site of pain origin during migraine attacks. *Cephalalgia* **1**(3): 143–147.

Bolay, H., U. Reuter, A. K. Dunn, Z. Huang, D. A. Boas and M. A. Moskowitz (2002). Intrinsic brain activity triggers trigeminal meningeal afferents in a migraine model. *Nature Medicine* **8**(2): 136–142.

Bove, G. M. and M. A. Moskowitz (1997). Primary afferent neurons innervating guinea pig dura. *Journal of Neurophysiology* **77**(1): 299–308.

Brennan, K. C. and A. Charles (2010). An update on the blood vessel in migraine. *Current Opinion in Neurology* **23**(3): 266–274.

Burstein, R., H. Yamamura, A. Malick and A. M. Strassman (1998). Chemical stimulation of the intracranial dura induces enhanced responses to facial stimulation in brain stem trigeminal neurons. *Journal of Neurophysiology* **79**(2): 964–982.

Burstein, R., M. Jakubowski and D. Levy (2005). Anti-migraine action of triptans is preceded by transient aggravation of headache caused by activation of meningeal nociceptors. *Pain* **115**(1–2): 21–28.

Burstein, R., M. Jakubowski, E. Garcia-Nicas, V. Kainz, Z. Bajwa, R. Hargreaves, L. Becerra and D. Borsook (2010). Thalamic sensitization transforms localized pain into widespread allodynia. *Annals of Neurology* **68**(1): 81–91.

Burstein, R., X. Zhang, D. Levy, K. R. Aoki and M. F. Brin (2014). Selective inhibition of meningeal nociceptors by botulinum neurotoxin type A: therapeutic implications for migraine and other pains. *Cephalalgia* **34**(11): 853–869.

Charbit, A. R., S. Akerman, P. R. Holland and P. J. Goadsby (2009). Neurons of the dopaminergic/calcitonin gene-related peptide A11 cell group modulate neuronal firing in the trigeminocervical complex: an electrophysiological and immunohistochemical study. *Journal of Neuroscience* **29**(40): 12532–12541.

Cuellar, J. M., N. A. Manering, M. Klukinov, M. I. Nemenov and D. C. Yeomans (2010). Thermal nociceptive properties of trigeminal afferent neurons in rats. *Molecular Pain* **6**: 39.

Daley, M. L., H. Pasupathy, M. Griffith, J. T. Robertson and C. W. Leffler (1995). Detection of loss of cerebral vascular tone by correlation of arterial and intracranial pressure signals. *IEEE Transactions on Biomedical Engineering* **42**(4): 420–424.

Davis, K. D. and J. O. Dostrovsky (1986). Activation of trigeminal brain-stem nociceptive neurons by dural artery stimulation. *Pain* **25**(3): 395–401.

Davis, K. D. and J. O. Dostrovsky (1988a). Cerebrovascular application of bradykinin excites central sensory neurons. *Brain Research* **446**(2): 401–406.

Davis, K. D. and J. O. Dostrovsky (1988b). Effect of trigeminal subnucleus caudalis cold block on the cerebrovascular-evoked responses of rostral trigeminal complex neurons. *Neuroscience Letters* **94**(3): 303–308.

Davis, K. D. and J. O. Dostrovsky (1988c). Properties of feline thalamic neurons activated by stimulation of the middle meningeal artery and sagittal sinus. *Brain Research* **454**(1–2): 89–100.

Davis, K. D. and J. O. Dostrovsky (1988d). Responses of feline trigeminal spinal tract nucleus neurons to stimulation of the middle meningeal artery and sagittal sinus. *Journal of Neurophysiology* **59**(2): 648–666.

Dodick, D. W (2008). Examining the essence of migraine – is it the blood vessel or the brain? A debate. *Headache* **48**(4): 661–667.

Dostrovsky, J. O., K. D. Davis and K. Kawakita (1991). Central mechanisms of vascular headaches. *Canadian Journal of Physiology and Pharmacology* **69**(5): 652–658.

Ebersberger, A., M. Ringkamp, P. W. Reeh and H. O. Handwerker (1997). Recordings from brain stem neurons responding to chemical stimulation of the subarachnoid space. *Journal of Neurophysiology* **77**(6): 3122–3133.

Ebersberger, A., H. G. Schaible, B. Averbeck and F. Richter (2001). Is there a correlation between spreading depression, neurogenic inflammation, and nociception that might cause migraine headache? *Annals of Neurology* **49**(1): 7–13.

Ekstein, D. and S. C. Schachter (2010). Postictal headache. *Epilepsy & Behavior* **19**(2): 151–155.

Fay, T (1935). The mechanism of headache. *Transactions of the American Neurological Association* **62**: 74–77.

Gallar, J., M. A. Pozo, R. P. Tuckett and C. Belmonte (1993). Response of sensory units with unmyelinated fibres to mechanical, thermal and chemical stimulation of the cat's cornea. *Journal of Physiology (London)* **468**: 609–622.

Harriott, A. M. and M. S. Gold (2008). Serotonin type 1D receptors (5HTR) are differentially distributed in nerve fibres innervating craniofacial tissues. *Cephalalgia* **28**(9): 933–944.

Harriott, A. M. and M. S. Gold (2009). Electrophysiological properties of dural afferents in the absence and presence of inflammatory mediators. *Journal of Neurophysiology* **101**(6): 3126–3134.

Hirata, H. and I. D. Meng (2010). Cold-sensitive corneal afferents respond to a variety of ocular stimuli central to tear production: implications for dry eye disease. *Investigative Ophthalmology & Visual Science* **51**(8): 3969–3976.

Holland, P. R., S. Akerman and P. J. Goadsby (2006). Modulation of nociceptive dural input to the trigeminal nucleus caudalis via activation of the orexin 1 receptor in the rat. *European Journal of Neuroscience* **24**(10): 2825–2833.

Ingvardsen, B. K., H. Laursen, U. B. Olsen and A. J. Hansen (1997). Possible mechanism of c-fos expression in trigeminal nucleus caudalis following cortical spreading depression. *Pain* **72**(3): 407–415.

Iversen, H. K. and J. Olesen (1996). Headache induced by a nitric oxide donor (nitroglycerin) responds to sumatriptan. A human model for development of migraine drugs. *Cephalalgia* **16**(6): 412–418.

Iversen, H. K., J. Olesen and P. Tfelt-Hansen (1989). Intravenous nitroglycerin as an experimental model of vascular headache. Basic characteristics. *Pain* **38**(1): 17–24.

Juhasz, G., T. Zsombok, E. A. Modos, S. Olajos, B. Jakab, J. Nemeth, J. Szolcsanyi, J. Vitrai and G. Bagdy (2003). NO-induced migraine attack: strong increase in plasma calcitonin gene-related peptide (CGRP) concentration and negative correlation with platelet serotonin release. *Pain* **106**(3): 461–470.

Karatas, H., S. E. Erdener, Y. Gursoy-Ozdemir, S. Lule, E. Eren-Kocak, Z. D. Sen and T. Dalkara (2013). Spreading depression triggers headache by activating neuronal Panx1 channels. *Science* **339**(6123): 1092–1095.

Kaube, H., K. L. Hoskin and P. J. Goadsby (1992). Activation of the trigeminovascular system by mechanical distension of the superior sagittal sinus in the cat. *Cephalalgia* **12**(3): 133–136.

Kaube, H., K. A. Keay, K. L. Hoskin, R. Bandler and P. J. Goadsby (1993). Expression of c-Fos-like immunoreactivity in the caudal medulla and upper cervical spinal cord following stimulation of the superior sagittal sinus in the cat. *Brain Research* **629**(1): 95–102.

Knight, Y. E. and P. J. Goadsby (2001). The periaqueductal grey matter modulates trigeminovascular input: a role in migraine? *Neuroscience* **106**(4): 793–800.

Knight, Y. E., T. Bartsch and P. J. Goadsby (2003). Trigeminal antinociception induced by bicuculline in the periaqueductal gray (PAG) is not affected by PAG P/Q-type calcium channel blockade in rat. *Neuroscience Letters* **336**(2): 113–116.

Kosaras, B., M. Jakubowski, V. Kainz and R. Burstein (2009). Sensory innervation of the calvarial bones of the mouse. *Journal of Comparative Neurology* **515**(3): 331–348.

Koulchitsky, S., M. J. Fischer, R. De Col, P. M. Schlechtweg and K. Messlinger (2004). Biphasic response to nitric oxide of spinal trigeminal neurons with meningeal input in rat –possible implications for the pathophysiology of headaches. *Journal of Neurophysiology* **92**(3): 1320–1328.

Koulchitsky, S., M. J. Fischer and K. Messlinger (2009). Calcitonin gene-related peptide receptor inhibition reduces neuronal activity induced by prolonged increase in nitric oxide in the rat spinal trigeminal nucleus. *Cephalalgia* **29**(4): 408–417.

Lambert, G. A., A. S. Zagami, N. Bogduk and J. W. Lance (1991). Cervical spinal cord neurons receiving sensory input from the cranial vasculature. *Cephalalgia* **11**(2): 75–85.

Lambert, G. A., A. J. Lowy, P. M. Boers, H. Angus-Leppan and A. S. Zagami (1992). The spinal cord processing of input from the superior sagittal sinus: pathway and modulation by ergot alkaloids. *Brain Research* **597**(2): 321–330.

Lambert, G. A., J. Michalicek, R. J. Storer and A. S. Zagami (1999). Effect of cortical spreading depression on activity of trigeminovascular sensory neurons. *Cephalalgia* **19**(7): 631–638.

Lambert, G. A., L. Truong and A. S. Zagami (2011). Effect of cortical spreading depression on basal and evoked traffic in the trigeminovascular sensory system. *Cephalalgia* **31**(14): 1439–1451.

Levy, D. and A. M. Strassman (2002a). Distinct sensitizing effects of the cAMP-PKA second messenger cascade on rat dural mechanonociceptors. *Journal of Physiology* **538**(Pt 2): 483–493.

Levy, D. and A. M. Strassman (2002b). Mechanical response properties of A and C primary afferent neurons innervating the rat intracranial dura. *Journal of Neurophysiology* **88**(6): 3021–3031.

Levy, D. and A. M. Strassman (2004). Modulation of dural nociceptor mechanosensitivity by the nitric oxide-cyclic GMP signaling cascade. *Journal of Neurophysiology* **92**(2): 766–772.

Levy, D., M. Jakubowski and R. Burstein (2004). Disruption of communication between peripheral and central trigeminovascular neurons mediates the antimigraine action of 5HT 1B/1D receptor agonists. *Proceedings of the National Academy of Sciences of the United States of America* **101**(12): 4274–4279.

Levy, D., R. Burstein and A. M. Strassman (2005). Calcitonin gene-related peptide does not excite or sensitize meningeal nociceptors: Implications for the pathophysiology of migraine. *Annals of Neurology* **58**(5): 698–705.

Levy, D., R. Burstein, V. Kainz, M. Jakubowski and A. M. Strassman (2007). Mast cell degranulation activates a pain pathway underlying migraine headache. *Pain* **130**(1–2): 166–176.

Levy, D., X. C. Zhang, M. Jakubowski and R. Burstein (2008). Sensitization of meningeal nociceptors: inhibition by naproxen. *European Journal of Neuroscience* **27**(4): 917–922.

Levy, D., V. Kainz, R. Burstein and A. M. Strassman (2012). Mast cell degranulation distinctly activates trigemino-cervical and lumbosacral pain pathways and elicits widespread tactile pain hypersensitivity. *Brain, Behavior, and Immunity* **26**(2): 311–317.

MacIver, M. B. and D. L. Tanelian (1993). Structural and functional specialization of A delta and C fiber free nerve endings innervating rabbit corneal epithelium. *Journal of Neuroscience* **13**(10): 4511–4524.

Martin, H. A., A. I. Basbaum, E. J. Goetzl and J. D. Levine (1988). Leukotriene B4 decreases the mechanical and thermal thresholds of C- fiber nociceptors in the hairy skin of the rat. *Journal of Neurophysiology* **60**(2): 438–445.

Messlinger, K., U. Hanesch, M. Baumgartel, B. Trost and R. F. Schmidt (1993). Innervation of the dura mater encephali of cat and rat: ultrastructure and calcitonin gene-related peptide-like and substance P-like immunoreactivity. *Anatomy and Embryology (Berlin)* **188**(3): 219–237.

Moskowitz, M. A (1984). The neurobiology of vascular head pain. *Annals of Neurology* **16**(2): 157–168.

Moskowitz, M.A (1991). The visceral organ brain: implications for the pathophysiology of vascular head pain. *Neurology* **41**(2 (Pt 1)): 182–186.

Moskowitz, M. A., K. Nozaki and R. P. Kraig (1993). Neocortical spreading depression provokes the expression of c-fos protein-like immunoreactivity within trigeminal nucleus caudalis via trigeminovascular mechanisms. *Journal of Neuroscience* **13**(3): 1167–1177.

Noseda, R., L. Constandil, L. Bourgeais, M. Chalus and L. Villanueva (2010a). Changes of meningeal excitability mediated by corticotrigeminal networks: a link for the endogenous modulation of migraine pain. *Journal of Neuroscience* **30**(43): 14420–14429.

Noseda, R., V. Kainz, M. Jakubowski, J. J. Gooley, C. B. Saper, K. Digre and R. Burstein (2010b). A neural mechanism for exacerbation of headache by light. *Nature Neuroscience* **13**(2): 239–245.

O'Connor, T. P. and D. van der Kooy (1986). Pattern of intracranial and extracranial projections of trigeminal ganglion cells. *Journal of Neuroscience* **6**(8): 2200–2207.

O'Connor, T. P. and D. van der Kooy (1988). Enrichment of a vasoactive neuropeptide (calcitonin gene related peptide) in the trigeminal sensory projection to the intracranial arteries. *Journal of Neuroscience* **8**(7): 2468–2476.

Petruska, J. C., J. Napaporn, R. D. Johnson, J. G. Gu and B. Y. Cooper (2000). Subclassified acutely dissociated cells of rat DRG: histochemistry and patterns of capsaicin-, proton-, and ATP-activated currents. *Journal of Neurophysiology* **84**(5): 2365–2379.

Potrebic, S., A. H. Ahn, K. Skinner, H. L. Fields and A. I. Basbaum (2003). Peptidergic nociceptors of both trigeminal and dorsal root ganglia express serotonin 1D receptors: implications for the selective antimigraine action of triptans. *Journal of Neuroscience* **23**(34): 10988–10997.

Pozo-Rosich, P., R. J. Storer, A. R. Charbit and P. J. Goadsby (2015). Periaqueductal gray calcitonin gene-related peptide modulates trigeminovascular neurons. *Cephalalgia* **35**(14): 1298–307.

Rau, K. K., N. Jiang, R. D. Johnson and B. Y. Cooper (2007). Heat sensitization in skin and muscle nociceptors expressing distinct combinations of TRPV1 and TRPV2 protein. *Journal of Neurophysiology* **97**(4): 2651–2662.

Ray, B. and H. Wolff (1940). Experimental studies on headache: pain-sensitive structures of the head and their significance in headache. *Archives of Surgery* **41**(4): 813–856.

Reuter, U., H. Bolay, I. Jansen-Olesen, A. Chiarugi, M. Sanchez del Rio, R. Letourneau, T. C. Theoharides, C. Waeber and M. A. Moskowitz (2001). Delayed inflammation in rat meninges: implications for migraine pathophysiology. *Brain* **124**(Pt 12): 2490–2502.

Reuter, U., A. Chiarugi, H. Bolay and M. A. Moskowitz (2002). Nuclear factor-kappaB as a molecular target for migraine therapy. *Annals of Neurology* **51**(4): 507–516.

Schlegel, T., S. K. Sauer, H. O. Handwerker and P. W. Reeh (2004). Responsiveness of C-fiber nociceptors to punctate force-controlled stimuli in isolated rat skin: lack of modulation by inflammatory mediators and flurbiprofen. *Neuroscience Letters* **361**(1–3): 163–167.

Schueler, M., K. Messlinger, M. Dux, W. L. Neuhuber and R. De Col (2013). Extracranial projections of meningeal afferents and their impact on meningeal nociception and headache. *Pain* **154**(9): 1622–1631.

Scroggs, R. S., S. M. Todorovic, E. G. Anderson and A. P. Fox (1994). Variation in IH, IIR, and ILEAK between acutely isolated adult rat dorsal root ganglion neurons of different size. *Journal of Neurophysiology* **71**(1): 271–279.

Simone, D. A. and K. C. Kajander (1997). Responses of cutaneous A-fiber nociceptors to noxious cold. *Journal of Neurophysiology* **77**(4): 2049–2060.

Strassman, A. M. and D. Levy (2004). The anti-migraine agent sumatriptan induces a calcium-dependent discharge in meningeal sensory neurons. *Neuroreport* **15**(9): 1409–1412.

Strassman, A. M. and D. Levy (2006). Response properties of dural nociceptors in relation to headache. *Journal of Neurophysiology* **95**(3): 1298–1306.

Strassman, A. M. and S. A. Raymond (1999). Electrophysiological evidence for tetrodotoxin-resistant sodium channels in slowly conducting dural sensory fibers. *Journal of Neurophysiology* **81**(2): 413–424.

Strassman, A., P. Mason, M. Moskowitz and R. Maciewicz (1986). Response of brainstem trigeminal neurons to electrical stimulation of the dura. *Brain Research* **379**(2): 242–250.

Strassman, A. M., S. Potrebic and R. J. Maciewicz (1994). Anatomical properties of brainstem trigeminal neurons that respond to electrical stimulation of dural blood vessels. *Journal of Comparative Neurology* **346**(3): 349–365.

Strassman, A. M., S. A. Raymond and R. Burstein (1996). Sensitization of meningeal sensory neurons and the origin of headaches. *Nature* **384**(6609): 560–564.

Strassman, A. M., W. Weissner, M. Williams, S. Ali and D. Levy (2004). Axon diameters and intradural trajectories of the dural innervation in the rat. *Journal of Comparative Neurology* **473**(3): 364–376.

Thomsen, L. L., C. Kruuse, H. K. Iversen and J. Olesen (1994). A nitric oxide donor (nitroglycerin) triggers genuine migraine attacks. *European Journal of Neurology* **1**(1): 73–80.

Vaughn, A. H. and M. S. Gold (2010). Ionic mechanisms underlying inflammatory mediator-induced sensitization of dural afferents. *Journal of Neuroscience* **30**(23): 7878–7888.

Williams, B (1976). Cerebrospinal fluid pressure changes in response to coughing. *Brain* **99**(2): 331–346.

Wolff, H (1963). *Headache and other head pain.* New York, Oxford University Press.

Zagami, A. S. and G. A. Lambert (1990). Stimulation of cranial vessels excites nociceptive neurones in several thalamic nuclei of the cat. *Experimental Brain Research* **81**(3): 552–566.

Zhang, X.-C., Levy, D. (2008). Modulation of meningeal nociceptors mechanosensitivity by peripheral proteinase-activated receptor-2: the role of mast cells. *Cephalalgia* **28**: 276–284.

Zhang, X. C., A. M. Strassman, R. Burstein and D. Levy (2007). Sensitization and activation of intracranial meningeal nociceptors by mast cell mediators. *Journal of Pharmacology and Experimental Therapeutics* **322**(2): 806–812.

Zhang, X., D. Levy, R. Noseda, V. Kainz, M. Jakubowski and R. Burstein (2010). Activation of meningeal nociceptors by cortical spreading depression: implications for migraine with aura. *Journal of Neuroscience* **30**(26): 8807–8814.

Zhang, X., D. Levy, V. Kainz, R. Noseda, M. Jakubowski and R. Burstein (2011a). Activation of central trigeminovascular neurons by cortical spreading depression. *Annals of Neurology* **69**(5): 855–865.

Zhang, X. C., V. Kainz, R. Burstein and D. Levy (2011b). Tumor necrosis factor-alpha induces sensitization of meningeal nociceptors mediated via local COX and p38 MAP kinase actions. *Pain* **152**(1): 140–149.

Zhang, X., R. Burstein and D. Levy (2012). Local action of the proinflammatory cytokines IL-1beta and IL-6 on intracranial meningeal nociceptors. *Cephalalgia* **32**(1): 66–72.

Zhang, X., V. Kainz, J. Zhao, A. M. Strassman and D. Levy (2013). Vascular extracellular signal-regulated kinase mediates migraine-related sensitization of meningeal nociceptors. *Annals of Neurology* **73**(6): 741–750.

Zhao, J. and D. Levy (2014). The sensory innervation of the calvarial periosteum is nociceptive and contributes to headache-like behavior. *Pain* **155**(7): 1392–1400.

Zhao, J. and D. Levy (2015). Modulation of intracranial meningeal nociceptor activity by cortical spreading depression: a reassessment. *Journal of Neurophysiology* **113**(7): 2778–2785.

3

Meningeal afferent ion channels and their role in migraine

Gregory Dussor

Behavioral and Brain Sciences, BSB-14, The University of Texas at Dallas, Richardson, Texas, USA

3.1   Meningeal afferents and migraine pain

Among the hypotheses proposed for the pain phase of migraine, activation of afferent nociceptors innervating the cranial meninges is the most widely accepted (Levy, 2010), but it is not clear what events lead to activation of these neurons. Prior preclinical studies show that dural afferents are mechanically sensitive (Kaube *et al.*, 1992; Strassman *et al.*, 1996; Levy and Strassman, 2002), consistent with the worsening of headaches due to changes in intracranial pressure. Receptors or structures on meningeal afferent endings that convey mechanical sensitivity to these neurons have yet to be fully described (though some potential candidates will be described below). Chemical sensitivity of dural afferents has also been described, and intracranial and circulating levels of various inflammatory mediators are significantly higher during migraine attacks (Sarchielli *et al.*, 2001; Perini *et al.*, 2005). Among the stimuli capable of activating or sensitizing dural afferents are capsaicin, mustard oil, hypotonic solutions, or an inflammatory soup (IS) (Strassman *et al.*, 1996; Bove and Moskowitz, 1997; Wei *et al.*, 2011; Edelmayer *et al.*, 2012). In addition, tumor necrosis factor-α (TNF-α), interleukin-6 (IL-6), and interleukin-1β (IL-1β) can also act to sensitize dural afferents (Zhang *et al.*, 2011, 2012; Yan *et al.*, 2012) (see Chapter 6).

This chapter will now focus on ion channels that may contribute to the activation and sensitization of dural afferents (Figure 3.1). Ion channels are responsible for generating and maintaining neuronal excitability, and dysfunction or dysregulation of ion channels on dural afferents can potentially contribute to the pathophysiology of migraine pain.

3.2   Transient receptor potential (TRP) channels and headache

TRP channels have been extensively studied for their role in pain, given their ability to detect stimuli such as temperature, changes in extracellular osmolarity, pH, and an extensive list of natural products (Liu *et al.*, 2003; Karai *et al.*, 2004; Ramsey *et al.*, 2006). Among the subtypes of TRP channels are TRPC, TRPM, TRPV, TRPA, TRPP,

Neurobiological Basis of Migraine, First Edition. Edited by Turgay Dalkara and Michael A. Moskowitz.

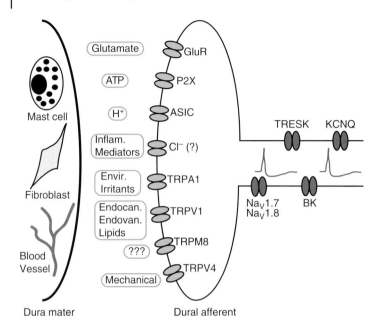

Figure 3.1 Ion channels expressed on dural afferents contribute to afferent signaling from the meninges. The dura mater is populated with a variety of cell types including mast cells, fibroblasts, and blood vessels. Release of substances from these cells can lead to sterile inflammation and recruitment of environmental irritants or other factors into the dura through blood vessels. Increased levels of pro-inflammatory mediators, endocannabinoids, endovanniloids, lipids, environmental irritants, glutamate, ATP, or H+ ions within the dura activate ion channels on trigeminal afferents innervating the dura. Mechanical stimuli can also act on the dura subsequent to changes in intracranial pressure. Channels activated by these stimuli include TRPs, ASICs, P2X, Glutamate, and Cl− channels. Depolarization of dural afferent terminals can lead to action potentials and afferent signaling through recruitment of voltage-gated Na+ channels. Action potential firing can be modulated in these neurons by the activity of K+ channels such as BK, KCNQ, and TRESK.

and TRPML members (Vriens *et al.*, 2009; Holzer and Izzo, 2014). TRP channels are generally excitatory, as they allow the influx of Na^+ and Ca^{++} into neurons (Ramsey *et al.*, 2006), and they have been investigated in the context of many sensory systems (Numazaki and Tominaga, 2004). Although much attention has been focused on TRP channels in pain outside the head, more recent studies have been building a case for these channels in headache disorders (Dussor *et al.*, 2014).

3.2.1 TRPA1

TRPA1 is thought to contribute to various forms of pain (Zygmunt and Hogestatt, 2014), and its expression on peripheral sensory neurons has been extensively documented (Jordt *et al.*, 2004). TRPA1 may be a sensor for extreme cold temperature (Story *et al.*, 2003), although this has been the subject of much debate (Caspani and Heppenstall, 2009). There was recently some degree of clinical validation given to a role for TRPA1 in human pain, following identification of a gain-of-function mutation in TRPA1 in humans with familial episodic pain syndrome (Kremeyer *et al.*, 2010). This condition is a rare disorder, characterized by upper limb pain but, unlike most other forms of pain (except migraine), this type of pain is often preceded by a prodrome phase, and triggered by fasting and physical stress.

One of the primary reasons for interest in TRPA1 for headache is its activation by environmental irritants such as formaldehyde (McNamara *et al.*, 2007), chlorine (Bessac and Jordt, 2008), cigarette smoke extract (Andre *et al.*, 2008), and acrolein (Bautista *et al.*, 2006), natural plant products, such as isothiocyanates from mustard (Jordt *et al.*, 2004), cinnamaldehyde from cinnamon (Bandell *et al.*, 2004), allicin from garlic (Bautista *et al.*, 2005), and endogenous oxidative and nitrative stress products such as 4-hydroxynonenal (Trevisani *et al.*, 2007), nitro-oleic acid (Taylor-Clark *et al.*, 2009), and reactive prostaglandins (Materazzi *et al.*, 2008). Many TRPA1 activators on this list are well-known migraine triggers (Wantke *et al.*, 2000; Irlbacher and Meyer, 2002; Kelman, 2007; Nassini *et al.*, 2012).

Several recent preclinical studies have suggested a role for TRPA1 in the pathophysiology of migraine. The findings that TRPA1 is expressed (Huang *et al.*, 2012) and functional (Edelmayer *et al.*, 2012) on dural afferents in rodents supports the possibility of a contribution from this channel in headache disorders. TRPA1 agonists, including mustard oil and acrolein, can increase dural blood flow in a CGRP-dependent manner when given intranasally (Kunkler *et al.*, 2011), and repetitive exposure to acrolein can sensitize these responses (Kunkler *et al.*, 2015). This suggests that activation of dural afferent nerve endings (the likely source of CGRP) can occur following environmental exposure to agents inhaled through the nose.

Using a behavioral model of migraine, dural application of mustard oil produced signs consistent with headache, including cutaneous facial allodynia and decreased exploratory locomotor behavior (Edelmayer *et al.*, 2012). Additionally, induction of CSD in rats leads to increased lipid peroxidation in the cortex, meninges, and TG, and application of hydrogen peroxide to the meninges activates afferent signaling via TRPA1 (Shatillo *et al.*, 2013). These studies provide preclinical data supporting a potential role for dural TRPA1 in increased blood flow, CGRP-dependent neurogenic inflammation, and headache.

Additional evidence supporting a role for TRPA1 in headache disorders comes from individuals who develop cluster-like headache attacks when exposed to the "headache tree" or *U. californica* (Nassini *et al.*, 2012). The volatile oils from this tree contain a substance known as umbellulone, an agonist of TRPA1, which can produce many of the same effects of mustard oil, including increased dural blood flow and CGRP release (Nassini *et al.*, 2012). Dural application of umbellulone also produced cutaneous facial allodynia and decreased exploratory behavior (Edelmayer *et al.*, 2012). How umbellulone is able to provoke headache in humans exposed to this substance is unclear. Two studies have shown effects of TRPA1 activators (including umbellulone) within the dura after nasal administration (Kunkler *et al.*, 2011; Nassini *et al.*, 2012), supporting a general concept where inhaled substances can promote headache either via access to the meninges, or via intraganglionic transmission in the trigeminal ganglia (Kunkler *et al.*, 2014).

These studies suggest that TRPA1 antagonists may have efficacy for environmental irritant-induced headaches, but there may also be potential for these therapeutics to treat migraine. Feverfew is a common herbal remedy for migraine, and one active ingredient in this herb, parthenolide, was recently found to be a TRPA1 partial agonist (Materazzi *et al.*, 2013). Rather than acting as an antagonist, parthenolide is capable of acting as a desensitizing agonist, leading to functional block of the channel. When rats were pre-treated with parthenolide to desensitize TRPA1, subsequent administration of mustard oil onto the dura produced significantly smaller headache-like responses than when mustard oil application was preceded by vehicle (Materazzi *et al.*, 2013). These studies lend further support to the potential of TRPA1 as a therapeutic headache target. Ultimately, efficacy of this approach awaits development of compounds suitable to test this hypothesis in human migraineurs.

3.2.2 TRPM8

Another TRP channel that has gained attention in the migraine literature recently is TRPM8. TRPM8 has long been known to be the sensor of cool temperatures (below 26°C), but it also responds to chemicals such as menthol and the supercooling agent icilin. Primary afferent sensory neurons express TRPM8 mRNA (McKemy *et al.*, 2002; Peier *et al.*, 2002) and, relevant to migraine, its expression is found in trigeminal ganglia (Nealen *et al.*, 2003). Within the trigeminal system, the most clear role for TRPM8 is in detection of cold stimuli in the oral cavity and head (Kim *et al.*, 2014) but, surprisingly, the channel may also participate in the detection of odorants (Lubbert *et al.*, 2013). Less clear is the endogenous function of TRPM8 expression on deep-tissue afferents, such as those in the colon and bladder (Mukerji *et al.*, 2006; Harrington *et al.*, 2011), as these nerve endings are, generally, not exposed to decreased temperature in the range of TRPM8 detection. These studies may imply an alternate sensory function for the channel. Although the endogenous activator is not clear, various lipids, or the growth factor artemin, have been proposed (Lippoldt *et al.*, 2013; Sousa-Valente *et al.*, 2014).

The interest in TRPM8 in relation to migraine is largely based on results of genome-wide association studies (GWAS) performed on migraine patients. Multiple studies have found variants in the TRPM8 gene in migraine patients (An *et al.*, 2013; Ghosh *et al.*, 2013; Chasman *et al.*, 2011,2014; Fan *et al.*, 2014; Freilinger *et al.*, 2012), which is highly suggestive of a role for this channel in migraine. It remains to be determined whether, and how, these genetic variants impact the function/expression of the channel, as studies have not yet been performed.

In terms of preclinical data supporting a role for TRPM8 in migraine, the studies are few in number. There is controversy surrounding whether TRPM8 is expressed in dural afferents, since little to no expression was observed in one study (Huang *et al.*, 2012), but another found expression to depend on the region of the dura examined (Newsom *et al.*, 2012). More recently, it was shown that application of the TRPM8 agonist icilin to the dura produced cutaneous facial allodynia in rats (Burgos-Vega *et al.*, 2015). This behavioral response was attenuated in the presence of sumatriptan, as well as a nitric oxide synthase (NOS) inhibitor. The ability of these agents to attenuate allodynia suggests that the state produced by TRPM8 activation within the dura is migraine-like, as sumatriptan is the gold standard in migraine treatment, and NOS inhibitors showed efficacy in a small human migraine trial (Lassen *et al.*, 1998, 2003). However, the endogenous role for TRPM8 activation during migraine is not clear.

3.2.3 TRPV1

TRPV1 is best known as the molecular sensor of noxious heat (above 42°C) and a sensor for plant extracts like capsaicin (Caterina and Julius, 2001). In addition to activation by heat and capsaicin, TRPV1 activity is potentiated by low pH (extracellular) (Jordt *et al.*, 2000), suggesting a broad role for the channel in pain due to injury or inflammation, and it can also be modulated downstream of other receptor signaling systems, including bradykinin, serotonin, prostaglandin and prokineticin receptors (Julius, 2013).

In relation to migraine, genetic variants in TRPV1 have been shown (Carreno *et al.*, 2012). However, like TRPM8, it is not yet clear how these variants contribute to channel expression and/or function. TRPV1 is expressed on dural afferent fibers (Shimizu *et al.*, 2007) and trigeminal ganglion neurons retrogradely labeled from the dura (Huang *et al.*, 2012). Functional activation of TRPV1 within the dura leads to dilation of dural vessels (Akerman *et al.*, 2003), initiation of afferent signaling (Strassman *et al.*, 1996; Bove and Moskowitz, 1997; Schepelmann *et al.*, 1999), activation of intracellular kinases in trigeminal ganglion neurons (Iwashita *et al.*, 2013), and headache-like behavioral responses (Yan *et al.*, 2011). Activity of TRPV1 is decreased following application of sumatriptan to cells (Evans *et al.*, 2012), and TRPV1-mediated behavioral responses are also sensitive to sumatriptan (Loyd *et al.*, 2012), suggesting TRPV1 modulation as one mechanism by which sumatriptan has efficacy for migraine. Also, recent studies in humans show increased expression of TRPV1 in arteries taken from the scalp of chronic migraine patients but not healthy controls (Del Fiacco *et al.*, 2015).

Similar to other TRP channels, the endogenous mechanisms that may activate TRPV1 during migraine are not known. Potential endogenous activators include endocannabinoids such as anandamide (Zygmunt *et al.*, 1999), endovanilloids such as N-arachidonoyl-dopamine (NADA) (Huang *et al.*, 2002), and lipid products of the lipoxygenase pathway (Hwang *et al.*, 2000), any of which may be present in the dura, and may contribute to migraine pain. TRPV1 is also modulated downstream of bradykinin (Chuang *et al.*, 2001), nerve-growth factor (Chuang *et al.*, 2001), and prostaglandin (Moriyama *et al.*, 2005) receptor signaling.

There have been several attempts to develop therapeutics based on modulation of TRPV1. Civamide, an intranasal TRPV1 agonist (presumably acting via desensitization of the channel or the entire nerve terminal), was found to be effective for both migraine and cluster headaches (Diamond *et al.*, 2000), and intranasal capsaicin is also efficacious for migraine (Fusco *et al.*, 2003). Preclinically, TRPV1 antagonists have shown variable results in several headache models. Systemic capsazepine, a TRPV1 antagonist, blocked capsaicin-induced vasodilation in the dura (Akerman *et al.*, 2003), and another systemic TRPV1 antagonist, SB-705498, also decreased dural afferent activity after stimulation of the dura (Lambert *et al.*, 2009). In other, similar experiments, however, the TRPV1 antagonist A993610 given systemically showed no efficacy (Summ *et al.*, 2011).

Most problematic for arguing a contribution of TRPV1 to migraine is the failure of a TRPV1 antagonist (SB-705498) against migraine in a human Phase II study (Palmer *et al.*, 2009). This compound also had no efficacy on photo- or phonophobia. The inconsistent results of TRPV1 antagonists in preclinical models, as well as the failed human trial, cast doubt on the future of this target for migraine therapeutics.

3.2.4 TRPV4

As mentioned above, dural afferents are mechanically sensitive (Ray and Wolff, 1940; Kaube *et al.*, 1992; Strassman *et al.*, 1996; Levy and Strassman, 2002). The additional sensitivity of dural afferents to changes in extracellular osmolarity (Strassman *et al.*, 1996) suggests a role for TRPV4 in afferent signaling, as this channel has been proposed to be both a mechano and an osmosensor (Liedtke *et al.*, 2000; Watanabe *et al.*, 2002; Liedtke *et al.*, 2003; Vriens *et al.*, 2004). Trigeminal ganglion neurons express the mRNA for TRPV4 (Kitahara *et al.*, 2005), and the channel appears to be functional on these neurons (Chen *et al.*, 2008a, 2008b). These studies suggest that TRPV4 may contribute to the mechanosensitivity of dural afferents but, until recently, preclinical headache experiments assessing a role for TRPV4 had not been conducted.

In a 2011 study, TRPV4-like currents were demonstrated on dural afferents *in vitro* in response to hypotonic solutions and the TRPV4 activator 4αPDD (Wei *et al.*, 2011). This study also showed headache-like behavioral responses in response to hypotonic stimulation of the dura, and effect blocked by a TRPV4 antagonist. These studies more directly implicate TRPV4 in processes contributing to headache, and suggest that this channel may contribute to mechanoactivation of dural afferents by changes in intracranial pressure, or other events known to worsen headache, such as coughing, sneezing, or routine physical activity (Burstein *et al.*, 2000).

3.3   Acid-sensing ion channels

Acid-sensing ion channels (ASICs) are cation channels, closely related to epithelial sodium channels (ENaC), that respond to decreased extracellular pH. There are four ASIC subunits and several splice variants (Deval *et al.*, 2010; Sherwood *et al.*, 2012; Wemmie *et al.*, 2013; Zha, 2013), and they are half-maximally activating by pHs between 4.0 and 6.8 (Deval *et al.*, 2010). There is expression of ASICs throughout the central (Grunder and Chen, 2010; Wemmie *et al.*, 2003) and peripheral nervous systems, including on primary afferent sensory neurons necessary for pain signaling (Alvarez de la Rosa *et al.*, 2002; Wemmie *et al.*, 2013). ASICs are thought to contribute to pain states such as angina, intermittent claudication, and arthritis.

Several prior studies implicate ASICs in migraine-related processes (for further review, see Dussor, 2015), and they may contribute to activation of dural afferents (Burstein, 2001). *In vivo* electrophysiological studies from the late 1990s found that dural afferents respond to pH 4.7 in rats (Burstein *et al.*, 1998), pH 5.0 in guinea pigs (Bove and Moskowitz, 1997), while another rat study examined responses to pH 6.1 in (Schepelmann *et al.*, 1999). Later studies examined the release of CGRP from both the dura and trigeminal ganglia in response to pH 5.4–5.9, and the ganglia release was blocked by the ASIC3 antagonist APETx2 (Zimmermann *et al.*, 2002; Durham and Masterson, 2013). Vasodilation in the meninges and afferent signaling in the TNC following electrical stimulation of the dura were both blocked by the ASIC antagonist amiloride (Holland *et al.*, 2012).

Recently, it was found that dural afferents generate ASIC currents at pH 6.0 and pH 7.0 (Yan *et al.*, 2011) that were blocked by amiloride. Further, dural afferents that respond to pH 6.0 also respond to the ASIC3 activator GMQ, and ASIC3 labeling was found on dural afferents (Yan *et al.*, 2013). Using a preclinical behavioral headache model, pH 5.0, 6.0, and 6.4 produced headache-like responses when applied to the dura, and both amiloride and APETx2 blocked these responses. These studies are some of the most direct evidence published thus far for a role of ASIC signaling within the meninges.

ASICs may also contribute to migraine-related processes, such as cortical spreading depression (CSD: for review of CSD see Pietrobon and Moskowitz, 2014). Holland and colleagues showed in preclinical studies that CSD events were blocked by amiloride, and the ASIC1a blocked PcTx1 (Holland *et al.*, 2012). However, this study went on to examine a potential contribution of ASICs to migraine in humans. In seven otherwise treatment-resistant migraine patients, four had substantial improvement in both headache severity and aura frequency. Although many questions remain from this small trial, these findings suggest that ASICs may contribute to migraine in humans, and they may be potential targets for novel therapeutics.

3.4 Glutamate-gated channels

Numerous studies suggest a role for glutamate-mediated signaling within the meninges and in the afferent system projecting from the meninges. In the dura, vasodilation following electrical or chemical stimulation was blocked by NMDA, AMPA, and kainate antagonists (Chan *et al.*, 2010). In the TG, glutamate is co-expressed on neurons that also express several serotonin 5-HT1 receptors (Ma, 2001) suggesting that triptans (acting on 5-HT1 receptors) may produce their therapeutic effects due to decreased glutamate release from TG afferents. 5-HT application inhibits the evoked release of glutamate from cultured TG neurons, an effect blocked by a 5HT1b/1d antagonist (Xiao *et al.*, 2008) and, in the TNC, multiple studies have shown a role for glutamate signaling related to migraine (Mitsikostas and Sanchez del Rio, 2001).

Glutamate receptors contribute to CGRP release within the TNC (Kageneck *et al.*, 2014). Activation of 5-HT1b and/or 5-HT1d receptors with sumatriptan or more selective agonists can inhibit glutamate release from pre-synaptic neurons (Jennings *et al.*, 2004; Choi *et al.*, 2012), while activation of TNC neurons following dural stimulation is inhibited in the presence of a kainate receptor antagonist (Andreou *et al.*, 2015). Finally, stimulation of the dura with an inflammatory cocktail causes an initial decrease in glutamate levels in the TNC, followed by a marked and prolonged increase (Oshinsky and Luo, 2006). Similarly, in animals subjected to repetitive stimulation of the dura with an inflammatory cocktail, there is a large increase in extracellular glutamate following administration of a nitric oxide donor (Oshinsky and Gomonchareonsiri, 2007). Together, these studies suggest that glutamate signaling at multiple sites throughout the dural afferent system can contribute to the pathophysiology of migraine.

3.5 ATP-gated channels

ATP acts as an extracellular neurotransmitter in part by signaling through ligand-gated ion channels known as P2X receptors (Burnstock, 2000). There are seven known subtypes of P2X channels. P2X3 has received a great deal of attention in the pain research field (Ford, 2012), as it is highly expressed on primary afferent nociceptors (Chen *et al.*, 1995; North, 2002; Burnstock, 2006). About half of dural afferents express $P2X_2$, $P2X_3$ or both (Staikopoulos *et al.*, 2007). Further, P2X3 can be upregulated by nerve growth factor (NGF), which is elevated in the cerebrospinal fluid of chronic daily headache patients (Sarchielli *et al.*, 2001).

In preclinical studies, NGF increases P2X3 currents in trigeminal ganglia (Simonetti *et al.*, 2006), and neutralization of tonic NGF levels decreases these currents (D'Arco *et al.*, 2007). Another migraine-related factor that can influence P2X3 is CGRP, which has been found to increase expression and currents (Fabbretti *et al.*, 2006). Finally, familial-hemiplegic migraine (FHM) Type 1 is a rare subtype of migraine due to mutations in voltage-gated calcium channels. In a mouse genetic model of FHM1, there was found to be increased membrane expression of P2X3 (Gnanasekaran *et al.*, 2011). These studies all suggest a contribution of P2X channels to migraine pathophysiology, but more work is needed to further explore this link.

3.6 K$^+$ channels

Preclinical studies have implicated several types of K$^+$ channels in migraine-related processes. Calcium-activated K$^+$ channels open following a rise in intracellular calcium (and, in some, cases a change in voltage). The large conductance calcium-activated K$^+$ channel, named BK or MaxiK, is widely expressed in the nervous system, and opening of this channel reduces neuronal excitability and neurotransmitter release (Gribkoff *et al.*, 2001). These channels are also expressed on primary sensory neurons, and BK knockout mice have increased pain behaviors (Lu *et al.*, 2013). In relation to migraine, BK mRNA and protein is found within the TG and TNC (Wulf-Johansson *et al.*, 2010). The BK blocker iberiotoxin caused an increase in CGRP release from TNC in this study. Another study found that the BK opener NS1619 inhibited vasodilation in the dura, and direct application of this compound to the TNC inhibited afferent activity, following dural stimulation (Akerman *et al.*, 2010). These studies suggest that targeting BK channels may have therapeutic potential for migraine.

Twin-pore or two-pore domain potassium channels are responsible for the leak K$^+$ currents that are the basis of the resting membrane potential (Enyedi and Czirjak, 2010). This family contains 15 members that are primarily voltage insensitive but can be modulated by intracellular pH, membrane stretch, lipids, and anesthetics. A recent study identified a mutation in KCNK18 (aka TRESK) in members of a family suffering from migraine with aura, but not in non-migraine family members (Lafreniere *et al.*, 2010), while another study found additional genetic variants in this channel in a distinct population of migraineurs (Rainero *et al.*, 2014).

TRESK is highly expressed in the TG of mice, as well as humans (Lafreniere *et al.*, 2010; Lafreniere and Rouleau, 2011). Functionally, expression of mutated TRESK channels in TG lowers the threshold for activation and increases the firing frequency of action potentials (Liu *et al.*, 2013). This occurs with mutations found migraine patients, but not in other channel mutants that are not associated with migraine (Guo *et al.*, 2014). Although these studies suggest a potential role for TRESK in afferent signaling from the meninges (and migraine pain), other studies have shown loss-of-function mutations in TRESK in both migraine patients and healthy controls (Andres-Enguix *et al.*, 2012). Thus, it remains unclear whether, and how, this channel contributes to migraine.

Another K$^+$ channel that may contribute to dural afferent signaling and migraine pain is KCNQ. KCNQ, also known as Kv7 (Kv7.1-Kv7.5) that generates M-current, is a K$^+$ channel opened at sub-threshold voltage that is non-inactivating, and decreases repetitive action potential firing (Brown and Passmore, 2009). Although this channel is found in sensory neurons, little attention has been paid to whether it may contribute to signaling in the trigeminal system. Recently however, systemic administration of ezogabine, a KCNQ opener, was found to decrease the spontaneous activity of dural afferents and to decrease their activation, if given before induction of CSD (Zhang *et al.*, 2013). Ezogabine is currently FDA-approved for partial onset seizures, and may offer an additional option for the treatment of migraine.

3.7 Other ion channels that may contribute to dural afferent signaling

A variety of other ion channels may contribute to dural afferent signaling, but these have been the subject of fewer focused studies. Although voltage-gated calcium channels may contribute to migraine, particularly FHM type 1, they have been reviewed elsewhere (Pietrobon, 2012) and are discussed in a separate chapter in this book. Several studies implicate changes in voltage-gated Na^+ channels in modulation of signaling from the dura. Exposure of dural afferents to interleukin-6 (IL-6), a cytokine elevated during migraine attacks (Fidan *et al.*, 2006; Sarchielli *et al.*, 2006), increases excitability of these neurons and increases association of extracellular signal-regulated protein kinase (ERK) with the Na^+ channel Nav1.7 (Yan *et al.*, 2012). ERK phosphorylation of Nav1.7 is known to sensitize the channel (Stamboulian *et al.*, 2010), suggesting that increased Na^+ channel activity in the presence of IL-6 contributes to enhanced signaling from the dura. Application of IL-6 to the dura of rats produced headache-like behavior that was blocked following inhibition of ERK (Yan *et al.*, 2012). Additionally, a cocktail of PGE2, bradykinin and histamine, applied to dural afferents, depolarized the resting membrane potential and decreased the action potential threshold (Harriott and Gold, 2009), the latter most likely mediated by an increase in tetrodotoxin-resistant voltage-gated Na^+ currents (Vaughn and Gold, 2010). However, this cocktail also activated a previously unrecognized depolarizing Cl^- current that may be responsible for the membrane depolarization (Vaughn and Gold, 2010).

Finally, $GABA_A$ has been implicated in migraine-related processes in the dura as well as the TNC. Plasma protein extravasation within the rat dura following stimulation of the TG was reduced by sodium valproate or muscimol, an effect blocked by the GABAA antagonist bicuculline (Lee *et al.*, 1995). Intracisternal capsaicin administration to guinea pigs caused c-fos expression in the TNC that was decreased by valproate administration and blocked by bicuculline (Cutrer *et al.*, 1995). These studies, together, show that numerous other ion channels may be modulated by the processes present within the dural afferent pathway during migraine, and these channels may be targets for novel therapeutics.

3.8 Conclusions

Migraine is one of the most prevalent disorders on the planet, and is one of the leading causes of pain and disability. Although triptans revolutionized the treatment of migraine when introduced several decades ago, they still leave most migraine patients with either residual symptoms, or completely untreated. CGRP-based therapeutics hold great promise, but it is yet unclear whether these agents will have efficacy in a larger fraction of migraine patients than triptans. Thus, there is a great need for additional novel therapeutics.

The studies described here make a compelling case that numerous ion channels contribute to the pathophysiology of migraine. Mutations in TRPM8 and TRESK identified by GWAS implicate these channels in common forms of migraine, and preclinical studies are beginning to uncover how these channels contribute to the disorder. Data from humans exposed to the "headache tree" and the efficacy (albeit limited) of natural products, such as feverfew, suggest that there may a contribution of TRPA1 to primary headache disorders. Preclinical studies support this concept, but more work is necessary to better understand how TRPA1 may play a role in migraine.

These examples of translation from human observations to animal studies are paralleled with studies examining a role for ASICs in migraine, which originated with animal experiments. These animal findings were translated into humans through the use and efficacy of amiloride in treatment-resistant migraine patients. This bi-directional translation between humans and animals is necessary for continued progress toward a greater understanding of the pathophysiology of migraine and development of new therapeutics. Although there is a clear contribution of the brain to migraine, the recent demonstration that antibodies against CGRP have efficacy for migraine, and the poor access of antibodies to the CNS, argue that mechanisms such as those described above, which can mediate a peripheral contribution to migraine pain, should continue to be the focus of future studies. Without these types of studies, migraine will remain one of the most disabling conditions on the planet, as increases in the understanding of the disorder will be slow.

3.9 Acknowledgements

This work was supported by funding from the NIH (NS072204) and the Migraine Research Foundation.

References

Akerman, S., H. Kaube and P. J. Goadsby (2003). Vanilloid type 1 receptors (VR1) on trigeminal sensory nerve fibres play a minor role in neurogenic dural vasodilatation, and are involved in capsaicin-induced dural dilation. *British Journal of Pharmacology* **140**(4): 718–724.

Akerman, S., P. R. Holland, M. P. Lasalandra and P. J. Goadsby (2010). Inhibition of trigeminovascular dural nociceptive afferents by Ca^{2+}-activated K^{+} (MaxiK/BK(Ca)) channel opening. *Pain* **151**(1): 128–136.

Alvarez de la Rosa, D., P. Zhang, D. Shao, F. White and C. M. Canessa (2002). Functional implications of the localization and activity of acid-sensitive channels in rat peripheral nervous system. *Proceedings of the National Academy of Sciences of the United States of America* **99**(4): 2326–2331.

An, X. K., Q. L. Ma, Q. Lin, X. R. Zhang, C. X. Lu and H. L. Qu (2013). PRDM16 rs2651899 variant is a risk factor for Chinese common migraine patients. *Headache* **53**(10): 1595–1601.

Andre, E., B. Campi, S. Materazzi, M. Trevisani, S. Amadesi, D. Massi, C. Creminon, N. Vaksman, R. Nassini, M. Civelli, P. G. Baraldi, D. P. Poole, N. W. Bunnett, P. Geppetti and R. Patacchini (2008). Cigarette smoke-induced neurogenic inflammation is mediated by alpha, beta-unsaturated aldehydes and the TRPA1 receptor in rodents. *Journal of Clinical Investigation* **118**(7): 2574–2582.

Andreou, A. P., P. R. Holland, M. P. Lasalandra and P. J. Goadsby (2015). Modulation of nociceptive dural input to the trigeminocervical complex through GluK1 kainate receptors. *Pain* **156**(3): 439–450.

Andres-Enguix, I., L. Shang, P. J. Stansfeld, J. M. Morahan, M. S. Sansom, R. G. Lafreniere, B. Roy, L. R. Griffiths, G. A. Rouleau, G. C. Ebers, Z. M. Cader and S. J. Tucker (2012). Functional analysis of missense variants in the TRESK (KCNK18) K channel. *Scientific Reports* **2**: 237.

Bandell, M., G. M. Story, S. W. Hwang, V. Viswanath, S. R. Eid, M. J. Petrus, T. J. Earley and A. Patapoutian (2004). Noxious cold ion channel TRPA1 is activated by pungent compounds and bradykinin. *Neuron* **41**(6): 849–857.

Bautista, D. M., P. Movahed, A. Hinman, H. E. Axelsson, O. Sterner, E. D. Hogestatt, D. Julius, S. E. Jordt and P. M. Zygmunt (2005). Pungent products from garlic activate the sensory ion channel TRPA1. *Proceedings of the National Academy of Sciences of the United States of America* **102**(34): 12248–12252.

Bautista, D. M., S. E. Jordt, T. Nikai, P. R. Tsuruda, A. J. Read, J. Poblete, E. N. Yamoah, A. I. Basbaum and D. Julius (2006). TRPA1 mediates the inflammatory actions of environmental irritants and proalgesic agents. *Cell* **124**(6): 1269–1282.

Bessac, B. F. and S. E. Jordt (2008). Breathtaking TRP channels: TRPA1 and TRPV1 in airway chemosensation and reflex control. *Physiology (Bethesda)* **23**: 360–370.

Bove, G. M. and M. A. Moskowitz (1997). Primary afferent neurons innervating guinea pig dura. *Journal of Neurophysiology* **77**(1): 299–308.

Brown, D. A. and G. M. Passmore (2009). Neural KCNQ (Kv7) channels. *British Journal of Pharmacology* **156**(8): 1185–1195.

Burgos-Vega, C. C., D. D. Ahn, C. Bischoff, W. Wang, D. Horne, J. Wang, N. Gavva and G. Dussor (2015). Meningeal transient receptor potential channel M8 activation causes cutaneous facial and hindpaw allodynia in a preclinical rodent model of headache. *Cephalalgia* **36**(2): 185–193.

Burnstock, G. (2000). P2X receptors in sensory neurones. *British Journal of Anaesthesia* **84**(4): 476–488.

Burnstock, G. (2006). Purinergic P2 receptors as targets for novel analgesics. *Pharmacology & Therapeutics* **110**(3): 433–454.

Burstein, R. (2001). Deconstructing migraine headache into peripheral and central sensitization. *Pain* **89**(2–3): 107–110.

Burstein, R., H. Yamamura, A. Malick and A. M. Strassman (1998). Chemical stimulation of the intracranial dura induces enhanced responses to facial stimulation in brain stem trigeminal neurons. *Journal of Neurophysiology* **79**(2): 964–982.

Burstein, R., M. F. Cutrer and D. Yarnitsky (2000). The development of cutaneous allodynia during a migraine attack clinical evidence for the sequential recruitment of spinal and supraspinal nociceptive neurons in migraine. *Brain* **123**(Pt 8): 1703–1709.

Carreno, O., R. Corominas, J. Fernandez-Morales, M. Camina, M. J. Sobrido, J. M. Fernandez-Fernandez, P. Pozo-Rosich, B. Cormand and A. Macaya (2012). SNP variants within the vanilloid TRPV1 and TRPV3 receptor genes are associated with migraine in the Spanish population. *American Journal of Medical Genetics Part B: Neuropsychiatric Genetics* **159B**(1): 94–103.

Caspani, O. and P. A. Heppenstall (2009). TRPA1 and cold transduction: an unresolved issue? *Journal of General Physiology* **133**(3): 245–249.

Caterina, M. J. and D. Julius (2001). The vanilloid receptor: a molecular gateway to the pain pathway. *Annual Review of Neuroscience* **24**: 487–517.

Chan, K. Y., S. Gupta, R. de Vries, A. H. Danser, C. M. Villalon, E. Munoz-Islas and A. Maassenvandenbrink (2010). Effects of ionotropic glutamate receptor antagonists on rat dural artery diameter in an intravital microscopy model. *British Journal of Pharmacology* **160**(6): 1316–1325.

Chasman, D. I., M. Schurks, V. Anttila, B. de Vries, U. Schminke, L. J. Launer, G. M. Terwindt, A. M. van den Maagdenberg, K. Fendrich, H. Volzke, F. Ernst, L. R. Griffiths, J. E. Buring, M. Kallela, T. Freilinger, C. Kubisch, P. M. Ridker, A. Palotie, M. D. Ferrari, W. Hoffmann, R. Y. Zee and T. Kurth (2011). Genome-wide association study reveals three susceptibility loci for common migraine in the general population. *Nature Genetics* **43**(7): 695–698.

Chasman, D. I., V. Anttila, J. E. Buring, P. M. Ridker, M. Schurks, T. Kurth and C. International Headache Genetics (2014). Selectivity in genetic association with sub-classified migraine in women. *PLOS Genetics* **10**(5): e1004366.

Chen, C. C., A. N. Akopian, L. Sivilotti, D. Colquhoun, G. Burnstock and J. N. Wood (1995). A P2X purinoceptor expressed by a subset of sensory neurons. *Nature* **377**(6548): 428–431.

Chen, L., C. Liu and L. Liu (2008a). Changes in osmolality modulate voltage-gated calcium channels in trigeminal ganglion neurons. *Brain Research* **1208**: 56–66.

Chen, L., C. Liu and L. Liu (2008b). The modulation of voltage-gated potassium channels by anisotonicity in trigeminal ganglion neurons. *Neuroscience* **154**(2): 482–495.

Choi, I. S., J. H. Cho, C. H. An, J. K. Jung, Y. K. Hur, J. K. Choi and I. S. Jang (2012). 5-HT(1B) receptors inhibit glutamate release from primary afferent terminals in rat medullary dorsal horn neurons. *British Journal of Pharmacology* **167**(2): 356–367.

Chuang, H. H., E. D. Prescott, H. Kong, S. Shields, S. E. Jordt, A. I. Basbaum, M. V. Chao and D. Julius (2001). Bradykinin and nerve growth factor release the capsaicin receptor from PtdIns(4,5)P2-mediated inhibition. *Nature* **411**(6840): 957–962.

Cutrer, F. M., V. Limmroth, G. Ayata and M. A. Moskowitz (1995). Attenuation by valproate of c-fos immunoreactivity in trigeminal nucleus caudalis induced by intracisternal capsaicin. *British Journal of Pharmacology* **116**(8): 3199–3204.

D'Arco, M., R. Giniatullin, M. Simonetti, A. Fabbro, A. Nair, A. Nistri and E. Fabbretti (2007). Neutralization of nerve growth factor induces plasticity of ATP-sensitive P2X3 receptors of nociceptive trigeminal ganglion neurons. *Journal of Neuroscience* **27**(31): 8190–8201.

Del Fiacco, M., M. Quartu, M. Boi, M. P. Serra, T. Melis, R. Boccaletti, E. Shevel and C. Cianchetti (2015). TRPV1, CGRP and SP in scalp arteries of patients suffering from chronic migraine. *Journal of Neurology, Neurosurgery & Psychiatry* **86**(4): 393–397.

Deval, E., X. Gasull, J. Noel, M. Salinas, A. Baron, S. Diochot and E. Lingueglia (2010). Acid-Sensing Ion Channels (ASICs): Pharmacology and implication in pain. *Pharmacology & Therapeutics* **128**(3): 549–558.

Diamond, S., F. Freitag, S. B. Phillips, J. E. Bernstein and J. R. Saper (2000). Intranasal civamide for the acute treatment of migraine headache. *Cephalalgia* **20**(6): 597–602.

Durham, P. L. and C. G. Masterson (2013). Two mechanisms involved in trigeminal CGRP release: implications for migraine treatment. *Headache* **53**(1): 67–80.

Dussor, G. (2015). ASICs as therapeutic targets for migraine. *Neuropharmacology* **94**: 64–71.

Dussor, G., J. Yan, J. Y. Xie, M. H. Ossipov, D. W. Dodick and F. Porreca (2014). Targeting TRP channels for novel migraine therapeutics. *ACS Chemical Neuroscience* **5**(11): 1085–1096.

Edelmayer, R. M., L. N. Le, J. Yan, X. Wei, R. Nassini, S. Materazzi, D. Preti, G. Appendino, P. Geppetti, D. W. Dodick, T. W. Vanderah, F. Porreca and G. Dussor (2012). Activation of TRPA1 on dural afferents: A potential mechanism of headache pain. *Pain* **153**(9): 1949–1958.

Enyedi, P. and G. Czirjak (2010). Molecular background of leak K^+ currents: two-pore domain potassium channels. *Physiological Reviews* **90**(2): 559–605.

Evans, M. S., X. Cheng, J. A. Jeffry, K. E. Disney and L. S. Premkumar (2012). Sumatriptan inhibits TRPV1 channels in trigeminal neurons. *Headache* **52**(5): 773–784.

Fabbretti, E., M. D'Arco, A. Fabbro, M. Simonetti, A. Nistri and R. Giniatullin (2006). Delayed upregulation of ATP P2X3 receptors of trigeminal sensory neurons by calcitonin gene-related peptide. *Journal of Neuroscience* **26**(23): 6163–6171.

Fan, X., J. Wang, W. Fan, L. Chen, B. Gui, G. Tan and J. Zhou (2014). Replication of migraine GWAS susceptibility loci in Chinese Han population. *Headache* **54**(4): 709–715.

Fidan, I., S. Yuksel, T. Ymir, C. Irkec and F. N. Aksakal (2006). The importance of cytokines, chemokines and nitric oxide in pathophysiology of migraine. *Journal of Neuroimmunology* **171**(1–2): 184–188.

Ford, A. P. (2012). In pursuit of P2X3 antagonists: novel therapeutics for chronic pain and afferent sensitization. *Purinergic Signalling* **8**(Suppl 1): 3–26.

Freilinger, T., V. Anttila, B. de Vries, R. Malik, M. Kallela, G. M. Terwindt, P. Pozo-Rosich, B. Winsvold, D. R. Nyholt, W. P. van Oosterhout, V. Artto, U. Todt, E. Hamalainen, J. Fernandez-Morales, M. A. Louter, M. A. Kaunisto, J. Schoenen, O. Raitakari, T. Lehtimaki, M. Vila-Pueyo, H. Gobel, E. Wichmann, C. Sintas, A. G. Uiterlinden, A. Hofman, F. Rivadeneira, A. Heinze, E. Tronvik, C. M. van Duijn, J. Kaprio, B. Cormand, M. Wessman, R. R. Frants, T. Meitinger, B. Muller-Myhsok, J. A. Zwart, M. Farkkila, A. Macaya, M. D. Ferrari, C. Kubisch, A. Palotie, M. Dichgans and A. M. van den Maagdenberg (2012). Genome-wide association analysis identifies susceptibility loci for migraine without aura. *Nature Genetics* **44**(7): 777–782.

Fusco, B. M., G. Barzoi and F. Agro (2003). Repeated intranasal capsaicin applications to treat chronic migraine. *British Journal of Anaesthesia* **90**(6): 812.

Ghosh, J., S. Pradhan and B. Mittal (2013). Genome-wide-associated variants in migraine susceptibility: a replication study from North India. *Headache* **53**(10): 1583–1594.

Gnanasekaran, A., M. Sundukova, A. M. van den Maagdenberg, E. Fabbretti and A. Nistri (2011). Lipid rafts control P2X3 receptor distribution and function in trigeminal sensory neurons of a transgenic migraine mouse model. *Molecular Pain* **7**: 77.

Gribkoff, V. K., J. E. Starrett, Jr, and S. I. Dworetzky (2001). Maxi-K potassium channels: form, function, and modulation of a class of endogenous regulators of intracellular calcium. *Neuroscientist* **7**(2): 166–177.

Grunder, S. and X. Chen (2010). Structure, function, and pharmacology of acid-sensing ion channels (ASICs): focus on ASIC1a. *International Journal of Physiology, Pathophysiology and Pharmacology* **2**(2): 73–94.

Guo, Z., P. Liu, F. Ren and Y. Q. Cao (2014). Nonmigraine-associated TRESK K$^+$ channel variant C110R does not increase the excitability of trigeminal ganglion neurons. *Journal of Neurophysiology* **112**(3): 568–579.

Harrington, A. M., P. A. Hughes, C. M. Martin, J. Yang, J. Castro, N. J. Isaacs, L. A. Blackshaw and S. M. Brierley (2011). A novel role for TRPM8 in visceral afferent function. *Pain* **152**(7): 1459–1468.

Harriott, A. M. and M. S. Gold (2009). Electrophysiological properties of dural afferents in the absence and presence of inflammatory mediators. *Journal of Neurophysiology* **101**(6): 3126–3134.

Holland, P. R., S. Akerman, A. P. Andreou, N. Karsan, J. A. Wemmie and P. J. Goadsby (2012). Acid-sensing ion channel 1: a novel therapeutic target for migraine with aura. *Annals of Neurology* **72**(4): 559–563.

Holzer, P. and A. A. Izzo (2014). The pharmacology of TRP channels. *British Journal of Pharmacology* **171**(10): 2469–2473.

Huang, D., S. Li, A. Dhaka, G. M. Story and Y. Q. Cao (2012). Expression of the transient receptor potential channels TRPV1, TRPA1 and TRPM8 in mouse trigeminal primary afferent neurons innervating the dura. *Molecular Pain* **8**: 66.

Huang, S. M., T. Bisogno, M. Trevisani, A. Al-Hayani, L. De Petrocellis, F. Fezza, M. Tognetto, T. J. Petros, J. F. Krey, C. J. Chu, J. D. Miller, S. N. Davies, P. Geppetti, J. M. Walker and V. Di Marzo (2002). An endogenous capsaicin-like substance with high potency at recombinant and native vanilloid VR1 receptors. *Proceedings of the National Academy of Sciences of the United States of America* **99**(12): 8400–8405.

Hwang, S. W., H. Cho, J. Kwak, S. Y. Lee, C. J. Kang, J. Jung, S. Cho, K. H. Min, Y. G. Suh, D. Kim and U. Oh (2000). Direct activation of capsaicin receptors by products of lipoxygenases: endogenous capsaicin-like substances. *Proceedings of the National Academy of Sciences of the United States of America* **97**(11): 6155–6160.

Irlbacher, K. and B. U. Meyer (2002). Nasally triggered headache. *Neurology* **58**(2): 294.

Iwashita, T., T. Shimizu, M. Shibata, H. Toriumi, T. Ebine, M. Funakubo and N. Suzuki (2013). Activation of extracellular signal-regulated kinase in the trigeminal ganglion following both treatment of the dura mater with capsaicin and cortical spreading depression. *Neuroscience Research* **77**(1–2): 110–119.

Jennings, E. A., R. M. Ryan and M. J. Christie (2004). Effects of sumatriptan on rat medullary dorsal horn neurons. *Pain* **111**(1–2): 30–37.

Jordt, S. E., M. Tominaga and D. Julius (2000). Acid potentiation of the capsaicin receptor determined by a key extracellular site. *Proceedings of the National Academy of Sciences of the United States of America* **97**(14): 8134–8139.

Jordt, S. E., D. M. Bautista, H. H. Chuang, D. D. McKemy, P. M. Zygmunt, E. D. Hogestatt, I. D. Meng and D. Julius (2004). Mustard oils and cannabinoids excite sensory nerve fibres through the TRP channel ANKTM1. *Nature* **427**(6971): 260–265.

Julius, D. (2013). TRP channels and pain. *Annual Review of Cell and Developmental Biology* **29**: 355–384.

Kageneck, C., B. E. Nixdorf-Bergweiler, K. Messlinger and M. J. Fischer (2014). Release of CGRP from mouse brainstem slices indicates central inhibitory effect of triptans and kynurenate. *Journal of Headache and Pain* **15**: 7.

Karai, L. J., J. T. Russell, M. J. Iadarola and Z. Olah (2004). Vanilloid receptor 1 regulates multiple calcium compartments and contributes to Ca^{2+}-induced Ca^{2+} release in sensory neurons. *Journal of Biological Chemistry* **279**(16): 16377–16387.

Kaube, H., K. L. Hoskin and P. J. Goadsby (1992). Activation of the trigeminovascular system by mechanical distension of the superior sagittal sinus in the cat. *Cephalalgia* **12**(3): 133–136.

Kelman, L. (2007). The triggers or precipitants of the acute migraine attack. *Cephalalgia* **27**(5): 394–402.

Kim, Y. S., J. H. Park, S. J. Choi, J. Y. Bae, D. K. Ahn, D. D. McKemy and Y. C. Bae (2014). Central connectivity of transient receptor potential melastatin 8-expressing axons in the brain stem and spinal dorsal horn. *PLoS One* **9**(4): e94080.

Kitahara, T., H. S. Li and C. D. Balaban (2005). Changes in transient receptor potential cation channel superfamily V (TRPV) mRNA expression in the mouse inner ear ganglia after kanamycin challenge. *Hearing Research* **201**(1–2): 132–144.

Kremeyer, B., F. Lopera, J. J. Cox, A. Momin, F. Rugiero, S. Marsh, C. G. Woods, N. G. Jones, K. J. Paterson, F. R. Fricker, A. Villegas, N. Acosta, N. G. Pineda-Trujillo, J. D. Ramirez, J. Zea, M. W. Burley, G. Bedoya, D. L. Bennett, J. N. Wood and A. Ruiz-Linares (2010). A gain-of-function mutation in TRPA1 causes familial episodic pain syndrome. *Neuron* **66**(5): 671–680.

Kunkler, P. E., C. J. Ballard, G. S. Oxford and J. H. Hurley (2011). TRPA1 receptors mediate environmental irritant-induced meningeal vasodilatation. *Pain* **152**(1): 38–44.

Kunkler, P. E., C. J. Ballard, J. J. Pellman, L. Zhang, G. S. Oxford and J. H. Hurley (2014). Intraganglionic signaling as a novel nasal-meningeal pathway for TRPA1-dependent trigeminovascular activation by inhaled environmental irritants. *PLoS One* **9**(7): e103086.

Kunkler, P. E., L. Zhang, J. J. Pellman, G. S. Oxford and J. H. Hurley (2015). Sensitization of the trigeminovascular system following environmental irritant exposure. *Cephalalgia* **35**(13): 1192–201.

Lafreniere, R. G. and G. A. Rouleau (2011). Migraine: Role of the TRESK two-pore potassium channel. *International Journal of Biochemistry & Cell Biology* **43**(11): 1533–1536.

Lafreniere, R. G., M. Z. Cader, J. F. Poulin, I. Andres-Enguix, M. Simoneau, N. Gupta, K. Boisvert, F. Lafreniere, S. McLaughlan, M. P. Dube, M. M. Marcinkiewicz, S. Ramagopalan, O. Ansorge, B. Brais, J. Sequeiros, J. M. Pereira-Monteiro, L. R. Griffiths, S. J. Tucker, G. Ebers and G. A. Rouleau (2010). A dominant-negative mutation in the TRESK potassium channel is linked to familial migraine with aura. *Nature Medicine* **16**(10): 1157–1160.

Lambert, G. A., J. B. Davis, J. M. Appleby, B. A. Chizh, K. L. Hoskin and A. S. Zagami (2009). The effects of the TRPV1 receptor antagonist SB-705498 on trigeminovascular sensitisation and neurotransmission. *Naunyn-Schmiedeberg's Archives of Pharmacology* **380**(4): 311–325.

Lassen, L. H., M. Ashina, I. Christiansen, V. Ulrich, R. Grover, J. Donaldson and J. Olesen (1998). Nitric oxide synthase inhibition: a new principle in the treatment of migraine attacks. *Cephalalgia* **18**(1): 27–32.

Lassen, L. H., I. Christiansen, H. K. Iversen, I. Jansen-Olesen and J. Olesen (2003). The effect of nitric oxide synthase inhibition on histamine induced headache and arterial dilatation in migraineurs. *Cephalalgia* **23**(9): 877–886.

Lee, W. S., V. Limmroth, C. Ayata, F. M. Cutrer, C. Waeber, X. Yu and M. A. Moskowitz (1995). Peripheral GABAA receptor-mediated effects of sodium valproate on dural plasma protein extravasation to substance P and trigeminal stimulation. *British Journal of Pharmacology* **116**(1): 1661–1667.

Levy, D. (2010). Migraine pain and nociceptor activation – where do we stand? *Headache* **50**(5): 909–916.

Levy, D. and A. M. Strassman (2002). Mechanical response properties of A and C primary afferent neurons innervating the rat intracranial dura. *Journal of Neurophysiology* **88**(6): 3021–3031.

Liedtke, W., Y. Choe, M. A. Marti-Renom, A. M. Bell, C. S. Denis, A. Sali, A. J. Hudspeth, J. M. Friedman and S. Heller (2000). Vanilloid receptor-related osmotically activated channel (VR-OAC), a candidate vertebrate osmoreceptor. *Cell* **103**(3): 525–535.

Liedtke, W., D. M. Tobin, C. I. Bargmann and J. M. Friedman (2003). Mammalian TRPV4 (VR-OAC) directs behavioral responses to osmotic and mechanical stimuli in Caenorhabditis elegans. *Proceedings of the National Academy of Sciences of the United States of America* **100**(Suppl 2): 14531–14536.

Lippoldt, E. K., R. R. Elmes, D. D. McCoy, W. M. Knowlton and D. D. McKemy (2013). Artemin, a glial cell line-derived neurotrophic factor family member, induces TRPM8-dependent cold pain. *Journal of Neuroscience* **33**(30): 12543–12552.

Liu, M., M. C. Liu, C. Magoulas, J. V. Priestley and N. J. Willmott (2003). Versatile regulation of cytosolic Ca^{2+} by vanilloid receptor I in rat dorsal root ganglion neurons. *Journal of Biological Chemistry* **278**(7): 5462–5472.

Liu, P., Z. Xiao, F. Ren, Z. Guo, Z. Chen, H. Zhao and Y. Q. Cao (2013). Functional Analysis of a Migraine-Associated TRESK K^+ Channel Mutation. *Journal of Neuroscience* **33**(31): 12810–12824.

Loyd, D. R., P. B. Chen and K. M. Hargreaves (2012). Anti-hyperalgesic effects of anti-serotonergic compounds on serotonin- and capsaicin-evoked thermal hyperalgesia in the rat. *Neuroscience* **203**: 207–215.

Lu, R., R. Lukowski, M. Sausbier, D. D. Zhang, M. Sisignano, C. D. Schuh, R. Kuner, P. Ruth, G. Geisslinger and A. Schmidtko (2013). BKCa channels expressed in sensory neurons modulate inflammatory pain in mice. *Pain* **155**(3): 556–65.

Lubbert, M., J. Kyereme, N. Schobel, L. Beltran, C. H. Wetzel and H. Hatt (2013). Transient receptor potential channels encode volatile chemicals sensed by rat trigeminal ganglion neurons. *PLoS One* **8**(10): e77998.

Ma, Q. P. (2001). Co-localization of 5-HT(1B/1D/1F) receptors and glutamate in trigeminal ganglia in rats. *Neuroreport* **12**(8): 1589–1591.

Materazzi, S., R. Nassini, E. Andre, B. Campi, S. Amadesi, M. Trevisani, N. W. Bunnett, R. Patacchini and P. Geppetti (2008). Cox-dependent fatty acid metabolites cause pain through activation of the irritant receptor TRPA1. *Proceedings of the National Academy of Sciences of the United States of America* **105**(33): 12045–12050.

Materazzi, S., S. Benemei, C. Fusi, R. Gualdani, G. De Siena, N. Vastani, D. A. Andersson, G. Trevisan, M. R. Moncelli, X. Wei, G. Dussor, F. Pollastro, R. Patacchini, G. Appendino, P. Geppetti and R. Nassini (2013). Parthenolide inhibits nociception and neurogenic vasodilatation in the trigeminovascular system by targeting the TRPA1 channel. *Pain* **154**(12): 2750–2758.

McKemy, D. D., W. M. Neuhausser and D. Julius (2002). Identification of a cold receptor reveals a general role for TRP channels in thermosensation. *Nature* **416**(6876): 52–58.

McNamara, C. R., J. Mandel-Brehm, D. M. Bautista, J. Siemens, K. L. Deranian, M. Zhao, N. J. Hayward, J. A. Chong, D. Julius, M. M. Moran and C. M. Fanger (2007). TRPA1 mediates formalin-induced pain. *Proceedings of the National Academy of Sciences of the United States of America* **104**(33): 13525–13530.

Mitsikostas, D. D. and M. Sanchez del Rio (2001). Receptor systems mediating c-fos expression within trigeminal nucleus caudalis in animal models of migraine. *Brain Research Reviews* **35**(1): 20–35.

Moriyama, T., T. Higashi, K. Togashi, T. Iida, E. Segi, Y. Sugimoto, T. Tominaga, S. Narumiya and M. Tominaga (2005). Sensitization of TRPV1 by EP1 and IP reveals peripheral nociceptive mechanism of prostaglandins. *Molecular Pain* **1**: 3.

Mukerji, G., Y. Yiangou, S. L. Corcoran, I. S. Selmer, G. D. Smith, C. D. Benham, C. Bountra, S. K. Agarwal and P. Anand (2006). Cool and menthol receptor TRPM8 in human urinary bladder disorders and clinical correlations. *BMC Urology* **6**: 6.

Nassini, R., S. Materazzi, J. Vriens, J. Prenen, S. Benemei, G. De Siena, G. la Marca, E. Andre, D. Preti, C. Avonto, L. Sadofsky, V. Di Marzo, L. De Petrocellis, G. Dussor, F. Porreca, O. Taglialatela-Scafati, G. Appendino, B. Nilius and P. Geppetti (2012). The 'headache tree' via umbellulone and TRPA1 activates the trigeminovascular system. *Brain* **135**(Pt 2): 376–390.

Nealen, M. L., M. S. Gold, P. D. Thut and M. J. Caterina (2003). TRPM8 mRNA is expressed in a subset of cold-responsive trigeminal neurons from rat. *Journal of Neurophysiology* **90**(1): 515–520.

Newsom, J., J. L. Holt, J. K. Neubert, R. Caudle and A. H. Ahn (2012). A high density of TRPM8 expressing sensory neurons in specialized structures of the head. *Abstract retrieved from Society for Neuroscience.*

North, R. A. (2002). Molecular physiology of P2X receptors. *Physiological Reviews* **82**(4): 1013–1067.

Numazaki, M. and M. Tominaga (2004). Nociception and TRP Channels. *Current Drug Targets. CNS and Neurological Disorders* **3**(6): 479–485.

Oshinsky, M. L. and S. Gomonchareonsiri (2007). Episodic dural stimulation in awake rats: a model for recurrent headache. *Headache* **47**(7): 1026–1036.

Oshinsky, M. L. and J. Luo (2006). Neurochemistry of trigeminal activation in an animal model of migraine. *Headache* **46**(Suppl 1): S39–44.

Palmer, C. B., R. Lai, F. Guillard, J. Bullman, A. Baines, A. Napolitano and J. Appleby (2009). *A randomised, two-period cross-over study to investigate the efficacy of the TRPV1 antagonist SB-705498 in acute migraine.* Pain in Europe VI, Lisbon, Portugal.

Peier, A. M., A. Moqrich, A. C. Hergarden, A. J. Reeve, D. A. Andersson, G. M. Story, T. J. Earley, I. Dragoni, P. McIntyre, S. Bevan and A. Patapoutian (2002). A TRP channel that senses cold stimuli and menthol. *Cell* **108**(5): 705–715.

Perini, F., G. D'Andrea, E. Galloni, F. Pignatelli, G. Billo, S. Alba, G. Bussone and V. Toso (2005). Plasma cytokine levels in migraineurs and controls. *Headache* **45**(7): 926–931.

Pietrobon, D. (2012). Calcium channels and migraine. *Biochimica et Biophysica Acta* **1828**(7): 1655–65.

Pietrobon, D. and M. A. Moskowitz (2014). Chaos and commotion in the wake of cortical spreading depression and spreading depolarizations. *Nature Reviews Neuroscience* **15**(6): 379–393.

Rainero, I., E. Rubino, S. Gallone, P. Zavarise, D. Carli, S. Boschi, P. Fenoglio, L. Savi, S. Gentile, P. Benna, L. Pinessi and G. Dalla Volta (2014). KCNK18 (TRESK) genetic variants in Italian patients with migraine. *Headache* **54**(9): 1515–1522.

Ramsey, I. S., M. Delling and D. E. Clapham (2006). An introduction to TRP channels. *Annual Review of Physiology* **68**: 619–647.

Ray, B. S. and H. G. Wolff (1940). Experimental studies on headache: Pain sensitive structures of the head and their significance in headache. *Archives of Surgery* **41**: 813–856.

Sarchielli, P., A. Alberti, A. Floridi and V. Gallai (2001). Levels of nerve growth factor in cerebrospinal fluid of chronic daily headache patients. *Neurology* **57**(1): 132–134.

Sarchielli, P., A. Alberti, A. Baldi, F. Coppola, C. Rossi, L. Pierguidi, A. Floridi and P. Calabresi (2006). Proinflammatory cytokines, adhesion molecules, and lymphocyte integrin expression in the internal jugular blood of migraine patients without aura assessed ictally. *Headache* **46**(2): 200–207.

Schepelmann, K., A. Ebersberger, M. Pawlak, M. Oppmann and K. Messlinger (1999). Response properties of trigeminal brain stem neurons with input from dura mater encephali in the rat. *Neuroscience* **90**(2): 543–554.

Shatillo, A., K. Koroleva, R. Giniatullina, N. Naumenko, A. A. Slastnikova, R. R. Aliev, G. Bart, M. Atalay, C. Gu, R. Khazipov, B. Davletov, O. Grohn and R. Giniatullin (2013). Cortical spreading depression induces oxidative stress in the trigeminal nociceptive system. *Neuroscience* **253**: 341–349.

Sherwood, T. W., E. N. Frey and C. C. Askwith (2012). Structure and activity of the acid-sensing ion channels. *American Journal of Physiology – Cell Physiology* **303**(7): C699–C710.

Shimizu, T., H. Toriumi, H. Sato, M. Shibata, E. Nagata, K. Gotoh and N. Suzuki (2007). Distribution and origin of TRPV1 receptor-containing nerve fibers in the dura mater of rat. *Brain Research* **1173**: 84–91.

Simonetti, M., A. Fabbro, M. D'Arco, M. Zweyer, A. Nistri, R. Giniatullin and E. Fabbretti (2006). Comparison of P2X and TRPV1 receptors in ganglia or primary culture of trigeminal neurons and their modulation by NGF or serotonin. *Molecular Pain* **2**: 11.

Sousa-Valente, J., A. P. Andreou, L. Urban and I. Nagy (2014). Transient receptor potential ion channels in primary sensory neurons as targets for novel analgesics. *British Journal of Pharmacology* **171**(10): 2508–2527.

Staikopoulos, V., B. J. Sessle, J. B. Furness and E. A. Jennings (2007). Localization of P2X2 and P2X3 receptors in rat trigeminal ganglion neurons. *Neuroscience* **144**(1): 208–216.

Stamboulian, S., J. S. Choi, H. S. Ahn, Y. W. Chang, L. Tyrrell, J. A. Black, S. G. Waxman and S. D. Dib-Hajj (2010). ERK1/2 mitogen-activated protein kinase phosphorylates sodium channel Na(v)1.7 and alters its gating properties. *Journal of Neuroscience* **30**(5): 1637–1647.

Story, G. M., A. M. Peier, A. J. Reeve, S. R. Eid, J. Mosbacher, T. R. Hricik, T. J. Earley, A. C. Hergarden, D. A. Andersson, S. W. Hwang, P. McIntyre, T. Jegla, S. Bevan and A. Patapoutian (2003). ANKTM1, a TRP-like channel expressed in nociceptive neurons, is activated by cold temperatures. *Cell* **112**(6): 819–829.

Strassman, A. M., S. A. Raymond and R. Burstein (1996). Sensitization of meningeal sensory neurons and the origin of headaches. *Nature* **384**(6609): 560–564.

Summ, O., P. R. Holland, S. Akerman and P. J. Goadsby (2011). TRPV1 receptor blockade is ineffective in different in vivo models of migraine. *Cephalalgia* **31**(2): 172–180.

Taylor-Clark, T. E., S. Ghatta, W. Bettner and B. J. Undem (2009). Nitrooleic acid, an endogenous product of nitrative stress, activates nociceptive sensory nerves via the direct activation of TRPA1. *Molecular Pharmacology* **75**(4): 820–829.

Trevisani, M., J. Siemens, S. Materazzi, D. M. Bautista, R. Nassini, B. Campi, N. Imamachi, E. Andre, R. Patacchini, G. S. Cottrell, R. Gatti, A. I. Basbaum, N. W. Bunnett, D. Julius and P. Geppetti (2007). 4-Hydroxynonenal, an endogenous aldehyde, causes pain and neurogenic inflammation through activation of the irritant receptor TRPA1. *Proceedings of the National Academy of Sciences of the United States of America* **104**(33): 13519–13524.

Vaughn, A. H. and M. S. Gold (2010). Ionic mechanisms underlying inflammatory mediator-induced sensitization of dural afferents. *Journal of Neuroscience* **30**(23): 7878–7888.

Vriens, J., H. Watanabe, A. Janssens, G. Droogmans, T. Voets and B. Nilius (2004). Cell swelling, heat, and chemical agonists use distinct pathways for the activation of the cation channel TRPV4. *Proceedings of the National Academy of Sciences of the United States of America* **101**(1): 396–401.

Vriens, J., G. Appendino and B. Nilius (2009). Pharmacology of vanilloid transient receptor potential cation channels. *Molecular Pharmacology* **75**(6): 1262–1279.

Wantke, F., M. Focke, W. Hemmer, R. Bracun, S. Wolf-Abdolvahab, M. Gotz, R. Jarisch, M. Tschabitscher, M. Gann and P. Tappler (2000). Exposure to formaldehyde and phenol during an anatomy dissecting course: sensitizing potency of formaldehyde in medical students. *Allergy* **55**(1): 84–87.

Watanabe, H., J. B. Davis, D. Smart, J. C. Jerman, G. D. Smith, P. Hayes, J. Vriens, W. Cairns, U. Wissenbach, J. Prenen, V. Flockerzi, G. Droogmans, C. D. Benham and B. Nilius (2002). Activation of TRPV4 channels (hVRL-2/mTRP12) by phorbol derivatives. *Journal of Biological Chemistry* **277**(16): 13569–13577.

Wei, X., R. M. Edelmayer, J. Yan and G. Dussor (2011). Activation of TRPV4 on dural afferents produces headache-related behavior in a preclinical rat model. *Cephalalgia* **31**(16): 1595–1600.

Wemmie, J. A., C. C. Askwith, E. Lamani, M. D. Cassell, J. H. Freeman and M. J. Welsh (2003). Acid-sensing ion channel 1 is localized in brain regions with high synaptic density and contributes to fear conditioning. *Journal of Neuroscience* **23**(13): 5496–5502.

Wemmie, J. A., R. J. Taugher and C. J. Kreple (2013). Acid-sensing ion channels in pain and disease. *Nature Reviews Neuroscience* **14**(7): 461–471.

Wulf-Johansson, H., D. V. Amrutkar, A. Hay-Schmidt, A. N. Poulsen, D. A. Klaerke, J. Olesen and I. Jansen-Olesen (2010). Localization of large conductance calcium-activated potassium channels and their effect on calcitonin gene-related peptide release in the rat trigemino-neuronal pathway. *Neuroscience* **167**(4): 1091–1102.

Xiao, Y., J. A. Richter and J. H. Hurley (2008). Release of glutamate and CGRP from trigeminal ganglion neurons: Role of calcium channels and 5-HT1 receptor signaling. *Molecular Pain* **4**: 12.

Yan, J., R. M. Edelmayer, X. Wei, M. De Felice, F. Porreca and G. Dussor (2011). Dural afferents express acid-sensing ion channels: a role for decreased meningeal pH in migraine headache. *Pain* **152**(1): 106–113.

Yan, J., O. K. Melemedjian, T. J. Price and G. Dussor (2012). Sensitization of dural afferents underlies migraine-related behavior following meningeal application of interleukin-6 (IL-6). *Molecular Pain* **8**: 6.

Yan, J., X. Wei, C. Bischoff, R. M. Edelmayer and G. Dussor (2013). pH-Evoked Dural Afferent Signaling Is Mediated by ASIC3 and Is Sensitized by Mast Cell Mediators. *Headache* **53**(8): 1250–1261.

Zha, X. M. (2013). Acid-sensing ion channels: trafficking and synaptic function. *Molecular Brain* **6**(1). doi: 10.1186/1756-6606-6-1.

Zhang, X. C., V. Kainz, R. Burstein and D. Levy (2011). Tumor necrosis factor-alpha induces sensitization of meningeal nociceptors mediated via local COX and p38 MAP kinase actions. *Pain* **152**(1): 140–149.

Zhang, X. C., R. Burstein and D. Levy (2012). Local action of the proinflammatory cytokines IL-1 beta and IL-6 on intracranial meningeal nociceptors. *Cephalalgia* **32**(1): 66–U109.

Zhang, X., M. Jakubowski, C. Buettner, V. Kainz, M. Gold and R. Burstein (2013). Ezogabine (KCNQ2/3 channel opener) prevents delayed activation of meningeal nociceptors if given before but not after the occurrence of cortical spreading depression. *Epilepsy & Behavior* **28**(2): 243–248.

Zimmermann, K., P. W. Reeh and B. Averbeck (2002). ATP can enhance the proton-induced CGRP release through P2Y receptors and secondary PGE(2) release in isolated rat dura mater. *Pain* **97**(3): 259–265.

Zygmunt, P. M. and E. D. Hogestatt (2014). Trpa1. *Handbook of Experimental Pharmacology* **222**: 583–630.

Zygmunt, P. M., J. Petersson, D. A. Andersson, H. Chuang, M. Sorgard, V. Di Marzo, D. Julius and E. D. Hogestatt (1999). Vanilloid receptors on sensory nerves mediate the vasodilator action of anandamide. *Nature* **400**(6743): 452–457.

4

Functional architecture of central pain pathways: focus on the trigeminovascular system

Rodrigo Noseda[1] and Luis Villanueva[2]

[1] *Department of Anesthesia, Critical Care and Pain Medicine, Beth Israel Deaconess Medical Center, Harvard Medical School, Boston, Massachusetts, USA*
[2] *Institut National de la Santé et de la Recherche Médicale/Université Paris Descartes, Centre de Psychiatrie et Neurosciences, Paris, France*

4.1 Introduction

This chapter describes our current understanding of the ascending and descending central nervous system pathways that are relevant for nociceptive processing in the trigeminal system. Such knowledge has emerged from a large body of pre-clinical and clinical evidence, showing complex interactions between bottom-up and top-down mechanisms that are essential for the discrimination of noxious information and pain perception. Special emphasis is given here to central components of the trigeminovascular system as neural substrates for migraine pain.

4.2 Ascending trigeminal nociceptive pathways

Activation of primary afferents by tissue-damaging events in the skin, muscle, joint and viscera, as well as in specialized structures of the cranio-facial and oral territories such as cornea, meninges and dental pulp, conveys nociceptive signals to second-order neurons in the spinal and medullary dorsal horn, respectively. Based on the anatomical and functional properties of such neurons, ascending pathways carrying nociceptive information to brainstem, midbrain, and forebrain regions have been associated with the ultimate experience of pain.

Such pathways originate mainly from two discrete laminated structures in both spinal and medullary dorsal horns: the superficial layer (lamina I) that contains neurons activated specifically by mechanical and thermal noxious inputs; and the deep layers (lamina V–VI) that contain neurons activated by noxious and innocuous inputs. Their anatomical and functional differences suggest that these neuronal populations play different roles in the processing of nociceptive information. Similarly, and depending on their higher order targets, the axonal fibers of projecting neurons travel along the spino/trigemino-bulbar, spino/trigemino-hypothalamic and spino/trigemino-thalamic

Neurobiological Basis of Migraine, First Edition. Edited by Turgay Dalkara and Michael A. Moskowitz.
© 2017 John Wiley & Sons, Inc. Published 2017 by John Wiley & Sons, Inc.

tracts, as well as indirect spino/trigemino-reticulo-thalamic tracts. While spinal and trigeminal inputs to the thalamus are mainly contralateral, projections to the pons and midbrain present contralateral dominance, and those to reticular areas are bilateral.

Spinal and trigeminal mechanisms involved in nociception share many structural and functional properties that are described below. There are, however, special features in the nociceptive processing from specialized structures innervated by trigeminal sources. For example, a higher level of complexity arises from the cornea, tooth pulp, and the meninges, mainly due to their dual representation and widespread afferent termination within the brainstem trigeminal sensory complex. As described in previous chapters, noxious input from these and other cranio-facial-oral tissues is conveyed through trigeminal ganglion neurons, whose central processes enter the brainstem via the trigeminal tract. These primary afferents reach the spinal trigeminal nucleus and upper cervical spinal cord to activate second-order neurons (Figure 4.1) (see Chapter 1).

4.2.1 Ascending nociceptive pathways from the superficial laminae of the dorsal horn

4.2.1.1 Spino/trigemino-bulbar projections

As illustrated in Figure 4.2, second-order neurons in lamina I project to several areas of the CNS that are important for sensory, affective, endocrine, and autonomic functions involved in homeostasis. A significant target in the brainstem, only described for trigeminal (but not spinal) projections, is the superior salivatory nucleus (SSN). This cluster of cholinergic preganglionic neurons provides parasympathetic innervation to cerebral vasculature, lacrimal glands, nasal and palatine mucosa, through the pterygopalatine ganglion (PPG) (Contreras *et al.*, 1980; Spencer *et al.*, 1990b). Accordingly, and critical for understanding the autonomic symptoms frequently seen in migraine and other primary headaches, activation of the SSN could contribute to protein extravasation and release of inflammatory mediators that activate and sensitize meningeal nociceptors, as suggested by the increased parasympathetic tone observed during migraine attacks (Yarnitsky *et al.*, 2003).

Other major brainstem areas receiving the densest projections from lamina I are the lateral parabrachial area (PB; about 50% of lamina I projecting neurons) and the ventrolateral periaqueductal gray matter (PAG, about 25% of lamina I projecting neurons). A large proportion of lateral PB neurons is driven by Aδ and C fibers, and responds to thermal and mechanical stimuli within noxious ranges (Bernard and Besson, 1990). A smaller proportion of these neurons is also responsive to cooling. The nociceptive (lateral) PB area projects densely to the central nucleus of the amygdala and the bed nucleus of the stria terminalis, which are probably involved in anxiety and reactions to fear. It also projects to the hypothalamic ventromedial nucleus, which participates in food intake (Bernard *et al.*, 1995).

In the context of migraine, it has been suggested that loss of appetite during an attack could be mediated by the trigeminal-PB circuit. Since noxious stimulation of the dura increases the number of c-fos-positive neurons in the Sp5C, PB, and hypothalamic ventromedial nucleus (VMH), and the involvement of this circuit in suppression of feeding behavior is possible. In addition, PB- and VMH-activated neurons express the anorectic peptide cholecystokinin (Malick *et al.*, 2001). More medial and dorsal areas of the PB also receive scarce ascending projections from the nucleus of the solitary tract, which is

Figure 4.1 Anatomical organization of the trigeminal brainstem sensory complex. After entering the trigeminal tract, most afferents pass caudally, while giving off collaterals that terminate in the subdivisions of the spinal trigeminal nucleus and upper cervical cord to activate second-order neurons. The spinal trigeminal sensory nucleus (Sp5) consists of three subnuclei (oralis, Sp5O; interpolaris, Sp5I; and caudalis, Sp5C). Aδ and C primary afferents fibers terminate somatotopically in a dorsal-ventral fashion, with mandibular afferents ending dorsally (V3), maxillary fibers projecting centrally (V2), and ophthalmic fibers innervating the ventral-most aspect of Sp5 (V1). At this level, convergence onto a single neuron receiving input from different primary afferents has been proposed to explain referral of pain and the difficulty in precisely localizing the painful focus. For example, migraine patients experiencing an attack commonly refer to their headaches as localized in the periorbital/frontal area; however, the precise source of pain is unknown, and can hypothetically originate from remote intracranial and/or extracranial pain-sensitive structures. C1 – first cervical segment of the spinal cord; Cu – cuneate nucleus; Pr5 – principal sensory trigeminal nucleus. Villanueva and Noseda (2012). Reproduced by permission of Elsevier.

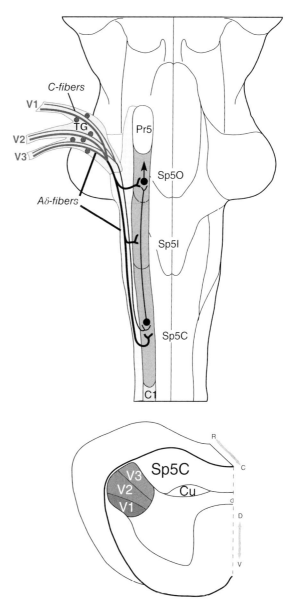

involved in visceral nociception and autonomic regulation, and which has been linked to nausea and vomiting during migraine (Hargreaves and Shepheard, 1999). Thus, PB pathways provide a substrate for integration of somatic/visceral nociceptive afferent activity and an indirect relay to higher forebrain regions involved in autonomic, emotional and neuroendocrine functions.

Closely related are the lateral and ventrolateral columns of the PAG. These receive mainly lamina I projections from spinal and trigeminal areas onto functionally different groups of neurons. Their activation produces antinociceptive, cardiovascular and defensive reactions, such as decrease in blood pressure, hyporeactive immobility, avoidance

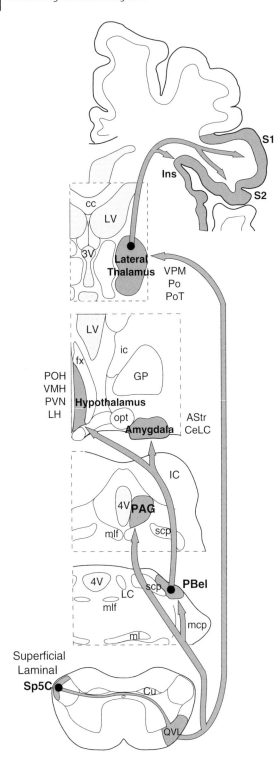

Figure 4.2 Schematic representation of the main ascending projections from superficial medullary trigeminal neurons. Lamina I trigeminal medullary neurons send nociceptive and thermal signals to the spinal, bulbar, and telencephalic regions implicated in autonomic, emotional, and somatosensory processing. Rather than subserving only pain processing, these circuits could contribute to sustaining basic emotional and motivational states. Abbreviations: AStr – amygdalostriatal transition area; cc – corpus callosum; CeLC – central amygdaloid nucleus – lateral capsular part; Cg – cingulate cortex; CL – centrolateral thalamic nucleus; CM – central medial thalamic nucleus; ECu – external cuneate nucleus; fx – fornix; GP – globus pallidus; Gr – gracile nucleus; ic – internal capsule; icp – inferior cerebellar peduncle; Ins – insular cortex; IOn – inferior olive nucleus; LC – locus coeruleus; LH – lateral hypothalamic nucleus; LRn – lateral reticular nucleus; LV – lateral ventricle; mcp – middle cerebellar peduncle; ml – medial lemniscus; mlf – medial longitudinal fasciculus; 7n – facial nucleus; opt – optic tract; PAG – periaqueductal gray; PBel – lateral parabrachial nucleus – external part; PBil – lateral parabrachial nucleus – internal part; PC – paracentral thalamic nucleus; pf – parafascicular thalamic nucleus; PF – prefrontal cortex; Po – posterior thalamic nuclear group; POH – preoptic hypothalamic region; PoT – posterior thalamic triangular nucleus; PVN – paraventricular hypothalamic nucleus; QVL – ventrolateral quadrant; S1 – primary somatosensory cortex; S2 – secondary somatosensory cortex; scp – superior cerebellar peduncle; SRD – subnucleus reticularis dorsalis; 3V – third ventricle; 4V – forth ventricle; Ve – vestibular nucleus; VMH – ventromedial hypothalamic nucleus; VMl – ventromedial thalamic nucleus, lateral part; VPM – ventral posteromedial thalamic nucleus. Villanueva and Noseda (2012). Reproduced by permission of Elsevier.

behavior, and vocalization, as well as a more general emotional state of fear and anxiety (Lovick, 1993; Bandler and Depaulis, 1991).

Ascending pathways from these areas to the hypothalamus and medial thalamus have also been described (Mantyh, 1983). Therefore, this lamina I-PAG pathway could participate in feedback mechanisms involved in the autonomic, aversive, and antinociceptive responses to strong nociceptive stimulation. In the context of migraine, activation of the PAG and nearby nuclei in the dorsolateral pons have been reported during attacks, and this is likely involved in descendent modulation of pain among other adaptive functions (see below).

4.2.1.2 Spino/trigemino-hypothalamic projections

The hypothalamus is associated with a variety of autonomic, neuroendocrine, and affective reactions to pain arising from any part of the body. Somatosensory and visceral ascending information from spinal and trigeminal sources likely influences these complex functions through direct pathways from brainstem nuclei, such as the nucleus of the solitary tract, medullary lateral reticular formation, PB and the PAG (Saper and Loewy, 1980; Sawchenko and Swanson, 1981; Beitz, 1982; Menetrey and Basbaum, 1987). Sparse, direct afferents from superficial and deep laminae of spinal and trigeminal dorsal horn have also been described using retrograde/anterograde labeling and antidromic mapping. Those areas receiving direct input are the anterior (AH), lateral (LH), posterior (PH) and mediodorsal (MDH) hypothalamic areas, as well as perifornical (PeF), paraventricular (PVN) and lateral preoptic (LPO) nuclei (Burstein *et al.*, 1987; Cliffer *et al.*, 1991; Newman *et al.*, 1996; Malick *et al.*, 2000; Gauriau and Bernard, 2004a). Thus, independently of the origin, hypothalamic activation through nociceptive ascending pathways likely disrupts the regular rhythmicity of sleep, food intake, thermoregulation, arousal and emotional reactions, among other functions.

In the context of migraine, the hypothalamus appears as a pivotal structure in the premonitory symptoms that precede the headache phase such as fatigue, yawning, sleepiness, irritability, hunger and craving, as they likely originate in the hypothalamus (see Chapter 12). Moreover, this diencephalic region appears to play an equally fundamental role in modulation of pain through its dense descending projections to the spinal and trigeminal dorsal horns (see below).

4.2.1.3 Spino/trigemino-thalamic projections

One of the most studied and relevant systems for pain perception is the spino/trigemino-thalamic pathway. Many anatomical areas of the rat, monkey and human thalamus are innervated by spinal and trigeminal lamina I neurons (around 15% of lamina I projecting neurons). In the rat, these thalamic targets include the posterior complex (Po), posterior triangular (PoT), ventral posterolateral (VPL), and ventral posteromedial (VPM) nuclei (Gauriau and Bernard, 2004c; Noseda *et al.*, 2008).

Axonal terminations are observed in the PoT, a caudal thalamic nucleus that conveys nociceptive input to the secondary somatosensory cortex, as well as tactile and nociceptive input to the insular cortex and amygdala (Gauriau and Bernard, 2004c). More rostrally, labeled terminals are distributed mainly in the dorsal aspect of Po, VPM and VPL thalamic nuclei. Early studies have shown that these regions convey tactile and nociceptive input to the primary and secondary somatosensory cortices, and could participate in the sensory-discriminative aspect of pain.

A more recent set of studies found that neurons located mainly in the dorsal aspect of the VPM and Po are activated by noxious stimulation of the trigeminally-innervated skin, dura (Burstein *et al.*, 2010; Noseda *et al.*, 2010b, 2011) and tooth pulp (Zhang *et al.*, 2006). Accordingly, individual trigeminovascular neurons in VPM project mainly to trigeminal areas of the primary (S1) and secondary (S2) somatosensory and insular cortices. Interestingly, populations of neurons responding to noxious stimulation of dural and facial receptive fields have also been recorded in other, non-VPM/Po thalamic nuclei (i.e., lateral posterior (LP) and lateral dorsal (LD) thalamic nuclei). Altogether, these dura-sensitive neurons in Po, LP and LD project to multiple cortical areas involved in sensory, motor, affective, associative, and cognitive functions.

Such extensive trigemino-thalamo-cortical network suggests that nociceptive signals are widely processed throughout the cortex, and consistent with the multiple symptoms experienced ictally by migraineurs (Noseda *et al.*, 2010b, 2011). This evidence is also in agreement with human functional imaging studies that showed activation of the VPM and dorsal thalamic areas following noxious thermal stimulation of the face (DaSilva *et al.*, 2002), and during spontaneous migraine (Burstein *et al.*, 2010).

In the monkey, thalamic regions receiving spinal and trigeminal input include an area within the suprageniculate/posterior complex named the posterior part of the ventro-medial nucleus (VMpo), the ventral caudal part of the medial dorsal/parafascicular nuclei (MDvc/Pf), and the VPM (Ralston and Ralston, 1992; Craig, 2004). Electrophysiological recordings in anesthetized and awake monkeys have revealed important differences between these thalamic lamina I targets. Accordingly, they not only encode different intensities of noxious stimuli, but also many neurons in the MDvc/Pf and VMpo present modality specificity and exhibit either nociceptive or thermal responses.

The cutaneous receptive fields of VMpo cells in monkeys are restricted (Craig *et al.*, 1994), whereas those from MDvc/Pf cells are often very large. Both the receptive fields boundary and the magnitude of their evoked responses change along with the monkey's behavioral state (Bushnell and Duncan, 1987, 1989; Bushnell *et al.*, 1993; Bushnell, 1995). These features may indicate that MDvc/Pf cells are better suited for the integration of behavioral reactions and, thus, are strongly implicated in the affective-emotional aspects of pain. This suggestion is supported by their cortical connectivity and by functional imaging studies.

Neurons in the VMpo project to the posterior insular cortex, the only brain area that, when stimulated, elicits pain in humans (Ostrowsky *et al.*, 2002; Craig, 2014), and have been implicated in the affective components of pain on the basis of its projections to various limbic structures, such as the amygdala and perirhinal cortex. Neurons in the MDvc/Pf nuclei project, in turn, to area 24 of the cingulate cortex, the activity of which appears to be more selectively modulated by noxious stimuli. In fact, this is a functionally heterogeneous area, constituted by adjacent zones implicated in attentional, motor, and autonomic reactions that might allow it to elicit various behavioral reactions (Vogt, 2005).

In contrast, clinical data have shown that other ventral posterior thalamic areas, not necessarily including the VMpo, also play a key role in relaying thermo-algesic signals along the spinothalamic system to the cortex (Montes *et al.*, 2005). This region, known as the ventral posterior thalamic complex (VP), projects to S1, and imaging studies have shown that noxious and innocuous stimuli similarly activate the contralateral S1, thus indicating the co-existence of pain and tactile representation in this area (Chen *et al.*,

2002). Furthermore, single-unit recordings from the VP in humans have shown that neurons could be activated by noxious stimuli, and that direct stimulation of this region induces thermal and/or painful sensations (Lenz and Dougherty, 1997). In the monkey, the VP area contains a majority of WDR neurons, whose receptive fields are not modified by the behavioral state and are smaller than those of spinal or medullary dorsal horn projecting neurons, suggesting a potential role in spatial discrimination (Bushnell *et al.*, 1993; Bushnell, 1995).

4.2.2 Ascending nociceptive signals from the deep laminae of the dorsal horn

4.2.2.1 Spino/trigemino-reticulo-thalamic projections

Except for a few anterograde studies (Gauriau and Bernard, 2004a; Noseda *et al.*, 2008), most of the data available on the precise projection sites of nociceptive neurons in laminae V–VI come from retrograde tracing. As illustrated in Figure 4.3, laminae V–VI neurons project to brainstem reticular areas, these being among their densest targets. A key role of the medullary reticular formation as a relay for nociceptive signals has been suggested, since the majority of anterolateral quadrant ascending axons in both animals and humans terminate within this area (see references in Villanueva and Nathan, 2000). Accordingly, numerous findings indicate that nociceptive input to the thalamus is relayed within the caudal medullary reticular formation (Villanueva *et al.*, 1998; Vogt, 2005).

The old proposal that the reticular formation does not play a specific role in the processing of pain was challenged by data obtained in the rat and monkey, showing that neurons within the medullary subnucleus reticularis dorsalis (SRD) respond selectively to the activation of Aδ and C fibers from the whole body surface. They also encode the intensity of noxious stimuli, and are activated via ascending pathways in the anterolateral quadrant (Villanueva *et al.*, 1990, 1996).

Axonal projections of SRD neurons terminate in the parafascicular and ventromedial thalamus (VMl) which, in turn, conveys nociceptive input from the entire body surface to layer I of the whole dorsolateral neocortex (Monconduit *et al.*, 1999; Desbois and Villanueva, 2001). VMl neurons have fine discriminative properties, as shown by their selective responsiveness to calibrated noxious stimuli. They have the ability to precisely encode different types of cutaneous stimuli within noxious ranges, and can be activated by innocuous stimuli only under conditions of experimental allodynia. Because the thalamic VMl lacks topographical discrimination, as illustrated by their "whole-body" receptive field to widespread noxious stimuli of cutaneous, muscular, or visceral origin, it may constitute an important nociceptive target of the originally termed "ascending reticular activating system" (Herkenham, 1986).

This spino/trigemino-reticulo-thalamo-cortical network could allow any painful stimuli to modify cortical activity in a widespread manner, since cortical interactions in layer I are considered to be a key substrate for the synchronization of large ensembles of neurons across cortical territories in association with conscious states. In this respect, layer I input may act as a "mode switch" by activating a spatially restricted low-threshold zone in the apical dendrites of layer V pyramidal neurons, evoking regenerative potentials propagating toward their somata which, in turn, could switch layer V neurons into burst-firing mode (Larkum and Zhu, 2002). This hypothesis fits with the facts that painful stimuli can elicit widespread cortical activation in humans, and that

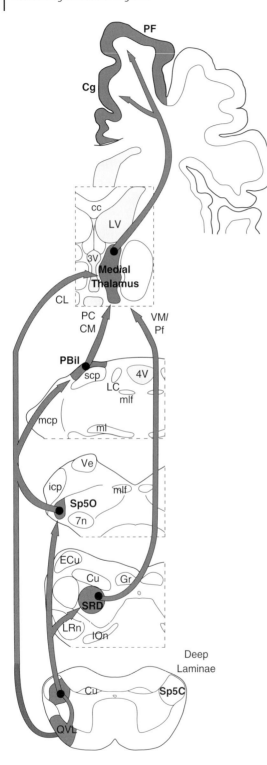

Figure 4.3 Schematic representation of the main ascending projections from deep medullary trigeminal neurons. Deep lamina trigeminal medullary neurons are able to convey a variety of signals, originating either from the external environment through the skin or from the internal organs. They send input to several regions implicated in somatosensory, motor, arousal, and attentional processing of nociceptive input. These deep medullary neurons appear to be implicated not only in pain processing, but also in creating the basic somesthetic activity that is necessary for homeostatic regulation. For abbreviations see Figure 4.2. Villanueva and Noseda (2012). Reproduced by permission of Elsevier.

increasing stimulus intensity increases the number of brain regions activated, including the ventral posterior and medial thalamic regions, as well as their targets in the pre-frontal, premotor, and motor cortices (Derbyshire *et al.*, 1997; Apkarian *et al.*, 2009).

4.3   Trigeminovascular pain is subject to descending control

A complex interplay between central neural networks involved in descending facilitatory and inhibitory responses to a given noxious stimulus is essential for the ultimate experience of pain. These endogenous systems, mainly originating from the brainstem, hypothalamus and cerebral cortex, are strongly influenced by behavioral, cognitive and emotional factors that are relevant for the survival of the individual. Under pathological conditions, however, dysfunctional engagement of these descending pathways certainly contributes to the transformation from acute to chronic pain states. In disorders such as migraine, this could contribute to the generation of episodic painful states in susceptible individuals, and to the evolution from acute to chronic migraine.

4.3.1   Descending modulation from the periaqueductal gray (PAG) and the rostral ventromedial medulla (RVM)

Early systematic studies of what was originally termed "stimulation-produced analgesia" in animals showed that localized microstimulation of the ventral PAG or RVM effectively elicited strong behavioral antinociceptive effects when noxious stimuli are applied anywhere in the body (Oliveras and Besson, 1988). Moreover, activation of the PAG by direct ascending lamina I projections produces cardiovascular and temperature changes, as well as defensive reactions, fear and anxiety (Oliveras and Besson, 1988; Bandler *et al.*, 1991). Since the PAG projects minimally to the spinal cord, but densely to the RVM, the latter constitutes the main direct link for descending modulation to all levels of spinal and trigeminal dorsal horns. RVM descending projections innervate superficial dorsal horn neurons which, in turn, modulate the activity of deep lamina cells at the origin of the spinal and trigeminal ascending nociceptive pathways, suggesting a broader modulatory role by the PAG-RVM system (Basbaum and Fields, 1978; Holstege and Kuypers, 1982; Suzuki *et al.*, 2002; Fields *et al.*, 1995; Mason, 2001; see Figure 4.4).

In the field of migraine, the role of this circuit is controversial, since early reports that described delayed migraine-like pain in patients undergoing electrode implantation near the PAG (Raskin *et al.*, 1987), and an imaging study showing activation of the brainstem in spontaneous migraine (Weiller *et al.*, 1995). These reports were used to propose the concept of the PAG as a "migraine generator". In theory, dysfunctional brainstem areas, including the PAG, could either enhance or suppress trigeminovascular neuronal activity at the origin of migraine-like pain via "on" and "off" cells in the RVM (Porreca *et al.*, 2002). In this regard, facilitatory influences mediated by RVM neurons have been reported in an animal model of migraine pain, through the assessment of cutaneous allodynia as a manifestation of central sensitization (Edelmayer *et al.*, 2009). Furthermore, it has been shown that evoked neuronal activity in Sp5C is inhibited by PAG stimulation (Knight and Goadsby, 2001), and that blocking the P/Q-type calcium channels in the PAG facilitates the activity of Sp5C nociceptive neurons (Knight *et al.*, 2002).

Conversely, several neuroimaging studies reporting brainstem activation in migraine patients do not include the PAG as an activated region during spontaneous or induced

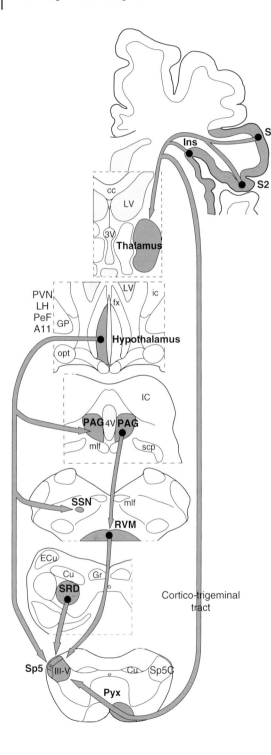

Figure 4.4 Schematic representation of the main central nervous system descending networks of pain modulation. A noxious stimulus activates bulbospinal and hypothalamic modulatory mechanisms by which nociceptive signals may attenuate or increase their own magnitudes. The most important widespread source of top-down modulation arises from the cortex, since both thalamic and pre-thalamic nociceptive relays are under corticofugal modulation (see text). A11 – dopaminergic cells group; Pef – perifornical hypothalamic nucleus; Pyx – pyramidal decussation; RVM – rostral ventral medulla; SSN – superior salivatory nucleus. For other abbreviations, see Figure 4.2. Villanueva and Noseda (2012). Reproduced by permission of Elsevier.

attacks. Activation has been found however, in nearby nuclei in the dorsolateral pons (DLP), which includes the mesencephalic trigeminal nucleus, principal sensory trigeminal nucleus, PB, vestibular nucleus, inferior colliculus, LC, and cuneiform nucleus (Weiller *et al.*, 1995; Bahra *et al.*, 2001; Afridi *et al.*, 2005; Moulton *et al.*, 2008; Stankewitz and May, 2011). This complex pattern of activation does not appear to be specific to migraine (Dunckley *et al.*, 2005; Becerra *et al.*, 2006; Keltner *et al.*, 2006; Linnman *et al.*, 2012), and reflects a potential role in facial and muscle tenderness, abnormal tactile sensation, motion sickness, nausea, altered auditory perception and, more importantly, modulation of pain. These functional and anatomical studies are consistent with a broader modulatory role of the PAG-RVM circuit, and suggest an absence of topographically specific modulation necessary for eliciting selectively migraine headache.

4.3.2 Diffuse noxious inhibitory controls (DNIC)

In contrast to segmental controls, heterosegmental controls are elicited mainly by noxious stimuli. These inhibitions are mediated by a supraspinal loop with signals that ascend to the brainstem and then descend again to effect inhibition in the spinal (Le Bars *et al.*, 1979) and trigeminal dorsal horn (Dickenson *et al.*, 1980; Villanueva *et al.*, 1984). More recently, in clinical contexts, DNIC has been termed "conditioned pain modulation" (CPM), since a number of studies have shown common anatomical and functional features in animals and humans. The supraspinal structures responsible for DNIC include the rat SRD in the caudal-dorsal medulla, which contains a homogeneous population of neurons activated exclusively by noxious stimuli applied to any region of the body, which precisely encode the intensity of these stimuli (Villanueva *et al.*, 1988, 1996). Moreover, lesions of the caudal medulla reduce DNIC in both animals and humans (De Broucker *et al.*, 1990).

DNIC mechanisms have been proposed to facilitate the extraction of nociceptive information by increasing the signal-to-noise ratio between a pool of dorsal horn neurons that are activated from a painful focus, and the remaining population of such neurons, which are simultaneously inhibited. DNIC appears to mediate noxious "counter-stimulation" phenomena ("pain inhibits pain") by mutual inhibition between pathways that generate sensation and by nocifensive responses, in the event that painful stimuli are applied simultaneously at two separate loci. For example, pain due to an injury on the foot is usually suppressed when the hand is immersed in painful ice-cold water. Likewise, DNIC reduces both spinal (Roby-Brami *et al.*, 1987) and trigeminal reflexes (Maillou and Cadden, 1997).

Human brain imaging studies, combined with psychophysics and electrophysiology, have shown an important contribution of cortical regions in the regulation of pain suppression by DNIC (Piche *et al.*, 2009; Sprenger *et al.*, 2011). Studies in chronic pain patients suggest that such higher-order CNS mechanisms, in addition to the brainstem loops associated with DNIC/CPM, could also be implicated in counter-stimulation phenomena. For example, the effects of counter-stimulation are altered in neuropathic pain patients, suggesting that DNIC mechanisms differ in health and disease (Bouhassira *et al.*, 2003).

Furthermore, the effects of DNIC on temporally and spatially summated pain are reduced from normal in dysfunctional pain states, such as painful trigeminal conditions, including temporomandibular disorder and trigeminal neuropathic pain (King *et al.*, 2009; Leonard *et al.*, 2009). Indeed, these observations suggest that the reduced ability of CPM to inhibit pain in chronic pain patients could be, in part, due to a dysfunction of the DNIC system itself (Yarnitsky, 2010). Moreover, some studies suggest that such disturbances could also contribute to head pain processing, as illustrated by a reduction in DNIC in patients with chronic tension-type headache (Pielsticker *et al.*, 2005; Cathcart *et al.*, 2010), and loss of DNIC acting on trigeminovascular Sp5C neurons in an animal model of medication overuse headache (Okada-Ogawa *et al.*, 2009).

4.3.3 Hypothalamic links for the descending control of trigeminovascular pain

In addition to the ascending pathways to the hypothalamus described above, many hypothalamic areas send back direct projections to the spinal and trigeminal dorsal horns, as well as indirect projections through brainstem structures involved in nociceptive processing, such as the PAG, LC, PB and RVM (Saper *et al.*, 1976; Holstege, 1987; Robert *et al.*, 2013). Inhibitory influences of hypothalamic stimulation on spinal nociception and pain behavior have been shown in various studies (Carstens, 1982, 1986; Carstens *et al.*, 1983; Carr and Uysal, 1985; Aimone and Gebhart, 1987; Tasker *et al.*, 1987; Aimone *et al.*, 1988). In recent years, the necessity to better understand these mechanisms has reemerged, due to the involvement of the hypothalamus in the pathophysiology of some primary headaches, as illustrated by functional imaging studies showing increased hypothalamic activity in patients experiencing trigeminal autonomic cephalalgias (TACs) (May *et al.*, 1998; Matharu *et al.*, 2004), and evidence suggesting that hypothalamic regions also become activated during migraine (Denuelle *et al.*, 2007).

Hypothalamic regulation of primary headaches has been linked to the characteristic cranial parasympathetic features of TACs, such as conjunctival injection, lacrimation, nasal congestion and ptosis (Goadsby and Lipton, 1997), and the premonitory symptoms frequently experienced by migraineurs, such as sleep-wake cycle disturbances, changes in mood, appetite, thirst, and urination (Giffin *et al.*, 2003). In this respect, animal studies have shown direct anatomical connections between the hypothalamus and Sp5C (Hancock, 1976; Malick *et al.*, 2000; Gauriau and Bernard, 2004b; Robert *et al.*, 2013), as well as the presence of neurons expressing c-fos in several hypothalamic nuclei mediating these functions after dural stimulation (Malick *et al.*, 2001; Benjamin *et al.*, 2004).

A recent study showed that the paraventricular hypothalamic nucleus (PVN), a key link of both neuroendocrine and autonomic integration of stress responses (hypothalamic-pituitary-adrenal; HPA axis) likely acts as a hub, simultaneously coordinating and regulating trigeminovascular pain and stress mechanisms (Robert *et al.*, 2013). Descending projections from the PVN are confined to laminae I/II of the Sp5C, the ventrolateral PAG and the SSN, which regulate lacrimal glands, nasal mucosa and cerebral vasculature via the PPG (Spencer *et al.*, 1990a).

During migraine and TACs attacks, PPG cells may reflexively stimulate lacrimation and mucous secretion in the nasal and oral cavities, and induce vasodilation and local release of inflammatory molecules in various intracranial structures. This, in turn, could activate meningeal nociceptors and drive Sp5C neurons, contributing to headache. Conversely, experimental depression of PVN cells using the $GABA_A$-receptor agonist muscimol inhibits both the basal activity of Sp5C neurons and activity evoked by nociceptive input from the meninges (Robert *et al.*, 2013). Interestingly, the cluster of PVN neurons that project to Sp5C/SSN cells is densely supplied with corticotrophin-releasing hormone (Simmons and Swanson, 2009).

Such evidence has led to the hypothesis that both HPA and trigeminovascular activities are processed in parallel by the PVN, which is further supported by data indicating that $GABA_A$-R-mediated inhibition of the excitatory output of PVN cells onto Sp5C neurons is significantly reduced in a model of acute restraint stress (Robert *et al.*, 2013). Indeed, acute stress reduces the potency of $GABA_A$-R inhibitory synapses impinging on parvocellular PVN neurons by downregulating the transmembrane anion transporter KCC2 (Hewitt *et al.*, 2009). Loss of inhibition due to changes in the expression of KCC2 could constitute a major maladaptive mechanism by which some primary headaches may be generated primarily within the PVN.

4.3.4   The cortex as a major source of descending modulation

Behavioral responses associated with endogenous feeling states (interoception), including processing of autonomic inputs related to homeostatic regulations, pain and emotions, are thought to be modulated in a hierarchical manner at multiple forebrain levels. A first level of regulation occurs within the hypothalamus, somatosensory cortices and insula. A second level involves prefrontal and cingulate cortices (Critchley *et al.*, 2001; Craig, 2005). The importance of behavioral context on pain perception suggests that powerful endogenous control of nociception originates in the cortex. Indeed, most nociceptive relays within the CNS are under corticofugal modulation. In contrast to descending controls from brainstem areas, cortical modulation often occurs in the absence of a painful stimulus, including effects of distraction, hypnosis, catastrophizing and anticipation/placebo (Apkarian *et al.*, 2005; Colloca and Benedetti, 2005; Tracey and Mantyh, 2007).

The main modulatory function of the cortex is highly dependent on its reciprocal interaction with thalamic relays, since there are nearly ten times as many fibers projecting downstream from the cortex to the thalamus as there are in the ascending direction from the thalamus to the cortex (Deschenes *et al.*, 1998). The function of this massive feedback network has not been fully elucidated, but it has been shown that inactivation of S1 results in rapid changes in the receptive field properties of somatosensory thalamic neurons, and a significant reduction in their ability to reorganize their receptive fields following reversible deafferentation of trigeminal primary afferents (Krupa *et al.*, 1999).

Under pathological circumstances, however, maladaptive changes induced by peripheral injury, deafferentation and progressive changes in both the chemistry and morphology of the brain may occur. This idea is supported by the fact that facial maps of the phantom hand may be present immediately after amputation (Borsook *et al.*, 1998), and by studies in healthy subjects showing that local anesthesia of the thumb increases the perceived size of the unanesthetized lips by approximately 50% (Gandevia and Phegan, 1999). Anatomo-functional studies also indicate that descending influences from S1 cortex are required to discriminate between innocuous and noxious somatosensory input at thalamic level by engaging specific, GABAergic-mediated, corticothalamic modulation (Monconduit *et al.*, 2006).

In addition to cortico-thalamic networks, early electrophysiological studies showed that stimulation of S1 cortex inhibits the evoked responses of a proportion of medullary nociceptive neurons in the Sp5C (Sessle *et al.*, 1981). Although the mediating pathways have not been identified, the seminal work of Dubner and colleagues has shown that corticofugal controls are likely involved in the modulation of neurons in the Sp5C by behaviorally significant stimuli in trained monkeys. This type of "task-related" modulation may produce a greater neuronal response than that produced by equivalent stimuli in the absence of the relevant behavioral state (Bushnell *et al.*, 1984). From the anatomical point of view, some studies have described direct, descending projections from the cerebral cortex to the spinal trigeminal sensory nucleus in the rat (Jacquin *et al.*, 1990; Desbois *et al.*, 1999; Noseda *et al.*, 2010a) and in humans (Kuypers, 1958; Figure 4.4).

A recent study in the rat reported that these projections are restricted within the S1 and insular cortices, and terminate in the Sp5C division innervated by the ophthalmic branch of the trigeminal nerve. This study also showed that cortical spreading depression (CSD)-related influences on insula and S1 produce, respectively, an enhancement and an inhibition of activity in Sp5C neurons evoked by the stimulation of meningeal nociceptors. These changes were shown to selectively affect meningeal (interoceptive) nociceptive input, rather than cutaneous (exteroceptive) tactile input onto Sp5C neurons. In this respect, the existence of a direct relationship between cortical excitability changes and modifications of brainstem trigeminovascular neuronal activities was established. Therefore, consistent with both the topographic localization (ophthalmic) of these networks and the painfulness of migraine attacks, it was hypothesized that such corticofugal influences could contribute to the development of migraine pain (Noseda *et al.*, 2010a).

More recently, Theriot and colleagues demonstrated that CSD induces also a reduction of both electrophysiological and hemodynamic activations in the somatosensory cortex evoked by somatosensory stimulation of the corresponding peripheral fields (Theriot *et al.*, 2012). Electrophysiological responses to somatosensory inputs were enhanced at the receptive field center, but suppressed in surround regions. Because such sharpening on chronic timescales could be used as a marker of sensory plasticity, these observations suggest that the profound alterations of sensory processing associated with CSD could contribute to chronic migraine-related sensitization. These findings shed new light on the role of corticofugal mechanisms and suggest that they may constitute a direct, topographically organized, "top-down" processing mechanism at the origin of migraine headache.

4.4 Conclusions

Taken together, these studies support the concept that CNS mechanisms that process trigeminovascular pain do not consist only of a bottom-up process, whereby a painful focus modifies the inputs to the next higher level. Indeed, a number of CNS regions mediate subtle forms of plasticity by adjusting neural maps downstream and, consequently, altering all the modulatory mechanisms as a result of sensory, autonomic, endocrine, cognitive and emotional influences. Disturbances in normal sensory processing within these loops could lead to maladaptive changes and impaired craniofacial functions at the origin of primary headaches.

References

Afridi SK, Giffin NJ, Kaube H, Friston KJ, Ward NS, Frackowiak RS, Goadsby PJ (2005). A positron emission tomographic study in spontaneous migraine. *Archives of Neurology* **62**(8): 1270–1275.

Aimone LD, Gebhart GF (1987). Spinal monoamine mediation of stimulation-produced antinociception from the lateral hypothalamus. *Brain Research* **403**(2): 290–300.

Aimone LD, Bauer CA, Gebhart GF (1988). Brain-stem relays mediating stimulation-produced antinociception from the lateral hypothalamus in the rat. *Journal of Neuroscience* **8**(7): 2652–2663.

Apkarian AV, Bushnell MC, Treede RD, Zubieta JK (2005). Human brain mechanisms of pain perception and regulation in health and disease. *European Journal of Pain* **9**(4): 463–484.

Apkarian AV, Baliki MN, Geha PY (2009). Towards a theory of chronic pain. *Progress in Neurobiology* **87**(2): 81–97.

Bahra A, Matharu MS, Buchel C, Frackowiak RS, Goadsby PJ (2001). Brainstem activation specific to migraine headache. *Lancet* **357**(9261): 1016–1017.

Bandler R, Depaulis A (1991). Midbrain periaqueductal gray control of defensive behavior in the cat and the rat. In: Depaulis A, Bandler R (eds). *The midbrain periaqueductal gray matter: functional, anatomical and neurochemical organization*, pp. 175–198. Plenum Press, New York.

Bandler R, Carrive P, Zhang SP (1991). Integration of somatic and autonomic reactions within the midbrain periaqueductal grey: viscerotopic, somatotopic and functional organization. *Progress in Brain Research* **87**: 269–305.

Basbaum AI, Fields HL (1978). Endogenous pain control mechanisms: review and hypothesis. *Annals of Neurology* **4**(5): 451–462.

Becerra L, Morris S, Bazes S, Gostic R, Sherman S, Gostic J, Pendse G, Moulton E, Scrivani S, Keith D, Chizh B, Borsook D (2006). Trigeminal neuropathic pain alters responses in CNS circuits to mechanical (brush) and thermal (cold and heat) stimuli. *Journal of Neuroscience* **26**(42): 10646–10657.

Beitz AJ (1982). The organization of afferent projections to the midbrain periaqueductal gray of the rat. *Neuroscience* **7**(1): 133–159.

Benjamin L, Levy MJ, Lasalandra MP, Knight YE, Akerman S, Classey JD, Goadsby PJ (2004). Hypothalamic activation after stimulation of the superior sagittal sinus in the cat: a Fos study. *Neurobiology of Disease* **16**(3): 500–505.

Bernard JF, Besson JM (1990). The spino(trigemino)pontoamygdaloid pathway: electrophysiological evidence for an involvement in pain processes. *Journal of Neurophysiology* **63**(3): 473–490.

Bernard JF, Dallel R, Raboisson P, Villanueva L, Le Bars D (1995). Organization of the efferent projections from the spinal cervical enlargement to the parabrachial area and periaqueductal gray: a PHA–L study in the rat. *Journal of Comparative Neurology* **353**(4): 480–505.

Borsook D, Becerra L, Fishman S, Edwards A, Jennings CL, Stojanovic M, Papinicolas L, Ramachandran VS, Gonzalez RG, Breiter H (1998). Acute plasticity in the human somatosensory cortex following amputation. *Neuroreport* **9**(6): 1013–1017.

Bouhassira D, Danziger N, Attal N, Guirimand F (2003). Comparison of the pain suppressive effects of clinical and experimental painful conditioning stimuli. *Brain* **126**(Pt 5): 1068–1078.

Burstein R, Cliffer KD, Giesler GJ, Jr, (1987). Direct somatosensory projections from the spinal cord to the hypothalamus and telencephalon. *Journal of Neuroscience* **7**(12): 4159–4164.

Burstein R, Jakubowski M, Garcia-Nicas E, Kainz V, Bajwa Z, Hargreaves R, Becerra L, Borsook D (2010). Thalamic sensitization transforms localized pain into widespread allodynia. *Annals of Neurology* **68**(1): 81–91.

Bushnell MC (1995). Thalamic processing of sensory-discriminative and affective-motivational dimensions of pain. In: Besson J M, Guilbaud G, Ollat H (eds). *Forebrain areas involved in pain processing*, p 63–77. John Libbey Eurotext, Paris.

Bushnell MC, Duncan GH (1987). Mechanical response properties of ventroposterior medial thalamic neurons in the alert monkey. *Experimental Brain Research* **67**(3): 603–614.

Bushnell MC, Duncan GH (1989). Sensory and affective aspects of pain perception: is medial thalamus restricted to emotional issues? *Experimental Brain Research* **78**(2): 415–418.

Bushnell MC, Duncan GH, Dubner R, He LF (1984). Activity of trigeminothalamic neurons in medullary dorsal horn of awake monkeys trained in a thermal discrimination task. *Journal of Neurophysiology* **52**(1): 170–187.

Bushnell MC, Duncan GH, Tremblay N (1993). Thalamic VPM nucleus in the behaving monkey. I. Multimodal and discriminative properties of thermosensitive neurons. *Journal of Neurophysiology* **69**(3): 739–752.

Carr KD, Uysal S (1985). Evidence of a supraspinal opioid analgesic mechanism engaged by lateral hypothalamic electrical stimulation. *Brain Research* **335**(1): 55–62.

Carstens E (1982). Inhibition of spinal dorsal horn neuronal responses to noxious skin heating by medial hypothalamic stimulation in the cat. *Journal of Neurophysiology* **48**(3): 808–822.

Carstens E (1986). Hypothalamic inhibition of rat dorsal horn neuronal responses to noxious skin heating. *Pain* **25**(1): 95–107.

Carstens E, Fraunhoffer M, Suberg SN (1983). Inhibition of spinal dorsal horn neuronal responses to noxious skin heating by lateral hypothalamic stimulation in the cat. *Journal of Neurophysiology* **50**(1): 192–204.

Cathcart S, Winefield AH, Lushington K, Rolan P (2010). Noxious inhibition of temporal summation is impaired in chronic tension-type headache. *Headache* **50**(3): 403–412.

Chen JI, Ha B, Bushnell MC, Pike B, Duncan GH (2002). Differentiating noxious- and innocuous-related activation of human somatosensory cortices using temporal analysis of fMRI. *Journal of Neurophysiology* **88**(1): 464–474.

Cliffer KD, Burstein R, Giesler GJ, Jr, (1991). Distributions of spinothalamic, spinohypothalamic, and spinotelencephalic fibers revealed by anterograde transport of PHA-L in rats. *Journal of Neuroscience* **11**(3): 852–868.

Colloca L, Benedetti F (2005). Placebos and painkillers: is mind as real as matter? *Nature Reviews Neuroscience* **6**(7): 545–552.

Contreras RJ, Gomez MM, Norgren R (1980). Central origins of cranial nerve parasympathetic neurons in the rat. *Journal of Comparative Neurology* **190**(2): 373–394.

Craig AD (2004). Distribution of trigeminothalamic and spinothalamic lamina I terminations in the macaque monkey. *Journal of Comparative Neurology* **477**(2): 119–148.

Craig AD (2005). Forebrain emotional asymmetry: a neuroanatomical basis? *Trends in Cognitive Sciences* **9**(12): 566–571.

Craig AD (2014). Topographically organized projection to posterior insular cortex from the posterior portion of the ventral medial nucleus in the long-tailed macaque monkey. *Journal of Comparative Neurology* **522**(1): 36–63.

Craig AD, Bushnell MC, Zhang ET, Blomqvist A (1994). A thalamic nucleus specific for pain and temperature sensation. *Nature* **372**(6508): 770–773.

Critchley HD, Mathias CJ, Dolan RJ (2001). Neuroanatomical basis for first- and second-order representations of bodily states. *Nature Neuroscience* **4**(2): 207–212.

DaSilva AFM, Becerra L, Makris N, Strassman AM, Gonzalez RG, Geatrakis N, Borsook D (2002). Somatotopic activation in the human trigeminal pain pathway. *Journal of Neuroscience* **22**(18): 8183–8192.

De Broucker T, Cesaro P, Willer JC, Le Bars D (1990). Diffuse noxious inhibitory controls in man. Involvement of the spinoreticular tract. *Brain* **113** (Pt 4): 1223–1234.

Denuelle M, Fabre N, Payoux P, Chollet F, Geraud G (2007). Hypothalamic activation in spontaneous migraine attacks. *Headache* **47**(10): 1418–1426.

Derbyshire SW, Jones AK, Gyulai F, Clark S, Townsend D, Firestone LL (1997). Pain processing during three levels of noxious stimulation produces differential patterns of central activity. *Pain* **73**(3): 431–445.

Desbois C, Villanueva L (2001). The organization of lateral ventromedial thalamic connections in the rat: a link for the distribution of nociceptive signals to widespread cortical regions. *Neuroscience* **102**(4): 885–898.

Desbois C, Le Bars D, Villanueva L (1999). Organization of cortical projections to the medullary subnucleus reticularis dorsalis: a retrograde and anterograde tracing study in the rat. *Journal of Comparative Neurology* **410**(2): 178–196.

Deschenes M, Veinante P, Zhang ZW (1998). The organization of corticothalamic projections: reciprocity versus parity. *Brain Research: Brain Research Reviews* **28**(3): 286–308.

Dickenson AH, Le Bars D, Besson JM (1980). Diffuse noxious inhibitory controls (DNIC). Effects on trigeminal nucleus caudalis neurones in the rat. *Brain Research* **200**(2): 293–305.

Dunckley P, Wise RG, Fairhurst M, Hobden P, Aziz Q, Chang L, Tracey I (2005). A comparison of visceral and somatic pain processing in the human brainstem using functional magnetic resonance imaging. *Journal of Neuroscience* **25**(32): 7333–7341.

Edelmayer RM, Vanderah TW, Majuta L, Zhang ET, Fioravanti B, De Felice M, Chichorro JG, Ossipov MH, King T, Lai J, Kori SH, Nelsen AC, Cannon KE, Heinricher MM, Porreca F (2009). Medullary pain facilitating neurons mediate allodynia in headache-related pain. *Annals of Neurology* **65**(2): 184–193.

Fields HL, Malick A, Burstein R (1995). Dorsal horn projection targets of ON and OFF cells in the rostral ventromedial medulla. *Journal of Neurophysiology* **74**(4): 1742–1759.

Gandevia SC, Phegan CM (1999). Perceptual distortions of the human body image produced by local anaesthesia, pain and cutaneous stimulation. *Journal of Physiology* **514** (Pt 2): 609–616.

Gauriau C, Bernard JF (2004a). A comparative reappraisal of projections from the superficial laminae of the dorsal horn in the rat: the forebrain. *Journal of Comparative Neurology* **468**(1): 24–56.

Gauriau C, Bernard JF (2004b). A comparative reappraisal of projections from the superficial laminae of the dorsal horn in the rat: the forebrain. *Journal of Comparative Neurology* **468**(1): 24–56.

Gauriau C, Bernard JF (2004c). Posterior triangular thalamic neurons convey nociceptive messages to the secondary somatosensory and insular cortices in the rat. *Journal of Neuroscience* **24**(3): 752–761.

Giffin NJ, Ruggiero L, Lipton RB, Silberstein SD, Tvedskov JF, Olesen J, Altman J, Goadsby PJ, Macrae A (2003). Premonitory symptoms in migraine: an electronic diary study. *Neurology* **60**(6): 935–940.

Goadsby PJ, Lipton RB (1997). A review of paroxysmal hemicranias, SUNCT syndrome and other short-lasting headaches with autonomic feature, including new cases. *Brain* **120**(Pt 1): 193–209.

Hancock MB (1976). Cells of origin of hypothalamo-spinal projections in the rat. *Neuroscience Letters* **3**(4): 179–184.

Hargreaves RJ, Shepheard SL (1999). Pathophysiology of migraine – new insights. *Canadian Journal of Neurological Sciences* **26**(Suppl 3): S12–S19.

Herkenham M (1986). New perspectives on the organization and evolution of nonspecific thalamocortical projections. In: Jones E G, Peters A (eds). *Cerebral cortex: sensory-motor areas and aspects of cortical connectivity*, vol **5**, p 403–445. Plenum Press, New York.

Hewitt SA, Wamsteeker JI, Kurz EU, Bains JS (2009). Altered chloride homeostasis removes synaptic inhibitory constraint of the stress axis. *Nature Neuroscience* **12**(4): 438–443.

Holstege G (1987). Some anatomical observations on the projections from the hypothalamus to brainstem and spinal cord: an HRP and autoradiographic tracing study in the cat. *Journal of Comparative Neurology* **260**(1): 98–126.

Holstege G, Kuypers HG (1982). The anatomy of brain stem pathways to the spinal cord in cat. A labeled amino acid tracing study. *Progress in Brain Research* **57**: 145–175.

Jacquin MF, Wiegand MR, Renehan WE (1990). Structure-function relationships in rat brain stem subnucleus interpolaris. VIII. Cortical inputs. *Journal of Neurophysiology* **64**(1): 3–27.

Keltner JR, Furst A, Fan C, Redfern R, Inglis B, Fields HL (2006). Isolating the modulatory effect of expectation on pain transmission: a functional magnetic resonance imaging study. *Journal of Neuroscience* **26**(16): 4437–4443.

King CD, Wong F, Currie T, Mauderli AP, Fillingim RB, Riley JL, 3rd, (2009). Deficiency in endogenous modulation of prolonged heat pain in patients with Irritable Bowel Syndrome and Temporomandibular Disorder. *Pain* **143**(3): 172–178.

Knight YE, Goadsby PJ (2001). The periaqueductal grey matter modulates trigeminovascular input: a role in migraine? *Neuroscience* **106**(4): 793–800.

Knight YE, Bartsch T, Kaube H, Goadsby PJ (2002). P/Q-type calcium-channel blockade in the periaqueductal gray facilitates trigeminal nociception: a functional genetic link for migraine? *Journal of Neuroscience* **22**(5): RC213.

Krupa DJ, Ghazanfar AA, Nicolelis MA (1999). Immediate thalamic sensory plasticity depends on corticothalamic feedback. *Proceedings of the National Academy of Sciences of the United States of America* **96**(14): 8200–8205.

Kuypers HG (1958). Corticobular connexions to the pons and lower brain-stem in man: an anatomical study. *Brain* **81**(3): 364–388.

Larkum ME, Zhu JJ (2002). Signaling of layer 1 and whisker-evoked Ca2+ and Na+ action potentials in distal and terminal dendrites of rat neocortical pyramidal neurons in vitro and in vivo. *Journal of Neuroscience* **22**(16): 6991–7005.

Le Bars D, Dickenson AH, Besson JM (1979). Diffuse noxious inhibitory controls (DNIC). *I. Effects on dorsal horn convergent neurones in the rat. Pain* **6**(3): 283–304.

Lenz FA, Dougherty PM (1997). Pain processing in the human thalamus. In: Steriade M, Jones E G, McCormick D A (eds). *Thalamus: experimental and clinical aspects*, p 617–651. Elsevier, New York.

Leonard G, Goffaux P, Mathieu D, Blanchard J, Kenny B, Marchand S (2009). Evidence of descending inhibition deficits in atypical but not classical trigeminal neuralgia. *Pain* **147**(1–3): 217–223.

Linnman C, Moulton EA, Barmettler G, Becerra L, Borsook D (2012). Neuroimaging of the periaqueductal gray: state of the field. *Neuroimage* **60**(1): 505–522.

Lovick TA (1993). Integrated activity of cardiovascular and pain regulatory systems: role in adaptive behavioural responses. *Progress in Neurobiology* **40**(5): 631–644.

Maillou P, Cadden SW (1997). Effects of remote deep somatic noxious stimuli on a jaw reflex in man. *Archives of Oral Biology* **42**(4): 323–327.

Malick A, Strassman RM, Burstein R (2000). Trigeminohypothalamic and reticulohypothalamic tract neurons in the upper cervical spinal cord and caudal medulla of the rat. *Journal of Neurophysiology* **84**(4): 2078–2112.

Malick A, Jakubowski M, Elmquist JK, Saper CB, Burstein R (2001). A neurohistochemical blueprint for pain-induced loss of appetite. *Proceedings of the National Academy of Sciences of the United States of America* **98**(17): 9930–9935.

Mantyh PW (1983). Connections of midbrain periaqueductal gray in the monkey. *I. Ascending efferent projections. Journal of Neurophysiology* **49**(3): 567–581.

Mason P (2001). Contributions of the medullary raphe and ventromedial reticular region to pain modulation and other homeostatic functions. *Annual Review of Neuroscience* **24**: 737–777.

Matharu MS, Cohen AS, McGonigle DJ, Ward N, Frackowiak RS, Goadsby PJ (2004). Posterior hypothalamic and brainstem activation in hemicrania continua. *Headache* **44**(8): 747–761.

May A, Bahra A, Buchel C, Frackowiak RS, Goadsby PJ (1998). Hypothalamic activation in cluster headache attacks. *Lancet* **352**(9124): 275–278.

Menetrey D, Basbaum AI (1987). Spinal and trigeminal projections to the nucleus of the solitary tract: A possible substrate for the somatovisceral and visceroviceral reflex activation. *Journal of Comparative Neurology* **255**: 439–450.

Monconduit L, Bourgeais L, Bernard JF, Le Bars D, Villanueva L (1999). Ventromedial thalamic neurons convey nociceptive signals from the whole body surface to the dorsolateral neocortex. *Journal of Neuroscience* **19**(20): 9063–9072.

Monconduit L, Lopez-Avila A, Molat JL, Chalus M, Villanueva L (2006). Corticofugal output from the primary somatosensory cortex selectively modulates innocuous and noxious inputs in the rat spinothalamic system. *Journal of Neuroscience* **26**(33): 8441–8450.

Montes C, Magnin M, Maarrawi J, Frot M, Convers P, Mauguiere F, Garcia-Larrea L (2005). Thalamic thermo-algesic transmission: ventral posterior (VP) complex versus VMpo in the light of a thalamic infarct with central pain. *Pain* **113**(1–2): 223–232.

Moulton EA, Burstein R, Tully S, Hargreaves R, Becerra L, Borsook D (2008). Interictal dysfunction of a brainstem descending modulatory center in migraine patients. *PLoS One* **3**(11): e3799.

Newman HM, Stevens RT, Apkarian AV (1996). Direct spinal projections to limbic and striatal areas: anterograde transport studies from the upper cervical spinal cord and the cervical enlargement in squirrel monkey and rat. *Journal of Comparative Neurology* **365**(4): 640–658.

Noseda R, Monconduit L, Constandil L, Chalus M, Villanueva L (2008). Central nervous system networks involved in the processing of meningeal and cutaneous inputs from the ophthalmic branch of the trigeminal nerve in the rat. *Cephalalgia* **28**(8): 813–824.

Noseda R, Constandil L, Bourgeais L, Chalus M, Villanueva L (2010a). Changes of meningeal excitability mediated by corticotrigeminal networks: a link for the endogenous modulation of migraine pain. *Journal of Neuroscience* **30**(43): 14420–14429.

Noseda R, Kainz V, Jakubowski M, Gooley JJ, Saper CB, Digre K, Burstein R (2010b). A neural mechanism for exacerbation of headache by light. *Nature Neuroscience* **13**(2): 239–245.

Noseda R, Jakubowski M, Kainz V, Borsook D, Burstein R (2011). Cortical projections of functionally identified thalamic trigeminovascular neurons: implications for migraine headache and its associated symptoms. *Journal of Neuroscience* **31**(40): 14204–14217.

Okada-Ogawa A, Porreca F, Meng ID (2009). Sustained morphine-induced sensitization and loss of diffuse noxious inhibitory controls in dura-sensitive medullary dorsal horn neurons. *Journal of Neuroscience* **29**(50): 15828–15835.

Oliveras JL, Besson JM (1988). Stimulation-produced analgesia in animals: behavioural investigations. *Progress in Brain Research* **77**: 141–157.

Ostrowsky K, Magnin M, Ryvlin P, Isnard J, Guenot M, Mauguiere F (2002). Representation of pain and somatic sensation in the human insula: a study of responses to direct electrical cortical stimulation. *Cerebral Cortex* **12**(4): 376–385.

Piche M, Arsenault M, Rainville P (2009). Cerebral and cerebrospinal processes underlying counterirritation analgesia. *Journal of Neuroscience* **29**(45): 14236–14246.

Pielsticker A, Haag G, Zaudig M, Lautenbacher S (2005). Impairment of pain inhibition in chronic tension-type headache. *Pain* **118**(1–2): 215–223.

Porreca F, Ossipov MH, Gebhart GF (2002). Chronic pain and medullary descending facilitation. *Trends in Neurosciences* **25**(6): 319–325.

Ralston HJ, 3rd,, Ralston DD (1992). The primate dorsal spinothalamic tract: evidence for a specific termination in the posterior nuclei (Po/SG) of the thalamus. *Pain* **48**(1): 107–118.

Raskin NH, Hosobuchi Y, Lamb S (1987). Headache may arise from perturbation of brain. *Headache* **27**(8): 416–420.

Robert C, Bourgeais L, Arreto CD, Condes-Lara M, Noseda R, Jay T, Villanueva L (2013). Paraventricular hypothalamic regulation of trigeminovascular mechanisms involved in headaches. *Journal of Neuroscience* **33**(20): 8827–8840.

Roby-Brami A, Bussel B, Willer JC, Le Bars D (1987). An electrophysiological investigation into the pain-relieving effects of heterotopic nociceptive stimuli. Probable involvement of a supraspinal loop. *Brain* **110**(Pt 6): 1497–1508.

Saper CB, Loewy AD (1980). Efferent connections of the parabrachial nucleus in the rat. *Brain Research: Brain Research Reviews* **197**(2): 291–317.

Saper CB, Loewy AD, Swanson LW, Cowan WM (1976). Direct hypothalamo-autonomic connections. *Brain Research* **117**(2): 305–312.

Sawchenko PE, Swanson LW (1981). Central noradrenergic pathways for the integration of hypothalamic neuroendocrine and autonomic responses. *Science* **214**(4521): 685–687.

Sessle BJ, Hu JW, Dubner R, Lucier GE (1981). Functional properties of neurons in cat trigeminal subnucleus caudalis (medullary dorsal horn). II. Modulation of responses to noxious and nonnoxious stimuli by periaqueductal gray, nucleus raphe magnus, cerebral cortex, and afferent influences, and effect of naloxone. *Journal of Neurophysiology* **45**(2): 193–207.

Simmons DM, Swanson LW (2009). Comparison of the spatial distribution of seven types of neuroendocrine neurons in the rat paraventricular nucleus: toward a global 3D model. *Journal of Comparative Neurology* **516**(5): 423–441.

Spencer SE, Sawyer WB, Wada H, Platt KB, Loewy AD (1990a). CNS projections to the pterygopalatine parasympathetic preganglionic neurons in the rat: a retrograde transneuronal viral cell body labeling study. *Brain Research* **534**(1–2): 149–169.

Spencer SE, Sawyer WB, Wada H, Platt KB, Loewy AD (1990b). CNS projections to the pterygopalatine parasympathetic preganglionic neurons in the rat: a retrograde transneuronal viral cell body labeling study. *Brain Research: Brain Research Reviews* **534**(1–2): 149–169.

Sprenger C, Bingel U, Buchel C (2011). Treating pain with pain: supraspinal mechanisms of endogenous analgesia elicited by heterotopic noxious conditioning stimulation. *Pain* **152**(2): 428–439.

Stankewitz A, May A (2011). Increased limbic and brainstem activity during migraine attacks following olfactory stimulation. *Neurology* **77**(5): 476–482.

Suzuki R, Morcuende S, Webber M, Hunt SP, Dickenson AH (2002). Superficial NK1-expressing neurons control spinal excitability through activation of descending pathways. *Nature Neuroscience* **5**(12): 1319–26.

Tasker RA, Choiniere M, Libman SM, Melzack R (1987). Analgesia produced by injection of lidocaine into the lateral hypothalamus. *Pain* **31**(2): 237–248.

Theriot JJ, Toga AW, Prakash N, Ju YS, Brennan KC (2012). Cortical sensory plasticity in a model of migraine with aura. *Journal of Neuroscience* **32**(44): 15252–15261.

Tracey I, Mantyh PW (2007). The cerebral signature for pain perception and its modulation. *Neuron* **55**(3): 377–391.

Villanueva L, Nathan P (2000). *Multiple pain pathways*. In: Devor M, Rowbotham MC, Wiesendfeld-Hallin Z (eds). Proceedings of the 9th World Congress on Pain, pp. 371–386.

Villanueva L, Noseda R (2012). Trigeminal Mechanisms of Nociception. In: McMahon S, Koltzenburg M, Tracey I, Turk D (eds.) *Wall and Melzack's Textbook of Pain*. Elsevier, 6th Edition.

Villanueva L, Cadden SW, Le Bars D (1984). Diffuse noxious inhibitory controls (DNIC): evidence for post-synaptic inhibition of trigeminal nucleus caudalis convergent neurones. *Brain Research* **321**(1): 165–168.

Villanueva L, Bouhassira D, Bing Z, Le Bars D (1988). Convergence of heterotopic nociceptive information onto subnucleus reticularis dorsalis neurons in the rat medulla. *Journal of Neurophysiology* **60**(3): 980–1009.

Villanueva L, Cliffer KD, Sorkin LS, Le Bars D, Willis WD, Jr, (1990). Convergence of heterotopic nociceptive information onto neurons of caudal medullary reticular formation in monkey (Macaca fascicularis). *Journal of Neurophysiology* **63**(5): 1118–1127.

Villanueva L, Bouhassira D, Le Bars D (1996). The medullary subnucleus reticularis dorsalis (SRD) as a key link in both the transmission and modulation of pain signals. *Pain* **67**(2–3): 231–240.

Villanueva L, Desbois C, Le Bars D, Bernard JF (1998). Organization of diencephalic projections from the medullary subnucleus reticularis dorsalis and the adjacent cuneate nucleus: a retrograde and anterograde tracer study in the rat. *Journal of Comparative Neurology* **390**(1): 133–160.

Vogt BA (2005). Pain and emotion interactions in subregions of the cingulate gyrus. *Nature Reviews Neuroscience* **6**(7): 533–544.

Weiller C, May A, Limmroth V, Juptner M, Kaube H, Schayck RV, Coenen HH, Diener HC (1995). Brain stem activation in spontaneous human migraine attacks. *Nature Medicine* **1**(7): 658–660.

Yarnitsky D (2010). Conditioned pain modulation (the diffuse noxious inhibitory control-like effect): its relevance for acute and chronic pain states. *Current Opinion in Anesthesiology* **23**(5): 611–615.

Yarnitsky D, Goor-Aryeh I, Bajwa ZH, Ransil BI, Cutrer FM, Sottile A, Burstein R (2003). 2003 Wolff Award: Possible parasympathetic contributions to peripheral and central sensitization during migraine. *Headache* **43**(7): 704–714.

Zhang S, Chiang CY, Xie YF, Park SJ, Lu Y, Hu JW, Dostrovsky JO, Sessle BJ (2006). Central sensitization in thalamic nociceptive neurons induced by mustard oil application to rat molar tooth pulp. *Neuroscience* **142**(3): 833–842.

Part II

Special features of migraine pain

5

Visceral pain

Michael S. Gold[1] and G.F. Gebhart[2]

[1] Center for Pain Research, Department of Neurobiology, School of Medicine, University of Pittsburgh, Pittsburgh, Pennsylvania, USA
[2] Center for Pain Research, Department of Anesthesiology, School of Medicine, University of Pittsburgh, Pittsburgh, Pennsylvania, USA

The role of trigeminal afferents, and specifically the durovascular innervation, has long been advanced as important to the neurobiology of vascular head pain, including the pathogenesis of migraine headaches (e.g., Moskowitz, 1984). In his influential paper on the visceral organ brain, Moskowitz (1991) emphasized similarities between visceral pain and migraine headache, and migraine is, indeed, more similar to pain arising from internal organs than pain arising from other tissues (Moskowitz, 1991). As discussed in the following sections, visceral pain and migraine share characteristics of referral of sensations and sensitization of receptive endings in their respective tissues, likely associated with similar underlying mechanisms. However, important differences highlight the fact that this analogy should be made with caution, as the differences will likely continue to dictate different therapeutic strategies for the treatment of migraine and visceral pain.

5.1 Organization of innervation

The internal organs are innervated by two sets of sensory nerves with cell bodies in dorsal root or vagal nodose/jugular ganglia, making the innervation of the viscera unique among tissues in the body. All organs in the thoracic and abdominal cavities are innervated by nerves with cell bodies located bilaterally in dorsal root ganglia (DRG) (i.e., they are innervated by "spinal nerves"). The spinal (central) terminations of these neurons are located principally in the superficial laminae of the spinal dorsal horn, but also in the intermediolateral cell column/sacral parasympathetic nucleus. All organs in the thoracic, and some organs in the abdominal cavities, are *also* innervated by the vagus nerve, the cell bodies of which are located in the nodose or jugular ganglia[1], with central terminations in the nucleus tractus solitarius (NTS) in the brainstem medulla.

In contrast to the relatively dense innervation of skin, the numbers of sensory (afferent) neurons innervating internal organs are few. However, their central terminations are more widely distributed than other somatic inputs, including spinal segments both

1 In primates, these ganglia are clearly distinguishable, the jugular being smaller and superior to the nodose, but in rodents they are not easily separable.

Neurobiological Basis of Migraine, First Edition. Edited by Turgay Dalkara and Michael A. Moskowitz.
© 2017 John Wiley & Sons, Inc. Published 2017 by John Wiley & Sons, Inc.

above and below the segment of entry and the contralateral spinal cord. The dual but sparse innervation of organs, coupled with significant central arborization in the spinal cord, contribute to several key features of visceral pain that distinguish it from most other types of pain, namely localization and referral.

Unlike innervation of internal organs by two nerves, the sensory innervation of the head is contained within the three divisions of one nerve – the trigeminal nerve. The divisions of the trigeminal nerve innervate all tissues in the head except the brain, but including the dura and dural vasculature. The cell bodies of their afferent terminals are located in trigeminal ganglia positioned bilaterally at the level of the pons. Furthermore, in contrast to visceral organs that receive bilateral innervation, the dura and dural vasculature, like the majority of other craniofacial structures on either size of midline, only receive innervation arising from the ipsilateral trigeminal ganglion. Several other features of the trigeminal system make innervation of the dura/dural vasculature distinct from that of the viscera.

First, the trigeminal ganglia are somatotopically organized, such that the somata of neurons innervating a particular area of the head are located within the ganglia in relatively close proximity to neurons innervating adjacent areas. This is in contrast to the spinal and nodose ganglia, which appear to have no somatotopic organization. Given evidence of intra-ganglionic communication via the release of transmitters within the ganglia following the activation of afferent terminals (Matsuka *et al.*, 2001), this form of cross-talk may become a source of signal amplification where, as hypothesized by Devor *et al.* (2002), this amplification may underlie a triggered attack of trigeminal neuralgia.

Second, while the axons of proprioceptive afferents are contained in branches of the trigeminal nerve, the somata giving rise to these axons are actually located in the brainstem, in the mesencephalic nucleus of the fifth cranial nerve. This is in contrast to spinal dorsal root ganglia, where the somata giving rise to proprioceptive afferents are co-localized with other types of sensory neurons. The functional implications of the spatial isolation of these two types of neurons in the trigeminal system, at least in the context of nociceptive processing, has yet to be elucidated. However, this organization does appear to facilitate the integration of sensory information arising from bi-lateral structures, such as the eyes and the muscles of mastication.

Third, the central terminals of trigeminal afferents are organized in a rostro-caudal orientation, with proprioceptive and non-nociceptive afferents terminating rostrally in the mesencephalic nucleus and primary or main sensory nucleus, respectively, and deep touch, pain and temperature-sensitive afferents, terminating in the spinal trigeminal nucleus. This latter structure is further subdivided, and spread rostral-caudally into nucleus oralis, interpolaris and caudalis; the majority of nociceptive afferents terminate in nucleus caudalis. This is in contrast to the dorsal-ventral termination pattern of sensory input to the spinal cord. The result is a significantly greater distance between the non-nociceptive and nociceptive terminals in the trigeminal system, which will necessarily change the timing of interactions between these afferent types thought to be necessary for phenomena such as mechanical allodynia and referred pain, as described below (see also Chapter 1).

Finally, somewhere between a difference and a similarity is the embryological origin of the sensory innervation of the head and viscera. That is, spinal ganglia are derived from neural crest cells, while the cells in the nodose ganglia are derived from ectodermal placode cells. The result is that the two nerves innervating most viscera are embryologically distinct. Similarly, the trigeminal ganglia are a mix of both neural crest and placode-derived cells. Unfortunately, it is not yet possible to identify these two cell types in the adult and, consequently, it is not possible to determine whether the two cell types give rise to distinct or overlapping patterns of innervation. As a result, the functional consequences of the mixed embryological origin of trigeminal ganglia have yet to be determined. However, differences between spinal and nodose ganglia, with respect to the dependence of afferent phenotype on specific trophic factors (i.e., many properties of peptidergic afferents in spinal ganglia depend on NGF (Bennett, 2001), while the properties of nodose ganglia neurons depend on BDNF (Winter, 1998)), suggest that changes in the trophic factor milieu may have very different consequences, depending on the embryological origin of the afferents present.

While pain is a sensory phenomenon, there is compelling evidence to suggest that autonomic efferent fibers contribute to the pain of injury. Because of their role in mediating components of both neuropathic (Perl, 1999) and inflammatory (Raja, 1995) pain, sympathetic efferents have received considerably more attention than parasympathetic efferents. This is not necessarily so in the context of migraine, where there is evidence that disruption of parasympathetic outflow can abort a migraine attack (Khan *et al.*, 2014). And while the vascular hypothesis of migraine has largely fallen under the weight of negative evidence (Goadsby, 2009; but see Karatas *et al.*, 2013), migraine attacks may be associated with "parasympathetic" features, such as congested sinuses and increased tearing (Gass and Glaros, 2013), as well as mast cell degranulation. Importantly, mast cell degranulation has been implicated in migraine (Levy, 2009), and can be driven by cholinergic receptor activation (Messlinger *et al.*, 2011). Nevertheless, in contrast to the relatively dense sympathetic innervation (at least in the rodent) of the dura, the parasympathetic innervation of this structure appears to be relatively sparse (Artico *et al.*, 1998).

Additional evidence in support of a potential role for sympathetic innervation of the dura in migraine comes from the observations that sympathetic postganglionic neuron terminals may be a rich source of prostaglandin E2 (PGE2), a mediator implicated in migraine. Prostaglandins are implicated in migraine both by the therapeutic efficacy of COX inhibitors and the increases in PGE2 detected in blood (Sarchielli *et al.*, 2000) and saliva (Tuca *et al.*, 1989) during a migraine attack. There is also evidence that PGE2 can sensitize dural afferents (Harriott and Gold, 2009). More recently, it has been shown that the serotonin 1D receptor, a target for the anti-migraine triptan drugs, is present on cranial sympathetic efferents (Harriott and Gold, 2008). Furthermore, there is also evidence that norepinephrine, a primary sympathetic mediator, can sensitize dural afferents (Wei *et al.*, 2015). Indirect support for the role of sympathetic efferents in migraine comes from the prophylactic efficacy of beta-adrenergic receptor antagonists and alpha-adrenergic receptor agonists for the treatment of migraine (Silberstein, 2009), as well as evidence of sympathetic dysregulation in migraineurs (Sauro and Becker, 2009).

While it has been hypothesized that dysregulation of parasympathetic efferent activity may contribute to the co-morbidity of visceral pain and headache, as well as the transition of cyclic vomiting in children and adolescents to migraine in adults (Han and Lee, 2009), evidence in support a role for either sympathetic or parasympathetic efferents in visceral pain is far less direct than that for their roles in migraine. Importantly, the efferent innervation of visceral structures is more complex than in cranial structures. Collateral branches of afferents can directly influence secretory and motor neurons in autonomic ganglia close to an organ, thus adding a layer of complexity to interpretation of the roles of sympathetic or parasympathetic efferents in visceral pain. For example, the celiac ganglia, one of the largest autonomic ganglia, not only receives cholinergic input from preganglionic fibers, but receives adrenergic fiber input as well.

5.2   Common features of visceral pain and headache

With respect to both visceral pain and migraine, because the principal sensations that arise from the internal organs and dura are discomfort and pain, nociceptors are considered the main class of sensory neurons innervating those tissues. Nociceptors respond to and encode noxious intensities of stimuli, and are characterized by their ability to sensitize (discussed below). Nociceptors do not uniformly have high thresholds for activation and, in fact, many are naturally activated by low, non-noxious intensities of stimulation but, uniquely, encode intensity into the noxious range.

This is clearly evident for visceral pain, which is commonly associated with discomfort and pain in response to normally non-noxious stimuli. However, this has been a more difficult feature to assess for dural afferents, both because of how little is known about what constitutes a physiologically relevant stimulus, and the difficulty in applying these stimuli to dural afferents without a significant amount of tissue injury needed to access their peripheral terminals. Nevertheless, the available evidence suggests that dural afferents are likely to normally encode chemical stimuli, such as a decrease in pH from the non-noxious, into the noxious range (Yan *et al.*, 2011).

5.2.1   Referred sensations

Visceral pain is typically diffuse in character and is difficult to localize. Importantly, it is not commonly felt at the source, but rather is referred (or "transferred") to other somatic structures. Referred sensations are generally described as "deep pains" that are generally, but not necessarily, present in somatic structures overlying the visceral organ. For example, pain associated with kidney stones is often described in the muscles of the lower back, whereas the pain of a heart attack may be present in the jaw, the left shoulder and/or the arm. Although innervation of the head is not as complex as that of the internal organs, the pain of migraine can be similarly diffuse, although laterality and periorbital localization are used as diagnostic criteria.

Additionally, both the location and the quality of referred visceral pain are generally quite different from that of the referred pain of migraine. The referred pain of migraine is generally cutaneous, and its character is commonly described as a tactile allodynia, or pain in response to normally non-painful mechanical stimulation of skin in the ophthalmic division of the trigeminal innervation. Interestingly, in further contrast to visceral pain (hypotheses concerning the basis for the comorbidity of IBS and fibromyalgia notwithstanding), the area of migraine-induced allodynia increases with increasing number and severity of migraines, such that some migraineurs may experience full body allodynia during their migraine attacks (Lipton *et al.*, 2008; Louter *et al.*, 2013). In addition, both headache and pain arising from internal organs are generally associated with exaggerated autonomic responses.

Referred visceral sensation arises in part due to convergence of independent visceral and somatic (i.e., non-visceral) inputs onto the same second order neurons in the spinal dorsal horn, a mechanism advanced by Ruch (1961) as the "convergence–projection" theory of referred visceral sensation. Most, if not virtually all, second order spinal neurons that receive input from one organ also receive input from either a non-visceral tissue (i.e., viscero-somatic convergence) and/or another organ (i.e., viscero-visceral convergence). There is considerable experimental evidence in support of such convergence, which is also advanced as contributing to the diffuse, difficult-to-localize character of visceral pain.

An earlier hypothesis proposed that referred visceral sensations arose from sensory axons derived from a single sensory neuron cell body in a dorsal root ganglion, one axon innervating skin and the other an internal organ. This so-called dichotomizing/bifurcating axon mechanism of referred sensation was initially dismissed for lack of convincing anatomical evidence, but it has gained new support, largely based on the availability of better nerve tracing tools. For example, innervation of two organs by one dorsal root ganglion neuron has been established in rodents for many organs, including colon and bladder, colon and uterus, and prostate and bladder. Although the reported proportion of visceral sensory neurons innervating two organs is small (10–20% of total organ innervation), there clearly exist two potential contributing mechanisms for referral of visceral sensations.

The referral and localization of migraine pain to the eye, forehead, temple and neck is likely due to a comparable convergence of inputs onto trigeminal subnucleus caudalis neurons in the brainstem, as suggested by the seminal observation of Penfield and McNaughton (1940) and Ray and Wolff (1940), whose patients described the pain associated with arterial and dural stimulation as pain in these regions of the ophthalmic division. Whether referral of headache pain can also arise from "dichotomizing axons" is less certain. Existing anatomical evidence is very limited, although there is also evidence to suggest that at least some of the "referral" may be due to unique features of the trigeminal nerve. One of these, as noted above, is the somatotopic organization of the ganglion, providing an anatomical substrate for the activation of neurons innervating adjacent structures.

Furthermore, while early anatomical tracing studies apparently failed to provide support for dichotomizing trigeminal axons, at least some evidence for this possibility was provided upon reevaluation. One study reported finding one trigeminal ganglion neuron per animal (rat) that innervated the middle cerebral artery (MCA) and the forehead (O'Connor and Van der Kooy, 1986). The authors did report, however, that a significant proportion of trigeminal ganglion neurons that innervated the MCA had collateral projections to branches of the middle meningeal artery and to surrounding dura. In addition, these and other authors (Borges and Moskowitz, 1983; O'Connor and Van der Kooy, 1986) noted that artery-innervating neurons in the trigeminal ganglion often had a forehead-innervating neuron nearby, which may provide a substrate for referred pain, as suggested above, and as has been suggested in the viscera (Brumovsky and Gebhart, 2010).

More recently, it has been demonstrated that a subpopulation of dural afferents give rise to branches that pass through the cranial sutures (Kosaras *et al.*, 2009). The differential distribution of these fibers has been hypothesized to account for the differing perceptions of the nature of the pain and, in particular, as to whether it is perceived as imploding or exploding (Kim *et al.*, 2010). More relevantly, the presence of these fibers has been suggested to account for the therapeutic efficacy of botulinum neurotoxin type A, which is thought to gain access to the relevant fibers through these branches (Burstein *et al.*, 2014). Notably, whether dichotomizing (bifurcating) axons and/or intraganglionic neuronal (satellite cell?) interactions underlie referred sensations from the viscera or in migraine, a peripheral mechanism(s) evidently plays a key role in referral of sensations (and in sensitization, as well).

All that said, the available evidence suggests that the tactile allodynia associated with a migraine attack necessarily involves changes in trigeminal subnucleus caudalis neurons (Sandkuhler, 2009; Peirs *et al.*, 2015) or higher brain centers (Burstein *et al.*, 2010) to enable low threshold sensory input to engage nociceptive circuitry. Thus, the differences between visceral pain and migraine with respect to the prevalence of allodynia suggests that there is a fundamental difference between the two with respect to the underlying neural circuitry engaged.

5.2.2 Sensitization

An essential property of nociceptors innervating all tissues is their ability to sensitize, defined as an increase in response magnitude to a noxious intensity of stimulation and a reduction in stimulus threshold for activation. Often, the size of the peripheral receptive field increases in area and, occasionally, spontaneous or ongoing activity may develop. Sensitization thus represents an increase in neuron excitability, which can be short in duration (e.g., during a migraine attack) or long-lasting (e.g., associated with many chronic visceral pain disorders).

There is a potentially important distinction to make here with respect to the time course of changes in afferent excitability – in particular, long lasting changes in excitability. That is, there is reasonable evidence to suggest that, at least for conditions such as post-infectious irritable bowel syndrome, persistent pain and sensitivity is due, at least in part, to the persistent sensitization of visceral afferents. In contrast, most cases of migraine are episodic, where there may be days, weeks, months or even years between attacks. This suggests that, in contrast to persistent sensitization of visceral afferents, the acute sensitization, necessary for the manifestation of the migraine, resolves between attacks.

On the other hand, there is clearly something unique about migraineurs, as stimuli such as nitroglycerine are able to generate a migraine in the majority of migraineurs, yet produce no comparable pain syndrome in non-migraineurs (Afridi *et al.*, 2004). Furthermore, severe stress, such as that sufficient to produce post-traumatic stress disorder (PTSD) and, even more commonly, the combination of a mild traumatic brain injury in combination with PTSD, results in the emergence of episodic, and even chronic, migraine-like headaches. This implies that there is a "threshold" that divides migraineurs from non-migraineurs, below which the acute sensitization of dural afferents results in a migraine attack. Whether this "threshold" is established by intrinsic properties of dural afferents remains to be determined. However, the available evidence would suggest that this is not likely to be the case.

Functional visceral pain disorders (e.g., irritable bowel syndrome, chronic pelvic pain syndrome, etc.) and migraine share several characteristics. Both are more common in women, with an onset at menarche and a reduction in prevalence and severity of symptoms (if not the complete elimination) with menopause. Both exist in the absence of an apparent pathobiology, where lesions, tissue inflammation, or obvious pathology are typically not evident. They are also episodic in nature, waxing and waning in both occurrence and intensity, but are commonly triggered by foods, or too little exercise or sleep, where stress is the most common trigger for both (although, in contrast to visceral pain, migraines triggered by a stressful event generally develop with a delay after stress resolution).

Peripheral contributions to chronic pain states are commonly discounted, despite growing evidence of their importance. For example, ongoing afferent input is present in chronic pain conditions, ranging from neuropathic pain (Ochoa *et al.*, 2005) to fibromyalgia (Serra *et al.*, 2014), and essential for most (e.g., Haroutounian *et al.*, 2014). With respect to chronic, functional visceral pain states, silencing afferent activity by intra-rectal instillation of a local anesthetic (lidocaine) significantly reduced reported patient discomfort and pain, their responses to provocative organ distension and hypersensitivity to palpation in the abdominal area of referred sensation for the duration of action of the local anesthetic (Verne *et al.*, 2003; Price *et al.*, 2009). Longer-lasting effects were produced by daily intra-vesical instillation of lidocaine for five consecutive days; significant attenuation of symptoms in interstitial cystitis/painful bladder syndrome (IC/PBS) patients were sustained for up to 15 days after initiating the daily intra-vesical treatment (Nickel *et al.*, 2009).

In a subsequent study, continuous intra-vesical infusion of lidocaine for two weeks produced clinically meaningful reductions in pain, urgency and voiding frequency in IC/PBS patients which, remarkably, were maintained for several months after the infusion device was removed (Nickel *et al.*, 2012). These experimental outcomes, in which a drug effect was restricted to a peripheral locus of action, confirm the significant contribution of persistent, on-going afferent activity to pain and discomfort in these visceral pain conditions. Notably, the results suggest that re-setting afferent excitability can lead to long-lasting effects, including relief of persistent pain.

Corresponding evidence is not available for migraine patients. However, indirect evidence, based on the efficacy of relatively recent therapeutic interventions, is consistent with an essential role for nociceptive durovascular afferents in the manifestation of migraine. First, while botulinum toxin A (BonTA) is approved for the treatment of chronic migraine, it only appears to work in a subpopulation of migraineurs – those who describe their migraines as "imploding" (Kim *et al.*, 2010). As noted above, Burstein and colleagues hypothesized that this subpopulation is enriched in dural afferents that penetrate cranial sutures, enabling the toxin access to the relevant afferent fibers.

Second, the recent success of the CGRP antibodies in the prevention of migraine (Wrobel Goldberg and Silberstein, 2015) argues for a peripheral pain generator, as the available evidence suggests that antibodies do not have access to the central nervous system (Vermeersch *et al.*, 2015). While the role of the persistently sensitized nociceptor in migraine is also not as well developed as that for visceral pain, evidence for rebound and medication overuse migraine suggest that a persistent increase in nociceptor excitability may contribute to the manifestation of migraine as well.

The concept of a "primed" nociceptor, where an inciting stimulus can drive persistent changes in the afferent that enable a dramatic increase in the duration of the response to a subsequent challenge (Reichling and Levine, 2009), is a relatively new concept in the pain community. Such a mechanism has been proposed to contribute to the emergence of chronic pain, where the altered signaling in the primed afferent enable the emergence of persistent pain, in response to what should normally be a transient episode of hypersensitivity. While such a change may contribute to the manifestation of persistent visceral pain, particularly in the context of a previous trauma or infection, it has yet to be determined whether comparable mechanisms underlie persistent sensitization of visceral afferents. However, with the exception of chronic migraine, which nevertheless appears to emerge via distinct processes other than those underlying nociceptor priming, the episodic nature of migraine argues against nociceptor priming as an under-lying mechanism of this pain syndrome.

In contrast, relatively transient sensitization of nociceptive afferents as a mechanism of pain and hypersensitivity was observed in some of the very first studies of this afferent population (Bessou *et al.*, 1971). This process clearly contributes to the manifestation of visceral hypersensitivity (Feng *et al.*, 2012b), and the available pre-clinical evidence suggests that this is also true for migraine. For example, in rats, bathing the dura with an inflammatory soup (IS; PGE2, histamine, serotonin, bradykinin and protons) produces, depending upon the concentration of IS constituents and pH, sensitization of meningial afferents (Strassman *et al.*, 1996) and a reduction in periorbital pressure thresholds (hypersensitivity) (Oshinsky and Gomonchareonsiri, 2007; Edelmayer *et al.*, 2012).

However, data from the study of isolated dural afferent cell bodies *in vitro* suggests that the mechanisms underlying IS-induced sensitization are relatively unique, and involve an increase in a Ca^{2+}-dependent Cl^- conductance, in addition to changes in Na^+ and K^+ currents (Vaughn and Gold, 2010). Also, while a similar Na^+ current appears to con-tribute to the sensitization of visceral afferents (Gold *et al.*, 2002), the extent to which comparable channels underlie the sensitization of dural and visceral afferents has yet to be fully evaluated.

5.2.3 Potential sensitizers

Given evidence reviewed above about sensitized input from the visceral and dural neu-rovascular innervations, the question arises as to what endogenous molecules in tissue contribute to and/or sustain altered afferent input? There is considerable documen-tation that serotonin, neuropeptides, post-ganglionic autonomic neurotransmitters, a variety of immune cell mediators and so on, play a role, either as activators or sensitiz-ers of afferent receptive endings. Serotonin receptor agonists and antagonists are used clinically in the treatment of IBS and nausea (5-HT3 antagonists, 5-HT4 agonist) and headache (5-HT1 agonists), as are substance-P/neurokinin and calcitonin gene-related peptide receptor antagonists. Both strategies can be effective in some cases, but neither is uniformly efficacious.

Just as there are "different" classes of IBS (constipation-predominant, diarrhea-predominant and alternating), not all migraines are alike (with and without aura, imploding and exploding), suggesting the likelihood of heterogeneity in the mecha-nisms underlying visceral hypersensitivity and migraine. However, the phenotyping of pain syndromes continues to improve. There is also an increased appreciation that the heterogeneity in phenotype is likely to reflect heterogeneity in mechanism which is, in turn, likely to account for the differential sensitivity to therapeutic interventions. As these trends take root, it will be interesting to determine the extent to which there is overlap in subpopulations of visceral pain and migraine patients.

5.2.4 Immune system involvement in visceral pain and migraine

In the gut, the role of immune-competent cells and their products have been long appre-ciated as likely sensitizers/primers of afferent endings and contributors to visceral pain. Most of the focus has been on pro- (e.g., IL-1, IL-6, IL-12, IL-18, TNF-α, IFNγ,)- and anti- (e.g., IL-4, IL-10) inflammatory cytokines, although it must be recognized that a given cytokine may be pro- or anti-inflammatory, depending on the target cell, activating signal and other factors (Cavaillon, 2001).

Several reviews have described the role(s) of immune cells in the viscera as contributing to visceral pain states (e.g., Van Nassauw *et al.*, 2007; Camilleri *et al.*, 2012; Feng *et al.*, 2012a; Murphy *et al.*, 2014), and there is a growing body of evidence to suggest that immune cells in the dura play a critical role in triggering a migraine attack. Immune cell mediators, such as TNFα and IL-1β, are increased in the internal jugular blood of migraineurs during a migraine attack (Perini *et al.*, 2005; Sarchielli *et al.*, 2006). Migraine-provocative stimuli, such as GTN drive mast cell degranulation and the activation of macrophages in the rat dura, have a delay comparable to that seen between GTN administration and the migraine attack in migraineurs (Reuter *et al.*, 2001). Degranulation of dural mast cells has been shown to sensitize dural afferents (Levy *et al.*, 2007).

We have recently demonstrated that the dura is enriched in a variety of both lymphoid-derived as well as myeloid-derived immune cells, and that the relative proportion of immune cells is increased by stress, as is the balance in the expression of pro- and anti-inflammatory mediators in these cells, which are shifted toward a pro-inflammatory phenotype (McIlvried *et al.*, 2015). Importantly, with receptors for a variety of mediators released during stress, as well as receptors for gonadal hormones, immune cells are ideally situated to contribute to the sex difference in the manifestation of migraine, in addition to the role of stress as a trigger for migraine attacks.

5.3   Summary and conclusions

The suggestion that visceral pain could be used as an analogy to enable us to understand migraine was provocative at the time. However, while there continues to be several lines of evidence in support of it, a growing body of evidence highlighting important differences between visceral pain and migraine suggest that this analogy should be made with caution. There are marked differences in the innervation of the underlying structures. There are also important differences in the mechanisms underlying sensitization of the respective nociceptive afferents, and the neural circuitry engaged during the manifestation of pain. Additional differences in mechanisms and neural circuitry are suggested by differences in the clinical presentation of visceral pain and migraine. Consequently, and probably most importantly, as we noted from the outset, these differences will likely continue to dictate different therapeutic strategies for the treatment of migraine and visceral pain.

5.4   Acknowledgement

This work is supported by 1R01NS083347 (MSG) and R01 DK093525 and R01 NS035790 (GFG).

References

Afridi SK, Kaube H, Goadsby PJ (2004). Glyceryl trinitrate triggers premonitory symptoms in migraineurs. *Pain* **110**: 675–680.

Artico M, De Santis S, Cavallotti C (1998). Cerebral dura mater and cephalalgia: relationships between mast cells and catecholaminergic nerve fibers in the rat. *Cephalalgia* **18**: 183–191.

Bennett DL (2001). Neurotrophic factors: important regulators of nociceptive function. *Neuroscientist* **7**: 13–17.

Bessou P, Burgess PR, Perl ER, Taylor CB (1971). Dynamic properties of mechanoreceptors with unmyelinated (C) fibers. *Journal of Neurophysiology* **34**: 116–131.

Borges LF, Moskowitz MA (1983). Do intracranial and extracranial trigeminal afferents represent divergent axon collaterals? *Neuroscience Letters* **35**: 265–270.

Brumovsky PR, Gebhart GF (2010). Visceral organ cross-sensitization – an integrated perspective. *Autonomic Neuroscience: Basic & Clinical* **153**: 106–115.

Burstein R, Jakubowski M, Garcia-Nicas E, Kainz V, Bajwa Z, Hargreaves R, Becerra L, Borsook D (2010). Thalamic sensitization transforms localized pain into widespread allodynia. *Annals of Neurology* **68**: 81–91.

Burstein R, Zhang X, Levy D, Aoki KR, Brin MF (2014). Selective inhibition of meningeal nociceptors by botulinum neurotoxin type A: therapeutic implications for migraine and other pains. *Cephalalgia* **34**: 853–869.

Camilleri M, Lasch K, Zhou W (2012). Irritable bowel syndrome: methods, mechanisms, and pathophysiology. The confluence of increased permeability, inflammation, and pain in irritable bowel syndrome. *American Journal of Physiology – Gastrointestinal and Liver Physiology* **303**: G775–785.

Cavaillon JM (2001). Pro- versus anti-inflammatory cytokines: myth or reality. *Cellular and Molecular Biology (Noisy-le-Grand, France)* **47**: 695–702.

Devor M, Amir R, Rappaport ZH (2002). Pathophysiology of trigeminal neuralgia: the ignition hypothesis. *Clinical Journal of Pain* **18**: 4–13.

Edelmayer RM, Ossipov MH, Porreca F (2012). An experimental model of headache-related pain. *Methods in Molecular Biology* **851**: 109–120.

Feng B, La JH, Schwartz ES, Gebhart GF (2012a). Irritable bowel syndrome: methods, mechanisms, and pathophysiology. Neural and neuro-immune mechanisms of visceral hypersensitivity in irritable bowel syndrome. *American Journal of Physiology – Gastrointestinal and Liver Physiology* **302**: G1085–1098.

Feng B, La JH, Schwartz ES, Tanaka T, McMurray TP, Gebhart GF (2012b). Long-term sensitization of mechanosensitive and -insensitive afferents in mice with persistent colorectal hypersensitivity. *American Journal of Physiology – Gastrointestinal and Liver Physiology* **302**: G676–683.

Gass JJ, Glaros AG (2013). Autonomic dysregulation in headache patients. *Applied Psychophysiology and Biofeedback* **38**: 257–263.

Goadsby PJ (2009). The vascular theory of migraine – a great story wrecked by the facts. *Brain* **132**: 6–7.

Gold MS, Zhang L, Wrigley DL, Traub RJ (2002). Prostaglandin E(2) Modulates TTX-R I(Na) in Rat Colonic Sensory Neurons. *Journal of Neurophysiology* **88**: 1512–1522.

Han DG, Lee CJ (2009). Headache associated with visceral disorders is "parasympathetic referred pain". *Medical Hypotheses* **73**: 561–563.

Haroutounian S, Nikolajsen L, Bendtsen TF, Finnerup NB, Kristensen AD, Hasselstrom JB, Jensen TS (2014). Primary afferent input critical for maintaining spontaneous pain in peripheral neuropathy. *Pain* **155**(7): 1272–9.

Harriott AM, Gold MS (2008). Serotonin type 1D receptors (5HTR) are differentially distributed in nerve fibres innervating craniofacial tissues. *Cephalalgia* **28**: 933–944.

Harriott AM, Gold MS (2009). Electrophysiological Properties of Dural Afferents in the Absence and Presence of Inflammatory Mediators. *Journal of Neurophysiology* **101**: 3126–3134.

Karatas H, Erdener SE, Gursoy-Ozdemir Y, Lule S, Eren-Kocak E, Sen ZD, Dalkara T (2013). Spreading depression triggers headache by activating neuronal Panx1 channels. *Science* **339**: 1092–1095.

Khan S, Schoenen J, Ashina M (2014). Sphenopalatine ganglion neuromodulation in migraine: what is the rationale? *Cephalalgia* **34**: 382–391.

Kim CC, Bogart MM, Wee SA, Burstein R, Arndt KA, Dover JS (2010). Predicting migraine responsiveness to botulinum toxin type A injections. *Archives of Dermatology* **146**: 159–163.

Kosaras B, Jakubowski M, Kainz V, Burstein R (2009). Sensory innervation of the calvarial bones of the mouse. *Journal of Comparative Neurology* **515**: 331–348.

Levy D (2009). Migraine pain, meningeal inflammation, and mast cells. *Current Pain and Headache Reports* **13**: 237–240.

Levy D, Burstein R, Kainz V, Jakubowski M, Strassman AM (2007). Mast cell degranulation activates a pain pathway underlying migraine headache. *Pain* **130**: 166–176.

Lipton RB, Bigal ME, Ashina S, Burstein R, Silberstein S, Reed ML, Serrano D, Stewart WF (2008). Cutaneous allodynia in the migraine population. *Annals of Neurology* **63**: 148–158.

Louter MA, Bosker JE, van Oosterhout WP, van Zwet EW, Zitman FG, Ferrari MD, Terwindt GM (2013). Cutaneous allodynia as a predictor of migraine chronification. *Brain* **136**: 3489–3496.

Matsuka Y, Neubert JK, Maidment NT, Spigelman I (2001). Concurrent release of ATP and substance P within guinea pig trigeminal ganglia in vivo. *Brain Research* **915**: 248–255.

McIlvried LA, Borghesi LA, Gold MS (2015). Sex-, Stress-, and Sympathetic Post-Ganglionic Neuron-Dependent Changes in the Expression of Pro- and Anti-Inflammatory Mediators in Rat Dural Immune Cells. *Headache* **55**: 943–957.

Messlinger K, Fischer MJ, Lennerz JK (2011). Neuropeptide effects in the trigeminal system: pathophysiology and clinical relevance in migraine. *The Keio Journal of Medicine* **60**: 82–89.

Moskowitz MA (1984). The neurobiology of vascular head pain. *Annals of Neurology* **16**: 157–168.

Moskowitz MA (1991). The visceral organ brain: implications for the pathophysiology of vascular head pain. *Neurology* **41**: 182–186.

Murphy SF, Schaeffer AJ, Thumbikat P (2014). Immune mediators of chronic pelvic pain syndrome. *Nature Reviews Urology* **11**: 259–269.

Nickel JC, Moldwin R, Lee S, Davis EL, Henry RA, Wyllie MG (2009). Intravesical alkalinized lidocaine (PSD597) offers sustained relief from symptoms of interstitial cystitis and painful bladder syndrome. *BJU International* **103**: 910–918.

Nickel JC, Jain P, Shore N, Anderson J, Giesing D, Lee H, Kim G, Daniel K, White S, Larrivee-Elkins C, Lekstrom-Himes J, Cima M (2012). Continuous intravesical lidocaine treatment for interstitial cystitis/bladder pain syndrome: safety and efficacy of a new drug delivery device. *Science Translational Medicine* **4**: 143ra100.

O'Connor TP, Van der Kooy D (1986). Cell death organizes the postnatal development of the trigeminal innervation of the cerebral vasculature. *Brain Research* **392**: 223–233.

Ochoa JL, Campero M, Serra J, Bostock H (2005). Hyperexcitable polymodal and insensitive nociceptors in painful human neuropathy. *Muscle Nerve* **32**: 459–472.

Oshinsky ML, Gomonchareonsiri S (2007). Episodic dural stimulation in awake rats: a model for recurrent headache. *Headache* **47**: 1026–1036.

Peirs C, Williams SP, Zhao X, Walsh CE, Gedeon JY, Cagle NE, Goldring AC, Hioki H, Liu Z, Marell PS, Seal RP (2015). Dorsal Horn Circuits for Persistent Mechanical Pain. *Neuron* **87**: 797–812.

Penfield W, McNaughton F (1940). Dural headache and innervation of the dura mater. *Archives of Neurology and Psychiatry* **44**: 43–75.

Perini F, D'Andrea G, Galloni E, Pignatelli F, Billo G, Alba S, Bussone G, Toso V (2005). Plasma cytokine levels in migraineurs and controls. *Headache* **45**: 926–931.

Perl ER (1999). Causalgia, pathological pain, and adrenergic receptors. *Proceedings of the National Academy of Sciences of the United States of America* **96**: 7664–7667.

Price DD, Craggs JG, Zhou Q, Verne GN, Perlstein WM, Robinson ME (2009). Widespread hyperalgesia in irritable bowel syndrome is dynamically maintained by tonic visceral impulse input and placebo/nocebo factors: evidence from human psychophysics, animal models, and neuroimaging. *NeuroImage* **47**: 995–1001.

Raja SN (1995). Role of the sympathetic nervous system in acute pain and inflammation. *Annals of Medicine* **27**: 241–246.

Ray BS, Wolff HG (1940). Experimental studies on headache. *Archives of Surgery* **41**: 813–856.

Reichling DB, Levine JD (2009). Critical role of nociceptor plasticity in chronic pain. *Trends in Neurosciences* **32**: 611–618.

Reuter U, Bolay H, Jansen-Olesen I, Chiarugi A, Sanchez del Rio M, Letourneau R, Theoharides TC, Waeber C, Moskowitz MA (2001). Delayed inflammation in rat meninges: implications for migraine pathophysiology. *Brain* **124**: 2490–2502.

Ruch TC (1961). Pathophysiology of pain. In: Ruch, TC *et al.* (eds). *Neurophysiology*, pp. 350–368 Philadelphia: Saunders.

Sandkuhler J (2009). Models and mechanisms of hyperalgesia and allodynia. *Physiological Reviews* **89**: 707–758.

Sarchielli P, Alberti A, Codini M, Floridi A, Gallai V (2000). Nitric oxide metabolites, prostaglandins and trigeminal vasoactive peptides in internal jugular vein blood during spontaneous migraine attacks. *Cephalalgia* **20**: 907–918.

Sarchielli P, Alberti A, Baldi A, Coppola F, Rossi C, Pierguidi L, Floridi A, Calabresi P (2006). Proinflammatory cytokines, adhesion molecules, and lymphocyte integrin expression in the internal jugular blood of migraine patients without aura assessed ictally. *Headache* **46**: 200–207.

Sauro KM, Becker WJ (2009). The stress and migraine interaction. *Headache* **49**: 1378–1386.

Serra J, Collado A, Sola R, Antonelli F, Torres X, Salgueiro M, Quiles C, Bostock H (2014). Hyperexcitable C nociceptors in fibromyalgia. *Annals of Neurology* **75**: 196–208.

Silberstein SD (2009). Preventive migraine treatment. *Neurologic Clinics* **27**: 429–443.

Strassman AM, Raymond SA, Burstein R (1996). Sensitization of meningeal sensory neurons and the origin of headaches. *Nature* **384**: 560–564.

Tuca JO, Planas JM, Parellada PP (1989). Increase in PGE2 and TXA2 in the saliva of common migraine patients. Action of calcium channel blockers. *Headache* **29**: 498–501.

Van Nassauw L, Adriaensen D, Timmermans JP (2007). The bidirectional communication between neurons and mast cells within the gastrointestinal tract. Autonomic Neuroscience: Basic & Clinical **133**: 91–103.

Vaughn AH, Gold MS (2010). Ionic mechanisms underlying inflammatory mediator-induced sensitization of dural afferents. *Journal of Neuroscience* **30**: 7878–7888.

Vermeersch S, Benschop RJ, Van Hecken A, Monteith D, Wroblewski VJ, Grayzel D, de Hoon J, Collins EC (2015). Translational Pharmacodynamics of Calcitonin Gene-Related Peptide Monoclonal Antibody LY2951742 in a Capsaicin-Induced Dermal Blood Flow Model. *Journal of Pharmacology and Experimental Therapeutics* **354**: 350–357.

Verne GN, Robinson ME, Vase L, Price DD (2003). Reversal of visceral and cutaneous hyperalgesia by local rectal anesthesia in irritable bowel syndrome (IBS) patients. *Pain* **105**: 223–230.

Wei X, Yan J, Tillu D, Asiedu M, Weinstein N, Melemedjian O, Price T, Dussor G (2015). Meningeal norepinephrine produces headache behaviors in rats via actions both on dural afferents and fibroblasts. *Cephalalgia* **35**(12): 1054–64.

Winter J (1998). Brain derived neurotrophic factor, but not nerve growth factor, regulates capsaicin sensitivity of rat vagal ganglion neurones. *Neuroscience Letters* **241**: 21–24.

Wrobel Goldberg S, Silberstein SD (2015). Targeting CGRP: A New Era for Migraine Treatment. *CNS Drugs* **29**: 443–452.

Yan J, Edelmayer RM, Wei X, De Felice M, Porreca F, Dussor G (2011). Dural afferents express acid-sensing ion channels: a role for decreased meningeal pH in migraine headache. *Pain* **152**: 106–113.

6

Meningeal neurogenic inflammation and dural mast cells in migraine pain

Dan Levy

Department of Anesthesia, Critical Care and Pain Medicine, Beth Israel Deaconess Medical Center, Harvard Medical School, Boston, Massachusetts, USA

6.1   Introduction

About 10% of the global adult population has active migraine (Stovner *et al.*, 2007). It is generally accepted that migraine headache is mediated by a cascade of nociceptive events – the persistent activation and increased sensitivity of pain sensitive afferents that innervate the intracranial meninges and their related large blood vessels (Levy, 2012; Olesen *et al.*, 2009), and the subsequent sensitization of nociceptive dorsal horn neurons in the upper cervical spinal cord and trigeminal nucleus caudalis, followed by the activation of pain centers in the thalamus and cortex (Noseda and Burstein, 2013). The endogenous factors that promote the activation and sensitization of meningeal nociceptors, the first step in this cascade, remain incompletely understood.

Tissue injury associated with local inflammation is a major driver of nociceptors' activation, sensitization and pain. Although migraine is not accompanied by any detectable tissue injury or pathology, a major migraine hypothesis implicates local meningeal inflammation as a key event that mediates the activation and sensitization of meningeal nociceptors (Burstein, 2001; Levy, 2010; Strassman and Raymond, 1997). Numerous clinical findings gathered over the years have provided key, yet indirect, support for the inflammatory hypothesis of migraine. Among those are higher levels of inflammatory mediators in the cephalic venous outflow (Perini *et al.*, 2005; Sarchielli *et al.*, 2006) and the ability of corticosteroids and non-steroidal-anti-inflammatory drugs to abort migraine pain (Klapper, 1993; Woldeamanuel *et al.*, 2015).

Landmark pre-clinical studies, including ours, provided further indirect support for this hypothesis by showing that meningeal nociceptors can become persistently activated and sensitized following stimulation with inflammatory mediators (Strassman *et al.*, 1996; Zhang *et al.*, 2007, 2010b), and that these nociceptive responses can promote the sensitization of central trigeminal and thalamic nociceptive neurons (Noseda and Burstein, 2013) with ensuing development of cephalic tactile hypersensitivity (Edelmayer *et al.*, 2009; Oshinsky and Gomonchareonsiri, 2007) – a major clinical feature of migraine (Lipton *et al.*, 2008).

Neurobiological Basis of Migraine, First Edition. Edited by Turgay Dalkara and Michael A. Moskowitz.
© 2017 John Wiley & Sons, Inc. Published 2017 by John Wiley & Sons, Inc.

6.2   The neurogenic inflammation hypothesis of migraine

The inflammatory hypothesis of migraine, originally proposed more than 35 years ago (Moskowitz *et al.*, 1979), implicates sterile meningeal inflammation as a key source of migraine headache. In their landmark hypothesis paper, Moskowitz *et al.* (1979) proposed that "*The headache phase of migraine may develop as a result of an abnormal interaction (and perhaps an abnormal release) of vasoactive neurotransmitters from the terminals of the trigeminal nerve with large intracranial and extracranial blood vessels*".

The meningeal process implicated in this hypothesis was neurogenic inflammation (NI), a peripheral response comprised primarily of increased capillary permeability, leading to plasma protein extravasation (PPE), arterial vasodilatation and activation of resident immune cells. NI results from activity-dependent release of vasoactive substances, in particular substance P (SP) and calcitonin gene-related peptide (CGRP) from peripheral nerve endings of primary afferent nociceptors. This release occurs through an "axon reflex" process, where action potentials from activated nociceptors are transmitted antidromically and invade peripheral end branches (Holzer, 1988). Key support for the NI hypothesis of migraine came from the early findings that dural and pial blood vessels are innervated by trigeminal sensory nerves that express vasoactive neuropeptides (Mayberg *et al.*, 1981) – findings which also led to the conceptualization of the trigeminovascular system and its role in migraine headache (Moskowitz, 1984). See Table 6.1.

6.3   Meningeal neurogenic plasma protein extravasation and migraine

A seminal study in animals described the development of meningeal PPE in the dura mater, following electrical stimulation of the trigeminal ganglion (Markowitz *et al.*, 1987). The subsequent findings that anti-migraine drugs, including ergot alkaloids and triptans, could block this experimental meningeal PPE (Buzzi *et al.*, 1995; Markowitz *et al.*, 1988), suggested a possible role for this process in mediating migraine headache. Currently, large clinical data supporting meningeal PPE during migraine are missing. However, one imaging study, conducted on a single migraine patient, has shown an increase in meningeal vascular permeability during an attack (Knotkova and Pappagallo, 2007). In agreement with studies on non-cranial tissues (Lynn, 1988), animal studies also implicated SP and its neurokinin 1 receptor (NK1-R) in mediating meningeal neurogenic PPE (Polley *et al.*, 1997; Shepheard *et al.*, 1993). However, available clinical data does not support a role for SP in migraine pain.

A small study reported the absence of SP release into the intracranial circulation during migraine (Friberg *et al.*, 1994). More importantly, in clinical trials, NK1-R antagonists did not abort migraine headache (Diener and Group, 2003; Goldstein *et al.*, 1997). While such negative data argues against the involvement of SP and meningeal neurogenic PPE in migraine pain, the possibility that the doses of NK1-R antagonists used in that studies were suboptimal and thus did not reach biologically active plasma levels was considered (Diener and Group, 2003; Moskowitz and Mitsikostas, 1997). The possibility that during migraine SP action does play a role in the NI response, but only during

Table 6.1 Major arguments for and against the contribution of meningeal NI to migraine headache.

Pros	Cons
Neurogenic meningeal PPE	
1) Meningeal afferents express SP, and its release promotes meningeal PPE	1) Limited evidence for meningeal PPE during migraine
2) Meningeal PPE is evoked by CSD, a putative migraine trigger	2) No evidence for intracranial release of SP during migraine
3) Meningeal PPE could, theoretically, lead to elaboration of pro-nociceptive molecules in the vicinity of meningeal nociceptors, promoting their activation and sensitization	3) NK1-R antagonists do not abort migraine pain
4) Experimental meningeal PPE is inhibited by abortive migraine drugs, which do not readily cross the BBB	4) In animal models, neurogenic PPE is not associated with activation or sensitization of nociceptors
Neurogenic meningeal vasodilatation	
1) Evidence for vasodilation of intracranial arteries during spontaneous migraine	1) Intracranial meningeal vasodilation is not always associated with the development of migraine headache
2) Some abortive anti-migraine drugs are vasoconstrictors	2) Inconsistent finding of elevated CGRP levels within the intracranial circulation during migraine
3) Meningeal afferents express CGRP and its release promotes meningeal vasodilatation	3) Anatomical localization of meningeal afferents does not support their activation by vasodilatation
4) CGRP infusion triggers migraine-like headache, accompanied by intracranial vasodilatation	4) CGRP and other vasodilators do not activate meningeal nociceptors
5) Meningeal vasodilatation is evoked by CSD, together with the activation of meningeal nociceptors	
6) CGRP-R antagonists, with limited BBB penetrability, are affective as abortive migraine drugs	
Meningeal MC degranulation	
1) Administration of the MC degranulating agent 48/80 into the cranial circulation promotes migraine-like headache	1) No data on SP evoked meningeal MC degranulation in humans, or NK1-R expression on human meningeal MCs
2) Inhibition of MC degranulation is prophylactic in some migraine patients	2) Human dural MCs do not express the required CGRP receptor component CLR
3) A sizable number of MC is localized to the dura mater, with many cells in close apposition to meningeal afferents that express CGRP and SP	3) Meningeal nociceptor activation requires an intense level of MC degranulation, which may be higher that that achieved during NI.
4) Evidence for dural MC degranulation following stimulation of TG afferents	
5) CGRP and SP degranulate meningeal MCs	
6) Dural MC degranulation can activate the migraine pain pathway	

its early stages, may also be entertained. Thus, blocking NK1-R at a later stage – when meningeal NI and migraine headache are already developed – may not serve as an affective abortive treatment regimen. A role for SP in more chronic migraine conditions may be worthy of further consideration.

6.4   Meningeal neurogenic vasodilatation and migraine

Arterial vasodilation – another major characteristic of experimental meningeal NI – has also been advocated for many years as a key cause of migraine headache. The theory that vasodilatation plays a role in migraine headache was largely based on the early observations of Graham and Wolff (1938), who described a close relationship between the decrease in pulsation amplitude of the temporal artery and the decline of headache intensity following treatment with the vasoconstrictor agent ergotamine. The later observation that intracranial arteries are pain-sensitive (Ray and Wolff, 1940) extended the extracranial vascular hypothesis to the intracranial vasculature – the idea that dilatation of meningeal arteries is a major source of migraine headache (Wolff, 1963). The earlier demonstration of migraine-related changes in middle cerebral artery blood flow, congruent with vasodilation, and which were reversed by sumatriptan (Friberg *et al.*, 1991), further added support to this hypothesis. A recent study was nevertheless less conclusive, demonstrating vasodilation of intracranial arteries, albeit not of substantial magnitude (Amin *et al.*, 2013).

Key studies in rodents have led researchers to suggest that peripheral CGRP release and its ensuing vascular action is the primary driver of neurogenic meningeal vasodilation (Edvinsson *et al.*, 1987). The view that cephalic vasodilatation in migraine is neurogenically mediated received strong support from the findings of Goadsby and colleagues (Goadsby and Edvinsson, 1993; Goadsby *et al.*, 1990); the study demonstrated elevated levels of CGRP in the extra-cerebral circulation during a migraine attack. These findings, however, could not be replicated in a later study (Tvedskov *et al.*, 2005).

Despite the inconclusive findings of increased CGRP levels within the intracranial circulation during a migraine attack (Friberg *et al.*, 1994; Sarchielli *et al.*, 2000), the findings that sumatriptan normalized the elevated CGRP levels observed in the extra-jugular vein, concomitant with headache relief (Goadsby and Edvinsson, 1993), further promoted the notion that CGRP, and possibly cranial neurogenic vasodilatation, contribute to migraine headache. That infusion of CGRP could trigger migraine-like headache (Asghar *et al.*, 2011; Hansen *et al.*, 2010; Lassen *et al.*, 2002), accompanied by a unilateral dilatation of the middle meningeal and middle cerebral arteries during unilateral headaches, and bilateral dilatation of these vessels during bilateral headaches (Asghar *et al.*, 2011; Hansen *et al.*, 2010; Lassen *et al.*, 2002), also suggested a peripheral role for CGRP and its related meningeal vasodilation in migraine headache – especially since, like SP, CGRP does not cross readily into the brain.

Whether meningeal vasodilatation plays a causative role in migraine, or is merely an epiphenomenon – a secondary event arising from the activation of intracranial trigeminal afferents and the ensuing meningeal release of vasodilatory neuropeptides – remains a hotly debated subject (Charles, 2013). According to the "vascular theory", intracranial vasodilatation (but possibly also extracranial) leads to the activation of nociceptors that innervate these vessels, with ensuing headache (Vecchia and Pietrobon, 2012).

A key process that could hypothetically mediate the activation of meningeal nociceptors by arterial vasodilatation is the stimulation of mechanosensitive stretch receptors located within the dilated vessels' wall. Anatomical studies in animals suggest, however, that most of the sensory innervation of the dura terminates in the connective tissue, far from the vessels (Messlinger *et al.*, 1993). The sensory innervation of the intracranial pia also predominantly terminates in the outermost layer of the adventitial leptomeninx of the pia (Fricke *et al.*, 1997) and, thus, is also unlikely to become activated by dilatation.

Our own animal studies, showing that administration of vasoactive agents, including CGRP, failed to activate nociceptors with dural peri-vascular receptive field (Levy *et al.*, 2005; Levy and Strassman, 2004; Zhang *et al.*, 2013), further suggesting that dural vasodilation *per se* is not nociceptive. While the nociceptive effect of pial vasodilation remains unknown, the demonstration of only a slight dilatation of intracranial arteries during migraine attacks, that was not reduced by effective treatment with sumatriptan (Amin *et al.*, 2013), further argues against the nociceptive effect of intracranial vasodilatation in migraine. Finally, the finding that infusion of vasoactive intestinal peptide to migraineurs evoked a marked cephalic vasodilatation, but not a migraineous headache (Rahmann *et al.*, 2008), is also congruent with the notion that a provoked intracranial vasodilation is not nociceptive in migraine.

6.5 Neurogenic mast cell activation in migraine

Another key feature of NI is the activation of immune cells (Chiu *et al.*, 2012). Of particular interest to migraine are mast cells (MCs) – resident cells which, during an inflammatory response, become activated and undergo degranulation (the extrusion and release of preformed granule-associated mediators). Activated MCs are pro-inflammatory: they release a host of mediators, such as histamine, serotonin, the pro-inflammatory cytokine TNF-alpha and proteases (Mekori and Metcalfe, 2000).

A role for MCs in meningeal NI is supported by the finding of a sizeable population of MCs within the intracranial dura mater of animals (Dimlich *et al.*, 1991; Keller and Marfurt, 1991; Strassman *et al.*, 2004) and humans (Artico and Cavallotti, 2001). In their original hypothesis, Moskowitz *et al.* (1979) proposed that the release of SP during migraine could also contribute to inflammation and headache by acting upon MCs. Indeed, later studies found that stimulation of the trigeminal ganglion, at a level that produces dural PPE (presumably mediated by meningeal SP action), also promoted morphological changes in dural MCs, suggestive of degranulation (Dimitriadou *et al.*, 1991, 1992).

These findings, together with data showing the presence of dural MCs in close apposition to terminals of dural afferents that express SP and CGRP (Rozniecki *et al.*, 1999; Strassman *et al.*, 2004), provided further indirect support for the ability of trigeminal axon reflex to activate intracranial dural MCs, and the notion of MC involvement in meningeal NI and headache. The activation of MCs' NK1-R is thought to promote their degranulation by SP (Foreman, 1987).

In animal studies related to migraine, SP action has been shown to activate dural MCs (Ottosson and Edvinsson, 1997; Rozniecki *et al.*, 1999). While it is not known whether SP can activate human dural MCs, the ineffectiveness of NK1-R antagonists in aborting migraine pain suggest that SP may not activate MCs in migraine, or that the levels of SP-evoked MC degranulation, if it occurs, may not contribute to migraine headache.

In addition to SP, CGRP also promotes MC degranulation in experimental animals, although with less potency than SP (Piotrowski and Foreman, 1986). In studies related to migraine, *in vitro* stimulation of rodent's meningeal MCs with CGRP induced 5-HT and histamine release (Ottosson and Edvinsson, 1997; Rozniecki *et al.*, 1999). The MC-degranulating effect of CGRP may, nonetheless, be rodent-specific. Rodent MCs express the required components of the CGRP receptor system, calcitonin receptor-like receptor (CLR) and receptor activity-modifying protein 1 (RAMP1 (Eftekhari *et al.*, 2013; Lennerz *et al.*, 2008; Rychter *et al.*, 2011). Human dural MCs were shown to express only RAMP1, however (Eftekhari *et al.*, 2013).

Pituitary adenylate cylcase-activating polypeptide (PACAP), another sensory neuropeptide, may also promote meningeal neurogenic MC degranulation (Baeres and Moller, 2004; Baun *et al.*, 2012). A recent clinical study demonstrated the expression of the PACAP receptor VPAC1R on human skin MCs (Seeliger *et al.*, 2010). Whether PACAP can promote the degranulation of human dural MCs is currently unknown.

While the notion that MCs degranulation is secondary to the nociceptive release of neuropeptides has been held for many years, the concept that MC degranulation itself, with or without NI, is pro-nociceptive has been considered in a variety of inflammatory pain models (Coelho *et al.*, 1998; Ribeiro *et al.*, 2000) and various painful inflammatory conditions (Barbara *et al.*, 2007; Nigrovic and Lee, 2007; Theoharides and Cochrane, 2004). While not directly related to meningeal NI, a causative role for MCs in migraine headache was already considered more than 50 years ago (Sicuteri, 1963). In that study, injection of a MC degranulating agent into the cranial circulation gave rise to a migrainous headache. In a later study, Monro and colleagues (Monro *et al.*, 1980, 1984) further implicated MCs in migraine by documenting potent migraine prophylactic action of the MC-stabilizing agent cromolyn in a subset of patients. Additional indirect lines of evidence further supporting the involvement of MCs in migraine came from studies showing elevated plasma levels of histamine, tryptase and TNF-alpha during migraine (Heatley *et al.*, 1982; Olness *et al.*, 1999; Perini *et al.*, 2005).

To explore the potential contribution of meningeal MCs to migraine headache, we examined in animals whether dural MC degranulation could promote the activation of peripheral and central nociceptive pathways implicated in migraine headache (Levy *et al.*, 2007). In that study, we found that the dural MC degranulation promoted persistent activation of the majority of meningeal nociceptors, as well as of nociceptive neurons in the trigeminal nucleus caudalis (Levy *et al.*, 2007). These findings indicated that dural MC degranulation could serve as a powerful peripheral pro-nociceptive stimulus, capable of triggering the activation of the peripheral and central components of the migraine pain pathway. Our finding that activation of dural MCs was also associated with the development of cephalic tactile hypersensitivity (Levy *et al.*, 2011) provided further indirect evidence for the role of dural MCs in migraine pain. Further exploration suggested that the MC mediators – serotonin, prostacyclin (PGI$_2$), tryptase, TNF-a and histamine – are likely to contribute to the MC-related meningeal nociception (Zhang *et al.*, 2007, 2010b; Zhang and Levy, 2008).

6.6 Endogenous events that could promote meningeal NI in migraine

One critical unknown aspect of the NI hypothesis of migraine is the identity of the endogenous event that leads to the initial activation of meningeal nociceptors. One event, which was hypothesized to promote this initial activation more than 30 years ago (Moskowitz, 1984), is cortical spreading depression (CSD) – a cortical event thought to mediate the aura phase of migraine. A landmark study in rodents provided support for this hypothesis, by showing the development of persistent dural vasodilatation and PPE following a single CSD event. These events were dependent upon an intact trigeminal nerve and activation of NK1-R, implicating a role for CSD in promoting meningeal NI (Bolay *et al.*, 2002).

The finding that, in the wake of CSD, meningeal vasodilatation was also linked to the activation of the sphenopalatine ganglion (Bolay *et al.*, 2002), contributed to the notion of confluence of action between trigeminal afferents and parasympathetic efferents in meningeal NI. More recently, CSD has been shown to promote dural MC degranulation in a mouse model (Karatas *et al.*, 2013), further suggesting the development of meningeal NI following CSD. Our recent studies provided direct evidence that a single CSD event, triggered in the visual or motor cortices, can indeed promote the activation of meningeal nociceptors (Zhang *et al.*, 2010a; Zhao and Levy, 2015). further suggesting that CSD may be the initial endogenous event that promotes meningeal NI.

6.7 Anti-migraine drugs and meningeal NI

As indicated above, support for the NI hypothesis of migraine came from studies showing the ability of migraine-aborting drugs to block experimentally evoked meningeal NI. One key mechanism that was proposed to underlie the actions of the anti-migraine agents tripans and dihydroergotamine is the inhibition of meningeal neuropeptide release from their dense core vesicles, through the activation of presynaptic $5HT1_{B/D}$ receptors on meningeal nociceptors (Buzzi and Moskowitz, 1991). Our own finding that administration of therapeutic doses of sumatriptan leads to the activation and sensitization of meningeal nociceptors, rather than inhibit them (Burstein *et al.*, 2005; Strassman and Levy, 2004), suggests, however, that the anti-migraine action of at least sumatriptan may not be related to inhibition of meningeal NI.

An alternative mechanism that was proposed to mediate the anti-migraine effects of triptans and ergots is their binding to presynaptic $5HT1_{B/D}$ receptors located on the central endings of meningeal nociceptors in the dorsal horn, and the subsequent inhibition of the central release of the vasoactive neuropeptides, which also serve as pain neurotransmitters (Arvieu *et al.*, 1996). This central inhibitory effect of sumatriptan has been suggested to arrest the communication between meningeal nociceptors and second-order dorsal horn neurons in the trigeminal nucleus caudalis (Levy *et al.*, 2004), thus blocking migraine headache.

While evidence for penetration of abortive migraine drugs such as sumatriptan into the brain is lacking in experimental animals and humans, the possibility that the blood-brain barrier is breached in migraine, for example because of CSD (Gursoy-Ozdemir *et al.*, 2004) or central neuroinflammation (Skaper *et al.*, 2014) and, therefore, allows the penetration of triptans, as well as other anti-migraine agents, should be entertained. Another peripheral mechanism that was attributed to anti-inflammatory effects of sumatriptan in the meninges is the inhibition of neurogenic dural MC degranulation (Buzzi *et al.*, 1992). The finding that MCs also express the $5HT1_{B/D}$ receptors (Kushnir-Sukhov *et al.*, 2006) points, nonetheless, to a potential direct inhibitory effect on MCs – one that does not necessary involve an axon reflex and release of neuropeptides.

The cumulative preclinical and clinical finding pointing to the involvement of CGRP in meningeal vasodilatation and migraine headache has greatly facilitated the development of novel CGRP receptor antagonists as potential anti-migraine drugs (Durham, 2004). The finding that such antagonists (the gepants olcegepant (Olesen *et al.*, 2004) and telcagepant (Ho *et al.*, 2010)) were effective in aborting migraine pain rekindled the notion of meningeal NI, in particular CGRP-evoked meningeal vasodilation and MC activation as critical mediators of migraine headache (Russo, 2015). While the role of CGRP in mediating meningeal vasodilatation has been considered most relevant to migraine (Asghar *et al.*, 2011), the pre-clinical findings of CGRP actions in numerous brain regions, some of which could potentially mediate migraine headache, including the trigeminal nucleus caudalis (Fischer *et al.*, 2005), the thalamus (Summ *et al.*, 2010) and periaqueductal gray (Pozo-Rosich *et al.*, 2015) raise the possibility of additional or alternative mechanisms of action for CGRP in migraine.

The relative small molecular size of the gepants, which could potentially penetrate the blood-brain barrier, and the high dose required to treat migraine, were suggested to indicate a possible central anti-migraine action of CGRP (Edvinsson, 2015; Tfelt-Hansen and Olesen, 2011). However, the finding that systemic administration of these agents at an efficacious dose achieved only low receptor occupancy within a human brain (Hostetler *et al.*, 2013), and that a high dose of these agents was also required to block cutaneous NI (Sinclair *et al.*, 2010), is congruent with peripheral CGRP action in migraine (Tfelt-Hansen and Olesen, 2011).

The very recent findings that monoclonal antibodies against CGRP – large molecules that do not readily cross the blood-brain barrier – block meningeal neurogenic vasodilatation (Zeller *et al.*, 2008) and, most importantly, are also affective as prophylactics in chronic migraine (Bigal *et al.*, 2015), provide a further argument for a peripheral role for CGRP, potentially as a mediator of meningeal NI and pain in migraine. The notion that chronic CGRP inhibition by antibodies serves to downregulate the expression of molecules that participate in triggering the process of migraine pain (including CGRP itself and its receptors) also requires some consideration.

6.8 Is meningeal NI a pro-nociceptive event in migraine?

A key, yet unanswered question, related to the role that meningeal NI might play in migraine, is whether this response is actually pro-nociceptive? Remarkably, the evidence for pro-nociceptive effects of NI in both animals and humans is patchy, at best.

In rodents, cutaneous NI evoked by antidromic electrical stimulation failed to activate or sensitize cutaneous nociceptors (Reeh *et al.*, 1986). However, electrical stimulation of skin nociceptors, which evoked a localized increase in blood flow, promoted cutaneous mechanical hyperalgesia (Doring *et al.*, 2014). The possibility that central changes related to the intense activation of nociceptors required for the elicitation of the axon reflex (i.e., central sensitization) (LaMotte *et al.*, 1992), rather than NI, contributed to this nociceptive effect, must also be entertained.

As indicated above, the pro-nociceptive effects of meningeal neurogenic vasodilatation and PPE are doubtful. The degranulation of a large number of dural MC undoubtedly is pro-nociceptive. A lower level of meningeal MC degranulation, provoked by meningeal axon reflex, may also be nociceptive. That a relatively lower level of meningeal MC degranulation, induced following systemic infusion of the migraine trigger nitroglycerin (Pedersen *et al.*, 2015; Reuter *et al.*, 2001), was not sufficient to promote activation of meningeal nociceptors (Zhang *et al.*, 2013), argues nonetheless otherwise. The possibility that neurogenic meningeal MC degranulation is pro-nociceptive should not be abandoned completely, however. In migraineurs, a higher density of meningeal MCs, potentially due to endocrine changes, such as fluctuation in female sex hormones (Boes and Levy, 2012), or increased propensity of these immune cells to become activated in response to meningeal axon reflex, could potentially result in a robust nociceptive effect that could contribute to the activation of meningeal nociceptors and the genesis of migraine headache.

In the wake of CSD, meningeal nociceptors become briefly activated during the passing of the CSD wave under their receptive field (Zhao and Levy, 2015). This is followed by a delayed and more persistent activation phase (Zhang *et al.*, 2010a; Zhao and Levy, 2015). It has been proposed that the initial brief nociceptor activation promotes meningeal NI (Bolay *et al.*, 2002; Karatas *et al.*, 2013), which is then responsible for the development of the delayed and persistent nociceptor activation (Bolay *et al.*, 2002; Levy, 2012). Our recent studies (Zhang *et al.*, 2011; Zhao and Levy, 2015) argue, however, against the role of meningeal NI, in particularly meningeal vasodilatation and MC degranulation, in mediating this nociceptive response following CSD. We found a similar persistent nociceptor activation following excision of the parasympathetic sphenopalatine ganglion – the ganglion whose activation was critical to the CSD-evoked meningeal neurogenic vasodilatation. In addition, CSD-evoked persistent nociceptor activation was also observed in craniotomized animals, a preparation in which the majority of dural MCs are already in a state of degranulation prior to the induction of CSD (Levy *et al.*, 2007).

6.9 Conclusions

The concept of NI undoubtedly had a tremendous impact on migraine research, and provided an important roadmap for the development of neuropeptide and receptor driven therapies for migraine (see Table 6.2). While meningeal NI continues to be regarded as a causal factor in migraine headache (Noseda and Burstein, 2013; Pietrobon and Moskowitz, 2012; Russo, 2015), direct evidence for the occurrence of NI during migraine and its role in meningeal nociception are limited at best. Future studies may provide better direct evidence for the presence of the various features of meningeal NI, or lack

Table 6.2 Impact of the neurogenic inflammation concept on migraine research progress.

Concepts/findings	References
The concept of NI inspired the discovery and conceptualization of the trigeminovascular system – the trigeminal sensory innervation of the cerebral meninges and their related large blood vessels	Moskowitz *et al.*, 1979; Mayberg *et al.*, 1981; Moskowitz, 1984
NI suggested neuropeptides as well as receptors on trigeminovascular afferents as therapeutic targets	Moskowitz *et al.*, 1979; Liu-Chen *et al.*, 1983a; Moskowitz *et al.*, 1983; Liu-Chen *et al.*, 1983b; Moskowitz, 1984
The concept that CSD depolarizes trigeminovascular neurons and promotes subsequent meningeal NI and headache	Moskowitz, 1984; Bolay *et al.*, 2002; Zhang *et al.*, 2010a
Experimental implication of neuropeptides in meningeal NI	Markowitz *et al.*, 1988
The notion that sensory neuropeptides as well as receptors on trigeminovascular afferents can be targeted for migraine therapy	Moskowitz *et al.*, 1979; Moskowitz, 1984; McCulloch *et al.*, 1986; Goadsby *et al.*, 1988; Goadsby *et al.*, 1990
Animal models of NI provided the first evidence for pre-junctional 5-HT1 (triptan) receptors on trigeminovascular afferents and that triptan action inhibited neuropeptide release and NI	Buzzi and Moskowitz, 1990; Buzzi and Moskowitz, 1991; Buzzi *et al.*, 1991
Called attention to the potential role of neurogenic dural MC degranulation in migraine	Moskowitz *et al.*, 1979; Dimitriadou *et al.*, 1991; Buzzi *et al.*, 1992
The notion of NI provided a confluence of action between trigeminal afferents and the parasympathetic efferent innervation.	Bolay *et al.*, 2002

thereof, during a migraine attack and, most importantly, whether they constitute active players in driving migraine pain, rather than simply epiphenomena.

References

Amin FM, Asghar MS, Hougaard A, Hansen AE, Larsen VA, *et al*. (2013). Magnetic resonance angiography of intracranial and extracranial arteries in patients with spontaneous migraine without aura: a cross-sectional study. *Lancet Neurology* **12**: 454–61.

Artico M, Cavallotti C (2001). Catecholaminergic and acetylcholine esterase containing nerves of cranial and spinal dura mater in humans and rodents. *Microscopy Research and Technique* **53**: 212–20.

Arvieu L, Mauborgne A, Bourgoin S, Oliver C, Feltz P, *et al*. (1996). Sumatriptan inhibits the release of CGRP and substance P from the rat spinal cord. *Neuroreport* 7: 1973–6.

Asghar MS, Hansen AE, Amin FM, van der Geest RJ, Koning P, *et al*. (2011). Evidence for a vascular factor in migraine. *Annals of Neurology* **69**: 635–45.

Baeres FM, Moller M (2004). Origin of PACAP-immunoreactive nerve fibers innervating the subarachnoidal blood vessels of the rat brain. *Journal of Cerebral Blood Flow & Metabolism* **24**: 628–35.

Barbara G, Wang B, Stanghellini V, de Giorgio R, Cremon C, *et al.* (2007). Mast cell-dependent excitation of visceral-nociceptive sensory neurons in irritable bowel syndrome. *Gastroenterology* **132**: 26–37.

Baun M, Pedersen MH, Olesen J, Jansen-Olesen I (2012). Dural mast cell degranulation is a putative mechanism for headache induced by PACAP-38. *Cephalalgia* **32**: 337–45.

Bigal ME, Walter S, Rapoport AM (2015). Therapeutic antibodies against CGRP or its receptor. *British Journal of Clinical Pharmacology* **79**(6) :886–95.

Boes T, Levy D (2012). Influence of sex, estrous cycle and estrogen on intracranial dural mast cells. *Cephalalgia* **32**(12): 924–31.

Bolay H, Reuter U, Dunn AK, Huang Z, Boas DA, Moskowitz MA (2002). Intrinsic brain activity triggers trigeminal meningeal afferents in a migraine model. *Nature Medicine* **8**: 136–42.

Burstein R (2001). Deconstructing migraine headache into peripheral and central sensitization. *Pain* **89**: 107–10.

Burstein R, Jakubowski M, Levy D (2005). Anti-migraine action of triptans is preceded by transient aggravation of headache caused by activation of meningeal nociceptors. *Pain* **115**: 21–8.

Buzzi MG, Moskowitz MA (1990). The antimigraine drug, sumatriptan (GR43175), selectively blocks neurogenic plasma extravasation from blood vessels in dura mater. *British Journal of Pharmacology* **99**: 202–06.

Buzzi MG, Moskowitz MA (1991). Evidence for 5-HT1B/1D receptors mediating the antimigraine effect of sumatriptan and dihydroergotamine. *Cephalalgia* **11**: 165–68.

Buzzi MG, Moskowitz MA, Peroutka SJ, Byun B (1991). Further characterization of the putative 5-HT receptor which mediates blockade of neurogenic plasma extravasation in rat dura mater. *British Journal of Pharmacology* **103**: 1421–28.

Buzzi MG, Dimitriadou V, Theoharides TC, Moskowitz MA (1992). 5-Hydroxytryptamine receptor agonists for the abortive treatment of vascular headaches block mast cell, endothelial and platelet activation within the rat dura mater after trigeminal stimulation. *Brain Research* **583**: 137–49.

Buzzi MG, Bonamini M, Moskowitz MA (1995). Neurogenic model of migraine. *Cephalalgia* **15**: 277–80.

Charles A (2013). Vasodilation out of the picture as a cause of migraine headache. *Lancet Neurology* **12**: 419–20.

Chiu IM, von Hehn CA, Woolf CJ (2012). Neurogenic inflammation and the peripheral nervous system in host defense and immunopathology. *Nature Neuroscience* **15**: 1063–7.

Coelho AM, Fioramonti J, Bueno L (1998). Mast cell degranulation induces delayed rectal allodynia in rats: role of histamine and 5-HT. *Digestive Diseases and Sciences* **43**: 727–37.

Diener HC, Group RPRS (2003). RPR100893, a substance-P antagonist, is not effective in the treatment of migraine attacks. *Cephalalgia* **23**: 183–5.

Dimitriadou V, Buzzi MG, Moskowitz MA, Theoharides TC (1991). Trigeminal sensory fiber stimulation induces morphological changes reflecting secretion in rat dura mater mast cells. *Neuroscience* **44**: 97–112.

Dimitriadou V, Buzzi MG, Theoharides TC, Moskowitz MA (1992). Ultrastructural evidence for neurogenically mediated changes in blood vessels of the rat dura mater and tongue following antidromic trigeminal stimulation. *Neuroscience* **48**: 187–203.

Dimlich RV, Keller JT, Strauss TA, Fritts MJ (1991). Linear arrays of homogeneous mast cells in the dura mater of the rat. *Journal of Neurocytology* **20**: 485–503.

Doring K, Best C, Birklein F, Kramer HH (2014). Zolmitriptan inhibits neurogenic inflammation and pain during electrical stimulation in human skin. *European Journal of Pain.* **19**(7): 966–972.

Durham PL (2004). CGRP-receptor antagonists – a fresh approach to migraine therapy? *The New England Journal of Medicine* **350**: 1073–5.

Edelmayer RM, Vanderah TW, Majuta L, Zhang ET, Fioravanti B, *et al*. (2009). Medullary pain facilitating neurons mediate allodynia in headache-related pain. *Annals of Neurology* **65**: 184–93.

Edvinsson L (2015). CGRP receptor antagonists and antibodies against CGRP and its receptor in migraine treatment. *British Journal of Clinical Pharmacology* **80**(2): 193–9.

Edvinsson L, Ekman R, Jansen I, McCulloch J, Uddman R (1987). Calcitonin gene-related peptide and cerebral blood vessels: distribution and vasomotor effects. *Journal of Cerebral Blood Flow & Metabolism* **7**: 720–8.

Eftekhari S, Warfvinge K, Blixt FW, Edvinsson L (2013). Differentiation of nerve fibers storing CGRP and CGRP receptors in the peripheral trigeminovascular system. *Journal of Pain* **14**: 1289–303.

Fischer MJ, Koulchitsky S, Messlinger K (2005). The nonpeptide calcitonin gene-related peptide receptor antagonist BIBN4096BS lowers the activity of neurons with meningeal input in the rat spinal trigeminal nucleus. *Journal of Neuroscience* **25**: 5877–83.

Foreman JC (1987). Peptides and neurogenic inflammation. *British Medical Bulletin* **43**: 386–400.

Friberg L, Olesen J, Iversen HK, Sperling B (1991). Migraine pain associated with middle cerebral artery dilatation: reversal by sumatriptan. *Lancet* **338**: 13–7.

Friberg L, Olesen J, Olsen TS, Karle A, Ekman R, Fahrenkrug J (1994). Absence of vasoactive peptide release from brain to cerebral circulation during onset of migraine with aura. *Cephalalgia* **14**: 47–54.

Fricke B, von During M, Andres KH (1997). Topography and immunocytochemical characterization of nerve fibers in the leptomeningeal compartments of the rat. A light- and electron-microscopical study. *Cell and Tissue Research* **287**: 11–22.

Goadsby PJ, Edvinsson L (1993). The trigeminovascular system and migraine: studies characterizing cerebrovascular and neuropeptide changes seen in humans and cats. *Annals of Neurology* **33**: 48–56.

Goadsby PJ, Edvinsson L, Ekman R (1988). Release of vasoactive peptides in the extracerebral circulation of humans and the cat during activation of the trigeminovascular system. *Annals of Neurology* **23**: 193–96.

Goadsby PJ, Edvinsson L, Ekman R (1990). Vasoactive peptide release in the extracerebral circulation of humans during migraine headache. *Annals of Neurology* **28**: 183–7.

Goldstein DJ, Wang O, Saper JR, Stoltz R, Silberstein SD, Mathew NT (1997). Ineffectiveness of neurokinin-1 antagonist in acute migraine: a crossover study. *Cephalalgia* **17**: 785–90.

Graham JR, Wolff HG (1938). Mechanism of migraine headache and action of ergotamine tatrate. *Archives of Neurology & Psychiatry* **39**: 737–63.

Gursoy-Ozdemir Y, Qiu J, Matsuoka N, Bolay H, Bermpohl D, *et al.* (2004). Cortical spreading depression activates and upregulates MMP-9. *The Journal of Clinical Investigation* **113**: 1447–55.

Hansen JM, Hauge AW, Olesen J, Ashina M (2010). Calcitonin gene-related peptide triggers migraine-like attacks in patients with migraine with aura. *Cephalalgia* **30**: 1179–86.

Heatley RV, Denburg JA, Bayer N, Bienenstock J (1982). Increased plasma histamine levels in migraine patients. *Clinical Allergy* **12**: 145–9.

Ho AP, Dahlof CG, Silberstein SD, Saper JR, Ashina M, *et al.* (2010). Randomized, controlled trial of telcagepant over four migraine attacks. *Cephalalgia* **30**: 1443–57.

Holzer P (1988). Local effector functions of capsaicin-sensitive sensory nerve endings: involvement of tachykinins, calcitonin gene-related peptide and other neuropeptides. *Neuroscience* **24**: 739–68.

Hostetler ED, Joshi AD, Sanabria-Bohorquez S, Fan H, Zeng Z, *et al.* (2013). *In vivo* quantification of calcitonin gene-related peptide receptor occupancy by telcagepant in rhesus monkey and human brain using the positron emission tomography tracer [11C]MK-4232. *Journal of Pharmacology and Experimental Therapeutics* **347**: 478–86.

Karatas H, Erdener SE, Gursoy-Ozdemir Y, Lule S, Eren-Kocak E, *et al.* (2013). Spreading depression triggers headache by activating neuronal Panx1 channels. *Science* **339**: 1092–5.

Keller JT, Marfurt CF (1991). Peptidergic and serotoninergic innervation of the rat dura mater. *The Journal of Comparative Neurology* **309**: 515–34.

Klapper J (1993). The pharmacologic treatment of acute migraine headaches. *Journal of Pain and Symptom Management* **8**: 140–7.

Knotkova H, Pappagallo M (2007). Imaging intracranial plasma extravasation in a migraine patient: a case report. *Pain Medicine* **8**: 383–7.

Kowalski ML, Kaliner MA (1988). Neurogenic inflammation, vascular permeability, and mast cells. *Journal of Immunology* **140**: 3905–11.

Kushnir-Sukhov NM, Gilfillan AM, Coleman JW, Brown JM, Bruening S, *et al.* (2006). 5-hydroxytryptamine induces mast cell adhesion and migration. *Journal of Immunology* **177**: 6422–32.

LaMotte RH, Lundberg LE, Torebjork HE (1992). Pain, hyperalgesia and activity in nociceptive C units in humans after intradermal injection of capsaicin. *Journal of Physiology* **448**: 749–64.

Lassen LH, Haderslev PA, Jacobsen VB, Iversen HK, Sperling B, Olesen J (2002). CGRP may play a causative role in migraine. *Cephalalgia* **22**: 54–61.

Lennerz JK, Ruhle V, Ceppa EP, Neuhuber WL, Bunnett NW, *et al.* (2008). Calcitonin receptor-like receptor (CLR), receptor activity-modifying protein 1 (RAMP1), and calcitonin gene-related peptide (CGRP) immunoreactivity in the rat trigeminovascular system: differences between peripheral and central CGRP receptor distribution. *The Journal of Comparative Neurology* **507**: 1277–99.

Levy D (2010). Migraine pain and nociceptor activation – where do we stand? *Headache* **50**: 909–16.

Levy D (2012). Endogenous mechanisms underlying the activation and sensitization of meningeal nociceptors: the role of immuno-vascular interactions and cortical spreading depression. *Current Pain and Headache Reports* **16**: 270–7.

Levy D, Strassman AM (2004). Modulation of Dural Nociceptor Mechanosensitivity by the Nitric Oxide – Cyclic GMP Signaling Cascade. *Journal of Neurophysiology* **92**(2): 766–72.

Levy D, Jakubowski M, Burstein R (2004). Disruption of communication between peripheral and central trigeminovascular neurons mediates the antimigraine action of 5HT 1B/1D receptor agonists. *Proceedings of the National Academy of Sciences of the United States of America* **101**: 4274–9.

Levy D, Burstein R, Strassman AM (2005). Calcitonin gene-related peptide does not excite or sensitize meningeal nociceptors: Implications for the pathophysiology of migraine. *Annals of Neurology* **58**: 698–705.

Levy D, Burstein R, Kainz V, Jakubowski M, Strassman AM (2007). Mast cell degranulation activates a pain pathway underlying migraine headache. *Pain* **130**: 166–76.

Levy D, Kainz V, Burstein R, Strassman AM (2011). Mast cell degranulation distinctly activates trigemino-cervical and lumbosacral pain pathways and elicits widespread tactile pain hypersensitivity. *Brain, Behavior, and Immunity* **26**(2): 311–7.

Lipton RB, Bigal ME, Ashina S, Burstein R, Silberstein S, *et al.* (2008). Cutaneous allodynia in the migraine population. *Annals of Neurology* **63**: 148–58.

Liu-Chen LY, Han DH, Moskowitz MA (1983a). Pia arachnoid contains substance P originating from trigeminal neurons. *Neuroscience* **9**: 803–8.

Liu-Chen LY, Mayberg MR, Moskowitz MA (1983b). Immunohistochemical evidence for a substance P-containing trigeminovascular pathway to pial arteries in cats. *Brain Research* **268**: 162–6.

Lynn B (1988). Neurogenic inflammation. *Skin Pharmacology* **1**: 217–24.

Markowitz S, Saito K, Moskowitz MA (1987). Neurogenically mediated leakage of plasma protein occurs from blood vessels in dura mater but not brain. *Journal of Neuroscience* **7**: 4129–36.

Markowitz S, Saito K, Moskowitz MA (1988). Neurogenically mediated plasma extravasation in dura mater: effect of ergot alkaloids. A possible mechanism of action in vascular headache. *Cephalalgia* **8**: 83–91.

Markowitz S, Saito K, Buzzi MG, Moskowitz MA (1989). The development of neurogenic plasma extravasation in the rat dura mater does not depend upon the degranulation of mast cells. *Brain Research* **477**: 157–65.

Mayberg M, Langer RS, Zervas NT, Moskowitz MA (1981). Perivascular meningeal projections from cat trigeminal ganglia: possible pathway for vascular headaches in man. *Science* **213**: 228–30.

McCulloch J, Uddman R, Kingman TA, Edvinsson L (1986). Calcitonin gene-related peptide: functional role in cerebrovascular regulation. *Proceedings of the National Academy of Sciences of the United States of America* **83**: 5731–5.

Mekori YA, Metcalfe DD (2000). Mast cells in innate immunity. *Immunological Reviews* **173**: 131–40.

Messlinger K, Hanesch U, Baumgartel M, Trost B, Schmidt RF (1993). Innervation of the dura mater encephali of cat and rat: ultrastructure and calcitonin gene-related peptide-like and substance P-like immunoreactivity. *Anatomy and Embryology (Berlin)* **188**: 219–37.

Monro J, Brostoff J, Carini C, Zilkha K (1980). Food allergy in migraine. Study of dietary exclusion and RAST. *Lancet* **2**: 1–4.

Monro J, Carini C, Brostoff J (1984). Migraine is a food-allergic disease. *Lancet* **2**: 719–21.

Moskowitz MA (1984). The neurobiology of vascular head pain. *Annals of Neurology* **16**: 157–68.

Moskowitz MA, Mitsikostas DD (1997). A negative clinical study in the search for a migraine treatment. *Cephalalgia* **17**: 720–1.

Moskowitz MA, Reinhard JF, Jr., Romero J, Melamed E, Pettibone DJ (1979). Neurotransmitters and the fifth cranial nerve: is there a relation to the headache phase of migraine? *Lancet* **2**: 883–5.

Moskowitz MA, Brody M, Liu-Chen LY (1983). *In vitro* release of immunoreactive substance P from putative afferent nerve endings in bovine pia arachnoid. *Neuroscience* **9**: 809–14.

Nigrovic PA, Lee DM (2007). Synovial mast cells: role in acute and chronic arthritis. *Immunological Reviews* **217**: 19–37.

Noseda R, Burstein R (2013). Migraine pathophysiology: anatomy of the trigeminovascular pathway and associated neurological symptoms, cortical spreading depression, sensitization, and modulation of pain. *Pain* **154**(Suppl 1): S44–53.

Olesen J, Diener HC, Husstedt IW, Goadsby PJ, Hall D, *et al.* (2004). Calcitonin gene-related peptide receptor antagonist BIBN 4096 BS for the acute treatment of migraine. *The New England Journal of Medicine* **350**: 1104–10.

Olesen J, Burstein R, Ashina M, Tfelt-Hansen P (2009). Origin of pain in migraine: evidence for peripheral sensitisation. *Lancet Neurology* **8**: 679–90.

Olness K, Hall H, Rozniecki JJ, Schmidt W, Theoharides TC (1999). Mast Cell Activation in Children With Migraine Before and After Training in Self-regulation. *Headache* **39**: 101–7.

Oshinsky ML, Gomonchareonsiri S (2007). Episodic dural stimulation in awake rats: a model for recurrent headache. *Headache* **47**: 1026–36.

Ottosson A, Edvinsson L (1997). Release of histamine from dural mast cells by substance P and calcitonin gene-related peptide. *Cephalalgia* **17**: 166–74.

Pedersen SH, Ramachandran R, Amrutkar DV, Petersen S, Olesen J, Jansen-Olesen I (2015). Mechanisms of glyceryl trinitrate provoked mast cell degranulation. *Cephalalgia* **35**(14): 1287–97.

Perini F, D'Andrea G, Galloni E, Pignatelli F, Billo G, *et al.* (2005). Plasma cytokine levels in migraineurs and controls. *Headache* **45**: 926–31.

Pietrobon D, Moskowitz MA (2012). Pathophysiology of Migraine. *Annual Review of Physiology* **75**: 365–91.

Piotrowski W, Foreman JC (1986). Some effects of calcitonin gene-related peptide in human skin and on histamine release. *British Journal of Dermatology* **114**: 37–46.

Polley JS, Gaskin PJ, Perren MJ, Connor HE, Ward P, Beattie DT (1997). The activity of GR205171, a potent non-peptide tachykinin NK1 receptor antagonist, in the trigeminovascular system. *Regulatory Peptides* **68**: 23–9.

Pozo-Rosich P, Storer RJ, Charbit AR, Goadsby PJ (2015). Periaqueductal gray calcitonin gene-related peptide modulates trigeminovascular neurons. *Cephalalgia* **35**(14): 1298–307.

Rahmann A, Wienecke T, Hansen JM, Fahrenkrug J, Olesen J, Ashina M (2008). Vasoactive intestinal peptide causes marked cephalic vasodilation, but does not induce migraine. *Cephalalgia* **28**: 226–36.

Ray BS, Wolff HG (1940). Experimental studies on headache: Pain sensitive structures of the head and their significance in headache. *Archives of Surgery* **41**: 813–56.

Reeh PW, Kocher L, Jung S (1986). Does neurogenic inflammation alter the sensitivity of unmyelinated nociceptors in the rat? *Brain Research* **384**: 42–50.

Reuter U, Bolay H, Jansen-Olesen I, Chiarugi A, Sanchez del Rio M, *et al.* (2001). Delayed inflammation in rat meninges: implications for migraine pathophysiology. *Brain* **124**: 2490–502.

Ribeiro RA, Vale ML, Thomazzi SM, Paschoalato AB, Poole S, *et al.* (2000). Involvement of resident macrophages and mast cells in the writhing nociceptive response induced by zymosan and acetic acid in mice. *European Journal of Pharmacology* **387**: 111–18.

Rozniecki JJ, Dimitriadou V, Lambracht-Hall M, Pang X, Theoharides TC (1999). Morphological and functional demonstration of rat dura mater mast cell-neuron interactions in vitro and in vivo. *Brain Research* **849**: 1–15.

Russo AF (2015). Calcitonin gene-related peptide (CGRP): a new target for migraine. *Annual Review of Pharmacology and Toxicology* **55**: 533–52.

Rychter JW, Van Nassauw L, Timmermans JP, Akkermans LM, Westerink RH, Kroese AB (2011). CGRP1 receptor activation induces piecemeal release of protease-1 from mouse bone marrow-derived mucosal mast cells. *Neurogastroenterology & Motility* **23**: e57–68.

Sarchielli P, Alberti A, Codini M, Floridi A, Gallai V (2000). Nitric oxide metabolites, prostaglandins and trigeminal vasoactive peptides in internal jugular vein blood during spontaneous migraine attacks. *Cephalalgia* **20**: 907–18.

Sarchielli P, Alberti A, Baldi A, Coppola F, Rossi C, *et al.* (2006). Proinflammatory cytokines, adhesion molecules, and lymphocyte integrin expression in the internal jugular blood of migraine patients without aura assessed ictally. *Headache* **46**: 200–7.

Seeliger S, Buddenkotte J, Schmidt-Choudhury A, Rosignoli C, Shpacovitch V, *et al.* (2010). Pituitary adenylate cyclase activating polypeptide: an important vascular regulator in human skin in vivo. *The American Journal of Pathology* **177**: 2563–75.

Shepheard SL, Williamson DJ, Hill RG, Hargreaves RJ (1993). The non-peptide neurokinin1 receptor antagonist, RP 67580, blocks neurogenic plasma extravasation in the dura mater of rats. *British Journal of Pharmacology* **108**: 11–2.

Sicuteri F (1963). Mast cell and their active substances: Their role in the pathogenesis of migraine. *Headache* **3**: 86.

Sinclair SR, Kane SA, Van der Schueren BJ, Xiao A, Willson KJ, *et al.* (2010). Inhibition of capsaicin-induced increase in dermal blood flow by the oral CGRP receptor antagonist, telcagepant (MK-0974). *British Journal of Clinical Pharmacology* **69**: 15–22.

Skaper SD, Facci L, Giusti P (2014). Mast cells, glia and neuroinflammation: partners in crime? *Immunology* **141**: 314–27.

Stovner L, Hagen K, Jensen R, Katsarava Z, Lipton R, *et al.* (2007). The global burden of headache: a documentation of headache prevalence and disability worldwide. *Cephalalgia* **27**: 193–210.

Strassman AM, Levy D (2004). The anti-migraine agent sumatriptan induces a calcium-dependent discharge in meningeal sensory neurons. *Neuroreport* **15**: 1409–12.

Strassman AM, Raymond SA (1997). On the origin of headaches. *Endeavour* **21**: 97–100.

Strassman AM, Raymond SA, Burstein R (1996). Sensitization of meningeal sensory neurons and the origin of headaches. *Nature* **384**: 560–64.

Strassman AM, Weissner W, Williams M, Ali S, Levy D (2004). Axon diameters and intradural trajectories of the dural innervation in the rat. *The Journal of Comparative Neurology* **473**: 364–76.

Summ O, Charbit AR, Andreou AP, Goadsby PJ (2010). Modulation of nociceptive transmission with calcitonin gene-related peptide receptor antagonists in the thalamus. *Brain* **133**: 2540–8.

Tfelt-Hansen P, Olesen J (2011). Possible site of action of CGRP antagonists in migraine. *Cephalalgia* **31**: 748–50.

Theoharides TC, Cochrane DE (2004). Critical role of mast cells in inflammatory diseases and the effect of acute stress. *Journal of Neuroimmunology* **146**: 1–12.

Tvedskov JF, Lipka K, Ashina M, Iversen HK, Schifter S, Olesen J (2005). No increase of calcitonin gene-related peptide in jugular blood during migraine. *Annals of Neurology* **58**: 561–8.

Vecchia D, Pietrobon D (2012). Migraine: a disorder of brain excitatory-inhibitory balance? *Trends in Neurosciences* **35**: 507–20.

Woldeamanuel Y, Rapoport A, Cowan R (2015). The place of corticosteroids in migraine attack management: A 65-year systematic review with pooled analysis and critical appraisal. *Cephalalgia* **35**(11): 996–1024.

Wolff HG (1963). Headache and other head pain. In: *Headache and other head pain*. New York: Oxford University Press.

Zeller J, Poulsen KT, Sutton JE, Abdiche YN, Collier S, *et al*. (2008). CGRP function-blocking antibodies inhibit neurogenic vasodilatation without affecting heart rate or arterial blood pressure in the rat. *British Journal of Pharmacology* **155**: 1093–103.

Zhang XC, Levy D (2008). Modulation of meningeal nociceptors mechanosensitivity by peripheral proteinase-activated receptor-2: the role of mast cells. *Cephalalgia* **28**: 276–84.

Zhang X, Strassman AM, Burstein R, Levy D (2007). Sensitization and activation of intracranial meningeal nociceptors by mast cell mediators. *Journal of Pharmacology and Experimental Therapeutics* **322**: 806–12.

Zhang X, Levy D, Noseda R, Kainz V, Jakubowski M, Burstein R (2010a). Activation of meningeal nociceptors by cortical spreading depression: implications for migraine with aura. *Journal of Neuroscience* **30**: 8807–14.

Zhang XC, Kainz V, Burstein R, Levy D (2010b). Tumor necrosis factor-alpha induces sensitization of meningeal nociceptors mediated via local COX and p38 MAP kinase actions. *Pain* **152**(1): 140–9.

Zhang X, Levy D, Kainz V, Noseda R, Jakubowski M, Burstein R (2011). Activation of central trigeminovascular neurons by cortical spreading depression. *Annals of Neurology* **69**: 855–65.

Zhang X, Kainz V, Zhao J, Strassman AM, Levy D (2013). Vascular extracellular signal-regulated kinase mediates migraine-related sensitization of meningeal nociceptors. *Annals of Neurology* **73**: 741–50.

Zhao J, Levy D (2015). Modulation of intracranial meningeal nociceptor activity by cortical spreading depression – A reassessment. *Journal of Neurophysiology* **113**(7):2778-85.

7

Sensitization and photophobia in migraine

Aaron Schain and Rami Burstein

Department of Anesthesia, Critical Care and Pain Medicine, Beth Israel Deaconess Medical Center, Harvard Medical School, Boston, Massachusetts, USA

7.1   Introduction

Migraine headache is commonly associated with signs of exaggerated intracranial and extracranial mechanical sensitivities, and photophobia. Patients exhibiting signs of intracranial hypersensitivity testify that their headache throbs, and that mundane physical activities that increase intracranial pressure (such as bending over or coughing) intensify the pain. Patients exhibiting signs of extracranial hypersensitivity report that, during migraine, their facial skin hurts in response to otherwise innocuous activities, such as combing, shaving, letting water run over their face in the shower, or wearing glasses or earrings (termed, here, cephalic cutaneous allodynia). Many of these patients also testify that, during migraine, their bodily skin is hypersensitive, and that wearing tight cloth, bracelets, rings, necklaces and socks, or using a heavy blanket, can be uncomfortable and/or painful (termed extracephalic cutaneous allodynia).

This review will summarize the evidence that supports the following cascade of events: the development of throbbing pain in the initial phase of migraine, mediated by sensitization of *peripheral* trigeminovascular neurons that innervate the meninges; the development of cephalic allodynia propelled by sensitization of second-order trigeminovascular neurons in the spinal trigeminal nucleus, which receive converging sensory input from the meninges as well as from the scalp and facial skin; and the development of extracephalic allodynia mediated by sensitization of third-order trigeminovascular neurons in the posterior thalamic nuclei, which receive converging sensory input from the meninges, facial and body skin. It will also summarize our current understanding of the neuronal substrate of photophobia.

7.2   Experimental activation of trigeminovascular pathways

About one-third of migraines are preceded by aura – a reversible, transient cortical event that reflects cortical spreading depression (CSD) (Lashley, 1941; Lauritzen, 1994). Direct electrophysiological evidence for the activation of trigeminovascular neurons by

Neurobiological Basis of Migraine, First Edition. Edited by Turgay Dalkara and Michael A. Moskowitz.
© 2017 John Wiley & Sons, Inc. Published 2017 by John Wiley & Sons, Inc.

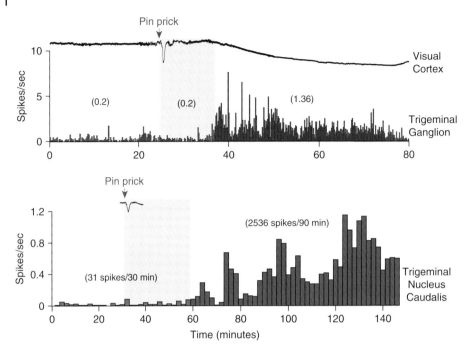

Figure 7.1 Electrophysiological recordings, showing delayed activation of meningeal nociceptors (top panel) and central trigeminovascular neurons (bottom panel) by cortical spreading depression. (Adapted from Zhang *et al.*, 2010, 2011).

CSD was reported recently (Zhang *et al.*, 2010, 2011; Figure 7.1). A potential explanation for how meningeal nociceptor activation begins after CSD has been proposed recently (Karatas *et al.*, 2013). In this study, various experimental approaches were performed in mice to demonstrate that CSD causes the opening of neuronal Panx1 megachannels, resulting in a cascade of events that leads to the release of proinflammatory molecules in the meninges.

The use of proinflammatory molecules in studying the pathophysiology of migraine gained popularity several years ago (Edelmayer *et al.*, 2012; Oshinsky and Gomonchareonsiri, 2007; Strassman *et al.*, 1996; Wieseler *et al.*, 2010), when it became apparent that, like many types of prolonged or chronic pain, migraine can also be associated with long-lasting activation and sensitization of peripheral nociceptors and central nociceptive neurons in the dorsal horn. This model involves prolonged activation and subsequent sensitization of the trigeminovascular system, in response to a brief exposure of the dura to a mixture of inflammatory agents, consisting of serotonin, bradykinin, histamine, and prostaglandin (Strassman *et al.*, 1996). These agents activate and sensitize somatic and visceral nociceptors in the rat (Beck and Handwerker, 1974; Davis *et al.*, 1993; Mizumura *et al.*, 1987; Neugebauer *et al.*, 1989; Steen *et al.*, 1992), and are potent algesics in humans (Armstrong *et al.*, 1957; Guzman *et al.*, 1962; Hollander *et al.*, 1957; Sicuteri, 1967), capable of inducing headache (Sicuteri, 1967).

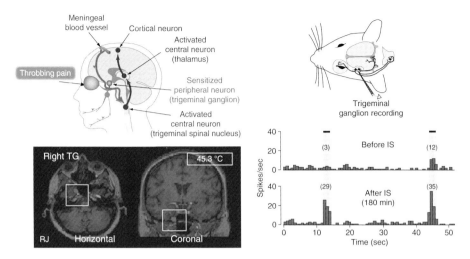

Figure 7.2 Sensitization of meningeal nociceptors believed to mediate the throbbing nature of migraine pain. Left panel: Schematic representation of peripheral sensitization and periorbital throbbing pain in human; fMRI evidence showing activation of the trigeminal ganglion during migraine. Right panel: Electrophysiological recording of a neuron in the rat TG, showing increased responsiveness to mechanical stimulation of the dura after topical application of inflammatory mediators (IS). (Adapted from Jakubowski *et al.*, 2005; Noseda and Burstein, 2013).

7.3 Peripheral sensitization

Using this animal model, it was found that a brief chemical irritation of the dura activates and sensitizes meningeal nociceptors (first-order trigeminovascular neurons) over a long period of time, rendering them responsive to mechanical stimuli to which they showed only minimal or no response prior to their sensitization (Figure 7.2) (Strassman *et al.*, 1996). During migraine, such *peripheral* sensitization is likely to mediate the throbbing pain and its aggravation during routine physical activities, such as coughing, sneezing, bending over, rapid head shake, holding one's breath, climbing up the stairs, or walking. By the end of migraine, when meningeal nociceptors are presumably no longer sensitized, their sensitivity to fluctuations in intracranial pressure returns to normal, and the patient no longer feels the throbbing.

7.4 Central sensitization: medullary dorsal horn

Brief stimulation of the dura with inflammatory agents also activates and sensitizes second-order trigeminovascular neurons located in the medullary dorsal horn that receive convergent input from the dura and the skin (Burstein *et al.*, 1998). In this paradigm, the central trigeminovascular neurons develop hypersensitivity in the periorbital skin, manifested as increased responsiveness to mild stimuli (brush, heat, cold), to which they showed only minimal or no response prior to their sensitization

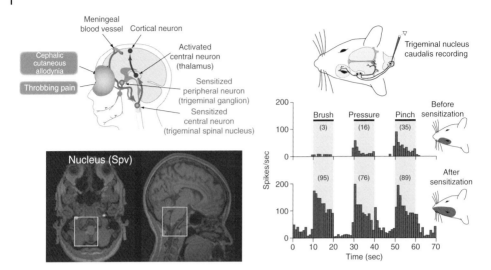

Figure 7.3 Sensitization of central trigeminovascular neurons in the spinal trigeminal nucleus, thought to mediate cephalic cutaneous allodynia during migraine. Left panel: schematic representation of central sensitization of spinal trigeminovascular neurons and cephalic cutaneous allodynia in the human; fMRI evidence showing activation of the spinal trigeminal nucleus during migraine. Right panel: electrophysiological recording of a neuron in the rat SpV, showing increased responsiveness to innocuous and noxious stimulation of the skin and the corresponding receptive field after induction of central sensitization. (Adapted from Burstein *et al.*, 1998; Noseda and Burstein, 2013).

(Figure 7.3, right panel). The induction of central sensitization by intracranial stimulation of the dura, and the ensuing extracranial hypersensitivity, is taken to suggest that a similar process may occur in patients during migraine (Figure 7.3).

Extracranial hypersensitivity during migraine was first noted in 1873 (Liveing, 1873) and later documented in the 1950s (Selby and Lance, 1960; Wolff *et al.*, 1953). At that time, extracranial hypersensitivity was ascribed to "hematomas that develop hours after onset of headache as a result of damage to vascular walls of blood vessels such as the temporal artery" (Wolff *et al.*, 1953), or "widespread distension of extracranial blood vessels or spasm of suboccipital scalp muscles" (Selby and Lance, 1960). The current view, however, is that extracranial hypersensitivity is a manifestation of central neuronal sensitization, rather than extracranial vascular pathophysiology.

Recent quantitative stimulation applied to the surface of the skin showed that pain thresholds to mechanical, heat, and cold skin stimuli decrease significantly during migraine in the majority of patients (Burstein *et al.*, 2000). This skin hypersensitivity, termed cutaneous allodynia, is typically found in the periorbital area on the side of the migraine headache. Patients commonly notice cutaneous allodynia during migraine when they become irritated by innocuous activities such as combing, shaving, taking a shower, wearing eyeglasses or earrings, or resting their head on the pillow on the headache side. Ipsilateral cephalic allodynia is likely to be mediated by sensitization of trigeminovascular neurons in the medullary dorsal horn that process sensory inputs from the dura and periorbital skin.

7.5   Central sensitization: thalamus

In the course of studying cephalic allodynia during migraine, we unexpectedly found clear evidence for allodynia in remote skin areas outside the innervation territory of the trigeminal nerve (Burstein *et al.*, 2000). In discussing of that study, we propose that ipsilateral cephalic allodynia is mediated by sensitization of dura-sensitive neurons in the medullary dorsal horn, because their cutaneous receptive field is confined to innervation territory of the ipsilateral trigeminal nerve (Burstein *et al.*, 1998; Craig and Dostrovsky, 1991; Davis and Dostrovsky, 1988; Ebersberger *et al.*, 1997; Strassman *et al.*, 1994; Yamamura *et al.*, 1999), and that extracephalic allodynia must be mediated by neurons that process sensory information that they receive from all levels of the spinal and medullary dorsal horn. Our search of such neurons focused on the thalamus, since an extensive axonal mapping of sensitized trigeminovascular neurons in the spinal trigeminal nucleus revealed projections to the posterior (PO), the ventral posteromedial (VPM) and the sub-parafascicular (PF) nuclei.

In 2010, we reported that topical administration of inflammatory molecules to the dura sensitized thalamic trigeminovascular neurons that process sensory information from the cranial meninges *and* cephalic and extracephalic skin (Burstein *et al.*, 2010). Sensitized thalamic neurons developed ongoing firing and exhibited hyper-responsiveness (increased response magnitude) and hypersensitivity (lower response threshold) to mechanical and thermal stimulation of extracephalic skin areas (Figure 7.4, right panels). Relevant to migraine pathophysiology was the finding that, in such neurons, innocuous extracephalic skin stimuli that did not induce neuronal firing before sensitization (e.g., brush) became as effective as noxious stimuli (e.g., pinch) in triggering large bouts of activity after sensitization was established.

To understand better the transformation of migraine headache into widespread, cephalic and extracephalic allodynia, we also studied the effects of extracephalic brush and heat stimuli on thalamic activation registered by fMRI during migraine in patients with whole-body allodynia (Burstein *et al.*, 2010). Functional assessment of blood oxygenation level-dependent (BOLD) signals showed that brush and heat stimulation at the skin of the dorsum of the hand produced larger BOLD responses in the posterior thalamus of subjects undergoing a migraine attack with extracephalic allodynia than the corresponding responses registered when the same patients were free of migraine and allodynia (Figure 7.4, left panel).

7.6   Temporal aspects of sensitization and their implications to triptan therapy

Central sensitization can be either activity-dependent or activity-independent (Ji *et al.*, 2003). The induction of sensitization in second-order trigeminovascular neurons, using chemical stimulation of the rat dura, is activity-dependent, as evidenced by lidocaine blockade of afferent inputs from the dura and subsequent sensitization. Once established, however, sensitization of the second-order trigeminovascular neurons

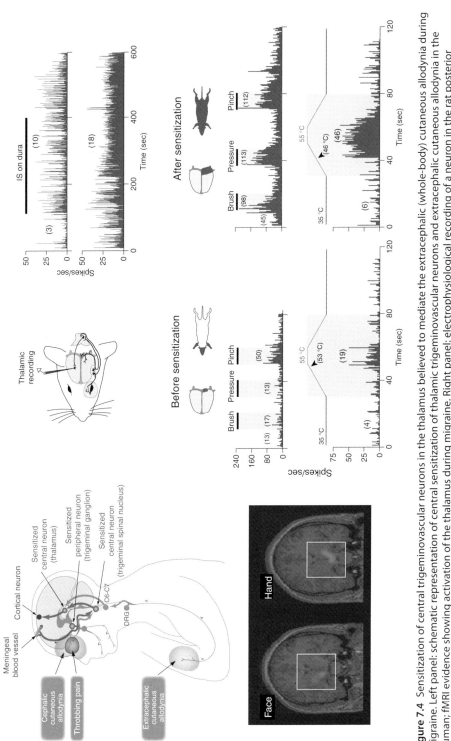

Figure 7.4 Sensitization of central trigeminovascular neurons in the thalamus believed to mediate the extracephalic (whole-body) cutaneous allodynia during migraine. Left panel: schematic representation of central sensitization of thalamic trigeminovascular neurons and extracephalic cutaneous allodynia in the human; fMRI evidence showing activation of the thalamus during migraine. Right panel: electrophysiological recording of a neuron in the rat posterior thalamus, showing enhanced spontaneous firing and increased responsiveness to mechanical and thermal stimulation of the skin, and the corresponding dural and cutaneous receptive fields after induction of central sensitization by application of inflammatory mediators (IS) to the dura. (Adapted from Noseda and Burstein, 2013 and Burstein et al. 2010).

becomes activity-independent, as it can no longer be interrupted by lidocaine on the dura (Burstein *et al.*, 1998).

Translating these findings in the context of migraine with allodynia, it appears that central sensitization depends on incoming impulses from the meninges in the early phase of the attack, and maintains itself in the absence of such sensory input later on. This view is strongly supported by the effects of the anti-migraine 5-HT$_{1B/1D}$ agonists, known as triptans, on the induction and maintenance of central sensitization in the rat (Burstein and Jakubowski, 2004), and the corresponding effects of early and late triptan therapy on allodynia during migraine (Burstein *et al.*, 2004).

In the rat, triptan administration concomitant with chemical irritation of the dura effectively prevents the development of central sensitization (Figure 7.5a). Similarly, treating patients with triptans early – within 60 minutes of the onset of migraine – effectively blocks the development of cutaneous allodynia (Figure 7.5c–d). However, neither central neuronal sensitization in the rat, nor cutaneous allodynia in patients, can be reversed by late triptan treatment (two hours after the application of sensitizing agent to the dura in the animal model, and four hours after the onset of migraine in allodynic patients) (Figure 7.5b–d). Most importantly, central sensitization appears to play a critical role in the management of migraine headache of allodynic patients. While non-allodynic patients can be rendered pain-free with triptans at any time during an attack, allodynic patients can be rendered pain-free only if treated with triptans early in the attack – namely, before the establishment of cutaneous allodynia (Burstein *et al.*, 2004) (Figure 7.5c–d).

7.7 Modulation of central sensitization

A growing body of evidence suggests that migraine patients are mostly non-allodynic during the first years of their migraine experience, yet are eventually destined to develop allodynia during their migraine attacks in later years (Burstein *et al.*, 2004; Burstein *et al.*, 2000; Mathew, 2003). It is, therefore, possible that repeated migraine attacks over the years have cumulative adverse consequences on the function of the trigeminovascular pathway, including a susceptibility to develop central sensitization.

The threshold for a central trigeminovascular neuron to enter a state of sensitization depends on the balance between incoming nociceptive signals and their modulation by spinal and suprabulber pathways. Many of the modulatory suprabulber pathways converge on the periaqueductal gray (PAG) and rostral ventromedial medulla (RVM) (Fields, 1999). Recent imaging studies have shown that the PAG is activated during migraine (Weiller *et al.*, 1995), and that it is deposited with abnormally high levels of iron in patients with a long history of migraine, suggesting abnormal neuronal functioning (Welch *et al.*, 2001).

Abnormal PAG functioning can either enhance activity of RVM neurons that *facilitate* pain transmission in the dorsal horn, or suppress activity of RVM neurons that *inhibit* pain transmission in the dorsal horn (Porreca *et al.*, 2002). This may enhance excitability and, therefore, promote responses of second-order trigeminovascular neurons to incoming nociceptive signals from the meninges, resulting in a reduced threshold for entering a state of central sensitization. Furthermore, the transition from episodic to chronic migraine that occurs in some patients over the years may involve a shift in the

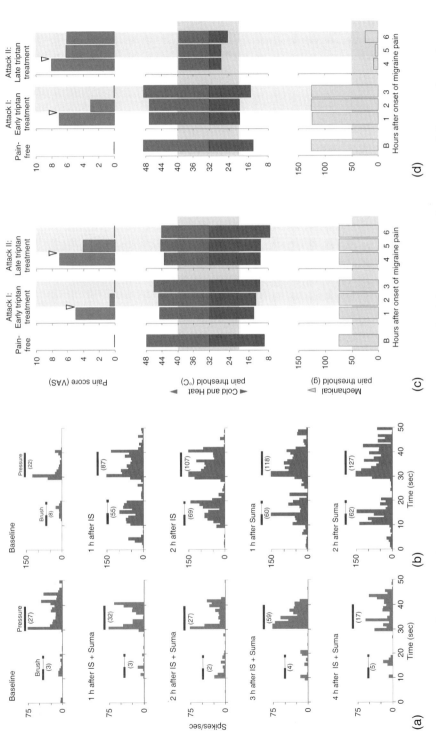

Figure 7.5 Sumatriptan effects on central sensitization, migraine pain intensity and periorbital skin sensitivity, in the presence and absence of central sensitization and cutaneous allodynia at the time of treatment. The development of central sensitization is prevented by early (a), but not by late (b) sumatriptan administration. Early and late sumatriptan treatment render a non-allodynic patient pain-free (c) whereas, in the allodynic patient (d), sumatriptan is effective in terminating the headache when administered early, but not when administered late. (Adapted from Burstein and Jakubowski, 2004 and Burstein *et al.* 2004).

underlying pathophysiology, from transient to a chronic state of sensitization. Altered functions of modulatory suprabulber pain pathways can contribute to this progression in migraine pathophysiology.

7.8   Neural substrate of migraine-type photophobia

There are few definitions of photophobia in the literature that refer to several light-induced neurological symptoms, including exacerbation of headache, hypersensitivity to light, and ocular discomfort/pain. These symptoms are not due to a fear of light, as the term "phobia" might suggest, but have been associated with intracranial pathologies such as migraine, meningitis, subdural hemorrhage, and intracranial tumors, as well as disorders of the anterior segment of the eye, such as uveitis, cyclitis, iritis, and blepharitis (Aurora *et al.*, 1999; Digre and Brennan, 2012; Kawasaki and Purvin, 2002; Lamonte *et al.*, 1995; Welty and Horner, 1990). In the last few years, new insights into the mechanisms of light-induced neurological symptoms have emerged.

The perception of migraine headache is uniquely intensified during exposure to ambient light (Kawasaki and Purvin, 2002; Liveing, 1873). This migraine-type photophobia, commonly described as exacerbation of the headache by light, is experienced by nearly 90% of migraineurs with normal eyesight (Drummond, 1986; Liveing, 1873; Miller, 1985; Selby and Lance, 1960). Clinical observations in partially blind migraineurs suggest that the exacerbation of headache by light depends on photic signals from the eye that converge on trigeminovascular neurons somewhere along its path.

The critical contribution of the optic nerve to migraine-type photophobia is best illustrated in migraine patients lacking any kind of visual perception due to complete damage of the optic nerve. Such patients report that light does not hurt them during migraine, that their sleep cycle is irregular, and that light does not induce pupillary response. Conversely, exacerbation of headache by light is preserved in blind migraineurs with an intact optic nerve, partial light perception but no sight, due to severe degeneration of rod and cone photoreceptors (Noseda *et al.*, 2010).

Retinal projections to the brain constitute two functionally different pathways. The first allows the formation of images by photoactivation of rods and cones, and the second allows regulation of biological functions, such as circadian photoentrainment, pupillary reflex, and melatonin release by activation of intrinsically photosensitive retinal ganglion cells (ipRGCs) containing melanopsin photoreceptors (Freedman *et al.*, 1999; Klein and Weller, 1972; Lucas *et al.*, 2001). Activation of ipRGCs is achieved not only by virtue of their unique photopigment, melanopsin (Berson *et al.*, 2002; Provencio *et al.*, 1998), but also extrinsically by rods and cones (Guler *et al.*, 2008). It is therefore likely that all retinal photoreceptors contribute to migraine-type photophobia in migraineurs with normal eyesight.

Integrating existing knowledge of the neurobiology of the trigeminovascular system and the anatomy of visual pathways, the following information is available:

a) Light enhances the activity of thalamic trigeminovascular neurons.
b) A subgroup of light/dura-sensitive neurons, located mainly in the LP/Po area of the posterior thalamus, receive direct input from RGCs.
c) The axons of these neurons project to cortical areas involved in the processing of pain and visual perception (Figure 7.6).

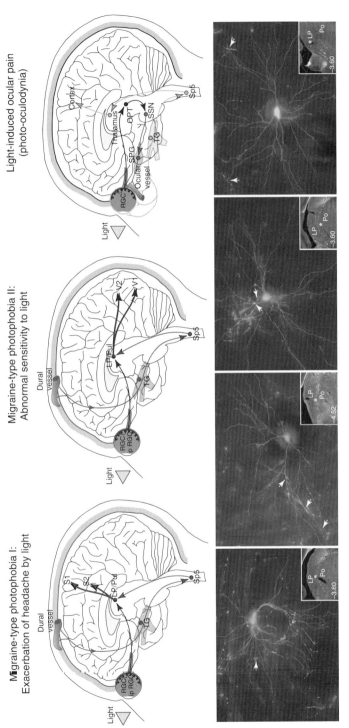

Figure 7.6 Mechanisms of photophobia. Top panel: proposed mechanism for exacerbation of headache by light, hypersensitivity to light in migraine patients and ocular pain induced by light (adapted from Noseda and Burstein, 2011). Bottom panel: dura/light-sensitive neurons (cell with clear counters) closely apposed to retinal afferents (faint processes; arrowheads point to potential axodendritic or axosomatic apposition) in the posterior thalamus. Adapted from Noseda *et al.* 2010 and Noseda and Burstein, 2011. Reproduced by permission of Nature Publishing Group.

Such convergence of photic signals from the retina onto the trigeminovascular thalamo-cortical pathway has been proposed as a neural mechanism for the exacerbation of migraine headache by light (Noseda *et al.*, 2010). Further evidence supporting the existence of such pathway in humans comes from imaging studies and probabilistic tractography that shows blood oxygen-level dependent (BOLD) responses in the pulvinar (LP/Po area in the rat) of patients undergoing a migraine attack with extracephalic allodynia (Burstein *et al.*, 2010), and direct pathways from the optic nerve to the pulvinar (Maleki *et al.*, 2012).

Some migraineurs describe photophobia as abnormal intolerance to light. Such a description of photo-hypersensitivity suggests that the flow of nociceptive signals along the trigeminovascular pathway converges on the visual cortex and alters its responsiveness to visual stimuli. Indeed, the visual cortex appears to be hyperexcitable in migraineurs, and may be the neural substrate of abnormal processing of light sensitivity (Denuelle *et al.*, 2011).

The discovery of light/dura-sensitive thalamic neurons, located outside the VPM nucleus, that project directly to the primary and secondary visual cortices (Noseda and Burstein, 2011; Noseda *et al.*, 2010), provides an anatomical substrate for the induction of abnormal intolerance to light during migraine (Figure 7.6). Additionally, a transgenic mouse model of migraine-related light-aversion or increased sensitivity to light has been recently developed. This genetically engineered model presents increased sensitivity to CGRP, due to overexpression of the human receptor activity-modifying protein 1 (hRAMP1), and provides strong behavioral evidence of aversion to light following intracerebroventricular administration of CGRP (Recober *et al.*, 2009, 2010).

Another clinical entity falling into the definition of photophobia is ocular discomfort or pain induced in the eye by exposure to bright light (Noseda and Burstein, 2011). More appropriately termed photo-oculodynia, this type of photophobia is thought to originate from indirect activation of intraocular trigeminal nociceptors. As proposed by Okamoto *et al.* (2010), bright light causes pain in the eye through activation of a complex neuronal pathway involving the olivary pretectal nucleus, the SSN and the sphenopalatine ganglion, which drives parasympathetically-controlled vasodilatation and mechanical deformation of ocular blood vessels. In turn, this activates trigeminal nociceptors and second-order nociceptive neurons in the SpVC. Lack of evidence for induction of vasodilatation by light in the human retina question this formulation.

References

Armstrong D, Jepson JB, Keele CA, Stewart JW (1957). Pain-producing substances in human inflammatory exudates and plasma. *Journal of Physiology (London)* **135**: 350–370.

Aurora SK, Cao Y, Bowyer SM, Welch KM (1999). The occipital cortex is hyperexcitable in migraine: experimental evidence. *Headache* **39**(7): 469–476.

Beck PW, Handwerker HO (1974). Bradykinin and serotonin effects on various types of cutaneous nerve fibers. *Pflügers Archiv* **347**(3): 209–222.

Berson DM, Dunn FA, Takao M (2002). Phototransduction by retinal ganglion cells that set the circadian clock. *Science* **295**(5557): 1070–1073.

Burstein R, Jakubowski M (2004). Analgesic triptan action in an animal model of intracranial pain: A race against the development of central sensitization. *Annals of Neurology* **55**(1): 27–36.

Burstein R, Yamamura H, Malick A, Strassman AM (1998). Chemical stimulation of the intracranial dura induces enhanced responses to facial stimulation in brain stem trigeminal neurons. *Journal of Neurophysiology* **79**(2): 964–982.

Burstein R, Yarnitsky D, Goor-Aryeh I, Ransil BJ, Bajwa ZH (2000). An association between migraine and cutaneous allodynia. *Annals of Neurology* **47**: 614–624.

Burstein R, Jakubowski M, Collins B (2004). Defeating migraine pain with triptans: A race against the development of cutaneous allodynia. *Annals of Neurology* **55**(1): 19–26.

Burstein R, Jakubowski M, Garcia-Nicas E, Kainz V, Bajwa Z, Hargreaves R, Becerra L, Borsook D (2010). Thalamic sensitization transforms localized pain into widespread allodynia. *Annals of Neurology* **68**(1): 81–91.

Craig AD, Dostrovsky JO (1991). Thermoreceptive lamina I trigeminothalamic neurons project to the nucleus submedius in the cat. *Experimental Brain Research* **85**(2): 470–474.

Davis KD, Dostrovsky JO (1988). Responses of feline trigeminal spinal tract nucleus neurons to stimulation of the middle meningeal artery and sagittal sinus. *Journal of Neurophysiology* **59**(2): 648–666.

Davis KD, Meyer RA, Campbell JN (1993). Chemosensitivity and sensitization of nociceptive afferents that innervate the hairy skin of monkey. *Journal of Neurophysiology* **69**(4): 1071–1081.

Denuelle M, Boulloche N, Payoux P, Fabre N, Trotter Y, Geraud G (2011). A PET study of photophobia during spontaneous migraine attacks. *Neurology* **76**(3): 213–218.

Digre KB, Brennan KC (2012). Shedding light on photophobia. *Journal of Neuro-Ophthalmology* **32**(1): 68–81.

Drummond PD (1986). A quantitative assessment of photophobia in migraine and tension headache. *Headache* **26**(9): 465–469.

Ebersberger A, Ringkamp M, Reeh PW, Handwerker HO (1997). Recordings from brain stem neurons responding to chemical stimulation of the subarachnoid space. *Journal of Neurophysiology* **77**(6): 3122–3133.

Edelmayer RM, Ossipov MH, Porreca F (2012). An experimental model of headache-related pain. *Methods in Molecular Biology* **851**: 109–120.

Fields HL (1999). Pain: an unpleasant topic. *Pain* (Suppl 6): S61–S69.

Freedman MS, Lucas RJ, Soni B, von Schantz M, Munoz M, David-Gray Z, Foster R (1999). Regulation of mammalian circadian behavior by non-rod, non-cone, ocular photoreceptors. *Science* **284**(5413): 502–504.

Guler AD, Ecker JL, Lall GS, Haq S, Altimus CM, Liao HW, Barnard AR, Cahill H, Badea TC, Zhao H, Hankins MW, Berson DM, Lucas RJ, Yau KW, Hattar S (2008). Melanopsin cells are the principal conduits for rod-cone input to non-image-forming vision. *Nature* **453**(7191): 102–105.

Guzman F, Braun C, Lim RKS (1962). Visceral pain and the pseudoaffective response to intra-arterial injection of bradykinin and other algesic agents. *Archives Internationales de Pharmacodynamie et de Thérapie* **136**: 353–384.

Hollander W, Michaelson AL, Wilkins RW (1957). Serotonin and antiserotonins. I. Their circulatory respiratory and renal effects in man. *Circulation* **16**: 246–255.

Jakubowski M, Levy D, Goor-Aryeh I, Collins B, Bajwa Z, Burstein R (2005). Terminating migraine with allodynia and ongoing central sensitization using parenteral administration of COX1/COX2 inhibitors. *Headache* **45**: 850–861.

Ji RR, Kohno T, Moore KA, Woolf CJ (2003). Central sensitization and LTP: do pain and memory share similar mechanisms? *Trends in Neurosciences* **26**(12): 696–705.

Karatas H, Erdener SE, Gursoy-Ozdemir Y, Lule S, Eren-Kocak E, Sen ZD, Dalkara T (2013). Spreading depression triggers headache by activating neuronal Panx1 channels. *Science* **339**(6123): 1092–1095.

Kawasaki A, Purvin VA (2002). Photophobia as the presenting visual symptom of chiasmal compression. *Journal of Neuro-Ophthalmology* **22**(1): 3–8.

Klein DC, Weller JL (1972). Rapid light-induced decrease in pineal serotonin N-acetyltransferase activity. *Science* **177**(48): 532–533.

Lamonte M, Silberstein SD, Marcelis JF (1995). Headache associated with aseptic meningitis. *Headache* **35**(9): 520–526.

Lashley KS (1941). Patterns of cerebral integration indicated by the scotomas of migraine. *Archives of Neurology & Psychiatry* **46**: 259–264.

Lauritzen M (1994). Pathophysiology of the migraine aura. The spreading depression theory. *Brain* **117**(Pt 1): 199–210.

Liveing E (1873). *On megrim, sick headache*. Nijmegen: Arts & Boeve, Publishers.

Lucas RJ, Douglas RH, Foster RG (2001). Characterization of an ocular photopigment capable of driving pupillary constriction in mice. *Nature Neuroscience* **4**(6): 621–626.

Maleki N, Becerra L, Upadhyay J, Burstein R, Borsook D (2012). Direct optic nerve pulvinar connections defined by diffusion MR tractography in humans: implications for photophobia. *Human Brain Mapping* **33**(1): 75–88.

Mathew NT (2003). Early intervention with almotriptan improves sustained pain-free response in acute migraine. *Headache* **43**(10): 1075–1079.

Miller NR (1985). Photophobia. In: Miller NR (ed). *Walsh and Hoyt's Clinical Neuro-ophthlmology*, 4th ed, pp. 1099–1106. Baltimore: Williams & Wilkins.

Mizumura K, Sato J, Kumazawa T (1987). Effects of prostaglandins and other putative chemical intermediaries on the activity of canine testicular polymodal receptors studied in vitro. *Pflügers Archiv* **408**(6): 565–572.

Neugebauer V, Schaible HG, Schmidt RF (1989). Sensitization of articular afferents to mechanical stimuli by bradykinin. *Pflügers Archiv* **415**(3): 330–335.

Noseda R, Burstein R (2011). Advances in understanding the mechanisms of migraine-type photophobia. *Current Opinion in Neurology* **24**(3): 197–202.

Noseda R, Burstein R (2013). Migraine pathophysiology: anatomy of the trigeminovascular pathway and associated neurological symptoms, cortical spreading depression, sensitization, and modulation of pain. *Pain* **154** (Suppl 1): S44–53.

Noseda R, Kainz V, Jakubowski M, Gooley JJ, Saper CB, Digre K, Burstein R (2010). A neural mechanism for exacerbation of headache by light. *Nature Neuroscience* **13**(2): 239–245.

Okamoto K, Tashiro A, Chang Z, Bereiter DA (2010). Bright light activates a trigeminal nociceptive pathway. *Pain* **149**(2): 235–242.

Oshinsky ML, Gomonchareonsiri S (2007). Episodic dural stimulation in awake rats: a model for recurrent headache. *Headache* **47**(7): 1026–1036.

Porreca F, Ossipov MH, Gebhart GF (2002). Chronic pain and medullary descending facilitation. [Review] [76 refs]. *Trends in Neurosciences* **25**(6): 319–325.

Provencio I, Jiang G, De Grip WJ, Hayes WP, Rollag MD (1998). Melanopsin: An opsin in melanophores, brain, and eye. *Proceedings of the National Academy of Sciences of the United States of America* **95**(1): 340–345.

Recober A, Kuburas A, Zhang Z, Wemmie JA, Anderson MG, Russo AF (2009). Role of calcitonin gene-related peptide in light-aversive behavior: implications for migraine. *Journal of Neuroscience* **29**(27): 8798–8804.

Recober A, Kaiser EA, Kuburas A, Russo AF (2010). Induction of multiple photophobic behaviors in a transgenic mouse sensitized to CGRP. *Neuropharmacology* **58**(1): 156–165.

Selby G, Lance JW (1960). Observations on 500 cases of migraine and allied vascular headache. *Journal of Neurology, Neurosurgery & Psychiatry* **23**: 23–32.

Sicuteri F (1967). Vasoneuractive substances and their implication in vascular pain. *Research and Clinical Studies in Headache* **1**: 6–45.

Steen KH, Reeh PW, Anton F, Handwerker HO (1992). Protons selectively induce lasting excitation and sensitization to mechanical stimulation of nociceptors in rat skin, *in vitro*. *Journal of Neuroscience* **12**(1): 86–95.

Strassman AM, Potrebic S, Maciewicz RJ (1994). Anatomical properties of brainstem trigeminal neurons that respond to electrical stimulation of dural blood vessels. *Journal of Comparative Neurology* **346**(3): 349–365.

Strassman AM, Raymond SA, Burstein R (1996). Sensitization of meningeal sensory neurons and the origin of headaches. *Nature* **384**(6609): 560–564.

Weiller C, May A, Limmroth V, Juptner M, Kaube H, Schayck RV, Coenen HH, Diener HC (1995). Brain stem activation in spontaneous human migraine attacks. *Nature Medicine* **1**(7): 658–660.

Welch KM, Nagesh V, Aurora SK, Gelman N (2001). Periaqueductal gray matter dysfunction in migraine: cause or the burden of illness? *Headache* **41**(7): 629–637.

Welty TE, Horner TG (1990). Pathophysiology and treatment of subarachnoid hemorrhage. *Clinical Pharmacology* **9**(1): 35–39.

Wieseler J, Ellis A, Sprunger D, Brown K, McFadden A, Mahoney J, Rezvani N, Maier SF, Watkins LR (2010). A novel method for modeling facial allodynia associated with migraine in awake and freely moving rats. *Journal of Neuroscience Methods* **185**(2): 236–245.

Wolff HG, Tunis MM, Goodell H (1953). Studies on migraine. *Archives of Internal Medicine* **92**: 478–484.

Yamamura H, Malick A, Chamberlin NL, Burstein R (1999). Cardiovascular and neuronal responses to head stimulation reflect central sensitization and cutaneous allodynia in a rat model of migraine. *Journal of Neurophysiology* **81**(2): 479–493.

Zhang X, Levy D, Kainz V, Noseda R, Jakubowski M, Burstein R (2011). Activation of central trigeminovascular neurons by cortical spreading depression. *Annals of Neurology* **69**(5): 855–865.

Zhang X, Levy D, Noseda R, Kainz V, Jakubowski M, Burstein R (2010). Activation of meningeal nociceptors by cortical spreading depression: implications for migraine with aura. *Journal of Neuroscience* **30**(26): 8807–8814.

8

Central circuits promoting chronification of migraine

Christopher W. Atcherley[1], Kelsey Nation[2], Milena De Felice[3], Jennifer Y. Xie[2],
Michael H. Ossipov[2], David W. Dodick[4] and Frank Porreca[1,2]

[1] Department of Collaborative Research and Neurology, Mayo Clinic, Scottsdale, Arizona, USA
[2] Department of Pharmacology, University of Arizona, Tucson, Arizona, USA
[3] School of Clinical Dentistry, University of Sheffield, South Yorkshire, United Kingdom
[4] Mayo Clinic Hospital, Phoenix, Arizona, USA

8.1 Introduction

The frequency of attacks in individuals with episodic migraine is predictive of the risk to eventual transformation to chronic migraine. Repeated or frequent activation of nociceptors can result in neural plasticity, which increases synaptic strength and amplification of innocuous signals – mechanisms commonly referred to as central sensitization. Central sensitization could contribute to migraine episodes, following exposure to normally sub-threshold migraine triggers. Dysfunction of descending pain modulatory circuits may promote the maintenance of states of central sensitization. Decreased descending inhibition, or possibly enhanced descending pain facilitation, has been repeatedly observed in patients with functional pain disorders, including migraine. It is now appreciated that neural plasticity in these circuits can also arise from overuse of drugs for acute migraine treatment, which can produce medication overuse headache. Collectively, both clinical and preclinical studies suggest that repeated episodic migraine, and medications used to acutely treat migraine, promote dysfunction in central pain modulation, to establish or maintain a "pain memory" that may lead to migraine chronification.

Here, we review the role of central pain modulatory circuits that may promote the pain associated with migraine, and how these circuits may be influenced by overuse of abortive medications, possibly resulting in medication overuse headache (MOH). We suggest that adaptations within central descending pain modulatory circuits amplify signals from the periphery promoting chronification of migraine. We review human data assessing conditioned pain modulation (CPM) responses in migraineurs, and in patients with MOH, and complement the interpretation of these findings with data from mechanistic investigations in preclinical models.

Neurobiological Basis of Migraine, First Edition. Edited by Turgay Dalkara and Michael A. Moskowitz.
© 2017 John Wiley & Sons, Inc. Published 2017 by John Wiley & Sons, Inc.

8.2 Pharmacotherapy of migraine

Successful pharmacological treatment of migraine is difficult to achieve. Acute treatment of migraine commonly relies on the use of over-the-counter (OTC) pain relievers, such as acetaminophen, ibuprofen, naproxen, and other non-steroidal anti-inflammatory drugs (NSAIDs). While these drugs have established clinical efficacy, many patients show little or no response to them, which is reflected in the high numbers needed to treat (NNT) values, ranging from 7 to 12, required in order to achieve a two-hour pain-free response (Becker, 2015). For patients who do not respond to OTC medications, the triptans are the drug of choice for treating acute migraine (Becker, 2015). While these drugs have demonstrated clinical efficacy, the NNT values to achieve a two-hour pain-free response for orally administered triptan formulations range from 3 to 12, suggestive of suboptimal efficacy for this class of drugs (Becker, 2015). In addition to the OTC drugs and the triptans, opioids and barbiturates are sometimes used to treat migraine, and have shown clinical efficacy (Marmura *et al.*, 2015), but with significant clinical drawbacks (see below).

Approximately 25 years after the triptan drugs revolutionized the treatment of migraine (Goadsby *et al.*, 2002; Lipton *et al.*, 2004), recent data from randomized clinical trials (RCTs) evaluating blockade of CGRP signaling promise a similar seismic shift in migraine therapy. RCTs have demonstrated that the CGRP antagonists olcagepant, telcagepant, and MK-3207 have all showed efficacy in acute treatment of migraine (Hoffmann and Goadsby, 2012; Silberstein, 2013) (see Chapter 9).

Although the precise mechanisms through which CGRP antagonists may block migraine are not completely understood, the use of [^{11}C]MK-4232 as a CGRP receptor PET tracer demonstrated that telcagepant achieved only low central receptor occupancy at efficacious doses (Hostetler *et al.*, 2013). This result suggests that the peripheral actions of CGRP are sufficient to promote migraine pain, a conclusion supported by the demonstrated clinical efficacy of anti-CGRP antibody strategies. Whether increased brain penetration of CGRP receptor antagonists during migraine attacks contributes to their efficacy remains to be evaluated (Hostetler *et al.*, 2013). Unfortunately, concerns about hepatic toxicity with repeated administration have currently delayed further development of small molecule CGRP antagonists for the long-term treatment of migraine (Olesen and Ashina, 2011; Silberstein, 2013). Recent studies with BI 44370 TA suggest that this toxicity may not be a class effect, and further clinical studies are ongoing (Hoffmann and Goadsby, 2012; Negro *et al.*, 2012).

The role of CGRP in migraine is also supported by multiple clinical trials with CGRP antibodies, directed either at the peptide or at the CGRP receptor. A recent RCT demonstrated that the monoclonal CGRP antibody ALD403 reduced the number of headache days in patients with frequent (i.e., 5–14 migraine days per 28-day period) episodic migraine (Dodick *et al.*, 2014a). The efficacy of ALD403 in preventing episodic migraine was confirmed in a recent Phase II RCT (Sun-Edelstein and Rapoport, 2016). A 12-week RCT demonstrated that LY2951742, also a monoclonal antibody to CGRP, reduced the frequency of episodic migraine (Dodick *et al.*, 2014b).

Phase II RCTs have also shown that the CGRP antibody TEV-48125 shows efficacy against episodic and chronic migraine, with acceptable safety and tolerability profiles (Bigal *et al.*, 2015a, 2015b). AMG 334 is a CGRP receptor antibody that was demonstrated to be effective in Phase II RCT (Sun *et al.*, 2016) for migraine prevention in patients with episodic migraine. Collectively, these RCTs have shown that blockade of CGRP activity is efficacious both for the acute and preventive treatment of migraine. Nonetheless, the continued examination of safety concerns should be of highest priority.

8.3   Medication overuse headache (MOH) and migraine chronification

MOH, formerly called rebound headache, is an important risk to consider during the management of episodic migraine. Although acute therapy may be effective, the frequency of migraine headache can increase over time, until episodic migraine transforms into chronic migraine ("chronification"). Chronic migraine is characterized by the occurrence of headache on 15 or more days per month (Olesen *et al.*, 2006), of which at least eight days per month meet criteria for migraine, with or without aura, and/or the headache responds to a migraine specific medication such as a triptan or ergot. Approximately 14% of episodic migraine sufferers can be expected to develop chronic migraine, representing 1.3% to 5.1% of the global population (Katsarava *et al.*, 2011; Diener, 2012).

Non-modifiable risk factors that are associated with chronic headache (>15 days per month) in those with migraine include female sex, age, low education, low socioeconomic status, and head injury (Diamond *et al.*, 2007; Bigal and Lipton, 2009; Ashina *et al.*, 2010). In addition, risk factors that can be modified, such as stressful life events, sleep disturbances, obesity, depression, and increased caffeine consumption have been identified (Bigal *et al.*, 2007; Bigal and Lipton, 2009; Ashina *et al.*, 2010). Importantly, not all therapeutics present similar risks of developing MOH.

Approximately 50–75% of patients with chronic migraine have a history of medication overuse (Bahra *et al.*, 2003; Diamond *et al.*, 2007; Bigal and Lipton, 2009; Diener, 2012). Opioids and products that contain barbiturates, such as butalbital, are commonly used in the abortive management of migraine, but present a high likelihood of development of MOH and should be avoided (Tepper, 2012). The use of butalbital for as little as five days per month, or of opioids for eight days per month, is associated with a high risk of MOH (Biagianti *et al.*, 2014). The odds ratios for developing MOH after a year of butalbital or of opioid use are 2.06 and 1.48, respectively (Tepper, 2012). While opioids and barbiturates present the highest risk, MOH also occurs with triptans after ten days of use per month, and with NSAIDS after 15 days of use per month (Tepper, 2012). The potential for small molecule CGRP antagonists to produce MOH when used in excess is not known.

There continues to be considerable debate as to whether patients should be initially managed with early discontinuation, early discontinuation plus preventive therapy, or preventive therapy without early discontinuation of the overused medication (Chiang *et al.*, 2015). The treatments employed in MOH are primarily a combination of patient information on the disease, and detoxification from the overused drug (Chiang *et al.*, 2015).

Discontinuation of the overused medication is a common treatment method for MOH. However, discontinuation is complicated by high rates of treatment failure and relapse because patients would have the same number of migraine headaches as they did initially, consequently repeating the same pattern of treatment that ultimately led to the development of MOH (Diener, 2012). Therefore, reducing the baseline frequency of migraine is important in order to prevent a recurrence of MOH. Recent RCTs have shown that migraine-preventive medications, especially onabotulinum toxin A and topiramate, may be effective in reducing headache and migraine days in patients with chronic migraine and MOH, but only onabotulinum toxin A is approved currently in the United States for chronic migraine (Diener *et al.*, 2011; Sun-Edelstein and Rapoport, 2016).

The prevalence of psychiatric disorders, such as obsessive-compulsive disorders, depression, and anxiety is increased in patients with MOH, complicating treatment and impacting the relapse rate (Diener *et al.*, 2011; Katsarava *et al.*, 2011; Diener, 2012). Indeed, a large proportion of patients with MOH meet the diagnostic criteria for substance dependence (Biagianti *et al.*, 2014; Fuh *et al.*, 2005). The complications of treating MOH and chronic migraine necessitate close evaluation of the pathophysiology and underlying mechanisms.

There is a growing awareness that the drugs used to treat migraine can, themselves, promote neural adaptations that affect susceptibility to initiating factors for migraine and subsequent pain processing. Consequently, there exists a need for multiple research strategies, including brain imaging (Lai *et al.*, 2015), in clinical and preclinical investigations (De Felice *et al.*, 2010a, b; Meng *et al.*, 2011), in order to understand better the underlying mechanisms of migraine and of MOH as brain disorders.

Brain imaging techniques, such as magnetic resonance imaging (MRI), magnetic resonance angiography (MRA) and positron emission topography (PET), have played a substantial role in advancing understanding of the neurological mechanisms involved in both primary and secondary headache syndromes. However, the use of functional imaging still faces technological challenges, due to the temporal limitations of the imaging techniques (seconds to minutes), and the duration of a single migraine, which ranges from hours to days (May, 2009).

The use of neuroimaging technology has facilitated the testing of hypotheses, and has increased our understanding. An early PET study showed increased cerebral blood flow in the brainstem and in the cingulate, auditory and visual cortices, during spontaneous migraine attacks (Weiller *et al.*, 1995). This increased blood flow was reduced in most areas, except the brainstem, by treatments with sumatriptan (Weiller *et al.*, 1995). Later studies, however, have established that primary headache syndromes are likely not related to vasodilation (Goadsby, 2009a, 2009b; Sprenger and Goadsby, 2010). No changes in cerebral artery diameters or cerebral blood flow were observed during induced (Schoonman *et al.*, 2008) or spontaneous migraine (Amin *et al.*, 2013). These, and other observations, have resulted in growing consensus that migraine is a disorder of the brain, with secondary changes in blood flow related to underlying brain activity (metabolic-flow coupling).

Consistent with the idea that migraine is a disorder of the central nervous system, cutaneous allodynia develops in about 80% of migraineurs during individual headaches (Burstein *et al.*, 2000a, 2000b). Additionally, in response to a cutaneous stimulation of the hand, migraineurs show larger fMRI BOLD (blood oxygenation level-dependent) signals in the posterior thalamus during a migraine attack, when compared to a migraine-free period (Burstein *et al.*, 2010). Similarly, preclinical observations have demonstrated hyperexcitability of sensory neurons in the posterior thalamus of rats, in response to innocuous and noxious stimulation of the paw following chemical stimulation of the dura mater (Burstein *et al.*, 2010). These findings suggest that sensitization of thalamic neurons mediates the spreading of cutaneous allodynia in migraineurs by processing nociceptive information from the cranial meninges with sensory information for the skin (Burstein *et al.*, 2010). Collectively, both clinical and preclinical findings demonstrate the contribution of central sensitization to migraine (see chapter 7).

8.4   Central circuits modulating pain

The experience of pain varies greatly between individuals, and has long been recognized to consist of sensory, affective and cognitive dimensions (see Navratilova and Porreca, 2014 for review). The pain experienced during the headache phase of migraine is multi-dimensional. Multiple regions of the brain are activated during migraine, including the primary and secondary somatosensory cortex (S1, S2), anterior cingulate cortex (ACC), prefrontal cortex (PFC), amygdala, thalamus, cerebellum and the mesolimbic reward circuit, which includes the ventral tegmental area (VTA) and nucleus accumbens (NAc) (Akerman *et al.*, 2011; Ossipov *et al.*, 2014).

The somatosensory cortices are believed to encode the sensory components of pain, while the cortical and limbic systems (ACC, PFC, amygdala, VTA and NAc) encode emotional and motivational responses, and are involved in the contextual features of pain. Importantly, while the activation of nociceptors usually elicits sensations of pain in humans, the relationship between nociception and pain is not linear (Fields, 1999; Price, 2000). It is now appreciated that many factors can influence pain, including emotional state, degree of anxiety, level of attentiveness, past experiences, memories, and context resulting in either enhancement or suppression of the pain experience (Fields, 2004). These factors engage central descending pain modulatory circuits that either positively or negatively influence sensory inputs, to determine the outcome of nociceptor activation.

Descending pain modulatory circuits have been shown to be opioid-sensitive, and relevant to the perception of pain and pleasure in normal and chronic pain states (Ossipov *et al.*, 2010, 2014). The actions of many non-opioid pain-relieving drugs, including anti-migraine medications, may ultimately depend on the release of endogenous opioids in cortical regions and engagement of descending pain inhibitory mechanisms (Navratilova *et al.*, 2015, 2016).

Neurons from the prefrontal cortex, anterior cingulate cortex, amygdala and sensory and motor cortices project significantly to the periaqueductal grey, which has reciprocal connections to the amygdala, hypothalamus, nucleus tractus solitarius, parabrachial nucleus, and rostral ventromedial medulla (RVM). The periaqueductal grey (PAG) also receives ascending nociceptive input from the dorsal horn and parabrachial nucleus (Heinricher and Fields, 2013). The input to the PAG from cortical and sub-cortical areas puts it in a prime position to merge the sensory, cognitive, and affective components of pain. The combination of inputs from higher brain areas and indirect output to the spinal and medullary dorsal horns makes the PAG the primary integration center for descending modulation of pain.

The output of the PAG is to the rostral ventromedial medulla (RVM, encompassing the nucleus raphe magnus, the nucleus reticularis gigantocellular-pars alpha, and the nucleus paragigantocellularis lateralis), and to the A7 noradrenergic nucleus, which both project directly to the dorsal horn of the spinal cord and to the trigeminocervical complex (Heinricher and Fields, 2013). The PAG also projects directly to the ventral horn of the spinal cord, where it exhibits control of defensive motor responses. Stimulating the periaqueductal grey causes a strong analgesic response, which can be reversed by naloxone; the antinociceptive activity of the PAG is thus mediated, at least in part, by opioid receptors (Fields, 2004). Activation of the PAG also activates RVM neurons, and produces nocifensive behaviors in rats. Activation of the PAG, therefore, directly controls motor responses to threatening stimuli, including noxious stimuli, and indirectly alters nociceptive input through projections to the RVM, serving a major role in pain onset and offset.

Projections from the RVM directly target the dorsal horn of the spinal cord and the trigeminal nucleus caudalis (Takemura *et al.*, 2006). In the RVM there are three well-characterized populations of neurons called ON, OFF, and NEUTRAL cells (Fields, 1999, 2000; Fields *et al.*, 1999). Animal studies using single unit electrophysiology recordings have shown that ON cells fire a burst of action potentials right before an animal responds to a noxious stimulus. OFF cells have high levels of tonic activity and cease firing right before a response to a noxious stimulus occurs. The NEUTRAL cells do not change firing rate during administration of noxious stimuli, and they are thought to modulate the other cells in the RVM.

Descending modulation of pain is bidirectional; pain signals can be inhibited or enhanced by these pathways. ON cells facilitate pain signals, whereas OFF cells inhibit pain signals. Mu (μ)-opioid receptors are mostly found on the ON cells, whereas kappa (κ)-opioid receptors are mainly found on OFF and NEUTRAL cells. Opioid analgesics directly inhibit ON cells, and they indirectly, through inhibition of GABAergic interneurons, excite OFF cells (De Felice *et al.*, 2011b; Heinricher and Fields, 2013). The region of the RVM includes the nucleus raphe magnus, which is a major source of serotonergic projections to the spinal cord, and it has generally been thought that these serotonergic projections may correspond to the functioning of RVM ON and OFF cells.

However, attempts to identify ON or OFF cells by neurotransmitter types have yielded contradictory results. Work from Dickenson and colleagues (Suzuki *et al.*, 2004; Bee and Dickenson, 2007, 2009; Asante and Dickenson, 2010; Sikandar *et al.*, 2012) has shown that descending serotonergic projections can modulate both inhibition and facilitation of nociceptive responses, although this has not been definitively tied to either ON or OFF cell activity and, indeed, may be secondary to such activity. Serotonin release in the spinal cord can be either pronociceptive or antinociceptive, depending on which serotonin receptors are activated. Activation of 5-HT1A, 5-HT1B, 5-HT1D, and 5-HT7 receptors tend to promote antinociception, whereas the 5-HT2A and 5-HT3 receptors are pronociceptive (Green *et al.*, 2000; Suzuki *et al.*, 2004; Sasaki *et al.*, 2006; Dogrul *et al.*, 2009; Rahman *et al.*, 2009).

Recent studies employing electrophysiology, retrograde tracers and siRNA have led to the conclusions that most OFF cells and neutral cells are GABAergic, as are approximately one-half of the ON cells (Foo and Mason, 2003; Kato *et al.*, 2006; Winkler *et al.*, 2006; Wei *et al.*, 2010). Moreover, only a small subset of neutral cells has been found to be serotonergic. Most recently, studies with viral vectors identified neurons projecting from the RVM, and coursing through the dorsal lateral funiculus and terminating in laminae I, II and V of the spinal dorsal horn, as expressing GABA and enkephalin (Zhang *et al.*, 2015). Activation of these neurons reduced behavioral responses to nociception, whereas silencing their activity enhanced nociceptive responses. Thus, these dual GABAergic/enkephalinergic neurons function in a manner consistent with OFF cells (Zhang *et al.*, 2015).

The clinical features of the premonitory phase of migraine, as well as imaging studies, have indicated the involvement of the hypothalamus (May, 2003; Maniyar *et al.*, 2014). A small number of neurons located in the lateral and posterior hypothalamus produce orexins, including orexin-A and orexin-B, which may contribute to migraine-related symptoms (Rainero *et al.*, 2011; Ebrahim *et al.*, 2002). The orexin receptors, orexin receptor 1 (OX1) and orexin receptor 2 (OX2), are G-protein coupled and are 64% homologous. Moreover, the rat and human OX1 and OX2 receptors demonstrate 94 and 95% homology, respectively. This suggests a high level of conservation across mammalian species, making this system a strong candidate for translational research (Sakurai *et al.*, 1998).

Orexin-B preferentially targets OX2 receptors, whereas orexin-A targets both OX1 and OX2 (Rainero *et al.*, 2011). OX1 and OX2 are found in the mesencephalic trigeminal nucleus, in addition to dorsal horn of the spinal cord (Holland *et al.*, 2005). Additionally, lamina I of the dorsal horn has a high density of orexin fibers, suggesting a role of orexin in pain transmission (Sarchielli *et al.*, 2008). OX1 and OX2 are also found in the VTA, NAc, and locus coeruleus, and are distributed throughout the descending pain modulatory circuits, including the PAG and RVM.

Orexin-A has been shown to induce analgesia in animal models of acute and inflammatory pain states, and when directly applied to the PAG, it reduces pain in the second, but not the first, phase of the formalin test (Yamamoto *et al.*, 2002). Importantly, activation of OX1 by orexin-A reduces neurogenic dural vasodilation, which in turn reduces release of CGRP (Holland *et al.*, 2005).

Taken together, these data indicate that orexins may play a role in central amplification related to the descending modulatory system. Measurements of orexin-A in patients with chronic migraine without MOH, and patients with MOH, showed significantly higher levels in the CSF of MOH patients and, to a lesser extent, in patients with chronic migraine, compared with control subjects (Sarchielli *et al.*, 2008). Additionally, in the MOH patients, there was a significant positive correlation of orexin-A levels and monthly drug intake. Elevated levels of orexin, and of corticotropin releasing factor suggested potential dysregulation of endocrine and autonomic regulation of migraine (Sarchielli *et al.*, 2008). Filorexant (MK-6069), a dual OX1/OX2 receptor antagonist, has been evaluated for potential migraine preventative effects. As orexin is important in maintaining wakefulness, the antagonist was evaluated as a once-daily dose taken at night. However, no significant difference between the active treatment and placebo was reported for the change from baseline in mean monthly migraine days (Chabi *et al.*, 2015; Diener *et al.*, 2015).

8.5 Evaluation of descending modulation: diffuse noxious inhibitory controls and conditioned pain modulation

Descending modulation is important for adaptive behaviors promoting survival. The connections between higher brain areas and the brainstem nuclei that modify pain signals allow evaluation of context and decisions that benefit survival of the organism. Inhibition of pain signals and escape is a preferred outcome in circumstances where further harm to the organism would occur if focus was directed to the injury. This is likely the neural correlate of stress-induced analgesia, and likely underlies the phenomenon of "pain inhibiting pain". This phenomenon was first described in animals (Le Bars *et al.*, 1979; Villanueva and Le Bars, 1995), and was termed "diffuse noxious inhibitory controls" or DNIC. Human studies refer to DNIC as conditioned pain modulation (CPM) (Nir and Yarnitsky, 2015).

CPM occurs in the absence of distraction, and the analgesic component of distraction is additive with CPM (Moont *et al.*, 2010). It is believed that CPM may help prevent further injury at the site of the most severe injury when multiple injuries are present. DNIC has been characterized with single unit electrophysiological recordings, showing that dorsal horn neurons that responded to noxious stimulation were inhibited when a second noxious stimulus was applied to a remote area of the body in rats (Dickenson and Le Bars, 1983).

Production of DNIC in animals involves an interaction between several brainstem structures, the dorsal reticular nucleus (DRt), the RVM, and the PAG. In humans, CPM is assessed by application of a noxious conditioning stimulus, combined with the application of a noxious test stimulus. The threshold to the test stimulus alone is first determined, and then the efficacy of the CPM response can be determined from the change in pain ratings to the test stimulus when the conditioning stimulus is co-administered. When the CPM response is efficient, the pain rating of the test stimulus will decrease. Deficiencies in this system are evident when there is a lack of change in pain rating to the test stimulus in the presence of the conditioning stimuli. Thus, CPM in humans, and DNIC in animals, can be used as a quantitative estimate of the efficiency of descending pain modulation.

Assessment of DNIC or CPM has important implications, particularly in functional pain conditions (i.e., pain states in which no obvious injury is identifiable), including migraine as well as in MOH. Clinical studies have shown that many chronic or recurrent pain conditions may be due, in part, to a dysfunction of endogenous pain modulation and CPM. Deficient or absent CPM has been demonstrated in idiopathic pain state, such as fibromyalgia, irritable bowel syndrome, temporomandibular joint disorders, whiplash injury, and chronic migraine and other headache disorders, as well as in the development of chronic pain after injury (Berman *et al.*, 2008; Jensen *et al.*, 2009; Yarnitsky, 2010; Lewis *et al.*, 2012; Loggia *et al.*, 2014).

Recently, it was shown that the efficacy of the DNIC response in rats after experimental neuropathic pain was predictive of recovery (Peters *et al.*, 2015). Rats with less efficient DNIC had a slower recovery from postoperative sensitivity, suggesting a role for endogenous descending inhibitory pathways in promoting recovery or limiting the central consequences of the injury (Peters *et al.*, 2015). Assessment of DNIC or of CPM may also prospectively predict the risk of development of chronic pain. Yarnitsky and colleagues were able to predict which patients were most likely to develop chronic post-thoracotomy pain by pre-operative assessment of CPM, and suggested that an inefficient CPM was likely responsible for contributing to the development of chronic pain (Yarnitsky *et al.*, 2008).

Numerous studies support the concept that a dysfunction of endogenous pain modulation and loss of CPM may be related to headache chronification. CPM has been shown to be impaired in chronic and/or widespread pain conditions, including chronic migraine (de Tommaso *et al.*, 2007; Perrotta *et al.*, 2010). A small study of female migraineurs and controls used a single CPM protocol and found no difference between the groups during the menstrual cycle (Teepker *et al.*, 2014). However, when a repeated testing protocol was used, in spite of normal initial responses, a waning of CPM was seen in patients with episodic migraine that was not observed in normal subjects (Nahman-Averbuch *et al.*, 2013). Patients with greater degrees of CPM waning also reported less pain reduction from migraine medication (Nahman-Averbuch *et al.*, 2013). It was suggested that migraine was associated with a subtle dysfunction of pain inhibitory systems, and may require more sophisticated testing protocols to test more accurately for loss of CPM (Nahman-Averbuch *et al.*, 2013).

Development of chronic tension-type headache has also been associated with dysfunctional CPM (Pielsticker *et al.*, 2005; Sandrini *et al.*, 2006). Serrao and colleagues found that the conditioned stimulus significantly depressed the nociceptive reflex area in normal individuals, indicative of a normal CPM response (Serrao *et al.*, 2004). In contrast, there was a significant increase in the RIII reflex area of individuals with chronic tension-type headache or episodic migraine, indicative of pain facilitation (Sandrini *et al.*, 2006).

Dysfunction of descending pain modulation may also promote medication overuse headache. Perrotta and colleagues found that patients with either MOH or episodic migraine without aura showed an altered CPM response when compared to normal control subjects (Perrotta *et al.*, 2010). CPM improved in MOH patients after withdrawal of the drug that produced MOH in the first place, suggesting that a propensity to developing MOH may be due to a dysfunction of endogenous pain inhibitory systems, and that this dysfunction may also contribute to episodic migraine as well (Perrotta *et al.*, 2010). It should be noted that patients with traumatic brain injuries (TBI) who also developed chronic post-traumatic headache (PTH) were demonstrated to have deficient CPM relative to TBI patients without headache (Defrin *et al.*, 2015).

Changes in CPM have generally been interpreted as a loss of descending inhibition. Boyer *et al.* (2014) found that repeated application of inflammatory mediator to the rat dura mater elicited a persistent cephalic and extracephalic allodynia, which was accompanied by increased Fos expression in the trigeminal system and impairment of the DNIC response. Importantly, the increase in central sensitization, and the loss of the DNIC response, was suggested to reflect a mechanism that could elevate the risk for developing chronic migraine (Boyer *et al.*, 2014). While the changes in CPM have been interpreted as an attenuation of descending inhibition, an equally plausible interpretation is that an apparent loss of inhibition could reflect enhanced descending facilitation, something that has been difficult to assess in humans.

Descending facilitation is highly adaptive, as it causes sensitivity to prevent further damage to an injured site (Porreca *et al.*, 2002; De Felice *et al.*, 2011a, 2011b). The likely contribution of dysfunction in descending pain modulation in cephalic pain, and MOH has also been supported in preclinical studies. Meng and colleagues found that rats with sustained morphine-induced sensitization, a model of MOH, had a loss of the DNIC response in medullary dorsal horn neurons (Okada-Ogawa *et al.*, 2009). Medullary dorsal horn neurons that responded to stimulation of the dura mater were inhibited by application of noxious stimulation of the tail of normal rats, indicating the presence of DNIC. After exposure to sustained morphine, however, the DNIC response of these dural-sensitive medullary dorsal horn neurons was absent. Administration of lidocaine into the RVM, which abolishes descending facilitation, restored the DNIC response in the morphine-exposed rats, suggesting that the apparent loss of inhibition was due to enhanced facilitation (Okada-Ogawa *et al.*, 2009).

Dysfunction of CPM/DNIC pain modulation, and increased facilitation from the RVM, may lead to sensitization of the trigeminovascular system, which can promote susceptibility to migraine pain. Rodent models of medication overuse headache have shown that the persistent exposure of rats to opioids or triptans promotes pronociceptive adaptations that can enhance pain signaling through descending pain modulatory circuits. The sustained exposure of morphine or of triptans (i.e., sumatriptan or naratriptan) to rats, either by constant infusion or repeated injections, produces enhanced sensitivity to light touch applied in the periorbital area, reflecting cutaneous allodynia (De Felice and Porreca, 2009; De Felice *et al.*, 2010a, 2010b; Okada-Ogawa *et al.*, 2009). Although response thresholds return to a normal baseline level after 14 days, a state of latent sensitization exists, since exposure to known triggers of migraine in humans (i.e., nitric oxide [NO] donor or bright light stress) will precipitate behavioral signs of cutaneous allodynia.

Treatment of rodents with opioids or triptans to induce enhanced susceptibility to putative migraine triggers may be analogous to hyperalgesic priming. The underlying consequence of exposure to the drug is to induce plasticity in primary afferent nociceptors, as well as within the central nervous system, resulting in increased susceptibility to normally subthreshold inputs.

Levine and colleagues developed the concept of "hyperalgesic priming" in order to explore the molecular mechanisms underlying the transition from acute to chronic pain (Reichling and Levine, 2009). Persistent exposure to opioids or triptans increased the expression of CGRP and of neuronal nitric oxide synthase (nNOS), but not of substance P, in the trigeminal ganglia (De Felice and Porreca, 2009; De Felice *et al.*, 2010a, 2010b). Importantly, the increased expression of CGRP and nNOS in trigeminal ganglion neurons persists long after discontinuation of either opiate or triptan exposure, and after behavioral responses to light touch have normalized.

Together, these findings suggest that these persistent changes in CGRP and nNOS expression could underlie latent sensitization (De Felice *et al.*, 2010a). The co-administration of an nNOS inhibitor, NXN-323, prevented the upregulation of nNOS and of CGRP, and the nNOS inhibitor given after induction of latent sensitization blocked the development of cutaneous allodynia induced by bright-light stress (De Felice *et al.*, 2010a). Plasticity within the central nervous system was suggested when triptan exposure reduced the stimulation threshold to elicit a CSD event, and this was blocked by topiramate (Green *et al.*, 2013). Taken together, these studies provide evidence that chronic headache conditions, including MOH and migraine, may be associated with dysfunction of endogenous pain modulatory systems.

8.6 Conclusions

It is recognized that the frequency of migraine attack is the best predictor of a transition to chronic migraine (Lipton, 2009), and that many migraineurs will progress from low-frequency episodic headache stage to high-frequency and, eventually, chronic migraine (Bigal and Lipton, 2008). The consequences of repeated attacks and nociceptive input to the central nervous system likely establish a state of sustained central sensitization that can result in amplification of subthreshold inputs (migraine triggers), resulting in a full-blown migraine attack. Such neural plasticity can be viewed as a type of "pain memory".

Multiple mechanisms of central sensitization and pain amplification have been demonstrated, including neural adaptations in descending pain modulatory mechanisms. Pre-clinical studies have demonstrated that enhanced descending facilitation promotes the expression of chronic neuropathic pain (Porreca *et al.*, 2002) and, importantly, descending inhibitory mechanisms protect against the expression of chronic neuropathic pain in injured animals (De Felice *et al.*, 2011b). The induction of latent sensitization by drugs promoting MOH also produces analogous neural adaptations that promote enhanced susceptibility to sub-threshold triggers, mediated through descending pain modulatory circuits, as demonstrated by prevention of stress- or NO-donor induced cutaneous allodynia following RVM blockade with bupivacaine (unpublished observations). Importantly, deficits in descending pain modulation have repeatedly translated across species, supporting the role of these circuits in chronification of pain and migraine, and revealing new approaches for development of novel therapies for migraine treatment.

References

Akerman S, Holland PR, Goadsby PJ (2011). Diencephalic and brainstem mechanisms in migraine. *Nature Reviews Neuroscience* **12**: 570–84.

Amin FM, Olesen J, Ashina M (2013). Intracranial and extracranial arteries in migraine –authors' reply. *Lancet Neurology* **12**: 848–9.

Asante CO, Dickenson AH (2010). Descending serotonergic facilitation mediated by spinal 5-HT3 receptors engages spinal rapamycin-sensitive pathways in the rat. *Neuroscience Letters* **484**: 108–112.

Ashina S, Lyngberg A, Jensen R (2010). Headache characteristics and chronification of migraine and tension-type headache: A population-based study. *Cephalalgia* **30**: 943–952.

Bahra A, Walsh M, Menon S, Goadsby PJ (2003). Does chronic daily headache arise de novo in association with regular use of analgesics? *Headache* **43**: 179–190.

Becker WJ (2015). Acute Migraine Treatment in Adults. *Headache* **55**: 778–793.

Bee LA, Dickenson AH (2007). Rostral ventromedial medulla control of spinal sensory processing in normal and pathophysiological states. *Neuroscience* **147**: 786–793.

Bee LA, Dickenson AH (2009). The importance of the descending monoamine system for the pain experience and its treatment. *F1000 Medicine Reports* **1**: 83.

Berman SM, Naliboff BD, Suyenobu B, Labus JS, Stains J, Ohning G, Kilpatrick L, Bueller JA, Ruby K, Jarcho J, Mayer EA (2008). Reduced brainstem inhibition during anticipated pelvic visceral pain correlates with enhanced *Brain Research*ponse to the visceral stimulus in women with irritable bowel syndrome. *Journal of Neuroscience* **28**: 349–59.

Biagianti B, Grazzi L, Usai S, Gambini O (2014). Dependency-like behaviors and pain coping styles in subjects with chronic migraine and medication overuse: results from a 1-year follow-up study. *BMC Neurology* **14**: 181.

Bigal ME, Lipton RB (2008). Clinical course in migraine: conceptualizing migraine transformation. *Neurology* **71**: 848–55.

Bigal ME, Lipton RB (2009). The epidemiology, burden, and comorbidities of migraine. *Neurologic Clinics* **27**: 321–334.

Bigal ME, Lipton RB, Holland PR, Goadsby PJ (2007). Obesity, migraine, and chronic migraine: possible mechanisms of interaction. *Neurology* **68**: 1851–1861.

Bigal ME, Dodick DW, Rapoport AM, Silberstein SD, Ma Y, Yang R, Loupe PS, Burstein R, Newman LC, Lipton RB (2015a). Safety, tolerability, and efficacy of TEV-48125 for preventive treatment of high-frequency episodic migraine: a multicentre, randomised, double-blind, placebo-controlled, phase 2b study. *Lancet Neurology* **14**: 1081–90.

Bigal ME, Edvinsson L, Rapoport AM, Lipton RB, Spierings EL, Diener HC, Burstein R, Loupe PS, Ma Y, Yang R, Silberstein SD (2015b). Safety, tolerability, and efficacy of TEV-48125 for preventive treatment of chronic migraine: a multicentre, randomised, double-blind, placebo-controlled, phase 2b study. *Lancet Neurology* **14**: 1091–1100.

Boyer N, Dallel R, Artola A, Monconduit L (2014). General trigeminospinal central sensitization and impaired descending pain inhibitory controls contribute to migraine progression. Pain **155**: 1196–205.

Burstein R, Cutrer MF, Yarnitsky D (2000a). The development of cutaneous allodynia during a migraine attack clinical evidence for the sequential recruitment of spinal and supraspinal nociceptive neurons in migraine. *Brain* **123**: 1703–1709.

Burstein R, Yarnitsky D, Goor-Aryeh I, Ransil BJ, Bajwa ZH (2000b). An association between migraine and cutaneous allodynia. *Annals of Neurology* **47**: 614–24.

Burstein R, Jakubowski M, Garcia-Nicas E, Kainz V, Bajwa Z, Hargreaves R, Becerra L, Borsook D (2010). Thalamic sensitization transforms localized pain into widespread allodynia. *Annals of Neurology* **68**: 81–91.

Chabi A, Zhang Y, Jackson S, Cady R, Lines C, Herring WJ, Connor KM, Michelson D (2015). Randomized controlled trial of the orexin receptor antagonist filorexant for migraine prophylaxis. *Cephalalgia* **35**(5): 379–88.

Chiang C-C, Schwedt TJ, Wang S-J, Dodick DW (2015). Treatment of medication-overuse headache: A systematic review. *Cephalalgia* **36**(4): 371–86.

De Felice M, Porreca F (2009). Opiate-induced persistent pronociceptive trigeminal neural adaptations: potential relevance to opiate-induced medication overuse headache. *Cephalalgia* **29**: 1277–84.

De Felice M, Ossipov MH, Porreca F (2011b). Persistent medication-induced neural adaptations, descending facilitation, and medication overuse headache. *Current Opinion in Neurology* **24**: 193–6.

De Felice M, Ossipov MH, Wang R, Dussor G, Lai J, Meng ID, Chichorro J, Andrews JS, Rakhit S, Maddaford S, Dodick D, Porreca F (2010a). Triptan-induced enhancement of neuronal nitric oxide synthase in trigeminal ganglion dural afferents underlies increased responsiveness to potential migraine triggers. *Brain* **133**: 2475–2488.

De Felice M, Ossipov MH, Wang R, Lai J, Chichorro J, Meng I, Dodick DW, Vanderah TW, Dussor G, Porreca F (2010b). Triptan-induced latent sensitization: a possible basis for medication overuse headache. *Annals of Neurology* **67**: 325–37.

De Felice M, Ossipov MH, Porreca F (2011a). Update on medication-overuse headache. *Current Pain and Headache Reports* **15**: 79–83.

De Felice M, Sanoja R, Wang R, Vera-Portocarrero L, Oyarzo J, King T, Ossipov MH, Vanderah TW, Lai J, Dussor GO, Fields HL, Price TJ, Porreca F (2011b). Engagement of descending inhibition from the rostral ventromedial medulla protects against chronic neuropathic pain. *Pain* **152**: 2701–9.

De Tommaso M, Sardaro M, Pecoraro C, Di Fruscolo O, Serpino C, Lamberti P, Livrea P (2007). Effects of the remote C fibres stimulation induced by capsaicin on the blink reflex in chronic migraine. *Cephalalgia* **27**: 881–90.

Defrin R, Riabinin M, Feingold Y, Schreiber S, Pick CG (2015). Deficient pain modulatory systems in patients with mild traumatic brain and chronic post-traumatic headache: implications for its mechanism. *Journal of Neurotrauma* **32**: 28–37.

Diamond S, Bigal ME, Silberstein S, Loder E, Reed M, Lipton RB (2007). Patterns of diagnosis and acute and preventive treatment for migraine in the United States: results from the American Migraine Prevalence and Prevention study. *Headache* **47**: 355–363.

Dickenson AH, Le Bars D (1983). Diffuse noxious inhibitory controls (DNIC) involve trigeminothalamic and spinothalamic neurones in the rat. *Experimental Brain Researchearch* **49**: 174–80.

Diener HC (2012). Detoxification for medication overuse headache is not necessary. *Cephalalgia* **32**: 423–427.

Diener HC, Holle D, Dodick D (2011). Treatment of chronic migraine. *Current Pain and Headache Reports* **15**: 64–69.

Diener H-C, Charles A, Goadsby PJ, Holle D (2015). New therapeutic approaches for the prevention and treatment of migraine. *Lancet Neurology* **14**: 1010–1022.

Dodick DW, Goadsby PJ, Silberstein SD, Lipton RB, Olesen J, Ashina M, Wilks K, Kudrow D, Kroll R, Kohrman B, Bargar R, Hirman J, Smith J (2014a). Safety and efficacy of ALD403, an antibody to calcitonin gene-related peptide, for the prevention of frequent episodic migraine: a randomised, double-blind, placebo-controlled, exploratory phase 2 trial. *Lancet Neurology* **13**: 1100–1107.

Dodick DW, Goadsby PJ, Spierings EL, Scherer JC, Sweeney SP, Grayzel DS (2014b). Safety and efficacy of LY2951742, a monoclonal antibody to calcitonin gene-related peptide, for the prevention of migraine: a phase 2, randomised, double-blind, placebo-controlled study. *Lancet Neurology* **13**: 885–892.

Dogrul A, Ossipov MH, Porreca F (2009). Differential mediation of descending pain facilitation and inhibition by spinal 5HT-3 and 5HT-7 receptors. *Brain Research* **1280**: 52–59.

Ebrahim IO, Howard RS, Kopelman MD, Sharief MK, Williams AJ (2002). The hypocretin/orexin system. *Journal of the Royal Society of Medicine* **95**: 227–30.

Fields HL (1999). Pain: an unpleasant topic. *Pain* (Suppl 6): S61–9.

Fields HL (2000). Pain modulation: expectation, opioid analgesia and virtual pain. *Progress in Brain Research* **122**: 245–253.

Fields H (2004). State-dependent opioid control of pain. *Nature Reviews Neuroscience* **5**: 565–75.

Fields HL, Basbaum AI, Wall PD, Melzack R (1999). Central nervous system mechanisms of pain modulation. In: *Textbook of Pain*, p. 309–329. Edinburgh: Churchill Livingstone.

Foo H, Mason P (2003). Brainstem modulation of pain during sleep and waking. *Sleep Medicine Reviews* **7**: 145–154.

Fuh JL, Wang SJ, Lu SR, Juang KD (2005). Does medication overuse headache represent a behavior of dependence? *Pain* **119**: 49–55.

Goadsby PJ (2009a). Pathophysiology of migraine. *Neurologic Clinics* **27**: 335–360.

Goadsby PJ (2009b). The vascular theory of migraine – a great story wrecked by the facts. *Brain* **132**: 6–7.

Goadsby PJ, Lipton RB, Ferrari MD (2002). Migraine – current understanding and treatment. *New England Journal of Medicine* **346**: 257–270.

Green GM, Scarth J, Dickenson A (2000). An excitatory role for 5-HT in spinal inflammatory nociceptive transmission; state-dependent actions via dorsal horn 5-HT(3) receptors in the anaesthetized rat. *Pain* **89**: 81–88.

Green AL, Gu P, De Felice M, Dodick D, Ossipov MH, Porreca F (2013). Increased susceptibility to cortical spreading depression in an animal model of medication-overuse headache. *Cephalalgia* **34**: 594–604.

Heinricher MM, Fields HL (2013). Central Nervous System Mechanisms of Pain Modulation. In: McMahon SB, Koltzenburg M, Tracey I, Turk DC (eds). *Wall & Melzack's Textbook of Pain*, pp. 129–142. Elsevier.

Hoffmann J, Goadsby PJ (2012). New Agents for Acute Treatment of Migraine: CGRP Receptor Antagonists, iNOS Inhibitors. *Current Treatment Options in Neurology* **14**: 50–59.

Holland PR, Akerman S, Goadsby PJ (2005). Orexin 1 receptor activation attenuates neurogenic dural vasodilation in an animal model of trigeminovascular nociception. *Journal of Pharmacology and Experimental Therapeutics* **315**: 1380–5.

Hostetler ED, Joshi AD, Sanabria-Bohórquez S, Fan H, Zeng Z, Purcell M, Gantert L, Riffel K, Williams M, O'Malley S, Miller P, Selnick HG, Gallicchio SN, Bell IM, Salvatore CA, Kane SA, Li C-C, Hargreaves RJ, de Groot T, Bormans G, Van Hecken A, Derdelinckx I, de Hoon J, Reynders T, Declercq R, De Lepeleire I, Kennedy WP, Blanchard R, Marcantonio EE, Sur C, Cook JJ, Van Laere K, Evelhoch JL (2013). *In vivo* quantification of calcitonin gene-related peptide receptor occupancy by telcagepant in rhesus monkey and human brain using the positron emission tomography tracer [11C]MK-4232. *Journal of Pharmacology and Experimental Therapeutics* **347**: 478–86.

Jensen KB, Kosek E, Petzke F, Carville S, Fransson P, Marcus H, Williams SCR, Choy E, Giesecke T, Mainguy Y, Gracely R, Ingvar M (2009). Evidence of dysfunctional pain inhibition in Fibromyalgia reflected in rACC during provoked pain. *Pain* **144**: 95–100.

Kato G, Yasaka T, Katafuchi T, Furue H, Mizuno M, Iwamoto Y, Yoshimura M (2006). Direct GABAergic and glycinergic inhibition of the substantia gelatinosa from the rostral ventromedial medulla revealed by in vivo patch-clamp analysis in rats. *Journal of Neuroscience* **26**: 1787–1794.

Katsarava Z, Manack A, Yoon M-S, Obermann M, Becker H, Dommes P, Turkel C, Lipton RB, Diener HC (2011). Chronic migraine: Classification and comparisons. *Cephalalgia* **31**: 520–529.

Lai T-H, Protsenko E, Cheng Y-C, Loggia ML, Coppola G, Chen W-T (2015). *Neural Plasticity*icity in Common Forms of Chronic Headaches. *Neural Plasticity* **2015**: 205985.

Le Bars D, Dickenson AH, Besson JM (1979). Diffuse noxious inhibitory controls (DNIC). I. Effects on dorsal horn convergent neurones in the rat. *Pain* **6**: 283–304.

Lewis GN, Rice DA, McNair PJ (2012). Conditioned pain modulation in populations with chronic pain: a systematic review and meta-analysis. *J Pain* **13**: 936–44.

Lipton RB (2009). Tracing transformation: chronic migraine classification, progression, and epidemiology. *Neurology* **72**: S3–7.

Lipton RB, Bigal ME, Goadsby PJ (2004). Double-blind clinical trials of oral triptans vs other classes of acute migraine medication – a review. *Cephalalgia* **24**: 321–32.

Loggia ML, Berna C, Kim J, Cahalan CM, Gollub RL, Wasan AD, Harris RE, Edwards RR, Napadow V (2014). Disrupted brain circuitry for pain-related reward/punishment in fibromyalgia. *Arthritis & Rheumatology (Hoboken, NJ)* **66**: 203–12.

Maniyar FH, Sprenger T, Monteith T, Schankin C, Goadsby PJ (2014). Brain activations in the premonitory phase of nitroglycerin-triggered migraine attacks. *Brain* **137**: 232–41.

Marmura MJ, Silberstein SD, Schwedt TJ (2015). The acute treatment of migraine in adults: the american headache society evidence assessment of migraine pharmacotherapies. *Headache* **55**: 3–20.

May A (2003). Headache: lessons learned from functional imaging. *British Medical Bulletin* **65**: 223–34.

May A (2009). New insights into headache: an update on functional and structural imaging findings. *Nature Reviews Neurology* **5**: 199–209.

Meng ID, Dodick D, Ossipov MH, Porreca F (2011). Pathophysiology of medication overuse headache: insights and hypotheses from preclinical studies. *Cephalalgia* **31**: 851–60.

Moont R, Pud D, Sprecher E, Sharvit G, Yarnitsky D (2010). "Pain inhibits pain" mechanisms: Is pain modulation simply due to distraction? *Pain* **150**: 113–120.

Nahman-Averbuch H, Granovsky Y, Coghill RC, Yarnitsky D, Sprecher E, Weissman-Fogel I (2013). Waning of "conditioned pain modulation": a novel expression of subtle pronociception in migraine. *Headache* **53**: 1104–1115.

Navratilova E, Porreca F (2014). Reward and motivation in pain and pain relief. *Nature Neuroscience* **17**: 1304–12.

Navratilova E, Atcherley CW, Porreca F (2015). Brain Circuits Encoding Reward from Pain Relief. *Trends in Neurosciences* **38**: 741–750.

Navratilova E, Morimura K, Xie JY, Atcherley CW, Ossipov MH, Porreca F (2016). Positive emotions and brain reward circuits in chronic pain. *Journal of Comparative Neurology* **524**(8): 1646–52.

Negro A, Lionetto L, Simmaco M, Martelletti P (2012). CGRP receptor antagonists: an expanding drug class for acute migraine? *Expert Opinion on Investigational Drugs* **21**: 807–818.

Nir R-R, Yarnitsky D (2015). Conditioned pain modulation. *Current Opinion in Supportive and Palliative Care* **9**: 131–7.

Okada-Ogawa A, Porreca F, Meng ID (2009). Sustained morphine-induced sensitization and loss of diffuse noxious inhibitory controls in dura-sensitive medullary dorsal horn neurons. *Journal of Neuroscience* **29**: 15828–35.

Olesen J, Ashina M (2011). Emerging migraine treatments and drug targets. *Trends in Pharmacological Sciences* **32**: 352–359.

Olesen J, Bousser MG, Diener HC, Dodick D, First M, Goadsby PJ, Gobel H, Lainez MJ, Lance JW, Lipton RB, Nappi G, Sakai F, Schoenen J, Silberstein SD, Steiner TJ (2006). New appendix criteria open for a broader concept of chronic migraine. *Cephalalgia* **26**: 742–746.

Ossipov MH, Dussor GO, Porreca F (2010). Central modulation of pain. *Journal of Clinical Investigation* **120**: 3779–87.

Ossipov MH, Morimura K, Porreca F (2014). Descending pain modulation and chronification of pain. *Current Opinion in Supportive and Palliative Care* **8**: 143–51.

Perrotta A, Serrao M, Sandrini G, Burstein R, Sances G, Rossi P, Bartolo M, Pierelli F, Nappi G (2010). Sensitisation of spinal cord pain processing in medication overuse headache involves supraspinal pain control. *Cephalalgia* **30**: 272–284.

Peters CM, Hayashida K-I, Suto T, Houle TT, Aschenbrenner CA, Martin TJ, Eisenach JC (2015). Individual differences in acute pain-induced endogenous analgesia predict time to resolution of postoperative pain in the rat. *Anesthesiology* **122**: 895–907.

Pielsticker A, Haag G, Zaudig M, Lautenbacher S (2005). Impairment of pain inhibition in chronic tension-type headache. *Pain* **118**: 215–223.

Porreca F, Ossipov MH, Gebhart GF (2002). Chronic pain and medullary descending facilitation. *Trends in Neurosciences* **25**: 319–25.

Price DD (2000). Psychological and Neural Mechanisms of the Affective Dimension of Pain. *Science* **288**(5472): 1769–1772.

Rahman W, Bauer CS, Bannister K, Vonsy JL, Dolphin AC, Dickenson AH (2009). Descending serotonergic facilitation and the antinociceptive effects of pregabalin in a rat model of osteoarthritic pain. *Molecular Pain* **5**: 45.

Rainero I, Rubino E, Gallone S, Fenoglio P, Picci LR, Giobbe L, Ostacoli L, Pinessi L (2011). Evidence for an association between migraine and the hypocretin receptor 1 gene. *Journal of Headache and Pain* **12**: 193–9.

Reichling DB, Levine JD (2009). Critical role of nociceptor plasticity in chronic pain. *Trends in Neurosciences* **32**: 611–8.

Sakurai T, Amemiya A, Ishii M, Matsuzaki I, Chemelli RM, Tanaka H, Williams SC, Richardson JA, Kozlowski GP, Wilson S, Arch JR., Buckingham RE, Haynes AC, Carr SA, Annan RS, McNulty DE, Liu W-S, Terrett JA, Elshourbagy NA, Bergsma DJ, Yanagisawa M (1998). Orexins and Orexin Receptors: A Family of Hypothalamic Neuropeptides and G Protein-Coupled Receptors that Regulate Feeding Behavior. *Cell* **92**: 573–585.

Sandrini G, Rossi P, Milanov I, Serrao M, Cecchini AP, Nappi G (2006). Abnormal modulatory influence of diffuse noxious inhibitory controls in migraine and chronic tension-type headache patients. *Cephalalgia* **26**: 782–789.

Sarchielli P, Rainero I, Coppola F, Rossi C, Mancini M, Pinessi L, Calabresi P (2008). Involvement of corticotrophin-releasing factor and orexin-A in chronic migraine and medication-overuse headache: findings from cerebrospinal fluid. *Cephalalgia* **28**: 714–22.

Sasaki M, Obata H, Kawahara K, Saito S, Goto F (2006). Peripheral 5-HT2A receptor antagonism attenuates primary thermal hyperalgesia and secondary mechanical allodynia after thermal injury in rats. *Pain* **122**: 130–136.

Schoonman GG, van der Grond J, Kortmann C, van der Geest RJ, Terwindt GM, Ferrari MD (2008). Migraine headache is not associated with cerebral or meningeal vasodilatation – a 3T magnetic resonance angiography study. *Brain* **131**: 2192–200.

Serrao M, Rossi P, Sandrini G, Parisi L, Amabile GA, Nappi G, Pierelli F (2004). Effects of diffuse noxious inhibitory controls on temporal summation of the RIII reflex in humans. *Pain* **112**: 353–60.

Sikandar S, Bannister K, Dickenson AH (2012). Brainstem facilitations and descending serotonergic controls contribute to visceral nociception but not pregabalin analgesia in rats. *Neuroscience Letters* **519**: 31–36.

Silberstein SD (2013). Emerging target-based paradigms to prevent and treat migraine. *Clinical Pharmacology & Therapeutics* **93**: 78–85.

Sprenger T, Goadsby PJ (2010). What has functional neuroimaging done for primary headache … and for the clinical neurologist? *Journal of Clinical Neuroscience* **17**: 547–53.

Sun H, Dodick DW, Silberstein S, Goadsby PJ, Reuter U, Ashina M, Saper J, Cady R, Chon Y, Dietrich J, Lenz R (2016). Safety and efficacy of AMG 334 for prevention of episodic migraine: a randomised, double-blind, placebo-controlled, phase 2 trial. *Lancet Neurology* **15**: 382–90.

Sun-Edelstein C, Rapoport AM (2016). Update on the Pharmacological Treatment of Chronic Migraine. *Current Pain and Headache Reports* **20**: 6.

Suzuki R, Rygh LJ, Dickenson AH (2004). Bad news from the brain: descending 5-HT pathways that control spinal pain processing. *Trends in Pharmacological Sciences* **25**: 613–617.

Takemura M, Sugiyo S, Moritani M, Kobayashi M, Yonehara N (2006). Mechanisms of orofacial pain control in the central nervous system. *Archives of Histology and Cytology* **69**: 79–100.

Teepker M, Kunz M, Peters M, Kundermann B, Schepelmann K, Lautenbacher S (2014). Endogenous pain inhibition during menstrual cycle in migraine. *European Journal of Pain* **18**: 989–998.

Tepper SJ (2012). Medication-overuse headache. *Continuum (Minneapolis, Minn)* **18**: 807–822.

Villanueva L, Le Bars D (1995). The activation of bulbo-spinal controls by peripheral nociceptive inputs: diffuse noxious inhibitory controls. *Biological Research* **28**: 113–25.

Wei F, Dubner R, Zou S, Ren K, Bai G, Wei D, Guo W (2010). Molecular depletion of descending serotonin unmasks its novel facilitatory role in the development of persistent pain. *Journal of Neuroscience* **30**: 8624–8636.

Weiller C, May A, Limmroth V, Jüptner M, Kaube H, Schayck R V, Coenen HH, Diener HC (1995). Brain stem activation in spontaneous human migraine attacks. *Nature Medicine* **1**: 658–60.

Winkler CW, Hermes SM, Chavkin CI, Drake CT, Morrison SF, Aicher SA (2006). Kappa opioid receptor (KOR) and GAD67 immunoreactivity are found in OFF and NEUTRAL cells in the rostral ventromedial medulla. *Journal of Neurophysiology* **96**: 3465–3473.

Yamamoto T, Nozaki-Taguchi N, Chiba T (2002). Analgesic effect of intrathecally administered orexin-A in the rat formalin test and in the rat hot plate test. *British Journal of Pharmacology* **137**: 170–6.

Yarnitsky D (2010). Conditioned pain modulation (the diffuse noxious inhibitory control-like effect): its relevance for acute and chronic pain states. *Current Opinion in Anesthesiology* **23**: 611–5.

Yarnitsky D, Crispel Y, Eisenberg E, Granovsky Y, Ben-Nun A, Sprecher E, Best LA, Granot M (2008). Prediction of chronic post-operative pain: pre-operative DNIC testing identifies patients at risk. *Pain* **138**: 22–28.

Zhang Y, Zhao S, Rodriguez E, Takatoh J, Han BX, Zhou X, Wang F (2015). Identifying local and descending inputs for primary sensory neurons. *Journal of Clinical Investigation* **125**: 3782–3794.

9

Triptans to calcitonin gene-related peptide modulators – small molecules to antibodies – the evolution of a new migraine drug class

Richard J. Hargreaves

Biogen, Cambridge, Massachusetts, USA

9.1   Introduction

Migraine is an heterogeneous disorder that affects 12–15% of the population [1]. Individual migraineurs try many different classes of compounds in order to find the drug that best ameliorates their migraine headaches. Over-the-counter analgesics provide benefit for some patients, but many still experience more severe or frequent migraine attacks that are ineffectively treated, leading them to prescription medicines for the acute treatment and prevention of migraines [2].

The serotonin 5-HT$_{1B/1D}$ receptor agonist drug class (Triptans) revolutionized the acute treatment of migraine. However, many migraine patients, especially those with co-existing cardiovascular risk factors, hesitated to take Triptans because of cardiovascular and cerebrovascular concerns [3] that the 5-HT1B receptor component in their pharmacology caused vasoconstriction, and the theoretical risk that the Triptans potentiate serotonin in the brain, causing serotonin syndrome. Reviews of clinical experience have, however, found that cardiovascular events, while present, are relatively rare [4], and there is inadequate evidence data to determine the real risk of serotonin syndrome [5].

It is estimated that 40% of migraine sufferers could benefit from prophylactic therapy, but only 13% are taking existing therapies. This is perhaps because currently approved preventative treatments have modest efficacy, and are often associated with safety or tolerability issues. Onabotulinum toxin A is the only drug approved to treat chronic migraine [6, 7].

Thus, there remains a large unmet medical need for migraineurs, and a need to have new classes of acute treatment and preventative anti-migraine drugs. This chapter discusses the evolution of the CGRP modulatory class of drugs that offers a unique solution for migraine patients.

9.2   Trigeminovascular system – migraine physiology and pharmacology

The pharmacology and physiology of the trigeminovascular systems that are activated during migraine pain, and the role of central pathways in modulating activity in the

Neurobiological Basis of Migraine, First Edition. Edited by Turgay Dalkara and Michael A. Moskowitz.
© 2017 John Wiley & Sons, Inc. Published 2017 by John Wiley & Sons, Inc.

trigeminal dorsal horn, are now well understood [8–11]. The sensory neuropeptide calcitonin gene-related peptide (CGRP) is a 37 amino acid peptide that exerts its biological action through activation of the CGRP receptor, a member of the family B G-protein-coupled receptors.

CGRP has been implicated strongly in the pathogenesis of migraine [12], and the journey to establish CGRP as a migraine target has recently been reviewed by Edvinsson, one of the pioneers in the field of neuropeptide research [13]. Intravenous infusion of human CGRP peptide induces migraine-like headache in migraineurs. It has been documented that CGRP levels are elevated in saliva, cerebrospinal fluid, and blood in the external jugular vein during migraine attacks. Moreover, elevated jugular vein blood CGRP levels have been reported to be normalized by Triptan treatment concomitant with migraine headache relief. Recent investigations have also provided some evidence that CGRP levels are elevated inter-ictally in migraineurs, raising the interesting possibility that the trigeminovascular system in patients could be "primed" to respond at a lower threshold than those individuals who do not suffer attacks [14, 15].

CGRP containing nerve fibers and CGRP receptors are widely distributed through the trigeminovascular sensory system, and are present peripherally in the pain-producing meningeal tissues on blood vessels, on trigeminal neurons, and centrally on neurons in the trigeminal dorsal horn pain signal relay centers of the brainstem. The physiological actions of CGRP include vasodilatation, trigeminal sensitization and activation of second order sensory neurons in the brain stem, as part of trigeminal sensory pain signal transmission [16, 17].

CGRP is released alongside substance P and glutamate when sensory nerves are activated. Seminal studies from the laboratories of Moskowitz [18] and Goadsby and Edvinsson [19, 20] have showed pre-clinically that the anti-migraine agents dihydroergotamine and sumatriptan attenuated elevated levels of CGRP in the saggital sinus and jugular vein plasma during electrical stimulation of the trigeminal ganglion and superior saggital sinus, respectively. Similarly, sumatriptan was also shown to reduce meningeal extravasation, mediated by substance P acting at neurokinin 1 receptors, evoked by electrical trigeminal ganglion stimulation [21]. This effect, on a proven biomarker of sensory nerve activation, has given further support to the peripheral trigeminal inhibitory effects of the serotonin agonist class.

Subsequent pharmacological studies focused on modulation of CGRP release in the meninges by the Triptan acute anti-migraine agents. Williamson, in the Merck Research Laboratories, developed an intra-vital microscopy model [22] to monitor meningeal blood vessel diameter in response to electrical stimulation of the dura mater [23]. In an elegant series of preclinical studies, he showed first that the vasodilatation was mediated exclusively by CGRP release from trigeminal sensory afferents as it was blocked by the antagonist peptide CGRP8-7 fragment, but not by a substance P receptor antagonist. Next, he showed that sumatriptan and rizatriptan inhibited electrically evoked vasodilatation, but not vasodilatation caused by exogenous administration of substance P or CGRP, proving that their mode of action was on trigeminal sensory nerve terminals to inhibit neuropeptide release [24, 25]. Subsequent, immuno-histochemical and preclinical pharmacological studies from the Merck labs supported the hypothesis that the inhibition of sensory neuropeptide release by Triptans in the meninges was likely to be mediated through activation of 5-HT1D receptors on trigeminal sensory nerve endings, and not the 5-HT1B receptors that predominated on blood vessels [26, 27].

In the late 1990s, Cumberbatch and Williamson [28] used the intravital meningeal microscopy technique, with electrophysiology recordings of second order sensory neurons in the trigeminal nucleus caudalis, to investigate whether circulating CGRP acting peripherally on a chronically sensitized trigeminal system could influence susceptibility to a migraine headache attack. In these experiments, they showed that exogenous intravenous administration of a 1 µg/kg bolus (at a concentration of 1 µg/ml) of CGRP (tracked using intravital microscopy of dilated meningeal blood vessels) could sensitize the trigeminal system, such that the responses to non-nociceptive sensory inputs (evoked by vibrissal stimulation) to convergent second order sensory neurons in the brain stem that received convergent sensory input from the dura became exaggerated. This enhanced response was blocked by a 5-HT1B/1D "triptan" agonist molecule.

At the time, it was suggested that these data supported the hypothesis that vasodilation in the meninges is capable of sensitizing the trigeminal system. However, subsequent research has suggested other potential explanations. First, there is no doubt that CGRP released or applied centrally will activate trigeminal neurons – the question is, can CGRP access its central receptors from the periphery? CGRP is a large polar peptide that is excluded from the brain by the blood-brain barrier, so it seems unlikely that it penetrates to central CGRP receptors to exert sensitizing effects. Second, it is known that there is no blood-brain barrier at the level of the trigeminal ganglion or peripheral cranial blood vessels, raising the possibility that the exogenous CGRP acts directly in the periphery to cause sensitization through activation of CGRP receptors on trigeminal neuronal cell bodies or perivascular trigeminal sensory nerves [29, 30].

A peripheral role for CGRP in migraine would be consistent with the trigeminal inhibitory action of clinically effective 5-HT1B/1D agonist Triptan molecules, and the observation that CGRP receptor antagonists that do not penetrate the brain give migraine headache pain relief (see below Section 5). To date, however, there is no direct evidence showing that CGRP does, or does not, activate trigeminal neurons, nor whether the observed effects of CGRP on trigeminal sensitivity are direct or indirect. These are areas for future study, especially as there are marked temporal differences in the effects seen in these short pre-clinical experiments, compared to the time taken for exogenous CGRP to trigger migraine in humans [31, 32].

9.3   Small molecule CGRP receptor antagonists

Understanding the pharmacology of trigeminal inhibition by the serotonin 5-HT$_{1B/1D/1F}$ receptor Triptan agonists that underpins their remarkable clinical efficacy [33], together with the lack of clinical efficacy of substance P neurokinin-1 receptor antagonists [34, 35], confirmed the pre-clinical and clinical physiological studies identifying CGRP, not substance P, as the critical sensory neuropeptide involved in migraine pain pathophysiology [36]. In addition to the promise of clinical efficacy, one of the great attractions of the CGRP modulatory approach was that it has the potential to avoid the cardiovascular risk associated with the Triptan class of drugs. Unlike the Triptans, CGRP antagonism is neutral on the vasculature in the absence of CGRP tone [37]. CGRP modulation thus held the promise of delivering a therapy that could be safe to use in migraine patients with Triptan contraindications (previous myocardial infarction, angina or stroke). These observations have provided the catalyst for many CGRP modulator drug discovery and development programs.

Pre-clinical studies *in vitro* in human coronary arteries [38, 39], and *in vivo* in cardiac physiology and models of myocardial ischemia [40] and chronic heart failure [41], showed that CGRP antagonism had no intrinsic action on cardiac vascular smooth muscle. Moreover, CGRP antagonism, unlike sumatriptan, had no effect on payback myocardial reactive hyperemic responses in conscious dogs [42]. It is noteworthy that the prototype serotonin 5-HT 1B/1D agonist sumatriptan also increased the severity of myocardial ischemia during atrial pacing in dogs with coronary artery stenosis [43].

Clinical studies with telcagepant (MK-0974) showed that it had no effect on spontaneous ischemia in cardiovascular patients [44], did not affect exercise time in patients with stable angina [45], did not affect nitroglycerin-induced vasodilatation in healthy men [46], nor have a hemodynamic interaction with sumatriptan [47]. A partially completed study of telcagepant in patients with migraine and stable coronary artery disease also supported the safety of the CGRP receptor antagonist mechanism [48].

The clinical efficacy of the small molecule CGRP receptor antagonists acutely against migraine has provided unequivocal support for the hypothesis that CGRP is a key player in migraine pathophysiology. To date, five different small molecule CGRP receptor antagonists have been tested for the acute treatment of migraine, and all have been shown to be effective (BIBN4096BS [49], MK-0974 [50], MK-3207 [51] BMS927711 [52], BI-44370TA [53].

The most extensively studied molecule to data is telcagepant [54], which today, through new publications, despite its discontinuation, continues to provide important insights into migraine mechanisms and the potential benefits and limitations of CGRP modulation for the treatment of migraine. In addition to acute migraine treatment, telcagepant has been studied with chronic daily dosing for migraine prevention [55] and seven days of dosing peri-menstrually for menstrual migraine [56]. The prevention studies showed similar efficacy, but with much improved tolerability to topiramate (as judged by comparison to a separate but similarly designed clinical trial of topiramate) and a reduction of peri-menstrual headaches (note: primary endpoint of monthly headache days was not significant with this dose regimen).

How, then, does the clinical efficacy of CGRP receptor antagonists in acute migraine compare to the Triptans that are now the current standard of care? Direct comparative randomized clinical trials of small molecule CGRP antagonists with the Triptans are very scarce. The only published studies to date have compared telcagepant with rizatriptan 10 mg [57] and zolmitriptan 5 mg [58] in acute migraine treatment, and have shown similar efficacy on the two-hour pain-free endpoint, but with markedly improved tolerability profile.

Tfelt-Hansen has, however, commented, on the basis of a "meta-analysis" of all CGRP antagonist trials, that the CGRP mechanism may be inferior in efficacy to the Triptans [59–61]. In a subsequent commentary on Triptans versus small molecule CGRP receptor antagonists Pascual, like Tfelt-Hansen, argued that there may be an inherent limit to the response one can expect from CGRP receptor antagonists [62], and that a meta-analysis of all "gepant" clinical trials suggests that the maximal acute anti-migraine efficacy of the small molecule CGRP receptor antagonists, as judged by the two-hour pain-free endpoint, is still "somewhat inferior to that of the most efficacious Triptans". These viewpoints were, however, countered by Ho and Bigal [63, 64] who suggested that the conclusions undervalued the potential usefulness of a new drug class with novel mechanism of action and the potential to help many patients with unmet medical needs.

9.4 Current status of small molecule CGRP receptor antagonist programs

Unfortunately, several of the small molecule CGRP receptor antagonists in development have been discontinued for safety, due to evidence of drug induced liver injury. Despite their structural chemical diversity, telcagepant (MK-0974) and MK-3207 showed increases in liver enzyme (ALT) levels several times the upper limit of normal and, with MK-3207, delayed liver-test abnormalities [51, 55, 56]. It should be noted that, with telcagepant, these effects were not seen during intermittent use for the acute treatment of migraine [65], but only after chronic or intensive use for migraine prevention or menstrual migraine. BI-44370 TA was also discontinued, but there has been speculation (but no formal reports) of whether this was also due to hepatotoxicity. These liver toxicity data has raised questions over whether the CGRP receptor blocking mechanism was inherently flawed as a therapeutic approach. However, the diverse presentation of the liver injury caused by the different CGRP molecules suggested that the hepatotoxicity could be due to the specific chemistry of each of these molecules.

In Merck, despite the setbacks, belief that the liver toxicity was structural, and not mechanism-based, drove the continuation of the CGRP receptor antagonist drug discovery programs, which eventually yielded the novel small molecule drug candidates MK-1602 (which has been evaluated in Phase 2 studies for acute migraine treatment) and MK-8031 (a candidate for phase 2 trials in migraine prevention). MK-1602 was shown on www.clinicalTrials.gov in 2012 to have enrolled 834 patients, and to have completed a dose-finding study in acute migraine treatment, using dosages of 1, 10, 25, 50 or 100 mg doses [66]. The results of this study have now been published [67].

The Merck CGRP antagonist small molecules have been licensed to Allergan/Pfizer who, it can only be assumed, evaluated the extent of hepatic de-risking as part of their diligence before making such a significant investment, and who will, no doubt, monitor liver function intensively in upcoming chronic dosing trials. The perception that drug-induced liver injury may be a predictable class effect of small molecule CGRP receptor antagonists persists, however, with a recent editorial from Gottshalk continuing to highlight potential mechanisms of liver toxicity [68]. This concern has, however, now been definitively addressed by long-term data from clinical studies, with the CGRP receptor blocking antibody AMG-334 after 52 weeks [69] where no liver abnormalities have been observed.

The relatively benign safety profile of AMG-334 [70] gives additional support for the suggestion that the drug-induced liver injury seen with the early CGRP receptor antagonists was molecule-based, not mechanism-based. These additional safety data were probably important in TEVA's decision to partner with Heptares on the development of small molecule CGRP receptor antagonists [71], in a strategic move into acute migraine treatment that is complimentary to TEV48125, their monoclonal antibody (see below), which is in Phase 3 clinical trials for migraine prevention.

The Triptan market for oral acute treatment of migraine will essentially be generic by the time a small molecule CGRP antagonist is launched. The CGRP mechanism is clearly differentiated from Triptans on the basis of improved tolerability and safety profile, as it is a non-vasoconstrictor non-serotonergic mechanism that will not have lingering concerns over cardiovascular side-effect liability and serotonin syndrome. To maximize success, it will be key to consider strategies to differentiate the efficacy, in addition to tolerability and safety, of the CGRP antagonist MK-1602 from the Triptans. These may include improvement over the 24-hour Triptan sustained efficacy profile, as well as use by Triptan non-responders and efficacy in Triptan-excluded populations.

Other acute anti-migraine approaches are now entering Phase 3 clinical trials. CoLucid Pharmaceutical's non-vasoconstrictor centrally acting serotonin 5-HT1F receptor selective agonist Lasmiditan faces a similar challenge to CGRP antagonism in differentiating from the Triptan class through efficacy, as well as CNS tolerability [72]. As a centrally acting serotonergic agonist it may, like the Triptans, have to address the issue of CNS serotonin syndrome. The development of small molecule orally administered CGRP receptor antagonists such as MK-8031 for migraine prevention has the potential to provide an alternative to current prophylactic medications, with flexibility in dosing compared to CGRP, modulating anti-body infusions or injections (see below). Thorough de-risking and monitoring for hepatic liability will no doubt have to be a feature of long-term exposure in prevention clinical trials.

9.5 Unraveling the site of action of small molecule CGRP receptor antagonists using clinical pharmacology and brain imaging

As with so many aspects of medical science, definitive clinical observations drive our interpretation and re-evaluation of experimental laboratory investigations that, in turn, generate new hypotheses for study. Let us consider how this cycle has played out for the CGRP modulator class.

CGRP receptors are distributed peripherally and centrally in the trigeminovascular system. Two important clinical pharmacodynamic assays were developed to assess the pharmacology of CGRP receptor antagonism and the relative roles of peripheral and central CGRP receptors in the anti-migraine therapeutic response to small molecule CGRP receptor antagonists. The first was the capsaicin-induced dermal vasodilatation assay (CIDV), in which capsaicin, applied to the intact forearm skin, triggers release of CGRP via activation of the TRPV1 receptor on sensory nerve fibers and, in turn, causes vasodilatation through its effects on CGRP receptors on blood vessels [73–75]. This response can be measured with laser Doppler, and its inhibition provides a measure of CGRP antagonism in the periphery. The second assay was enabled by the development of a novel PET imaging tracer, [^{11}C]MK-4232, as a key pharmacological tool to visualize CGRP receptors in the brain. This tracer, which is highly specific for CGRP receptors, was used to determine whether a small molecule CGRP antagonist, telcagepant (MK-0974), engaged central CGRP receptor sites at clinically effective anti-migraine doses [76].

The PET data, together with CIDV-based estimates of the peripheral activity of CGRP receptor antagonists, showed that small molecule CGRP receptor antagonists that effectively saturated (>90% inhibition) peripheral responses, but did not engage central sites at and significantly above clinically effective anti-migraine doses, could relieve migraine pain [77, 78]. This observation had three potentially important implications for our understanding of migraine pain:

- First, that migraine pain is, at least in part, peripheral in origin, since non-brain penetrant drugs could relieve it.
- Second that, as a consequence, it was likely that the key site of action for the Triptans was most probably trigeminal inhibition, with consequent prevention of CGRP release in the periphery, not centrally – despite the fact that the adverse event profile of Triptans showed evidence for some CNS effects.
- Third, preliminary case reports of $[^{11}C]$MK-4232 PET studies of the occupancy of central CGRP receptors by telcagepant (MK-0974), between and during migraine attacks, showed no evidence for increased occupancy by telcagepant during an attack, suggesting that the blood-brain barrier remains intact during migraine, and does not allow drug entry to CNS target sites [79].

It remains unknown whether accessing central sites will deliver greater efficacy as today's CGRP modulator drugs are generally excluded from reaching therapeutic levels in the brain.

9.6 Biologic approaches to CGRP modulation

Concerns over the hepatotoxic liability of small molecule CGRP receptor antagonists, and the demonstration that peripherally restricted molecules were clinically efficacious against acute and chronic migraine, has added huge impetus to the development of biologic antibody approaches to CGRP modulation as potential migraine therapeutics. This area has been intensely reviewed in the recent literature [see 80, 81, 82, 83, 84, 85].

9.6.1 Early experimental studies with CGRP antibodies

In the late 1980s, immuno-neutralization studies with CGRP antisera conducted in Graham Dockray's laboratory highlighted the central role of the of CGRP in neurogenic inflammation [86–88]. Subsequently, in 1993–1995, Keith Tan conducted immune-blockade studies *in vitro* and *in vivo* with an anti-calcitonin gene-related peptide monoclonal antibody and its Fab' fragment in the Merck Research Laboratories at Terling's Park in the UK. His *in vitro* experiments [89] first selected antibody candidates that could block the neurotransmitter role of CGRP *in vitro*, and these were then subsequently examined *in vivo* [90] for their ability to inhibit skin vasodilatation evoked by CGRP released from sensory nerve fibers as a result of anti-dromic stimulation of the saphenous nerve.

This assay has similar pharmacology to the activation of sensory nerves and consequent CGRP release thought to occur in migraine, and to the capsaicin-induced dermal vasodilatation studies that were more recently used to study the peripheral pharmacodynamic modulation of CGRP clinically by small molecule and CGRP antibodies. Tan's *in vivo* studies showed that a Fab' CGRP antibody fragment was most active, producing a blockade of vasodilatation equivalent to that produced by the CGRP receptor peptide antagonist $CGRP_{8-37}$, whereas the full-length CGRP mAb was inactive over the short time course of his experiments.

These findings proved that neutralizing approaches could be used to modulate the peripheral activity of the CGRP peptide and, interestingly, that the size of the biologic agent could affect the time-course of pharmacological activity, presumably by differential rate of access to the high levels of CGRP released into the synaptic cleft during the short acute time course (30 minutes) of these experiments. This pharmacodynamic observation indicated that full-length CGRP mAbs would be unlikely to have value in acute, compared to chronic, settings where there is more time for equilibration, allowing them to realize their pharmacological effects. This interpretation aligns with the investigation of CGRP mAbs for chronic migraine prevention, rather than acute migraine reversal.

9.6.2 CGRP antibody therapeutics

Antibody drug administration is invasive, being either subcutaneous or intravenous and, as such, they are not well suited to frequent administration – for example, as acute symptomatic therapies, where small molecules are generally preferred especially when speed of onset is important.

Antibody drugs, however, have several important advantages over small molecule drug candidates, especially in chronic indications:

1) They have long-circulating plasma half lives leading to monthly/infrequent administration improving adherence.
2) Unlike small molecules, they lack active metabolites, as they are not degraded in the liver.
3) As antibodies are not hepatically metabolized, they have no metabolic drug-drug interactions to contend with.
4) Their exquisite target selectivity minimizes off-target pharmacology, leading to low toxicity and relatively benign tolerability profiles.

There are currently four CGRP antibody drug candidates that have shown efficacy in the prevention of frequent episodic migraine. These are the CGRP ligand neutralizing antibodies TEV48125 (previously Labrys LBR-101) [91], LY2951742 [92] and ALD-403 [93], and the CGRP receptor antibody AMG-334 [70]. TEV48125 has completed and published successful Phase 2B clinical trials in chronic migraine, using SC monthly administration [94]. Positive topline Phase 2B results were also recently released by Alder for ALD-403, given IV quarterly in chronic migraine [95]. The other antibody candidates have included the chronic migraine indication in their Phase 3 clinical programs. LY 2951742 is the only candidate currently in Phase 3 clinical trials for the treatment of episodic [96] and chronic cluster headache [97].

TEV48125 was discovered at Rinat as RN-307, and was subsequently transferred to Pfizer in a 2006 buyout of the company, before being spun out from Pfizer to Labrys, where it became LBR101. Teva acquired LBR101 in a 2014 buyout of Labrys, after it had completed only Phase 1 clinical studies, reflecting their confidence in the mechanism delivering meaningful efficacy. In an interesting approach, Arteus, a biotech funded by Atlas Ventures and Orbimed, licensed the Eli Lilly program for LY2951742 and obtained clinical proof of concept for migraine prevention, resulting in Lilly exercising their option to take the drug back for late stage development. In contrast, ALD-403 and AMG-334 have been discovered and developed by their parent companies Alder Pharmaceuticals and Amgen, respectively.

9.6.3 Comparing the CGRP modulators clinically

The latest disclosed clinical data for the four antibody candidates confirm their efficacy in preventing frequent episodic migraine [70, 91–93]. To date, only Alder have studied intravenous administration in frequent episodic and chronic migraine with quarterly administration [93, 95] and only Teva have successfully completed Phase 2B trials SC with monthly dosing in chronic migraine [97].

It is too early to tell which of the antibodies will have the best clinical efficacy profile, as the clinical trials for each are different, which makes true comparisons between them impossible. Factors to watch out for when comparing the emerging efficacy profiles of the CGRP antibodies are summarized in Table 9.1. It is also worthwhile remembering that the clinical efficacy data for all the antibodies uses placebo-adjusted responses in migraine day reductions, and this is that this is effectively a "double delta" readout, with subtraction first from baseline headache days and then from placebo.

Table 9.1 Factors to consider when comparing clinical trials with CGRP antibodies.

Mechanism	CGRP ligand neutralizing vs. CGRP receptor neutralizing Differences in tolerability and safety profiles
Dosing route	Intravenous vs. subcutaneous – monthly or quarterly • How frequent – how many injections to deliver active doses
Headache definitions	Frequent episodic migraine and chronic migraine ICDH-2 or ICDH3 • Migraine days vs. headache days
Severity	Baseline number of migraine days at entry • Important for hyper-responder analyses
Study periods	Lead-in and baseline periods, long-term data • Potential to affect placebo and drug response, long term efficacy
Inclusion criteria	Baseline headache days • More or less severe migraine population being treated • Use of standard preventatives
Exclusion Criteria	Previous use of anti-CGRP antibodies or Botox – common • Lack of response to preventatives, limited exposure to opiates and barbiturates
Concomitant medications	Use of rescue and other prophylaxis medications • Clinical trial restrictions vs. likely real life scenarios
Placebo	Size and variability of placebo response • Use of non-placebo adjusted response data to describe trial outcomes
Response	Reduction in moderate to severe migraine days • Reduction in migraine hours • Responder rate • Reduction in use of preventative medications
Hyper-responders	Contribution of hyper-responders to overall clinical benefit • Response data without patients with > 75% and 100% reduction in migraine days

Perhaps the most remarkable finding in the clinical trials of all the CGRP anti-bodies has been evidence for a significant number of migraine patients who are hyper-responders to prolonged CGRP modulation. In these trials, some patients have had an unprecedented drop of > 75% in their migraine headache days or, amazingly, complete resolution of their migraine headache attacks. Interestingly, too, recent data from Lilly suggests that the onset of action of LY2951742 is as early as one week after dosing [98], and treated patients meeting < 50% response criteria after one month could go on to continue their improvement in subsequent months, with a proportion becoming hyper-responders [99].

Data with AMG334 also showed a significant percentage of hyper-responders. Company communications [100] have reported that 62% of the AMG334 patients demonstrated a greater than 50% reduction in migraine days after monthly treatment for 52 weeks, with 38% getting a 75% or better response and one in five declaring that they were free of migraines. We need now to do more research to deconstruct migraine and the characteristics of the patients in the clinical trials in order to understand the reasons underlying these hyper-responders further.

It remains to be proved whether the three CGRP neutralizing anti-bodies (TEV48125, LY2951742 and ALD-403) are more similar than different. It is worth remembering that, for the CGRP ligand antibodies, the doses required for efficacy will be a product of the drug concentration needed to give sustained neutralization of CGRP and the clearance rate, or plasma half-life, of the antibody-ligand conjugate. For the neutralizing antibodies, it is therefore differences in half-life and bioavailability by SC or IM routes, rather than affinity for CGRP (as all are reported to have similarly high binding, despite never having been tested head-to-head) that will be the key to dose, duration of action and dosing intervals.

Other key differentiators may ultimately relate to their pharmaceutical, rather than pharmacological, properties (viscosity, needle size required for delivery, and suitability for novel delivery devices) that drive the ability to deliver the drug in different formats, IV versus SC/IM and, consequently, whether quarterly, as well as monthly dosing, is possible to pursue. In contrast, the clinical pharmacodynamic profile of the CGRP receptor anti-body AMG-334 may well differ, due to its alternative mechanism of action. For the CGRP receptor antibody, duration of action will be a function of the dose required to sustain blocking concentrations above the turnover rate of the drug-CGRP receptor complex, and this is likely to differ from the plasma half-life of the drug itself. The turnover rate of the CGRP receptor complex is currently unknown, but higher doses of AMG-334 than those studied to date may be required to saturate this CGRP receptor turnover process and give improved efficacy. Similar to the neutralizing antibodies, the pharmaceutical properties of the antibody will also be important for dosing and delivery.

It is a rare and exciting time for patients to have four novel antibody therapeutics directed at the same pathophysiology and therapeutic indication competing for a first-to-market advantage. The race is now on for the three CGRP ligand-neutralizing antibodies TEV48125, LY2951742 and ALD-403, which will attempt to differentiate themselves from one another and the CGRP receptor antibody AMG-334 in late phase clinical trials. From public company disclosures, it is very likely that, in 2016–2017, all the mAbs will be in the midst of Phase 3 clinical trials in frequent episodic and chronic migraine using SC monthly dosing regimens and, additionally, will be exploring the possibility of dosing every three months on a quarterly schedule. To date, only ALD403 is being developed for the IV route with quarterly administration. On these timelines, it is conceivable that these molecules could be filed and launched in 2018–2019.

9.6.4 Safety and tolerability of the CGRP antibodies

The consequences of long-term CGRP system blockade were previously unknown but, to date, all four CGRP antibodies look generally safe and well tolerated [70, 91–94]. The final profiles await the outcome of longer-term studies, with greater numbers of patients, to see whether there are differences between the CGRP-ligand neutralizing and CGRP receptor antibodies. To date, there is no evidence for the hepatotoxicity liability that was seen with small molecule CGRP antagonists in chronic daily use, indicating that this adverse safety finding was, indeed, most likely to have been molecule-based and not mechanism-based in nature. Moreover, there is no evidence for the cardiovascular adverse effects, whose specter plagued the Triptan drug class [101].

Notably, the unremarkable 12-month open label extension safety data recently released by AMGEN on their CGRP receptor antibody AMG334 [100] given at 70 mg, was very reassuring for the prospects of all the Phase 3 trials, given that it has a similar mode of action to the receptor blocking small molecule antagonists. In the Phase 3 studies it will be important to watch for signals of immunogenicity, and the presence of neutralizing and anti-drug antibodies that could underlie increased clearance or inactivation of the therapeutic antibody, leading to inefficacy. These properties may vary between the CGRP ligand and receptor antibody candidates since, for circulating peptides such as CGRP, rather than receptors that are not shed into the circulation, neutralizing antibodies may well exist before drug administration. In Phase 2 studies reported to date, if anti-drug antibodies have been found, then these were detectable before drug administration and did not generally increase in titer significantly after exposure – but more data is required from optimized immunoassays run on larger numbers of samples from the Phase 3 trials.

9.7 Summary and conclusion

It is now 25 years since the discovery of the Triptans, the last new class of drugs to advance the treatment of migraine headaches. The physiological and clinical pharmacological evidence implicating CGRP in the trigeminovascular system in migraine pain is now proven. The need for better migraine preventative agents has long been unsatisfied, as inefficacy and lack of tolerability drive poor adherence to therapy [102, 103].

The journal *Science* recently featured CGRP as the molecule at the heart of migraine science [104]. CGRP modulators have the potential to provide differentiated, effective and improved therapy for acute migraine treatment and prevention of frequent episodic and chronic migraine. The availability of injectable biologics and small molecule oral CGRP modulators will provide flexible dosing options for patients, physicians and payers.

References

1 Victor TW, Hu X, Campbell JC *et al.* (2010). Migraine prevalence by age and sex in the United states: A life span study. *Cephalagia* **30**: 1065–1072.
2 Miller S and Matharu MS (2014). Migraine is underdiagnosed and undertreated. *Practitioner* **258**; 19–24.
3 Bigal ME, Golden W, Buse D *et al.* (2010). Triptan use as a function of cardiovascular risk. A population based study. *Headache* **50**: 256–263.
4 Roberto G, Raschi E, Piccinni C *et al.* (2015). Adverse cardiovascular events associated with Triptans and ergotamines for treatment of migraine: systematic review of observational studies. *Cephalagia* **35**: 118–131.
5 Evans RW, Tepper SJ, Shapiro RE *et al.* (2010). The FDA alert on serotonin syndrome with use of Triptans combined with selective serotonin reuptake inhibitors or selective serotonin-norepinephrine reuptake inhibitors: American headache society position paper. *Headache* **50**: 1089–1099.
6 Jackson JL, Cogbill E, Santana-Devial R *et al.* (2015). A comparative effectiveness meta-analysis of drugs for the prophylaxis of migraine headache. *PLoS One* **10**: e0130733.
7 Lipton RB and Silberstein SD (2015). Episodic and chronic migraine headache: breaking down barriers to optimal treatment and prevention. *Headache* **55**(Suppl. 2): 103–122.
8 Moskowitz MA (1991). The visceral organ brain: implications for the pathophysiology of vascular head pain. *Neurology* **41**: 182–186.
9 Hargreaves RJ and Shepheard SL (1999). Pathophysiology of migraine – New Insights. *Canadian Journal of Neurological Sciences* **26**(Suppl 3): S12–S19.
10 Goadsby PJ, Lipton RB and Ferrari MD (2002). Migraine: current understanding and treatment. *New England Journal of Medicine* **346**: 257–270.
11 Hargreaves RJ (1999). Receptor Pharmacology in the trigeminovascular system: A window to understanding migraine mechanism and treatment. *Seminars in Headache Management Migraine Pathophysiology* **4**: 10–15.
12 Salvatore CA and Kane SA (2011). CGRP receptor antagonists: toward a novel migraine therapy. *Current Pharmaceutical Biotechnology* **12**: 1671–1680.
13 Edvinsson L (2015). The journey to establish CGRP as a migraine target: A retrospective view. *Headache* **55**: 1249–1255.
14 Cernuda-Morolion E, Larossa D, Ramon C, Vega J, Martinez-Camblor P, Pascual J (2013). Interictal increase of CGRP levels in peripheral blood as a biomarker for chronic migraine. *Neurology* **81**: 1191–1196.
15 Silberstein SD and Edvinsson L (2013). Is CGRP a marker for chronic migraine? *Neurology* **81**: 1184–1185.
16 Hargreaves RJ (2007). New migraine and pain research. *Headache* **47**(Suppl 1): S26–S43.
17 Ho, TW, Edvinsson L and Goadsby PJ (2010). CGRP and its receptors provide new insights into migraine pathophysiology. *Nature Reviews Neurology* **6**: 573–582.
18 Buzzi MG, Carter WB, Shimizu T, Heath H, Moskowitz MA (1991). Dihydroergotomine and sumatriptan attenuate levels of CGRP in plasma in rat superior sagittal sinus during electrical stimulation of the trigeminal ganglion. *Neuropharmacology* **30**: 1193–1200.

19 Goadsby PJ and Edvinsson L (1993). The trigeminovascular system and migraine: studies characterizing cerebrovascular and neuropeptide changes seen in humans and cats. *Annals of Neurology* **33**: 48–56.

20 Knight YE, Edvinsson L and Goadsby PJ (1999). Blockade of calcitonin gene-related peptide release after superior saggital sinus stimulation in the cat: a comparison of avitriptan and CP122,288. *Neuropeptides* **33**: 41–46.

21 Buzzi MG, Moskowitz MA (1991). Evidence for 5-HT1B/1D receptors mediating the antimigraine effect of sumatriptan and dihydroergotamine. *Cephalalgia* **11**: 165–168.

22 Williamson DJ, Hargreaves RJ (2001). Neurogenic inflammation in the context of migraine. *Microscopy Research and Techniques* **53**: 167–178.

23 Williamson DJ, Hargreaves RJ, Hill RG, Shepheard SL (1997). Intravital microscope studies on the effects of neurokinin agonists and calcitonin gene-related peptide on dural vessel diameter in the anaesthetised rat. *Cephalalgia* **17**: 518–524.

24 Williamson DJ, Hargreaves RJ, Hill RG, Shepheard SL (1997). Sumatriptan inhibits neurogenic vasodilation of dural blood vessels in the anaesthetised rat – Intravital microscope studies. *Cephalalgia* **17**: 525–531.

25 Williamson DJ, Shepheard SL, Hill RG, Hargreaves RJ (1997). The novel anti-migraine agent, rizatriptan, inhibits neurogenic dural vasodilation and extravasation. *European Journal of Pharmacology* **328**: 61–64.

26 Longmore J, Shaw D, Smith D *et al*. (1997). Differential distribution of 5-HT1D and 5-HT1B-immunoireactivity within the human trigemino-cerebrovascular system: implications for the discovery of new anti-migraine drugs. *Cephalalgia* **17**: 833–842.

27 Shepheard SL, Williamson DJ, Beer MS, Hill RG, Hargreaves RJ (1997). Differential effects of 5-HT$_{1B/1D}$ receptor agonists on neurogenic dural vasodilation and plasma extravasation in anaesthetised rats. *Neuropharmacology* **36**: 525–533.

28 Cumberbatch MJ, Williamson DJ, Mason GS, Hill RG, Hargreaves RJ (1999). Dural vasodilatation causes a sensitization of rat caudal trigeminal neurones *in vivo* that is blocked by a 5-HT$_{1B/1D}$ agonist. *British Journal of Pharmacology* **126**: 1478–1486.

29 Eftekhari S and Edvinsson L (2010). Possible sites of action of the new calcitonin gene-related peptide receptor antagonists. *Therapeutic Advances in Neurological Disorders* **3**: 369–378

30 Eftekhari S, Salvatore CA, Chen TB *et al*. (2013). Trigeminal ganglion – a site of action for CGRP receptor antagonists. *Cephalalgia* **33**: 954. Program Late Abstracts (Supplement).

31 Lassen LH, Haderslev PA, Jacobsen VB *et al*. (2002). CGRP may play a causative role in migraine. *Cephalalgia* **22**: 54–61.

32 Hansen JM, Hauge AW, Olesen J and Ashina M (2010). Calcitonin gene-related peptide triggers migraine-like attacks in patients with migraine with aura. *Cephalalgia* **30**: 1179–1186.

33 Goadsby PJ and Hargreaves RJ (2000). Mechanisms of action of serotonin 5-HT1B/1D agonists: insights into migraine pathophysiology using rizatriptan. *Neurology* **55**(9 Suppl 2): S8–S14.

34 Goldstein DJ, Offen WW, Klein EG *et al*. (2001). Lanepitant an NK-1 antagonist in migraine prevention. *Cephalagia* **21**: 102–16

35 Goldstein DJ, Wang O, SAper JG *et al.* (1997). Ineffectiveness of neurokinin antagonist in acute migraine: a cross over study. *Cephalalgia* **17**: 785–790.

36 Edvinsson L, Hargreaves, R (2006). CGRP Involvement in Migraines. In: Olesen J, Goadsby PJ, Ramadan NM, Tfelt-Hansen, P, Welch KMA (eds). *The Headaches*, 3rd Edition, Chapter 31, pp. 289–299. Lippincott Williams and Wilkins, Philadelphia, PA.

37 Edvinsson L, Chan KY, Eftekhari S, *et al.* (2010). Effect of the calcitonin gene-related peptide (CGRP) receptor antagonist telcagepant in human cranial arteries. *Cephalalgia* **30**: 1233–1240.

38 Lynch JJ, Regan CP, Edvinsson L, Hargreaves RJ, Kane SA (2010). Comparison of the vasoconstrictor effects of the calcitonin gene-related peptide (CGRP) receptor antagonist telcagepant (MK-0974) and zolmitriptan in human isolated coronary arteries. *Journal of Cardiovascular Pharmacology* **55**: 518–521.

39 Chan KY, Edvinsson L, Eftekhari S *et al.* (2011). Characterization of the Calcitonin Gene-Related Peptide Receptor Antagonist Telcagepant (MK-0974) in Human Isolated Coronary Arteries. *Journal of Pharmacology and Experimental Therapeutics* **334**: 746–752.

40 Regan CP, Stump GL, Kane SA, Lynch JJ (2009). Calcitonin gene-related peptide receptor antagonism does not affect the severity of myocardial ischemia during atrial pacing in dogs with coronary artery stenosis. *Journal of Pharmacology and Experimental Therapeutics* **328**: 571–578.

41 Shen Y, Hong X, Malleee JJ *et al.* (2003). Effects of inhibition of alpha CGRP receptors on cardiac and peripheral vascular dynamics in conscious dogs with chronic heart failure. *Journal of Cardiovascular Pharmacology* **42**: 656–661.

42 Lynch JJ, Shen YT, Pittman TJ, *et al.* (2009). Effects of the prototype serotonin 5-HT (1B/1D) receptor agonist sumatriptan and calcitonin gene-related peptide (CGRP) receptor antagonist CGRP (8-37) on myocardial reactive hyperemic response in conscious dogs. *European Journal of Pharmacology* **623**: 96–102.

43 Lynch JJ, Stump GL, Kane SA, Regan CP (2009). The prototype serotonin 5-HT 1B/1D agonist sumatriptan increases the severity of myocardial ischemia during atrial pacing in dogs with coronary artery stenosis. *Journal of Cardiovascular Pharmacology* **53**: 474–479.

44 Behm MO, Blanchard RL, Murphy MG, *et al.* (2011). Effect of telcagepant on spontaneous ischemia in cardiovascular patients in a randomized study. *Headache* **51**: 954–960.

45 Chaitman BR, Ho AP, Behm MO, *et al.* (2012). A randomized, placebo-controlled study of the effects of telcagepant on exercise time in patients with stable angina. *Clinical Pharmacology & Therapeutics* **91**: 459–466.

46 Van der Schueren BJ, Blanchard R, Murphy MG *et al.* (2011). The potent calcitonin gene-related peptide receptor antagonist, telcagepant, does not affect nitroglycerin-induced vasodilation in healthy men. *British Journal of Clinical Pharmacology* **71**: 708–717.

47 Depre M, Macleod C, Palcza J *et al.* (2013). Lack of hemodynamic interaction between CGRP-receptor antagonist telcagepant (MK-0974) and sumatriptan: results from a randomized study in patients with migraine. *Cephalagia* **33**: 1292–1301.

48 Ho TW, Ho AP, Chaitman BR *et al.* (2012). Randomized, controlled study of telcagepant in patients with migraine and coronary artery disease. *Headache* **52**: 224–235.

49 Olesen J, Diener HC, Husstedt IW *et al.* (2004). Calcitonin gene-related peptide receptor antagonist BIBN 4096 BS for the acute treatment of migraine. *New England Journal of Medicine* **350**: 1104–1110.

50 Connor KM, Shapiro RE, Diener HC *et al.* (2009). Randomized controlled trial of telcagepant for the acute treatment of migraine. *Neurology* **73**: 970–977.

51 Hewitt DJ, Aurora SK, Dodick DW, *et al.* (2011). Randomized controlled trial of the CGRP receptor antagonist MK-3207 in the acute treatment of migraine. *Cephalalgia* **31**: 712–722.

52 Marcus R, Goadsby PJ, Dodick D, Stock D, Manos G, Fischer TZ (2014). BMS-927711 for the acute treatment of migraine: a double-blind, randomized, placebo controlled, dose-ranging trial. *Cephalalgia* **34**: 114–125.

53 Diener HC, Barbanti P, Dahlof C, Reuter U, Habeck J, Podhorna J (2010). BI 44370 TA, an oral CGRP antagonist for the treatment of acute migraine attacks: results from a phase II study. *Cephalalgia* **31**: 573–584.

54 Bell IM (2014). Calcitonin Gene-Related peptide receptor antagonists?: New therapeutic agents for migraine. *Journal of Medicinal Chemistry* **57**: 7838–7858.

55 Ho TW, Connor KM, Zhang Y, *et al.* (2014). Randomized controlled trial of the CGRP receptor antagonist telcagepant for migraine prevention. *Neurology* **83**: 958–66.

56 Ho TW, Ho AP, Tang G *et al.* (2016). Randomized controlled clinical trial of CGRP antagonist telcagepant for prevention of headache in women with perimenstrual migraine. *Cephalagia* **36**: 148–161.

57 Ho TW, Mannix LK, Fan X *et al.* (2008). Randomized controlled trial of an oral CGRP antagonist, MK-0974 in acute treatment of migraine. *Neurology* **70**: 1304–1312.

58 Ho TW, Ferrari MD, Dodick DW *et al.* (2008). Efficacy and tolerability of MK-0974 (telcagepant) a new oral antagonist of the calcitonin gene related peptide receptor compared with zolmitriptan for acute migraine: a randomized, placebo controlled parallel treatment trial. *Lancet* **372**: 2115–2123.

59 Tflet-Hansen P (2009). Is there an inherent limit to the efficacy of calcitonin-gene related peptide receptor antagonists in the acute treatment of migraine? A comment. *Journal of Headache and Pain* **10**: 389–391.

60 Tfelt-Hansen P (2011). Excellent tolerability but relatively low clinical efficacy of telcagepant in migraine. *Headache* **51**: 118–123.

61 Tfelt-Hansen P (2011). Optimal balance of efficacy and tolerability of oral Triptans and telcagepant: a review and a clinical comment. *Journal of Headache and Pain* **12**: 275–280.

62 Pascual J (2014). Efficacy of BMS-927711 and other gepants vs triptans: There seem to be other players beside CGRP. *Cephalagia* **34**: 1028–1029.

63 Bigal ME and Ho TW (2009). Is there an inherent limit to acute migraine treatment efficacy? *Journal of Headache and Pain* **10**; 393–394.

64 Ho TW and Bigal ME (2011). Excellent tolerability but relatively low initial clinical efficacy of telcagepant in migraine: a response. *Headache* **51**: 617–618.

65 Connor KM, Aurora SK, Loeys T *et al.* (2011). Long-term tolerability of telcagepant for acute treatment of migraine in a randomized trial. *Headache* **51**: 73–84.

66 MK-1602: https: and clinicaltrials.gov/ct2/show/NCT01613248, 2012

67 Voss T, Lipton RB, Dodick DW, Dupre N, Ge JY, Bachman R, Assaid C, Aurora SK, Michelson D (2016). A phase IIb randomized, double-blind, placebo-controlled trial of ubrogepant for the acute treatment of migraine. *Cephalalgia* **36**: 887–898.

68 Gottschalk PGH (2016). Telcagepant – almost gone, but not to be forgotten. *Cephalalgia* **36**; 103–105.

69 AMG-334: AMGEN company communication http: //www.fiercebiotech.com/story/amgens-migraine-drug-gains-momentum-crowded-race/2015-06-19

70 Sun H, Dodick DW, Silberstein S *et al.* (2016) Safety and efficacy of AMG 334 for prevention of episodic migraine; a randomized double-blind, placebo-controlled phase 2 trial. *Lancet Neurology* **15**; 382–390.

71 Heptares-Teva: (http: //www.fiercebiotech.com/story/teva-wagers-410m-heptares-migraine-program/2015-11-25

72 Reuter U, Israel H and Neeb L (2015). The pharmacological profile and clinical prospects of the oral 5-HT1F agonist lasmiditan in the acute treatment of migraine. *Therapeutic Advances in Neurological Disorders* **8**: 46–54..

73 Hershey JC, Corcoran HA, Baskin EP *et al.* (2005). Investigation of the species selectivity of a non-peptide CGRP receptor antagonist using a novel pharmacodynamic assay. *Regulatory Peptides* **127**: 71–77.

74 Buntinx L, Vermeersch S and de Hoon J (2015). Development of anti-migraine therapeutics using the capsaicin-induced dermal blood flow model. *British Journal of Clinical Pharmacology* **80**: 992–1000.

75 Sinclair SR, Kane SA, Van der Schueren BJ *et al.* (2010). Inhibition of capsaicin-induced increase in dermal blood flow by the oral CGRP receptor antagonist, telcagepant (MK-0974). *British Journal of Clinical Pharmacology* **69**: 15–22

76 Bell IM, Gallicchio SN, Stump CA *et al.* (2013). [11C]MK-4232; The first positron emission tomography tracer for the calcitonin-genrelated peptide receptor. *ACS Medicinal Chemistry Letters* **18**: 863–868.

77 Ho AP, Dahlof CG, Silberstein S *et al.* (2010). Randomized controlled trial of telcagepant over four migraine attacks. *Cephalalgia* **30**: 1443–1457.

78 Hostetler ED, Joshi AD, Sanabria-Bohórquez S *et al.* (2013) *In vivo* quantification of calcitonin gene-related peptide (CGRP) receptor occupancy by telcagepant in rhesus monkey and human brain using the positron emission tomography(PET) tracer $[^{11}C]$MK-4232. *Journal of Pharmacology and Experimental Therapeutics* **347**: 478–486.

79 Vermeersch S, De Hoon JN, De Saint-Hubert B *et al.* (2012). *PET imaging in healthy subjects and migraineurs suggests CGRP receptor antagonists do not have to act centrally to achieve clinical efficacy.* Presentation at: European Headache and Migraine Trust 3rd International Congress, London, United Kingdom, 09/20/2012.

80 Bigal ME, Walter S, Rapoport AM (2013). Calcitonin gene-related peptide (CGRP) and migraine current understanding and state of development. *Headache* **53**: 1230–1244.

81 Bigal ME, Walter S (2014). Monoclonal antibodies for migraine: preventing calcitonin gene-related peptide activity. *CNS Drugs* **28**: 389–399.

82 Diener HC, Charles A, PJ and Holle D (2015). New therapeutic approaches for the prevention and treatment of migraine. *Lancet Neurology* **14**: 1010–1022

83 Karsan N and Goadsby PJ (2015). Calcitonin gene related peptide and migraine. Current opinion in *Neurology* **28**: 250–254.

84 Edvinsson L (2015). CGRP antagonists and antibodies against CGRP and its receptor in migraine treatment. *British Journal of Clinical Pharmacology* **80**: 193–199.

85 Diener HC and Dodick DW (2016). Headache research in 2015: progress in migraine treatment. *Lancet Neurology* **15**: 4–5.

86 Louis SM, Jamihin A, Russell NJW, Dockray GJ (1989). The role of substance P and calcitonin gene related peptide in neurogenic plasma extravasation and vasodilatation in the rat. *Neuroscience* **32**: 581–586

87 Louis SM, Johnstone D, Russell *et al.* (1989). Antibodies to calcitonin gene related peptide reduce inflammation induced by topical mustard oil but not that due to carrageenan in the rat. *Neuroscience Letters* **102**; 257–260.

88 Dockray GJ, Forster ER, Louis SM *et al.* (1992). Immunoneutralization studies with calcitonin gene-related peptide. *Annals of the New York Academy of Sciences* **657**: 258–267.

89 Tan KKC, Brown MJ, Longmore *et al.* (1994). Demonstration of the neurotransmitter role of calcitonin-gene related peptide (CGRP) by immunoblockade with anti-CGRP monoclonal antibodies. *British Journal of Pharmacology* **111**: 703–710.

90 Tan K, Brown MJ, Hargreaves RJ, Shepheard SL, Cook DA, Hill RG (1995). Calcitonin gene related peptide (CGRP) as an endogenous vasodilator: immunoblockade studies *in vivo* with an anti-CGRP monoclonal antibody and its Fab fragment. *Clinical Science* **89**: 565–573.

91 Bigal ME, Dodick DW, Rapoport AM *et al.* (2015). Safety, tolerability, and efficacy of TEV-48125 for preventive treatment of high-frequency episodic migraine: a multicentre, randomised, double-blind, placebo-controlled, phase 2b study. *Lancet Neurology* **14**; 1081–1090.

92 Dodick DW, Goadsby PJ, Spierings EL, Scherer JC, Sweeney SP, Grayzel DS (2014). Safety and efficacy of LY2951742, a monoclonal antibody to calcitonin gene-related peptide, for the prevention of migraine: a phase 2, randomized double-blind, placebo-controlled study. *Lancet Neurology* **13**: 885–892

93 Dodick DW, Goadsby PJ, Silberstein SD, *et al*, for the ALD403 study investigators (2014). Safety and efficacy of ALD403, an antibody to calcitonin gene-related peptide, for the prevention of frequent episodic migraine: a randomised, double-blind, placebo-controlled, exploratory phase 2 trial. *Lancet Neurology* **13**: 1100–1107.

94 Bigal ME, Edvinsson E, Rapoport AM *et al.* (2015). Safety, tolerability, and efficacy of TEV-48125 for preventive treatment of chronic migraine: a multicentre, randomised, double-blind, placebo-controlled, phase 2b study. *Lancet Neurology* **14**: 1091–1100.

95 ALD-403 Chronic migraine: (http: //investor.alderbio.com/releasedetail.cfm? ReleaseID=962238)

96 LY 2951742 episodic cluster headache: https: //clinicaltrials.gov/ct2/show/ NCT02397473?term=LY2951742+and+cluster+headache&rank=2

97 LY 2951742 chronic cluster headache: (https: //clinicaltrials.gov/ct2/show/ NCT02438826?term=LY2951742+and+cluster+headache&rank=1)

98 Goadsby PJ, Dodick DW, Martinez J *et al*. (2015). Onset of efficacy of LY2951742 in migraine prevention. Data from a Phase2a randomized double blind placebo controlled study of a monoclonal antibody to calcitonin gene-related peptide (a post-hoc analysis). *Headache* **55**(suppl S3): 177–178.

99 Dodick DW, Goadsby PJ, Ferguson M *et al*. (2015). Sustained response outcomes from a Phase 2a randomized double blind placebo controlled study of a monoclonal antibody to calcitonin gene-related peptide (a post-hoc analysis). **Headache** 55: (suppl S3): 177.

100 AMG-334 hyper-responders: http: //www.fiercebiotech.com/story/amgens-migraine-drug-gains-momentum-crowded-race/2015-06-19

101 Walter S and Bigal ME (2015). TEV-48125: a review of a monoclonal CGRP antibody in development for the preventive treatment of migraine. *Current Pain and Headache Reports* **19**: 6

102 Lipton RB, Bigal ME, Diamond M, Freitag F, Reed ML, Stewart WF, AMPP Advisory group (2007). Migraine prevalence, disease burden and the need for preventative therapy. *Neurology* **68**: 343–349.

103 Berger A, Bloudek LM, Varon SF, Oster G (2012). Adherence with migraine prophylaxis in clinical practice. *Pain Practice* **12**: 541–549.

104 Underwood E (2016). A shot at migraine. *Science* **351**: 116–119.

10

Lessons learned from CGRP mutant mice

Levi P. Sowers[1,2], Annie E. Tye[3] and Andrew F. Russo[1–3]

[1] *Department of Molecular Physiology and Biophysics, University of Iowa, Iowa City, IA 52242*
[2] *VA Center for the Prevention and Treatment of Visual Loss, Iowa City, IA 52242*
[3] *Neuroscience Program, University of Iowa, Iowa City, IA 52242*

10.1   Introduction

Calcitonin gene-related peptide (CGRP) plays a pivotal role in migraine pathogenesis, and the development of CGRP-mutant mouse models has been fruitful in the ongoing delineation of the role of CGRP in migraine (Villalon, 2009; Ho, 2010; Russo, 2015a). Here, we review the current mouse models with altered CGRP signaling, and the lessons learned from each of these models.

10.2   Modeling migraine

Modeling migraine in a mouse poses unique challenges, not the least of which is the question: how can we tell if a mouse has a migraine? At present, we cannot know for sure that a mouse has a headache. However, we *can* measure the headache-associated symptoms, such as sensitivity to light and touch.

The past decade has witnessed the development of animal models designed to study migraine-related processes. These models can be broadly categorized in two paradigms: those using anesthetizing agents to elucidate the relevant molecular pathways and anatomical networks; and those assessing behavioral output in response to experimental manipulation in awake animals (Romero-Reyes, 2014).

Of course, the obvious drawback of models using anesthesia is the inability to assess pain-related behavior. Behavioral tests have been developed to measure sensitivity to touch and light, and both tests have their advantages and disadvantages. Touch sensitivity is measured by fairly straightforward von Frey filament applications but is limited, in that it is a nociceptive reflex response. On the other hand, light sensitivity is an operant response that likely involves higher brain integration, but the assay is more subject to experimental confounders. Both touch and light sensitivity will be emphasized in the following discussion of CGRP mouse models.

10.3 Calcitonin gene-related peptide (CGRP) in migraine

CGRP is a widely expressed neuropeptide that has a potent vasodilatory effect. It functions as a regulator of cardiovascular tone, with a specific role in protecting tissues against ischemic damage (Benarroch, 2011; Russell, 2014; Russo, 2015a). In addition, CGRP plays a major role both in the development of peripherally-mediated neurogenic inflammation and in centrally-mediated neuromodulation of nociceptive inputs (Moskowitz, 1979, 1984, 1993; Mayberg, 1981, Liu-Chen, 1983; van Rossum, 1997; Benarroch, 2011; Raddant, 2011; Russo, 2015a; and see Figure 10.1).

Two isoforms of CGRP, αCGRP and βCGRP, are expressed from neighboring genes (Amara, 1985; Mulderry, 1988). The peptides have nearly identical sequences and functions. αCGRP is the isoform implicated in migraine, due to its relative prevalence in the trigeminal nerve. The remainder of this chapter will refer to αCGRP simply as CGRP, unless noted otherwise.

It is now well accepted that CGRP contributes to migraine pathophysiology. Serum CGRP levels are elevated during migraine, and this increase can be reversed with sumatriptan (Goadsby, 1990, 1993; Juhasz, 2005). CGRP is also elevated in people with chronic migraine (Cernuda-Morollon, 2013). Injection of CGRP causes delayed onset of headache, but this is only seen in migraineurs (Lassen, 2002; Hansen, 2010).

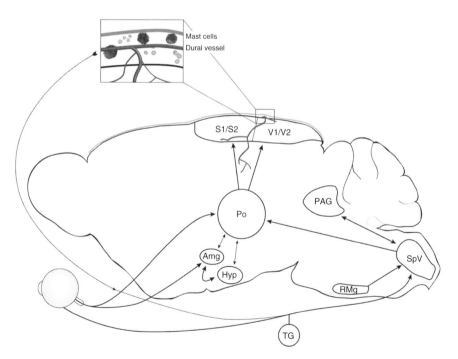

Figure 10.1 Potential sites of CGRP action. CGRP could be acting at both peripheral and central sites. CGRP release in the periphery may act during migraine to activate the spinal trigeminal nucleus leading to pain. CGRP release in the brain could be acting on a number of possible target nuclei to induce both sensory abnormalities and pain. Abbreviations: Amg – amygdala; Hyp – hypothalamus; TG – trigeminal ganglion; PAG – periaqueductal gray; Po – posterior thalamus; Rmg – raphe magnus; SpV – spinal trigeminal nucleus; S1, S2 – somatosensory cortex; V1, V2 – visual cortex.

Notably, while there are other vasodilators that may be sufficient to induce headache (e.g., PACAP and nitroglycerin), this is not a property of all vasodilators, specifically VIP (Rahmann, 2008).

Finally, CGRP has become a target for the treatment of migraine (Olesen, 2004; Ho, 2008; Connor, 2009; Diener, 2011; Hewitt, 2011; Marcus, 2014). Small-molecule CGRP receptor antagonists have been shown to be quite effective in treating migraine but, although promising, production of these inhibitors was discontinued, due to liver toxicity following daily doses over two months (Ho, 2014). Recent developments in humanized monoclonal antibodies have been more fruitful (Dodick, 2014a, 2014b; Bigal, 2015a, 2015b; Sun, 2016). Promising data indicate that these antibodies have the potential to be used as a prophylactic treatment for migraine (see Chapter 9).

10.4   What has CGRP manipulation in mice taught us about migraine?

The objective of this section is to review the current state of migraine research, using mouse models that affect CGRP signaling (Table 10.1). The CGRP mutants include both loss and gain of function models that affect either the CGRP ligand or CGRP receptor.

10.4.1   CGRP ligand mouse models

To date, several lines of αCGRP knockout mice have been generated, which are described below. However, to our knowledge, there have not been any βCGRP knockouts, nor have there been any lines that overexpress CGRP.

A handful of CGRP knockout mouse models have been developed, with a few key differences that can help hone in on the functional roles played by CGRP in migraine pathophysiology. CGRP and calcitonin (CT) are alternative splicing products of the *CALCA* gene, so creative engineering of the mouse *Calca* gene has created both αCGRP- and calcitonin (CT)/αCGRP-knockout models. In addition, the functionally indistinct βCGRP is expressed from a separate gene. Although migraine-specific studies have yet to be undertaken in CGRP knockout models, other phenotypes, including pain, have been characterized to some degree (Zhang, 2001).

Nociceptive responses in two lines of CGRP knockout mice have been reported. CT/αCGRP knockout display normal baseline responses to noxious heat stimuli (Zhang, 2001). However, prolonged peripheral inflammation induced by kaolin/carrageenan has resulted in no secondary hyperalgesia to heat in the knockout mice, while a significant decrease in paw withdrawal latency has been observed in wild type counterparts (Zhang, 2001). These results are interesting in terms of migraine, because they suggest that CGRP may underlie central sensitization in migraine pain.

Likewise, another strain of αCGRP knockout mice, made by targeted disruption of exon 5 of the CT/αCGRP gene, display reduced edema formation and nociception in response to chemical pain associated with inflammation (Salmon, 2001). Moreover, these mice display a lack of ATP-induced *in vivo* thermal hyperalgesia and reduced morphine analgesia (Salmon, 1999; Devesa, 2014). These data suggest that CGRP is involved with the transmission of pain associated with neurogenic inflammation.

Table 10.1 Mouse models that affect CGRP signaling.

Model	Background	Phenotype	Reference
αCGRP$^{-/-}$	129Sv	Reduced sound-evoked activity and vestibulo-ocular reflex; bone loss due to decreased formation; normal cardiovascular and neuromuscular development; enhanced colitis in a model of inflammatory bowel disease	Lu 1999, Maison 2003, Schinke 2004, Thompson 2008, Luebke 2014
αCGRP$^{-/-}$	129Sv x C57Bl/6	Increased HR and high BP due to increased peripheral vascular resistance; antigen challenge decreased bronchial hyperresponsiveness; reduced leukotrienes in lungs; decreased insulin-like growth factor release; impaired blood flow after hind limb ischemia	Oh-hashi 2001, Aoki-Nagase 2002, Zhao 2010, Mishima 2011
αCGRP$^{-/-}$	129Sv x C57Bl/6	Suppressed wound healing; reduced tumor-angiogenesis	Toda 2008a, Toda 2008b
αCGRP$^{-/-}$	C57Bl/6	Reduced morphine analgesia; attenuated pain response to chemical pain and inflammation; reduced morphine withdrawal signs; prevented ATP-induced thermal hyperalgesia; increased angiotensin II-induced hypertension and oxidative stress	Salmon 1999, Salmon 2001, Devesa 2014, Smillie 2014
CT/αCGRP$^{-/-}$	129Sv x C57Bl/6	Increased BP; decreased β-CGRP mRNA; increased bone formation	Gangula 2000, Hoff 2002
RAMP1$^{-/-}$	C57Bl/6 x BALBc	Hypertensive but normal HR; increased serum CGRP and pro-inflammatory cytokines	Tsujikawa 2007
RAMP1$^{-/-}$	BALBc	Increased LPS-induced inflammation	Mikami 2014
hRAMP1 over-expression	C57Bl/6 x 129Sv	Global hRAMP1 overexpression resulted in increased CGRP-induced vasodilation; decreased angiotensin II-induced hypertension and endothelial dysfunction. Nervous system hRAMP1 overexpression (nestin/hRAMP1) resulted in light-aversive behavior; mechanical allodynia; reduced motility in the dark; lean body mass due to increased sympathetic activation of brown fat	Recober 2009, Marquez de Prado 2009, Recober 2010, Sabharwal 2010, Chrissobolis 2010, Zhang 2011, Fernandes-Santos 2013
RAMP2$^{-/-}$	129Sv	Die in utero due to intersitial lymphedema	Dackor 2007, Fritz-Six 2008
RAMP2$^{-/-}$	C57Bl/6	Die in utero due to abnormal angiogenesis (edema/hemorrhage)	Yamauchi 2014
RAMP2$^{+/-}$	C57Bl/6	Reduced neovascularization; increased vascular permeability; delay in CBF recovery; increased inflammation/oxidative stress; increased neuronal death	Ichikawa-Shindo 2008, Igarashi 2014

(Continued)

Table 10.1 (Continued)

Model	Background	Phenotype	Reference
RAMP2 over-expression	B6D2F1	Smooth muscle overexpression resulted in normal basal BP and HR; enhanced response to AM; not protected from angiotensin II-induced hypertension and cardiac hypertrophy	Tam 2006, Liang 2009
DI-VE-RAMP2$^{-/-}$ DI-LE-RAMP2$^{-/-}$	C57Bl/6 x BALBc	Vascular structural abnormalities; spontaneous vascular inflammation and organ fibrosis	Yamauchi 2014
RAMP3$^{-/-}$	C57Bl/6 x BALBc	Delayed lymphatic drainage; intestinal lymphatic vessels reduced in size; more severe lymphedema; increased leukocytes and mast cells	Yamauchi 2014, Dackor 2007
CTR$^{+/-}$	C57Bl/6	Increased bone formation and mass	Davey 2008
Calclr$^{-/-}$	129s6/SvEv	Die in urtero due to extreme hydrops fetalis; display extreme interstitial edema	Dackor 2006

Other neurological abnormalities arise in mice lacking CGRP. A recent report showed the loss of αCGRP resulted in vestibular abnormalities. Specifically, the mice showed a reduced vestibulo-ocular reflex (Luebke, 2014). In addition, these mice displayed abnormal growth of cochlear neural responses with increasing stimulus levels (Maison, 2003). These results are interesting, because many migraine patients can display vestibular abnormalities during migraine (Stolte, 2015).

In contrast to pain phenotypes, the effect of CGRP loss on the cardiovascular system has yielded conflicting results in different knockout strains. Two lines showed a deleterious effect on resting parameters. A αCGRP knockout strain showed increased arterial pressure, heart rate, and peripheral vascular resistance (Oh-hashi, 2001). In addition, these mice displayed decreased bronchial hyper-responsivity to an antigen challenge and decreased insulin-like growth factor release (Aoki-Nagase, 2002; Zhao, 2010). Similarly, mice that lacked both CT and αCGRP had increased resting blood pressure (Gangula, 2000). Conversely, two other strains lacking αCGRP had no changes in resting cardiovascular parameters (Lu, 1999; Smillie, 2014).

The reason for these differences is not known, but may be due to different approaches used to knockout αCGRP or genetic backgrounds. However, one of the latter CGRP knockout mice did have enhanced hypertension and aortic hypertrophy following angiotensin II-induced hypertension, suggesting that CGRP helps maintain vascular health in response to physiological challenges (Smillie, 2014). These phenotypes are important to note concerning migraine, due to the development of monoclonal antibodies targeted against CGRP, which will reduce CGRP levels over the long-term.

Interestingly, the CGRP knockout strain that showed a resting cardiovascular phenotype (Oh-hashi, 2001) also had elevated sympathetic nervous activity. This phenotype is possibly consistent with elevated CGRP contributing to sympathetic nervous hypoactivity in migraine (Peroutka, 2004). This same CGRP knockout strain showed other vascular phenotypes. Upon unilateral limb ischemia, CGRP knockout mice displayed impaired blood flow recovery and decreased capillary density. These data suggest that CGRP contributes to angiogenesis in response to ischemia (Mishima, 2011).

Other phenotypes may or may not be important for migraine research, but should be noted. Specifically, one $\alpha CGRP^{-/-}$ mouse line displayed an abnormal bone phenotype, along with enhanced colitis, in a model of inflammatory bowel disease (Schinke, 2004; Thompson, 2008). Another showed decreased wound healing and reduced tumor-associated angiogenesis (Toda, 2008a, 2008b). Finally, the $\alpha CGRP^{-/-}$ mice developed by Oh-hashi *et al.* (2001) were shown to have decreased insulin-like growth factor release in multiple areas of the body (Harada, 2007).

10.4.2 CGRP receptor mutant mouse models: CLR, CTR, and the RAMPs

The classical receptor for CGRP consists of a heteromeric complex of calcitonin receptor-like receptor (CLR), receptor activity-modifying protein 1 (RAMP1), and receptor component protein (RCP) (Poyner, 2002). Recent evidence shows that CGRP also binds to the amylin receptor, which is composed of RAMP1 and the calcitonin receptor (CTR) (Walker, 2015). Two receptors that bind the CGRP-like peptide adrenomedullin can be formed by the binding of CLR with RAMP2 or RAMP3 (Poyner, 2002). Although these receptors can also bind CGRP, the binding occurs with much lower affinities. It is likely that these interactions are less important in migraine pathophysiology, as clinically effective antagonists specifically target CLR/RAMP1 and not CLR/RAMP2 or CLR/RAMP3. Furthermore, injection of adrenomedullin into human migraineurs fails to induce migraine (Petersen, 2009).

10.4.2.1 Calcitonin receptor-like receptor (CLR)
Calcitonin receptor-like receptor knockout ($Calcrl^{-/-}$) mice have major defects, including in the cardiovascular system, but die *in utero* so, therefore, migraine-like symptoms have not been studied (Dackor, 2006).

10.4.2.2 Calcitonin receptor (CTR)
Although the CT receptor is not viewed as the canonical receptor for CGRP, CGRP can bind the CTR/RAMP1 complex with comparable affinity, as seen with CLR/RAMP1 (Walker, 2015). Given the presence of CTR/RAMP1 complexes in the rodent and human trigeminal ganglion, the possibility that CTR may contribute to migraine remains an open question, although no link has been discovered (Walker, 2015). To date, the only phenotype reported for CTR knockout mice involved abnormal calcium homeostasis (Davey, 2008).

10.4.2.3 hRAMP1 overexpressing mice
Studies suggest that migraineurs are particularly sensitive to CGRP, which led our laboratory to speculate whether CGRP receptor overexpression in mice could recapitulate a migraine-like phenotype. Our lab developed a CGRP-sensitized mouse model by overexpressing the rate-limiting component of the CGRP receptor, RAMP1 (Russo, 2015b). Gene transfer studies using human RAMP1 (hRAMP1) in cultured trigeminal neurons and vascular smooth muscle cells demonstrated that RAMP1 is functionally rate-limiting (Zhang, 2006, 2007). In contrast, overexpression of RCP did not have any detectable effect on CGRP receptor activity (unpublished data).

To generate a mouse model, the approach was to use double-transgenic mice that express hRAMP1 under the control of the neuronal and glial-specific nestin promoter in a Cre-dependent manner. The transgenic nestin/hRAMP1 mice had an up to twofold increase in the level of RAMP1 (combination of endogenous mouse RAMP1 and transgenic hRAMP1) in the nervous system (Zhang, 2007).

The nestin/hRAMP1 mice have proven to be a valuable tool in the elucidation of CGRP's role in migraine symptomology. The mice showed two migraine relevant phenotypes in the light aversion assay (Recober, 2009a, 2010; Kaiser, 2012):

1) intracerebroventricular injection of CGRP caused nestin/hRAMP1 mice to go into the dark; and
2) once in the dark, they displayed reduced motility, which was not seen in the light side of the chamber.

The latter observation is reminiscent of the behavior of human migraineurs, who will actively seek out a darkened room where they can rest quietly.

It was then asked whether intracerebroventricular CGRP in combination with a bright light stimulus (27 000 lux, which approximates a sunny day) would be sufficient to induce light aversion in wild type (C57Bl/6J) mice. After a habituation period, which served to reduce the natural exploratory drive, a significant reduction in time spent in the light by wild type mice was seen, similar to that with nestin/hRAMP1 mice (Recober, 2009a; Kaiser, 2012).

To support the idea that these mice were experiencing migraine-like phenotypes, rizatriptan was used to treat light-aversive behaviors in both the nestin/hRAMP1 mice and C57Bl/6J mice. Pre-treatment led to a significant reduction in light-aversive behaviors and also restored normal motility in these mice (Recober, 2009b; Kaiser, 2012).

In addition to the light-dark assay, mechanical allodynia was tested in order to assess pain thresholds in the nestin/hRAMP1 mice. Mechanical allodynia is a problem for many migraineurs. In fact, 40–50% of patients experience sensitization to cutaneous stimuli (Burstein, 2000; LoPinto, 2006) (see Chapter 7). While this mechanical allodynia is predominant in the facial region, 36% of patients report having allodynia in extracephalic regions. Following intrathecal CGRP administration in nestin/hRAMP1 mice, there was a significant decrease in withdrawal thresholds to von Frey filaments (Marquez de Prado, 2009). Moreover, capsaicin increased mechanical responses in both wild type and nestin/hRAMP1 mice, but a higher dose was required in wild type mice (Marquez de Prado, 2009).

Cardiovascular phenotypes were also observed in these mice. In mice with global hRAMP1 overexpression, the mice displayed increased CGRP-induced vasodilation and decreased angiotensin II-induced hypertension and endothelial dysfunction (Chrissobolis, 2010; Sabharwal, 2010). It was also found that the nestin/hRAMP1 mice displayed an unexpected lean body mass phenotype, which was likely caused by increased sympathetic activation of brown fat metabolism, due to increased amylin and CGRP activity (Zhang, 2011; Fernandes-Santos, 2013).

From the nestin/hRAMP1 mice, it was determined that CGRP and its receptor could induce migraine-like phenotypes, including reduced motility, light-aversive behaviors, and mechanical allodynia (Marquez de Prado, 2009; Recober, 2010). When taken together, these data demonstrate that CGRP may be a significant player in migraine pathophysiology, and suggests that CGRP could contribute to central sensitization in migraine.

10.4.2.4 RAMP1 knockout

Ramp1$^{-/-}$ mice appear normal and display normal fertility. *Ramp1*$^{-/-}$ mice do not display a vasodilatory response to CGRP, compared with wild type counterparts, which confirms that CGRP's effects are mainly through receptors containing RAMP1. As with some of the CGRP knockout mice, the *Ramp1*$^{-/-}$ mice show elevated blood pressure, relative to controls (Tsujikawa, 2007). These data illustrate the importance of RAMP1 in maintaining normal blood pressure. In addition, experiments in *Ramp1*$^{-/-}$ mice suggest that CGRP could act as an anti-inflammatory agent in response to lipopolysaccharide injection in mice (Tsujikawa, 2007). Another pedigree of *Ramp1*$^{-/-}$ mice also had an impaired immune phenotype, with attenuated asthma-like responses (Li, 2014). Like the CGRP knockout mice, the *Ramp*$^{-/-}$ strains show conflicting cardiovascular phenotypes. Li *et al.* showed that their *Ramp1*$^{-/-}$ mice had normal blood pressure indistinguishable from wild type controls.

10.4.2.5 RAMP2 overexpression

Mice overexpressing RAMP2 in vascular smooth muscle had normal basal arterial blood pressure and heart rate; relative to wild type controls; but were not protected from Angiotensin II-induced hypertension and cardiac hypertrophy (Tam, 2006; Liang, 2009). CLR/RAMP2 forms a receptor that mainly binds adrenomedullin, although CGRP can bind weakly to CLR/RAMP2. Treating the RAMP2 overexpressing mice with adrenomedullin resulted in increased vasodilation when compared to wild type mice. In contrast, CGRP injection in these mice did not show any differences compared to wild type mice.

10.4.2.6 RAMP2 knockout

Multiple lines of *Ramp2*$^{-/-}$ mice are embryonic-lethal. These mice fail to form proper vasculature, and die early in embryonic development (Dackor, 2007; Fritz-Six, 2008; Ichikawa-Shindo, 2008). To overcome this, drug-inducible tissue specific *Ramp2* knockouts were developed to examine the role of RAMP2 in vascular and lymphatic endothelial cells (DI-VE-RAMP2$^{-/-}$ and DI-LE-RAMP2$^{-/-}$, respectively) (Yamauchi, 2014). Both models displayed structural abnormalities in the vasculature, spontaneous vascular inflammation, and organ fibrosis.

These data are in agreement with a number of studies that strongly link RAMP2 to vascular development (Yamauchi, 2014). Heterozygous *Ramp2*$^{+/-}$ mice had a slight increase in baseline blood pressure and blunted vasodilatory responses to adrenomedullin, and normal CGRP responses (Ichikawa-Shindo, 2008). In contrast, a heterozygous *Ramp2*$^{+/-}$ model displayed an outwardly normal phenotype, although reduced fertility (Igarashi, 2014). After experimentally induced occlusion of the middle cerebral artery, these mice showed delayed recovery of cerebral blood flow, increased inflammation and oxidative stress, and increased neuronal death (Igarashi, 2014).

10.4.2.7 RAMP3 knockout

Ramp3$^{-/-}$ mice are normal at birth, and have and show no developmental problems or aberrations in blood pressure or heart rate. However, in a model of post-operative lymphedema (Yamauchi, 2014), *Ramp3*$^{-/-}$ mice exhibited delayed lymphatic drainage, possibly due to reduced lymphatic vessel diameter, as well as increased lymphedema with concurrent increases in leukocyte and mast cell populations (Yamauchi, 2014).

10.5   Conclusions

In general, the phenotypes of CGRP mutant mice are consistent with CGRP being a key player in hypersensitivity to some stimuli that are associated with migraine. With respect to nociceptive stimuli, mice lacking CGRP and mice with elevated CGRP receptors show decreased and increased responses, respectively. Likewise, mice with elevated CGRP receptors show increased sensitivity to light. CGRP mutant mice also tend to show a lack of compensation to vascular challenges in the absence of CGRP activity, which is mirrored by increased resilience to some of those same challenges when the receptor is overexpressed. Whether, or how, these vascular functions contribute to migraine remains an open question. Future studies on CGRP mouse models will allow us to define the mechanisms by which CGRP is acting in migraine pathophysiology.

References

Amara, S. G., J. L. Arriza, S. E. Leff, L. W. Swanson, R. M. Evans and M. G. Rosenfeld (1985). Expression in brain of a messenger RNA encoding a novel neuropeptide homologous to calcitonin gene-related peptide. *Science* **229**(4718): 1094–1097.

Aoki-Nagase, T., T. Nagase, Y. Oh-Hashi, T. Shindo, Y. Kurihara, Y. Yamaguchi, *et al.* (2002). Attenuation of antigen-induced airway hyperresponsiveness in CGRP-deficient mice. *American Journal of Physiology. Lung Cellular and Molecular Physiology* **283**(5): L963–970.

Benarroch, E. E. (2011). CGRP: sensory neuropeptide with multiple neurologic implications. *Neurology* **77**(3): 281–287.

Bigal, M. E., D. W. Dodick, A. M. Rapoport, S. D. Silberstein, Y. Ma, R. Yang, *et al.* (2015a). Safety, tolerability, and efficacy of TEV-48125 for preventive treatment of high-frequency episodic migraine: a multicentre, randomised, double-blind, placebo-controlled, phase 2b study. *Lancet Neurology* **14**(11): 1081–1090.

Bigal, M. E., L. Edvinsson, A. M. Rapoport, R. B. Lipton, E. L. Spierings, H. C. Diener, *et al.* (2015b). Safety, tolerability, and efficacy of TEV-48125 for preventive treatment of chronic migraine: a multicentre, randomised, double-blind, placebo-controlled, phase 2b study. *Lancet Neurology* **14**(11): 1091–1100.

Burstein, R., D. Yarnitsky, I. Goor-Aryeh, B. J. Ransil and Z. H. Bajwa (2000). An association between migraine and cutaneous allodynia. *Annals of Neurology* **47**(5): 614–624.

Cernuda-Morollon, E., D. Larrosa, C. Ramon, J. Vega, P. Martinez-Camblor and J. Pascual (2013). Interictal increase of CGRP levels in peripheral blood as a biomarker for chronic migraine. *Neurology* **81**(14): 1191–1196.

Chrissobolis, S., Z. Zhang, D. A. Kinzenbaw, C. M. Lynch, A. F. Russo and F. M. Faraci (2010). Receptor activity-modifying protein-1 augments cerebrovascular responses to calcitonin gene-related peptide and inhibits angiotensin II-induced vascular dysfunction. *Stroke* **41**(10): 2329–2334.

Connor, K. M., R. E. Shapiro, H. C. Diener, S. Lucas, J. Kost, X. Fan, *et al.* (2009). Randomized, controlled trial of telcagepant for the acute treatment of migraine. *Neurology* **73**(12): 970–977.

Dackor, R. T., K. Fritz-Six, W. P. Dunworth, C. L. Gibbons, O. Smithies and K. M. Caron (2006). Hydrops fetalis, cardiovascular defects, and embryonic lethality in mice lacking the calcitonin receptor-like receptor gene. *Molecular and Cellular Biology* **26**(7): 2511–2518.

Dackor, R., K. Fritz-Six, O. Smithies and K. Caron (2007). Receptor activity-modifying proteins 2 and 3 have distinct physiological functions from embryogenesis to old age. *Journal of Biological Chemistry* **282**(25): 18094–18099.

Davey, R. A., A. G. Turner, J. F. McManus, W. S. Chiu, F. Tjahyono, A. J. Moore, *et al.* (2008). Calcitonin receptor plays a physiological role to protect against hypercalcemia in mice. *Journal of Bone and Mineral Research* **23**(8): 1182–1193.

Devesa, I., C. Ferrandiz-Huertas, S. Mathivanan, C. Wolf, R. Lujan, J. P. Changeux and A. Ferrer-Montiel (2014). alphaCGRP is essential for algesic exocytotic mobilization of TRPV1 channels in peptidergic nociceptors. *Proceedings of the National Academy of Sciences of the United States of America* **111**(51): 18345–18350.

Diener, H. C., P. Barbanti, C. Dahlof, U. Reuter, J. Habeck and J. Podhorna (2011). BI 44370 TA, an oral CGRP antagonist for the treatment of acute migraine attacks: results from a phase II study. *Cephalalgia* **31**(5): 573–584.

Dodick, D. W., P. J. Goadsby, E. L. Spierings, J. C. Scherer, S. P. Sweeney and D. S. Grayzel (2014a). Safety and efficacy of LY2951742, a monoclonal antibody to calcitonin gene-related peptide, for the prevention of migraine: a phase 2, randomised, double-blind, placebo-controlled study. *Lancet Neurology* **13**(9): 885–892.

Dodick, D. W., P. J. Goadsby, S. D. Silberstein, R. B. Lipton, J. Olesen, M. Ashina, *et al.* (2014b). Safety and efficacy of ALD403, an antibody to calcitonin gene-related peptide, for the prevention of frequent episodic migraine: a randomised, double-blind, placebo-controlled, exploratory phase 2 trial. *Lancet Neurology* **13**(11): 1100–1107.

Fernandes-Santos, C., Z. Zhang, D. A. Morgan, D. F. Guo, A. F. Russo and K. Rahmouni (2013). Amylin acts in the central nervous system to increase sympathetic nerve activity. *Endocrinology* **154**(7): 2481–2488.

Fritz-Six, K. L., W. P. Dunworth, M. Li and K. M. Caron (2008). Adrenomedullin signaling is necessary for murine lymphatic vascular development. *Journal of Clinical Investigation* **118**(1): 40–50.

Gangula, P. R., H. Zhao, S. C. Supowit, S. J. Wimalawansa, D. J. Dipette, K. N. Westlund, *et al.* (2000). Increased blood pressure in alpha-calcitonin gene-related peptide/calcitonin gene knockout mice. *Hypertension* **35**(1 Pt 2): 470–475.

Goadsby, P. J. and L. Edvinsson (1993). The trigeminovascular system and migraine: studies characterizing cerebrovascular and neuropeptide changes seen in humans and cats. *Annals of Neurology* **33**(1): 48–56.

Goadsby, P. J., L. Edvinsson and R. Ekman (1990). Vasoactive peptide release in the extracerebral circulation of humans during migraine headache. *Annals of Neurology* **28**(2): 183–187.

Hansen, J. M., A. W. Hauge, J. Olesen and M. Ashina (2010). Calcitonin gene-related peptide triggers migraine-like attacks in patients with migraine with aura. *Cephalalgia* **30**(10): 1179–1186.

Harada, N., K. Okajima, H. Kurihara and N. Nakagata (2007). Stimulation of sensory neurons by capsaicin increases tissue levels of IGF-I, thereby reducing reperfusion-induced apoptosis in mice. *Neuropharmacology* **52**(5): 1303–1311.

Hewitt, D. J., S. K. Aurora, D. W. Dodick, P. J. Goadsby, Y. J. Ge, R. Bachman, *et al.* (2011). Randomized controlled trial of the CGRP receptor antagonist MK-3207 in the acute treatment of migraine. *Cephalalgia* **31**(6): 712–722.

Ho, T. W., M. D. Ferrari, D. W. Dodick, V. Galet, J. Kost, X. Fan, *et al.* (2008). Efficacy and tolerability of MK-0974 (telcagepant), a new oral antagonist of calcitonin gene-related peptide receptor, compared with zolmitriptan for acute migraine: a randomised, placebo-controlled, parallel-treatment trial. *Lancet* **372**(9656): 2115–2123.

Ho, T. W., L. Edvinsson and P. J. Goadsby (2010). CGRP and its receptors provide new insights into migraine pathophysiology. *Nature Reviews Neurology* **6**(10): 573–582.

Ho, T. W., K. M. Connor, Y. Zhang, E. Pearlman, J. Koppenhaver, X. Fan, *et al.* (2014). Randomized controlled trial of the CGRP receptor antagonist telcagepant for migraine prevention. *Neurology* **83**(11): 958–966.

Ichikawa-Shindo, Y., T. Sakurai, A. Kamiyoshi, H. Kawate, N. Iinuma, T. Yoshizawa, *et al.* (2008). The GPCR modulator protein RAMP2 is essential for angiogenesis and vascular integrity. *Journal of Clinical Investigation* **118**(1): 29–39.

Igarashi, K., T. Sakurai, A. Kamiyoshi, Y. Ichikawa-Shindo, H. Kawate, A. Yamauchi, *et al.* (2014). Pathophysiological roles of adrenomedullin-RAMP2 system in acute and chronic cerebral ischemia. *Peptides* **62**: 21–31.

Juhasz, G., T. Zsombok, B. Jakab, J. Nemeth, J. Szolcsanyi and G. Bagdy (2005). Sumatriptan causes parallel decrease in plasma calcitonin gene-related peptide (CGRP) concentration and migraine headache during nitroglycerin induced migraine attack. *Cephalalgia* **25**(3): 179–183.

Kaiser, E. A., A. Kuburas, A. Recober and A. F. Russo (2012). Modulation of CGRP-induced light aversion in wild-type mice by a 5-HT(1B/D) agonist. *Journal of Neuroscience* **32**(44): 15439–15449.

Lassen, L. H., P. A. Haderslev, V. B. Jacobsen, H. K. Iversen, B. Sperling and J. Olesen (2002). CGRP may play a causative role in migraine. *Cephalalgia* **22**(1): 54–61.

Li, M., S. E. Wetzel-Strong, X. Hua, S. L. Tilley, E. Oswald, M. F. Krummel and K. M. Caron (2014). Deficiency of RAMP1 attenuates antigen-induced airway hyperresponsiveness in mice. *PLoS One* **9**(7): e102356.

Liang, L., C. W. Tam, G. Pozsgai, R. Siow, N. Clark, J. Keeble, *et al.* (2009). Protection of angiotensin II-induced vascular hypertrophy in vascular smooth muscle-targeted receptor activity-modifying protein 2 transgenic mice. *Hypertension* **54**(6): 1254–1261.

Liu-Chen, L. Y., D. H. Han and M. A. Moskowitz (1983). Pia arachnoid contains substance P originating from trigeminal neurons. *Neuroscience* **9**(4): 803–808.

LoPinto, C., W. B. Young and A. Ashkenazi (2006). Comparison of dynamic (brush) and static (pressure) mechanical allodynia in migraine. *Cephalalgia* **26**(7): 852–856.

Lu, J. T., Y. J. Son, J. Lee, T. L. Jetton, M. Shiota, L. Moscoso, *et al.* (1999). Mice lacking alpha-calcitonin gene-related peptide exhibit normal cardiovascular regulation and neuromuscular development. *Molecular and Cellular Neuroscience* **14**(2): 99–120.

Luebke, A. E., J. C. Holt, P. M. Jordan, Y. S. Wong, J. S. Caldwell and K. E. Cullen (2014). Loss of alpha-calcitonin gene-related peptide (alphaCGRP) reduces the efficacy of the Vestibulo-ocular Reflex (VOR). *Journal of Neuroscience* **34**(31): 10453–10458.

Maison, S. F., R. B. Emeson, J. C. Adams, A. E. Luebke and M. C. Liberman (2003). Loss of alpha CGRP reduces sound-evoked activity in the cochlear nerve. *Journal of Neurophysiology* **90**(5): 2941–2949.

Marcus, R., P. J. Goadsby, D. Dodick, D. Stock, G. Manos and T. Z. Fischer (2014). BMS-927711 for the acute treatment of migraine: a double-blind, randomized, placebo controlled, dose-ranging trial. *Cephalalgia* **34**(2): 114–125.

Marquez de Prado, B., D. L. Hammond and A. F. Russo (2009). Genetic enhancement of calcitonin gene-related Peptide-induced central sensitization to mechanical stimuli in mice. *Journal of Pain* **10**(9): 992–1000.

Mayberg, M., R. S. Langer, N. T. Zervas and M. A. Moskowitz (1981). Perivascular meningeal projections from cat trigeminal ganglia: possible pathway for vascular headaches in man. *Science* **213**(4504): 228–230.

Mikami, N., K. Sueda, Y. Ogitani, I., Otani, M., Takatsuji, Y., Wada, *et al*. (2014). Calcitonin Gene-Related Peptide Regulates Type IV Hypersensitivity through Dendritic Cell Functions. *PLOS ONE* **9**(1).

Mishima, T., Y. Ito, K. Hosono, Y. Tamura, Y. Uchida, M. Hirata, *et al*. (2011). Calcitonin gene-related peptide facilitates revascularization during hindlimb ischemia in mice. *American Journal of Physiology: Heart and Circulatory Physiology* **300**(2): H431–439.

Moskowitz, M. A. (1984). The neurobiology of vascular head pain. *Annals of Neurology* **16**(2): 157–168.

Moskowitz, M. A., J. F. Reinhard, Jr., J. Romero, E. Melamed and D. J. Pettibone (1979). Neurotransmitters and the fifth cranial nerve: is there a relation to the headache phase of migraine? *Lancet* **2**(8148): 883–885.

Moskowitz, M. A., K. Nozaki and R. P. Kraig (1993). Neocortical spreading depression provokes the expression of c-fos protein-like immunoreactivity within trigeminal nucleus caudalis via trigeminovascular mechanisms. *Journal of Neuroscience* **13**(3): 1167–1177.

Mulderry, P. K., M. A. Ghatei, R. A. Spokes, P. M. Jones, A. M. Pierson, Q. A. Hamid, *et al*. (1988). Differential expression of alpha-CGRP and beta-CGRP by primary sensory neurons and enteric autonomic neurons of the rat. *Neuroscience* **25**(1): 195–205.

Oh-hashi, Y., T. Shindo, Y. Kurihara, T. Imai, Y. Wang, H. Morita, *et al*. (2001). Elevated sympathetic nervous activity in mice deficient in alphaCGRP. *Circulation Research* **89**(11): 983–990.

Olesen, J., H. C. Diener, I. W. Husstedt, P. J. Goadsby, D. Hall, U. Meier, *et al*. (2004). Calcitonin gene-related peptide receptor antagonist BIBN 4096 BS for the acute treatment of migraine. *New England Journal of Medicine* **350**(11): 1104–1110.

Peroutka, S. J. (2004). Migraine: a chronic sympathetic nervous system disorder. *Headache* **44**(1): 53–64.

Petersen, K. A., S. Birk, K. Kitamura and J. Olesen (2009). Effect of adrenomedullin on the cerebral circulation: relevance to primary headache disorders. *Cephalalgia* **29**(1): 23–30.

Poyner, D. R., P. M. Sexton, I. Marshall, D. M. Smith, R. Quirion, W. Born, *et al*. (2002). International Union of Pharmacology. XXXII. The Mammalian Calcitonin Gene-Related Peptides, Adrenomedullin, Amylin, and Calcitonin Receptors. *Pharmacological Reviews* **54**(2): 233–246.

Raddant, A. C. and A. F. Russo (2011). Calcitonin gene-related peptide in migraine: intersection of peripheral inflammation and central modulation. *Expert Reviews in Molecular Medicine* **13**: e36.

Rahmann, A., T. Wienecke, J. M. Hansen, J. Fahrenkrug, J. Olesen and M. Ashina (2008). Vasoactive Intestinal Peptide Causes Marked Cephalic Vasodilation, but does not Induce Migraine. *Cephalalgia* **28**(3): 226–236.

Recober, A., A. Kuburas, Z. Zhang, J. A. Wemmie, M. G. Anderson and A. F. Russo (2009a). Role of calcitonin gene-related peptide in light-aversive behavior: implications for migraine. *Journal of Neuroscience* **29**(27): 8798–8804.

Recober, A., Kaiser, E.A., Kuburas, A., Wemmie, J.A., Anderson, M.G., Russo, A.F. (2009b). CGRP-induced photophobia blocked by olcegepant and rizatriptan in a transgenic migraine model. *Cephalalgia* **29(suppl 1)** 1.

Recober, A., E. A. Kaiser, A. Kuburas and A. F. Russo (2010). Induction of multiple photophobic behaviors in a transgenic mouse sensitized to CGRP. *Neuropharmacology* **58**(1): 156–165.

Romero-Reyes, M. and S. Akerman (2014). Update on animal models of migraine. *Current Pain and Headache Reports* **18**(11): 462.

Russell, F. A., R. King, S. J. Smillie, X. Kodji and S. D. Brain (2014). Calcitonin gene-related peptide: physiology and pathophysiology. *Physiological Reviews* **94**(4): 1099–1142.

Russo, A. F. (2015a). Calcitonin gene-related peptide (CGRP): a new target for migraine. *Annual Review of Pharmacology and Toxicology* **55**: 533–552.

Russo, A. F. (2015b). CGRP as a neuropeptide in migraine: lessons from mice. *British Journal of Clinical Pharmacology* **80**(3): 403–414.

Sabharwal, R., Z. Zhang, Y. Lu, F. M. Abboud, A. F. Russo and M. W. Chapleau (2010). Receptor activity-modifying protein 1 increases baroreflex sensitivity and attenuates Angiotensin-induced hypertension. *Hypertension* **55**(3): 627–635.

Salmon, A. M., I. Damaj, S. Sekine, M. R. Picciotto, L. Marubio and J. P. Changeux (1999). Modulation of morphine analgesia in alphaCGRP mutant mice. *Neuroreport* **10**(4): 849–854.

Salmon, A. M., M. I. Damaj, L. M. Marubio, M. P. Epping-Jordan, E. Merlo-Pich and J. P. Changeux (2001). Altered neuroadaptation in opiate dependence and neurogenic inflammatory nociception in alpha CGRP-deficient mice. *Nature Neuroscience* **4**(4): 357–358.

Schinke, T., S. Liese, M. Priemel, M. Haberland, A. F. Schilling, P. Catala-Lehnen, *et al*. (2004). Decreased bone formation and osteopenia in mice lacking alpha-calcitonin gene-related peptide. *Journal of Bone and Mineral Research* **19**(12): 2049–2056.

Smillie, S. J., R. King, X. Kodji, E. Outzen, G. Pozsgai, E. Fernandes, *et al*. (2014). An ongoing role of alpha-calcitonin gene-related peptide as part of a protective network against hypertension, vascular hypertrophy, and oxidative stress. *Hypertension* **63**(5): 1056–1062.

Stolte, B., D. Holle, S. Naegel, H. C. Diener and M. Obermann (2015). Vestibular migraine. *Cephalalgia* **35**(3): 262–270.

Sun, H., D. W. Dodick, S. Silberstein, P. J. Goadsby, U. Reuter, M. Ashina, *et al*. (2016). Safety and efficacy of AMG 334 for prevention of episodic migraine: a randomised, double-blind, placebo-controlled, phase 2 trial. *Lancet Neurology* **15**(4): 382–390.

Tam, C. W., K. Husmann, N. C. Clark, J. E. Clark, Z. Lazar, L. M. Ittner, *et al*. (2006). Enhanced vascular responses to adrenomedullin in mice overexpressing receptor-activity-modifying protein 2. *Circulation Research* **98**(2): 262–270.

Thompson, B. J., M. K. Washington, U. Kurre, M. Singh, E. Y. Rula and R. B. Emeson (2008). Protective roles of alpha-calcitonin and beta-calcitonin gene-related peptide in spontaneous and experimentally induced colitis. *Digestive Diseases and Sciences* **53**(1): 229–241.

Toda, M., T. Suzuki, K. Hosono, I. Hayashi, S. Hashiba, Y. Onuma, *et al.* (2008a). Neuronal system-dependent facilitation of tumor angiogenesis and tumor growth by calcitonin gene-related peptide. *Proceedings of the National Academy of Sciences of the United States of America* **105**(36): 13550–13555.

Toda, M., T. Suzuki, K. Hosono, Y. Kurihara, H. Kurihara, I. Hayashi, *et al.* (2008b). Roles of calcitonin gene-related peptide in facilitation of wound healing and angiogenesis. *Biomedicine & Pharmacotherapy* **62**(6): 352–359.

Tsujikawa, K., K. Yayama, T. Hayashi, H. Matsushita, T. Yamaguchi, T. Shigeno, *et al.* (2007). Hypertension and dysregulated proinflammatory cytokine production in receptor activity-modifying protein 1-deficient mice. *Proceedings of the National Academy of Sciences of the United States of America* **104**(42): 16702–16707.

van Rossum, D., U. K. Hanisch and R. Quirion (1997). Neuroanatomical localization, pharmacological characterization and functions of CGRP, related peptides and their receptors. *Neuroscience & Biobehavioral Reviews* **21**(5): 649–678.

Villalon, C. M. and J. Olesen (2009). The role of CGRP in the pathophysiology of migraine and efficacy of CGRP receptor antagonists as acute antimigraine drugs. *Pharmacology & Therapeutics* **124**(3): 309–323.

Walker, C. S., S. Eftekhari, R. L. Bower, A. Wilderman, P. A. Insel, L. Edvinsson, *et al.* (2015). A second trigeminal CGRP receptor: function and expression of the AMY1 receptor. *Annals of Clinical and Translational Neurology* **2**(6): 595–608.

Yamauchi, A., T. Sakurai, A. Kamiyoshi, Y. Ichikawa-Shindo, H. Kawate, K. Igarashi, *et al.* (2014). Functional differentiation of RAMP2 and RAMP3 in their regulation of the vascular system. *Journal of Molecular and Cellular Cardiology* **77**: 73–85.

Zhang, L., A. O. Hoff, S. J. Wimalawansa, G. J. Cote, R. F. Gagel and K. N. Westlund (2001). Arthritic calcitonin/alpha calcitonin gene-related peptide knockout mice have reduced nociceptive hypersensitivity. *Pain* **89**(2–3): 265–273.

Zhang, Z., I. M. Dickerson and A. F. Russo (2006). Calcitonin gene-related peptide receptor activation by receptor activity-modifying protein-1 gene transfer to vascular smooth muscle cells. *Endocrinology* **147**(4): 1932–1940.

Zhang, Z., C. S. Winborn, B. Marquez de Prado and A. F. Russo (2007). Sensitization of calcitonin gene-related peptide receptors by receptor activity-modifying protein-1 in the trigeminal ganglion. *Journal of Neuroscience* **27**(10): 2693–2703.

Zhang, Z., X. Liu, D. A. Morgan, A. Kuburas, D. R. Thedens, A. F. Russo and K. Rahmouni (2011). Neuronal receptor activity-modifying protein 1 promotes energy expenditure in mice. *Diabetes* **60**(4): 1063–1071.

Zhao, J., N. Harada, H. Kurihara, N. Nakagata and K. Okajima (2010). Cilostazol improves cognitive function in mice by increasing the production of insulin-like growth factor-I in the hippocampus. *Neuropharmacology* **58**(4–5): 774–783.

Part III

Clinical characteristics of migraine

11

The clinical characteristics of migraine

F. Michael Cutrer[1], Ryan Smith[2] and David W. Dodick[3]

[1] Department of Neurology, Mayo Clinic, Rochester, Minnesota, USA
[2] Department of Molecular Physiology and Biophysics, VA Center for the Prevention and Treatment of Visual Loss, Iowa City, Iowa, USA
[3] Mayo Clinic Hospital, Phoenix, Arizona, USA

11.1   Overview of migraine

Migraine is a collection of symptoms that may include headache, malaise, nausea, vomiting, hypersensitivity to several modes of sensory input (light, sound smell), and often disquieting focal neurological symptoms. Migraine attacks can be variable from one sufferer to another, or even within a given individual, with some attacks predominated by neurological symptoms and others by severe head pain. It is clear that migraine is a brain disorder that, at its essence, reflects lowered activation thresholds for the trigeminocervical pain system and for a human form of cortical spreading depression, which underlies the transient focal neurological symptoms of migraine. Migraine is common, with an estimated one-year prevalence of 7% of men and 18% of women in the USA. [1]. Migraine may appear in early childhood, but most often starts in late childhood or early adolescence, gradually increasing to peak prevalence in the 30s or 40s, and decreasing as age increases [2].

The disorder occurs in both episodic and chronic forms, as established by the International Headache Society. The occurrence of headaches for 15 or more days per month for three months or more constitutes chronic migraine, if the headaches are classifiable as migraine for at least eight days per month. In episodic migraine, there are less than 15 headache days per month. In our experience, the most common presentation of chronic migraine is daily or almost daily low-grade headaches, with full-blown migrainous attacks superimposed for two or more headache days per week. The centerpiece of the migraine syndrome is a headache that occurs in most attacks.

11.2   Migraine prodrome

About 60% of migraineurs report that at least some of their attacks are preceded by neck stiffness, food cravings, vague symptoms such as fatigue and yawning, or mood changes

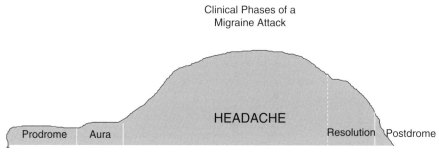

Figure 11.1 Classical progression of the migraine attack (Modified from Blau 1992) [9].

from two up to 48 hours prior to the onset of migraine headache (see Figure 11.1) [3, 4]. In a prospective electronic diary-based study, the most common prodromal symptoms were a feeling of tiredness, difficulty concentrating and neck stiffness [5].

11.3 The migraine headache is the centerpiece of the syndrome

Migraine patients have varied descriptions of their headaches. In most cases, the pain is sufficient to disrupt normal activities, although the intensity ranges from merely annoying to disabling. Headache intensity may vary to some degree from attack to attack. The severity of a migraine headache is often worsened by routine physical activity. Migraine headaches are typically unilateral, or at least more severe on one side. However up to 40% of patients have attacks in which the pain is bilateral, or even holocephalic, from the beginning.

When unilateral, the pain consistently occurs on the same side in only about 20% of patients. The quality of the pain may be pressure-like, throbbing, or a combination of both. In many patients, the throbbing appears only as the intensity of the pain reaches a moderately severe level. In patients with chronic migraine, there may also be intermittent jabbing pain, which is usually experienced in the area where the pain has been most intense.

When occurring episodically, the headache generally escalates from mild pain to a more severe level over an hour or two. In many patients, the more severe headaches are accompanied by nausea, which may range from mild queasiness and anorexia, to severe prolonged vomiting and retching. Vomiting occurs in about one third of patients [4].In addition, migraine headaches are also frequently associated with heightened sensitivity to light, sound and smells.

In adults, untreated episodic attacks persist for at least four hours, and may continue for up to three days. In the chronic form of migraine, the patient has some degree of low-grade headache, with or without nausea or light/sound sensitivity, every day or almost every day, with less common full-blown migraine attacks superimposed on a background of daily headaches. As a result, when asked the duration of their headaches, patients with chronic migraine may respond that their headaches last for weeks or months. In addition to head pain, patients also frequently experience a feeling of malaise or extreme fatigue during an attack. These symptoms are often unresponsive to acute migraine treatments, and may be misinterpreted by the patient as a side-effect of their abortive headache medication.

Migraine headache is based on recurrent activation of the trigeminocervical pain system (TCPS). In migraineurs, the activation threshold for head pain is altered, to the extent that the TCPS can be falsely and repeatedly activated by triggering factors in the internal or external environment that represent no immediate threat to the brain (see (Table 11.1)).

The International Headache Society has codified the characteristics of the migraine headache into a set of diagnostic criteria for migraine without aura [4].

Table 11.1 Common environmental triggers for migraine.

- Certain foods or food additives
- Menstrual cycle
- Barometric pressure or weather change
- Sleep pattern disturbance
- Bright or glaring light
- Loud noises
- Strong smells
- Fasting or missing a meal
- Physical exertion
- Stress or release from stress
- Alcohol

A) At least five attacks fulfilling criteria B–D
B) Headache attacks lasting 4–72 hours (untreated or unsuccessfully treated)
C) Headache has at least two of the following four characteristics:
   1) unilateral location
   2) pulsating quality
   3) moderate or severe pain intensity
   4) aggravation by or causing avoidance of routine physical activity (e.g. walking or climbing stairs)
D) During headache at least one of the following:
   1) nausea and/or vomiting
   2) photophobia and phonophobia
E) Not better accounted for by another ICHD-3 diagnosis

Figure 11.2 Migraine without aura [4].

11.4 Migraine aura

Approximately 30% of migraine sufferers experience one or more transient focal neurological symptoms, known as the migraine aura [6]. The migraine aura develops gradually (in more than four minutes), and persists for up to one hour. The typical aura emanates most often from the cerebral cortex. New aura types proposed in the IHCD 3 beta [4] would arise from brain stem and retina. The classical aura types include: visual, sensory, language and motor symptoms (see Figure 11.3).

Typical auras include transient visual, sensory and language disturbance.

11.4.1 Visual aura

The classical migraine visual aura begins with a small area of visual disturbance lateral to the point of visual fixation. This disturbance is homonomous, and may be an area of visual loss or a bright spot. The visual disturbance has a positive phase, followed by a negative phase. The positive phenomena include a visual disturbance that slowly expands, over five minutes to one hour, to involve a hemifield or quadrant of vision [7]. The expanding margin of the visual disturbance may have the appearance of zigzagging lines or geometric shapes, known as fortification spectra because of their similarity to walls of a medieval town, in which fortification lines were arranged at right angles to one another.

As the aura progresses, it may assume a sickle or "C" shape, with shimmering edges (scintillations), with or without color. The negative phase consists of a complete lack of image left in the wake of the expanding scintillations – an area of visual loss called a scotoma [8]. Colored dots, bean-like forms, bright bars, simple flashes (phosphenes), specks, white dots, curved lines, or other geometric forms may also be seen [6, 8]. Vision returns centrally as the disturbance spreads to the periphery [7] (See Figure 11.4).

11.4.2 Sensory aura

Just as in the visual aura, the sensory usually has both positive symptoms (spreading or migratory paresthesias), followed by numbness, a negative symptom [7]. The classic

---

A) At least two attacks fulfilling criteria B and C
B) One or more of the following fully reversible aura symptoms:
   1) Visual
   2) Sensory
   3) Speech and/or language
   4) Motor
   5) Brain stem
   6) Retinal
C) At least two of the following four characteristics:
   1) At least one aura symptom spreads gradually over five minutes, and/or two or more symptoms occur in succession
   2) Each individual aura symptom lasts 5–60 minutes
   3) At least one aura symptom is unilateral
   4) The aura is accompanied, or followed within 60 minutes, by headache
D) Not better accounted for by another ICHD-3 diagnosis, and transient ischemic attack has been excluded

Figure 11.3 Migraine with aura [4].

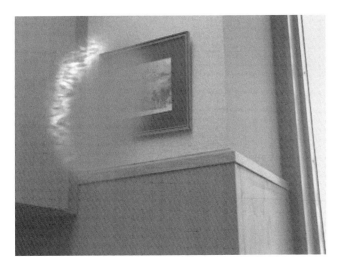

Figure 11.4 Representation of the classical migraine visual aura. Note the positive visual hallucination (fortification spectra), followed by negative visual phenomena (scotoma).

term for sensory aura, cheiro-oral, describes the typical appearance of tingling, followed by numbness that starts in the hand and then migrates up the arm to involve the face, lips, and tongue. Sensory aura may also involve the leg, foot, or body as well [10]. In many instances, what a patient is calling "weakness" in an arm or leg by the patient may actually be clumsiness that arises when proprioception is lost in the context of a sensory aura. Therefore, it is very important, whenever a patient complains of "weakness", to clarify whether it is clumsiness associated with the sensory aura, or true weakness which is much rarer [7].

11.4.3 Language aura

Almost as common as sensory aura is language disturbance, the third type of migraine aura. This symptom can be quite distressing for the patient, given the impact it has on comprehension and communication due to word-finding difficulties, and a decreased ability to read or write [10]. It should be remembered that cheiro-oral sensory changes can cause a slurring speech disturbance arising from loss of sensation in the tongue, and should not be confused with a language aura [10].

Word-finding difficulty is the most common type of language aura, but expressive and receptive language impairment can certainly occur [11]. Apraxia, proper name agnosia, transient amnesia, and prosopagnosia have all been attributed to language aura in the literature [12]. When headache patients are asked if they have any trouble thinking or talking during an attack, they may report non-specific cognitive issues that do not meet the criteria for language aura. Cognitive symptoms, such as impairment of attentional performance, lack of concentration, mental "cloudiness" or "fuzziness" may be separate from language aura, and can also be seen in migraine without aura (and other headache types) [13]. Therefore, in order to assign the correct diagnosis, the astute clinician will need to evaluate the details of the language disturbance carefully.

11.4.4 Duration of typical aura

Typical migraine aura gradually appears, spreads and resolves over a period of 5–60 minutes for each aura symptom. If a patient has more than one type of typical aura, they typically occur in succession, and not simultaneously. If a typical migraine aura persists for longer than an hour (but less than one week), it is then termed probable migraine with aura [4]. However, a recent review found that 12–37% of migraine aura sufferers report that at least some of their aura symptoms last longer than an hour [14]. In addition, cases of aura lasting days and weeks have been well documented [15]. Such prolonged auras have formerly been called "complicated migraine"; however the ICHD-3 beta classification refers to them as persistent aura without infarction when they persist for more than a week [4].

11.4.5 Motor aura or hemiplegic migraine

In the past, episodes of unilateral motor weakness during migraine attacks were referred to as motor aura, until the term motor aura was replaced by the *Hemiplegic migraine aura* subtype in ICHD-2, soon after genetic mutations underlying motor aura were identified. Motor aura differs from the typical aura types, in that there is a much longer average duration of motor weakness in hemiplegic migraine. In attacks of hemiplegic migraine, unilateral weakness frequently lasts from hours to days – much longer than the 60 minutes or less associated with the other aura types. In addition, the symptoms of motor aura do not have obvious positive and negative phases that spread with time, and no twitching or migratory spasm is noted prior to weakness by patients with hemiplegic migraine. However, there does seem to be sequential weakness of body areas during attacks of hemiplegic migraine [10]. It is also important to note that all patients with hemiplegic migraine also have typical auras in the context of their attacks (See Figure 11.5).

Migraine with motor aura (hemiplegic migraine)

A) At least two attacks fulfilling criteria B and C
B) Aura consisting of both of the following:
    1) Fully reversible motor weakness
    2) Fully reversible visual, sensory and/or speech/ language symptoms
C) At least two of the following four characteristics:
    1) At least one aura symptom spreads gradually over five minutes, and/or two or more symptoms occur in succession.
    2) Each individual non-motor aura symptom lasts 5–60 minutes, and motor symptoms last < 72 hours.
    3) At least one aura symptom is unilateral.
    4) The aura is accompanied, or followed within 60 minutes, by headache
D) Not better accounted for by another ICHD-3 diagnosis, and transient ischemic attack and stroke have been excluded.

Figure 11.5 The ICHD3 beta lists the following criteria for the diagnosis of migraine with motor aura (hemiplegic migraine) [4].

Migraine with brainstem aura (previously basilar migraine)

A) At least two attacks fulfilling criteria B–D
B) Aura consisting of visual, sensory and/or speech/ language symptoms, each fully reversible, but no motor or retinal symptoms
C) At least two of the following brainstem symptoms:
   1) Dysarthria
   2) Vertigo
   3) Tinnitus
   4) Hyperacusis
   5) Diplopia
   6) Ataxia
   7) Decreased level of consciousness
D) At least two of the following four characteristics:
   1) At least one aura symptom spreads gradually over five minutes, and/or two or more symptoms occur in succession
   2) Each individual aura symptom lasts 5–60 minutes
   3) At least one aura symptom is unilateral
   4) The aura is accompanied, or followed within 60 minutes, by headache
E) Not better accounted for by another ICHD-3 diagnosis, and transient ischemic attack has been excluded.

Figure 11.6 Migraine with brainstem aura (previously basilar migraine) [4].

11.5 Proposed aura types

11.5.1 Brainstem aura

The proposed IHCD3 criteria include aura symptoms arising from the brainstem, as opposed to the cortex [4]. Weakness is not a feature of migraine with brainstem aura. Most patients with this type of aura present in early adolescence, and their aura reverts to a more typical aura in their 40s and 50s [16]. This subtype of aura was previously termed basilar migraine, as it was thought to be related to spasm and/or compromised blood flow in the basilar artery territory [17]. As a result, patients with hemiplegic and basilar-type migraine were excluded from clinical trials involving triptans and, as such, triptans are contraindicated in these patients. Multiple small case series have been performed showing these drugs may be safe in this condition, but determining risk would require the exposure of large numbers of patients [18] (See Figure 11.6).

11.5.2 Retinal aura

The most recent proposed criteria also include an aura type consisting of symptoms of monocular visual loss. This type of aura would be termed retinal aura [4] . Patients may have difficulty distinguishing a hemianopia from vision loss from one eye. It is critical to ask patients if they alternately covered one eye. This type of aura is extremely rare, and other causes of monocular vision loss should be investigated before making this diagnosis. Proposed pathophysiology for this aura type is thought to be a spreading depression

Retinal aura

A) At least two attacks fulfilling criteria B and C
B) Aura consisting of fully reversible monocular positive and/or negative visual phenomena (e.g., scintillations, scotomata or blindness) confirmed during an attack by either or both of the following:
   1) Clinical visual field examination
   2) The patient's drawing (made after clear instruction) of a monocular field defect
C) At least two of the following three characteristics:
   1) The aura spreads gradually over five minutes
   2) Aura symptoms last 5–60 minutes
   3) The aura is accompanied, or followed within 60 minutes, by headache
D) Not better accounted for by another ICHD-3 diagnosis and other causes of amaurosis fugax have been excluded.

Figure 11.7 Retinal aura [4].

of the retina, or vasospasm of retinal arterioles [19]. Permanent vision loss has been described in some patients meeting the criteria [20] (See Figure 11.7).

11.5.3 Migraine aura versus other causes of neurological deficit

There are characteristics of visual and sensory auras that are helpful in differentiating migrainous aura from symptoms related to cerebral ischemia. Both sensory and visual auras have a slow migratory or spreading quality, in which symptoms slowly spread across the affected body part or the visual field, followed by a gradual return to normal function in the areas first affected after 20–60 minutes. This spreading quality is not characteristic of an ischemic event [7], in which neurological deficits tend to appear suddenly and are simultaneously experienced in several body parts.

The recognition of these characteristics was a seminal observation that led to the formulation of the neurogenic theory of migraine aura [22]. In addition, although a migratory pattern may also be seen in partial seizure disorders, the progression of symptoms in a partial seizure is much more rapid. It is also notable that neither ischemia nor seizure-based symptoms are associated with the return of function in the areas of the cortex which were first affected, even as symptoms are simultaneously appearing in newly affected areas. Lastly, in contrast to transient ischemic attacks, migrainosus aura is stereotypic and repetitive.

In migraine aura where more than one aura symptom occurs, different neurological symptoms occur one after the other, and not simultaneously (e.g., visual and sensory symptoms). Some patients experience all three typical auras in sequence during a single attack [7]. In over 20 years of asking patients to describe their aura, none have reported the appearance of all aura types at the same time [7]. In contrast to migraine aura, the simultaneous appearance of multiple types of neurological symptoms is, however, fairly common in cerebral ischemia.

11.6 Postdrome

In the majority of patients, the resolution of the migraine headache, often occurring during a period of sleep, is followed by a wide constellation of continuing symptoms.

Patients report malaise, fatigue, and variable mood changes, including both depressed and euphoric moods, persistent soreness in the area affected by the headache (hypersensitivity), or transient pain with sudden head movement or trivial stimulations, such as shaving or combing of hair (allodynia), impaired or slowed thinking, or gastrointestinal symptoms [21]. These symptoms can last hours to days, and can vary from one attack to the other, both in intensity and quality. This final phase is termed the migraine postdrome, although patients often refer to it as the migraine "hangover."

11.7 Status migrainosus

Some individuals are prone to have migraine attacks that persist for longer than 72 hours despite treatment. These attacks are classified as *status migrainosus*. During status migrainosus, headache-free periods of less than four hours (sleep not included) may occur infrequently, and often follow treatment with analgesics. Status migrainosus is frequently associated with prolonged analgesic use, which occasionally necessitates in-patient treatment for the control of pain and associated symptoms. Success in effectively treating status migrainous is inconsistent and, despite aggressive medical therapy with serotonin agonists, antiemetics, analgesics and even sedation, patients may leave the hospital with the headache resolving spontaneously at a later time. This pattern suggests that, in some patients, the migraine attacks reverberate and persist within the central nervous system until an intrinsic inhibitory system finally suppresses them.

Summary

The clinical features of migraine represent a wide array of symptoms, including pain activation, focal neurological deficits, vegetative dysfunction and mood alteration. The most successful lines of research into the neurobiology of migraine originate in, and must always return for validation, to the clinical migraine syndrome as it occurs in humans.

References

1 Lipton, R.B., *et al*. (2001). Prevalence and burden of migraine in the United States: data from the American Migraine Study II. *Headache* **41**(7): 646–57.

2 Stewart, W.F., *et al*. (1992). Prevalence of migraine headache in the United States. Relation to age, income, race, and other sociodemographic factors. *JAMA* **267**(1): 64–9.

3 Aminoff, R.P.S., D.A. Greenberg, M.J (2009). *Clinical neurology*, 7th Edition, New York, NY, Lange Medical Books/McGraw-Hill.

4 The International Classification of Headache Disorders, 3rd edition (beta version) (2013). *Cephalalgia* **33**(9): 629–808.

5 Giffin, N.J., *et al*. (2003). Premonitory symptoms in migraine: an electronic diary study. *Neurology* **60**(6): 935–40.

6 Queiroz, L.P., *et al*. (2011). Characteristics of migraine visual aura in Southern Brazil and Northern USA. *Cephalalgia* **31**(16): 1652–8.

7 Cutrer, F.M. and K. Huerter (2007). Migraine aura. *The Neurologist* **13**(3): 118–25.

8 Evans, R.W. (2014). The clinical features of migraine with and without aura. *Practical Neurology* **13**: 26–32.

9 Blau, J.N. (1992). Migraine: theories of pathogenesis. *Lancet* **339**(8803): 1202–7.

10 Foroozan, R. and F.M. Cutrer (2009). Transient neurologic dysfunction in migraine. *Neurologic Clinics* **27**(2): 361–78.

11 Russell, M.B. and J. Olesen (1996). A nosographic analysis of the migraine aura in a general population. *Brain* **119**(Pt 2): 355–61.

12 Vincent, M.B. and N. Hadjikhani (2007). Migraine aura and related phenomena: beyond scotomata and scintillations. *Cephalalgia* **27**(12): 1368–77.

13 Moore, D.J., E. Keogh, and C. Eccleston (2013). Headache impairs attentional performance. *Pain* **154**(9): 1840–5.

14 Viana, M., *et al.* (2013). The typical duration of migraine aura: a systematic review. *Cephalalgia* **33**(7): 483–90.

15 Haas, D.C. (1982). Prolonged migraine aura status. *Annals of Neurology* **11**(2): 197–9.

16 Kuhn, W.F., S.C. Kuhn, and L. Daylida (1997). Basilar migraine. *European Journal of Emergency Medicine* **4**(1): 33–8.

17 Bickerstaff, E.R. (1961). Impairment of consciousness in migraine. *Lancet* **2**(7211): 1057–9.

18 Sturzenegger, M.H. and O. Meienberg (1985). Basilar artery migraine: a follow-up study of 82 cases. *Headache* **25**(8): 408–15.

19 Grosberg, B.M., *et al.* (2006). Retinal migraine reappraised. *Cephalalgia* **26**(11): 1275–86.

20 Codeluppi, L., *et al.* (2015). Optic nerve involvement in retinal migraine. *Headache* **55**(4): 562–4.

21 Kelman, L. (2006). The postdrome of the acute migraine attack. *Cephalalgia* **26**(2): 214–20.

22 Lashley K (1941). Patterns of cerebral integration indicated by scotomas of migraine. *Archives of Neurology and Psychiatry* **46**: 331–339.

12

The premonitory phase of migraine

Michele Viana[1] and Peter J. Goadsby[2]

[1] *Headache Science Center, C. Mondino National Neurological Institute, Pavia, Italy*
[2] *Headache Group – NIHR-Wellcome Trust King's Clinical Research Facility, King's College, London, UK*

Migraine is a highly disabling disorder of the brain (Akerman *et al.*, 2011; Global Burden of Disease Study, 2015), characterized by episodes of moderate to severe headache, often accompanied by a constellation of non-headache symptoms (Headache Classification Committee of the International Headache Society, 2013). Excluding migraine aura, non-headache symptoms have been associated with three phases of attack: the premonitory phase; the headache phase; and the postdrome. Sometimes, the term prodrome has been used, although, since this includes the premonitory phase and the aura phase (Headache Classification Committee of the International Headache Society, 2013), it is both misleading and unhelpful in terms of understanding the pathophysiology of migraine. Characterization of the phenotype of the premonitory phase, and understanding its neurobiology, would provide a very significant step towards understanding migraine better *in toto*.

12.1 What is the premonitory phase? Towards a definition

Premonitory symptoms are defined in ICHD-3-beta as: "symptoms preceding and fore-warning of a migraine attack by 2–48 hours occurring before the aura in migraine with aura and before the onset of pain in migraine without aura" (Headache Classification Committee of the International Headache Society, 2013). This definition is clearly fundamentally flawed, as it means all symptoms between two hours and headache onset are in limbo, which can account for nearly half of patients (Kelman, 2004). Moreover, when the premonitory phase is triggered, the symptoms occur well within two hours (Afridi *et al.*, 2004), consistent with the Kelman (2004) timeline.

Operationally, we have considered premonitory symptoms to be those appearing before pain that are not clearly aura symptoms (Maniyar *et al.*, 2015). A further complexity is that the symptoms are not limited to the premonitory phase, but can also last during the headache and postdromal phases (Giffin *et al.*, 2003). This illustrates the parallel nature of the biology of the migraine attack (Goadsby, 2002), and the potential independence from the pain of symptoms such as photophobia and phonophobia. The most frequent symptoms present in the headache phase, excluding symptoms mentioned in the ICHD criteria of migraine, are: tiredness; stiff neck; blurred vision; irritability; difficulty with thoughts; difficulty with reading and writing; and difficulty with concentration (Giffin *et al.*, 2003). Most frequent premonitory symptoms present in the postdromal phase are: asthenia; tiredness; stiff neck; light sensitivity; noise sensitivity; thirst; difficulty with concentration; and difficulty with thoughts (Giffin *et al.*, 2005; Quintela *et al.*, 2006).

12.2   How common are premonitory symptoms?

Although premonitory symptoms that warn of an impending migraine headache have been recognized for many years, their population prevalence is uncertain. Early estimates of premonitory symptoms have varied from below 10% to 88% (Drummond and Lance, 1984; Waelkens, 1985; Rasmussen and Olesen, 1992; Russell *et al.*, 1996; Kelman, 2004; Schoonman *et al.*, 2006). The most comprehensive large scale adult study has recently reported that 77% of a cohort of 2223 migraine patients reported premonitory symptoms (Laurell *et al.*, 2015). Similarly, it is reported that two-thirds of a pediatric cohort had one or more premonitory symptoms (Cuvellier *et al.*, 2009). While these studies were cross-sectional, and the adult study was questionnaire-based, the prevalence fits with the authors' experience that at least 80% of patients in tertiary clinics have the symptoms. Sometimes they occur with the headache phase, and this can obfuscate their identification. A major limitation of these studies has been the retrospective nature of the approaches.

12.3   Do premonitory symptoms reliably predict a migraine attack?

Giffin and colleagues (2003) used hand-held diaries to study prospectively premonitory symptoms heralding headache attacks. Seventy-six subjects completed a four-center clinic-based study. Participants were instructed to keep diaries for three months, and they recorded a total of 803 attacks, recording potential premonitory symptoms. The investigators evaluated how often premonitory symptoms were followed by headache over the next 72 hours. The most common premonitory symptom was tiredness, reported in 72% of sessions with premonitory symptoms, followed by difficulty with concentration (51%), and stiff neck (50%). We summarize the prevalence of all symptoms in figure 12.1. When premonitory symptoms were reported in the electronic diaries, they were followed on 72% of occasions by a migraine headache within 72 hours. For 82% of patients, premonitory features were followed by a migraine headache within 72 hours more than 50% of the time.

   To assess the probability of headache following a symptom, the authors calculated prevalence ratios, the proportion of time a symptom was followed by headache over 72 hours, and the proportion of time that they were not followed by headache. Interestingly, yawning, emotional changes and difficult in reading and writing were the most predictive for a migraine headache. In a prospective study with a paper diary, Quintela *et al.* (2006) assessed the predictive value of premonitory symptoms, defining "true" premonitory symptoms as those experienced the day before the headache had started, but only

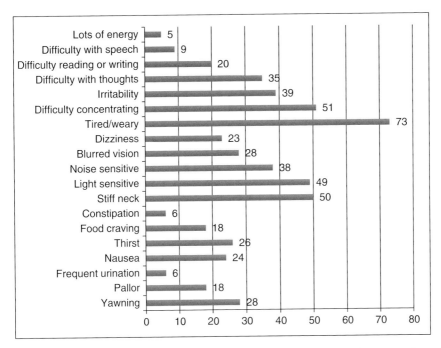

Figure 12.1 Proportion of attack with a non-headache feature reported in the "premonitory phase" (*n* = 803, based on Giffin *et al.*, 2003. Reproduced by permission of Wolters Kluwer Health, Inc.).

if they were not reported as present in a questionnaire completed in a pain-free period. The most common individual true symptoms were anxiety (46%), phonophobia (44%), irritability (42%), unhappiness and yawning (40%) and asthenia (38%).

12.4 Premonitory symptoms in individuals

The mean number of premonitory symptoms reported per person varied from 0–21, with a median of 10, in a study by Schoonman *et al.* (2006). It is notable that Schoonman and colleagues inquired about the presence of 12 symptoms, while Quintela and colleagues used a checklist with 28 symptoms (Quintela *et al.*, 2006). In the Schoonman study, only gender influenced the number of premonitory symptoms (women reported a mean of 3.3 symptoms, compared with a mean of 2.5 in men (*P* = 0.01)), while the effects of age, education, migraine subtype, and mean attack frequency did not alter the symptom frequencies. In the Quintela study, "true" premonitory symptoms were more frequent in patients experiencing migraine with aura episodes, and less in those who were not using preventives. The median duration of premonitory symptoms was reported as two hours in a large clinic-based study (Kelman, 2004).

12.5 Intra-patient variability of the premonitory phase

It has been demonstrated that the features of a migraine attack, including the number and type of premonitory symptoms, are not stereotyped in patients (Viana *et al.*, 2016).

In the study by Quintela *et al.* (2006), the consistency of premonitory symptoms in the 60 patients who had completed the questionnaire for three attacks was analyzed. Consistency was reviewed only for those premonitory symptoms which were present in at least one attack in more than 25% of patients. In these patients, premonitory symptom consistency in at least two out of three migraine attacks ranged from 25–83% (mean 63%) and, in three out of three, attacks ranged from 6–53% (mean 30%). Concentration difficulties, unhappiness, anxiety and yawning were the most consistent premonitory symptoms.

12.6 Difference between patients with and without premonitory symptoms

Kelman (2004) studied a total of 893 migraine patients, of which 33% reported prodrome (*sic* – i.e., premonitory) symptoms. Patients with premonitory symptoms differed from patients without them in having more triggers as a whole, and more individual triggers, including alcohol, hormones, light, not eating, perfume, stress, and weather changes. They also had longer duration of aura, a longer time between aura and headache, and more aura with no headache. Regarding headache, they had longer time to peak of headache, longer time to respond to triptan, longer maximum duration of headache, and more headache-associated nausea. With regard to other symptoms, they had headache-associated running of the nose or tearing of the eyes, more postdromal symptoms, and longer duration of postdromal symptoms.

12.7 Premonitory symptoms in children

Cuvellier *et al.* (2009) retrospectively studied with a questionnaire the prevalence of 15 predefined premonitory symptoms in a clinic-based population. In 103 children and adolescents fulfilling the ICHD-2 criteria for pediatric migraine (Headache Classification Committee of The International Headache Society, 2004), at least one premonitory symptom was reported by 69 (67%). The most frequently reported premonitory symptoms were face changes, fatigue and irritability, and the median number of premonitory symptoms reported per subject was two. Age, migraine subtype, with or without aura, and mean attack frequency per month had no effect on the number of premonitory symptoms reported per subject. the authors concluded that premonitory symptoms are frequently reported by children and adolescents with migraine, and that face changes seem to be a premonitory symptom peculiar to pediatric migraine. The latter needs consideration as a cranial autonomic symptom (Goadsby and Lipton, 1997).

12.8 Premonitory symptoms and migraine triggers

Some premonitory symptoms raise challenging questions regarding the nature of migraine triggers.

Chocolate is considered one of the most common food that can trigger a migraine attack. Yet, when compared to carob in a double-blind study, chocolate failed to demonstrate any significant triggering effect (Marcus *et al.*, 1997). Food cravings are clearly present as premonitory symptoms (Giffin *et al.*, 2003), so is the attribution of the trigger, because the behavior or eating is linked to migraine. The latter is plausibly linked to hypothalamic region activation in the premonitory phase of migraine (Maniyar *et al.*, 2014b). Moreover, as an example, hypothalamic feeding and thirst mechanisms related to neuropeptide Y (NPY – Stanley and Leibowitz, 1984, 1985; Bellinger and Bernardis, 2002) may play a role in the early disengagement of descending brain modulatory mechanisms that are facilitating the attack. It can be shown that NPY inhibits nociceptive trigeminovascular activation in the trigeminocervical complex (Martins-Oliveira *et al.*, 2013), which may be at the basis of this link to behavioral change.

Similarly, light is considered by many patients to be a trigger yet, when patients claiming light triggering were carefully studied, no patients could be triggered (Hougaard *et al.*, 2013). Given photophobia occurs in the premonitory phase (Giffin *et al.*, 2003), and can be shown to be associated with excess activation of the visual cortex, compared to patients without photophobia (Maniyar *et al.*, 2014a), it is again plausible that the patient mistakes the premonitory phase photic sensitivity for light as a trigger. An understanding of these phenomena may be greatly useful to patients and biologists alike (Goadsby and Silberstein, 2013).

12.9 Premonitory symptoms and pathophysiological studies

As the premonitory phase is the first segment of a migraine attack, evaluating the activity of central nervous system in this frame time is of vital importance to understand the pathophysiology of migraine.

Electrophysiological studies have consistently shown lack of habituation of cortical responses to various stimuli, that increases progressively in the period before the headache and normalizes with headache, consistent with the notion that the premonitory phase is likely to entail events key to migraine generation (Schoenen *et al.*, 2003).

Maniyar and colleagues (2014b) performed positron emission tomography (PET) scans with $H_2^{15}O$ in eight patients to measure cerebral blood flow as a marker of neuronal. They conducted scans at baseline, in the premonitory phase without pain, and during migraine headache, in eight patients. They used glyceryl trinitrate (nitroglycerin) to trigger premonitory symptoms (Thomsen *et al.*, 1994; Afridi *et al.*, 2004) and migraine headache in patients with episodic migraine without aura, who habitually experienced premonitory symptoms during spontaneous attacks. By comparing the first premonitory scans in all patients to baseline scans in all patients, it was found there were activations in the posterolateral hypothalamus, midbrain tegmental area, periaqueductal grey, dorsal pons and various cortical areas, including occipital, temporal and prefrontal cortex. The authors concluded that brain activations, in particular in the hypothalamic region, seen in the premonitory phase of migraine attacks, can explain many of the premonitory symptoms, and may provide some insight into why migraine is commonly activated by a change in homeostasis.

12.10   Treatment during the premonitory phase

There have been few clinical trials where the ability of a medication taken during pre-monitory symptoms to prevent the expected migraine attack has been tested. Such tri-als are obviously difficult to do, as patients with premonitory symptoms must first be recruited, the reliability of their premonitory symptoms determined, and then the med-ication must be tested.

The classically quoted study in this area is of Waelkens (1982), who studied dom-peridone taken during the premonitory phase in a double-blind, placebo-controlled, crossover fashion. Nineteen patients, all with what was termed "classical" migraine that included "sensory or psychic intolerance" prior to pain, treated 76 attacks during the study. Patients had warning symptoms 7–48 hours (median 24) before headache onset, and all had severe headache. Medication was taken at the first warning sign, and each patient treated four attacks, two with placebo and two with domperidone 30 mg, in random order. No aura or headache was experienced in 66% of attacks treated with domperidone, compared with 5% of attacks treated with placebo ($P < 0001$).

In second study, Waelkens (1984) examined further the ability of domperidone taken during the premonitory phase to prevent migraine attacks. The study included 19 patients, 18 of whom had migraine with aura. The patients took three doses of domperidone (20, 30 or 40 mg) in a blind fashion and in random order. Each patient treated two attacks with each dose. Taken at the very first appearance of the early warning symptoms, the 20 mg, 30 mg and 40 mg doses prevented, respectively, 30%, 58% and 63% of the expected attacks. There was a suggestion that domperidone was more effective when taken early, even 12 hours, before attack onset. It did not seem to work nearly as well when taken within one hour of attack onset. Waelkens (1985) subsequently noted that, whether symptoms continued during the attack or ceased as headache began, the domperidone effect was no different.

Luciani *et al.* (2000) assessed naratriptan for efficacy when taken in response to premonitory symptoms, performing an open-label study in 20 patients. In the trial, patients recorded diaries for three episodes of premonitory symptoms, and these were followed by headache 100% of the time. During the treatment phase of the trial, patients were instructed to take naratriptan 2.5 mg during the premonitory phase when they felt headache was inevitable. Each patient treated up to six premonitory phases. While headache followed the premonitory phase 100% of the time during the baseline phase, during the open-label treatment phase, only 40% of the treated premonitory phases were followed by headache. Moreover, the results suggested that headache prevention seemed to be more reliable when medication was taken more than two hours before headache onset, and those headaches that did occur appeared milder than those during the baseline phase.

12.11   Conclusion

The premonitory phase of migraine offers a very rich opportunity to study the biology of the condition in the attack's earliest phase. It has the distinct advantage of not having pain, so mechanisms identified and explored do not have the simple explanation of being a response to pain. The premonitory phase further offers insights to patients in terms of differentiating triggering from the earliest stages of their attacks. Even if we have no treatments, if it is clear an attack is possible, the patient can prepare by minimizing aggravating factors and making sure treatments are available when headache strikes. As we understand the biology of this phase, we will no doubt develop therapies that, for many, will enable patients to avoid the disabling suffering of the pain of migraine.

References

Afridi S, Kaube H, Goadsby PJ (2004). Glyceryl trinitrate triggers premonitory symptoms in migraineurs. *Pain* **110**: 675–80.

Akerman S, Holland P, Goadsby PJ (2011). Diencephalic and brainstem mechanisms in migraine. *Nature Reviews Neuroscience* **12**: 570–84.

Bellinger LL, Bernardis LL (2002). The dorsomedial hypothalamic nucleus and its role in ingestive behavior and body weight regulation. Lessons learned from lesioning studies. *Physiology & Behavior* **76**: 431–42.

Cuvellier JC, Mars A, Vallee L (2009). The prevalence of premonitory symptoms in paediatric migraine: a questionnaire study in 103 children and adolescents. *Cephalalgia* **29**(11): 1197–201.

Drummond PD, Lance JW (1984). Neurovascular disturbances in headache patients. *Clinical and Experimental Neurology* **20**: 93–9.

Giffin NJ, Ruggiero L, Lipton RB, Silberstein S, Tvedskov JF, Olesen J, *et al.* (2003). Premonitory symptoms in migraine: an electronic diary study. *Neurology* **60**: 935–40.

Giffin NJ, Lipton RB, Silberstein SD, Tvedskov JF, Olesen J, Goadsby PJ (2005). The migraine postdrome: an electronic diary study. *Cephalalgia* **25**: 958.

Global Burden of Disease Study (2015). Global, regional, and national incidence, prevalence, and years lived with disability for 301 acute and chronic diseases and injuries in 188 countries, 1990–2013: a systematic analysis for the Global Burden of Disease Study 2013. *Lancet* **386**(9995): 743–800.

Goadsby PJ (2002). Parallel concept of migraine pathogensis. *Annals of Neurology* **51**: 140.

Goadsby PJ, Lipton RB (1997). A review of paroxysmal hemicranias, SUNCT syndrome and other short-lasting headaches with autonomic features, including new cases. *Brain* **120**: 193–209.

Goadsby PJ, Silberstein SD (2013). Migraine triggers – harnessing the messages of clinical practice. *Neurology* **80**: 424–5.

Headache Classification Committee of The International Headache Society (2004). The International Classification of Headache Disorders (second edition). *Cephalalgia* **24**(Suppl 1): 1–160.

Headache Classification Committee of the International Headache Society (2013). The International Classification of Headache Disorders, 3rd edition (beta version). *Cephalalgia* **33**: 629–808.

Hougaard A, Amin F, Hauge AW, Ashina M, Olesen J (2013). Provocation of migraine with aura using natural trigger factors. *Neurology* **80**: 428–31.

Kelman L (2004). The premonitory symptoms (prodrome): a tertiary care study of 893 migraineurs. *Headache* **44**: 865–72.

Laurell K, Artto V, Bendtsen L, Hagen K, Haggstrom J, Linde M, *et al.* (2015). Premonitory symptoms in migraine: A cross-sectional study in 2714 persons. *Cephalalgia* **36**(10), 951–9.

Luciani R, Carter D, Mannix L, Hemphill M, Diamond M, Cady R (2000). Prevention of migraine during prodrome with naratriptan. *Cephalalgia* **20**: 122–6.

Maniyar FH, Sprenger T, Goadsby PJ (2014a). Photic hypersensitivity in the premonitory phase of migraine – A PET study. *European Journal of Neurology* **21**: 1178–83.

Maniyar FH, Sprenger T, Monteith T, Schankin C, Goadsby PJ (2014b). Brain activations in the premonitory phase of nitroglycerin triggered migraine attacks. *Brain* **137**: 232–42.

Maniyar FH, Sprenger T, Monteith T, Schankin CJ, Goadsby PJ (2015). The premonitory phase of migraine – what can we learn from it? *Headache* **45**: 609–20.

Marcus DA, Scharff L, Turk D, Gourley LM (1997). A double-blind provocative study of chocolate as a trigger of headache. *Cephalalgia* **17**: 855–62.

Martins-Oliveira M, Akerman S, Goadsby PJ (2013). Neuropeptide Y Inhibits Neuronal Activation in the Trigeminocervical Complex: Implications in Pain Processing in Migraine Pathophysiology. *Cephalalgia* **33**(Suppl 8): 212.

Quintela E, Castillo J, Munoz P, Pascual J (2006). Premonitory and resolution symptoms in migraine: a prospective study in 100 unselected patients. *Cephalalgia* **26**(9): 1051–60.

Rasmussen BK, Olesen J (1992). Migraine with aura and migraine without aura: an epidemiological study. *Cephalalgia* **12**: 221–8.

Russell MB, Rassmussen BK, Fenger K, Olesen J (1996). Migraine without aura and migraine with aura are distinct clinical entities: a study of four hundred and eight-four male and female migraineurs from the general population. *Cephalalgia* **16**: 239–45.

Schoenen J, Ambrosini A, Sandor PS, Maertens de Noordhout A (2003). Evoked potentials and transcranial magnetic stimulation in migraine: published data and viewpoint on their pathophysiologic significance. *Clinical Neurophysiology* **114**: 955–72.

Schoonman GG, Evers DJ, Terwindt GM, van Dijk JG, Ferrari MD (2006). The prevalence of premonitory symptoms in migraine: a questionnaire study in 461 patients. *Cephalalgia* **26**: 1209–13.

Stanley BG, Leibowitz SF (1984). Neuropeptide Y: stimulation of feeding and drinking by injection into the paraventricular nucleus. *Life Sciences* **35**(26): 2635–42.

Stanley BG, Leibowitz SF (1985). Neuropeptide Y injected in the paraventricular hypothalamus: a powerful stimulant of feeding behavior. *Proceedings of the National Academy of Sciences of the United States of America* **82**(11): 3940–3.

Thomsen LL, Kruuse C, Iversen HK, Olesen J (1994). A nitric oxide donor (nitroglycerine) triggers genuine migraine attacks. *European Journal of Neurology* **1**: 73–80.

Viana M, Sances G, Ghiotto N, Guaschino E, Allena M, Nappi G, Goadsby PJ, Tassorelli C (2016). Variability of the characteristics of a migraine attack within patients. *Cephalalgia* **36**(9): 825–30.

Waelkens J (1982). Domperidone in the prevention of complete classical migraine. *British Medical Journal* **284**: 944.

Waelkens J (1984). Dopamine blockade with domperidone: bridge between prophylactic and abortive treatment of migraine? A dose-finding study. *Cephalalgia* **4**: 85–90.

Waelkens J (1985). Warning symptoms in migraine: characteristics and therapeutic implications. *Cephalalgia* **5**: 223–8.

Part IV

Migraine genetics and CSD

13

The genetic borderland of migraine and epilepsy

Isamu Aiba and Jeffrey Noebels

Developmental Neurogenetics Laboratory, Department of Neurology, Baylor college of Medicine, Houston, Texas, USA

13.1   Introduction

"While migraine is to be classed with the epilepsies, provisionally, as a 'discharging lesion', it would be as absurd to classify it as ordinary epilepsy as to classify whales with other mammals. A whale is in law a fish, and in zoology a mammal."
                    J. Hughlings Jackson, Lecture before the Harveian Society, 1879.

Over a century has elapsed since Jackson exhorted neurologists to divide these two episodic disorders, whose overlapping clinical features made their diagnosis "by no means an easy matter", into separate phenomena for scientific study. Gowers, his contemporary, agreed they were co-occupants of a clinical "borderland" of epilepsy, yet emphasized the large difference between them in the tempo of their transcerebral spread (Gowers, 1906). Leao later described the wave of cortical depression and vasoreaction in cortex (Leao, 1947) that matched the speed of the expanding scotoma mapped by Lashley during his own migraine (Milner, 1958), and clinical imaging studies since that time have cemented this relationship (Hadjikhani *et al.*, 2001).

While the naturally occurring sequence of molecular events that trigger the human phenomenon remain unclear to this day, animal studies have pinpointed the early phase of neuronal hyperexcitability due to rises in extracellular potassium and glutamate in the seconds preceding the leading edge of the wave, thereby identifying a brief moment of molecular overlap between the electrogenesis of epileptic discharges and the dramatic silencing of neurons in a migrainous aura. Within this framework, recent genetic discoveries have now positioned these network excitability shifts into a common molecular borderland, and raise fascinating questions regarding their shared pathogenesis.

13.2   Gene-linked comorbidity

Long considered a major island in the archipelago of epilepsy comorbidity, migraine headache, with particular emphasis on the clinical aura as a prodrome or aftermath of a seizure, is now a key entry point into the search for the additional genes and molecular mechanisms underlying both disorders. As might be expected of two of the most

Neurobiological Basis of Migraine, First Edition. Edited by Turgay Dalkara and Michael A. Moskowitz.
© 2017 John Wiley & Sons, Inc. Published 2017 by John Wiley & Sons, Inc.

common diagnoses made in pediatric and adult neurology clinics, headache and seizures each feature a broad spectrum of diagnostic subtypes and rich individual clinical variation, while their distinction may still be arrived at with difficulty. Whether of primary therapeutic or simply anecdotal clinical interest, comorbid syndromes have dramatically escalated the isolation of single gene-linked epilepsy phenotypes (Noebels, 2015a).

It is noteworthy that the very first gene isolated for epilepsy, the syndrome of myoclonic epilepsy with ragged-red fiber myopathy (MERRF), bearing a mitochondrial DNA tRNA-Lys mutation (Shoffner *et al.*, 1990), is also linked to migraine (Zeviani *et al.*, 1993), pointing to a shared metabolic substrate. Interestingly, in both migraine and epilepsy syndromes, it is the characteristic aura and its cerebral localization, rather than the subsequent headache or convulsive episode, that facilitated the initial genetic discoveries. For example, in migraine, the frontal lobe aura of hemiplegia, known since the 19th century (see Whitty, 1953), ultimately led to cloning the first migraine with aura gene, a pore-forming subunit of the voltage-activated calcium channel, *CACNA1A*, for familial hemiplegic migraine (FHM1) (Ophoff *et al.*, 1996). In epilepsy, the unusual auditory aura reported in cases of autosomal dominant lateral temporal lobe epilepsy (ADLTE) led to isolation of the first gene for epilepsy with aura, the secreted protein LGI1 that interacts with the KCNA1 potassium channel, a key gene for temporal lobe seizures (Kalachikov *et al.*, 2002; Schulte *et al.*, 2006).

While auras feature prominently in the classification of headache (Headache Classification Committee of the International Headache, 2013), they are less emphasized in the epilepsy classification (Berg *et al.*, 2010) and, unlike migraine, the electrophysiology of auras preceding seizure is relatively unexplored. The pathophysiology of an aura in migraine now centers on concurrent alterations in network excitability and blood flow, culminating in spreading depolarization (SD) (Pietrobon and Moskowitz, 2013). However, this relationship is not well established in the auras of epilepsy, which are assumed to represent local irritability in, or near, a seizure focus prior to its spread. Why an aura is not a consistent feature of epilepsy is not known, but cortical recruitment at the onset of a seizure ranges from nearly instantaneous in primary generalized epilepsies to a speed of ≈ 4mm/sec in secondary recruitment from a cortical seizure focus – about 60 times faster than SD (Martinet *et al.*, 2015).

13.3   The challenge of dissecting seizure and aura excitability defects

Ictal events of migraine and epilepsy are considered separable, since extracellular K^+ ceiling levels attained during an experimental seizure (12–15 mM) fall far short of those typically found during experimental SD (30–50 mM) (Somjen, 2002). However, these *in vivo* values are obtained from artificially triggered events in normal adult cortex, rather than spontaneous seizures or migraine aura in brains with the chronic disorder. Similarly, an *in silico* model of the intervening excitability spectrum using physiological parameters and a Hodgkin-Huxley formalism has been proposed (Wei *et al.*, 2014).

However, cellular excitability, oxygen extraction, and neurovascular coupling are not monotonically linked, and display non-linear tipping points that are mediated by aberrant vasoreactivity, membrane depolarization block, mitochondrial function, and failed homeostasis of the extracellular milieu. These parameters are all altered in a mutant, anesthetized or injured brain or injured brain. Dynamic interactions between SD and experimental seizure foci represent a complex function of reverberating waves and reentrant thresholds (Koroleva and Bures, 1979, 1980, 1983). More realistic disease models of human pathophysiology are needed to compare the spectrum of underlying mechanisms directly.

Even with a broader range of appropriate models, deciphering the aura mechanisms of epilepsy and migraine poses numerous challenges to dissect early phase pathophysiology from other network synchronization defects. Spreading depolarization may lead to a seizure, or may appear following one, and the amplitudes and propagation distances of the depolarizing wave vary. When examined in patients, extensive monitoring is required to capture a spontaneous attack (Hartl *et al.*, 2015), DC-coupled EEG recordings requiring intracranial electrodes are not feasible, and non-invasive indirect assays may be ambiguous.

When reproduced in experimental models, the thresholds for SD and seizures depend on the stimuli and metabolic substrates selected, and are subject to other experimental variables (see Chapter 19). Finally, aura thresholds, whether due to a single gene mutation or acquired brain injury, are not static, but vary with brain maturity and tissue remodeling. Given the pleiotrophic effects of channel mutations in different neuronal circuits, one can anticipate that different genes and vascular lesions contributing to the biology of migraine aura will ultimately explain the spectrum of individual patterns and triggers, as found in stroke (Dreier and Reiffurth, 2015) and epilepsy (Noebels, 2015b).

Despite this complexity, once a monogenic disorder is isolated, tracing the cellular and functional expression of the mutated gene in experimental models is a reliably informative route to elucidate causative mechanisms and therapeutic targets. Conditional expression of epilepsy gene mutations within cortical microcircuitry is a new approach to define essential determinants of network synchronization. For example, cell type specific ablation of *CACNA1A*, the gene encoding the P/Q-type calcium channel that underlies both seizures and FHM1, reveals that at least two interneuron populations – parvalbumin and somatostatin – collaborate to structure an EEG seizure pattern into convulsive or spike-wave absence phenotypes, depending on the balance of transmitter release at their synapses (Rossignol *et al.*, 2013). The *SCN1A* sodium channel has been conditionally mutated in these same interneuron types, producing alternative temperature-sensitive seizure and behavioral phenotypes (Rubinstein *et al.*, 2015a). Since SD also shows laminar and regional properties (Gniel and Martin, 2010), similar strategies, using selective knockin mutations of migraine genes in cortical glia and neuronal cell types, may help to further pinpoint critical network excitability threshold relationships.

In this chapter, we review the remarkable genetic overlap emerging between human migraine with aura and various monogenic ion channel epilepsies. We also describe new insights into mechanisms linking SD in the brainstem to a novel "aura" comorbidity phenotype, sudden unexpected death, the most common cause of premature lethality in epilepsy. In models of this syndrome, two genes for hemiplegic migraine (*CACNA1A*, *SCN1A*) lead to SD-linked postictal collapse of cardiorespiratory homeostasis in experimental models, and *in vitro* studies reveal a lower SD threshold in the mutant brainstem. Finally, we draw attention to MAPT, a shared protective gene for epilepsy and SD. Ablation of MAPT, the gene encoding Tau, a microtubule binding protein, corrects the SD threshold and prolongs survival in SUDEP mutant mouse models.

13.4   Clinical overlap of migraine with aura and epilepsy phenotypes

13.4.1   Classification and co-prevalence

Relationships between these entities have been recently reviewed (Verrotti *et al.*, 2011; Rogawski, 2012; Nye and Thadani, 2015). Migraine and seizures are episodic events, defined by their differing patterns of abnormal neuronal excitability, speed of onset, spread, and predilection for specific brain regions. While individual syndromes have distinct ages of onset, individuals with epilepsy have a 4.5 times higher lifetime risk of developing migraine over the general population (Toldo *et al.*, 2010), resulting in an approximately 20% prevalence rate in this group (Oakley and Kossoff, 2014). Likewise, the risk of epilepsy among those with migraine is strongly associated, and a history of migraine with aura (but not without aura) increases the risk of epilepsy over three-fold in later life (Ludvigsson *et al.*, 2006). Up to 25% of children with epilepsy experience migraine (Kelley *et al.*, 2012). In contrast, seizures are uncommon in the younger migraine population, and most cases of migraine (>80%) occur in the absence of routine EEG abnormality (Martens *et al.*, 2012).

13.4.2   Timing

The definition of "ictal headache" is being refined (Parisi *et al.*, 2015). Migraine in epilepsy patients may occur either in the absence of an ongoing seizure ("interictal migraine") or as a headache accompanying one ("peri-ictal migraine"). Given the subjective symptoms and the possibility of concurrent interictal EEG spiking or subclinical seizure discharges, these entities cannot be firmly dissociated without electrographic evidence. The incidence of peri-ictal migraine is high (>60%) in individuals with epilepsy (Kanemura *et al.*, 2013). Headache arises at various phases; it appears during the pre-ictal phase in about 5–15% of cases, during the postictal phase in 40–70% of cases, and overlaps in the remainder (Yankovsky *et al.*, 2005; Parisi *et al.*, 2012). Like the ictal phase, the pre-ictal period of a cortical seizure may be associated with transient hyperemia and vascular inflammation (Cai *et al.*, 2008).

The syndromic classification system of the epilepsies centers on age of onset, electroclinical seizure semiology, relation to fever, imaging findings, cognitive dysfunction, genetics, and drug profile (Berg *et al.*, 2010). There are over 20 recognized epilepsy syndromes and seizure types, but many more epilepsies are now recognized and defined genetically, often by their comorbid status with developmental cognitive delay (over 160 entries in OMIM for "epileptic encephalopathy"). The fraction of seizures with premonitory auras depends on the region affected and consistency of the symptomatic description. In temporal lobe epilepsies, about 23/40 patients have reported aura-like subclinical seizures, and half of those showed electroclinical correlates (Sperling and O'Connor, 1990). In a second study, 67% of 244 patients reliably reported an aura, and 80% of these lasted one minute or less. In occipital epilepsies, visual symptoms are present in only half of patients, while no TLE patients reported visual auras (Appel *et al.*, 2015; Punia *et al.*, 2015).

13.4.3   Migraine aura and headache arise from distinct pathways and triggers

Migraine auras are typically congruent with the pain in terms of laterality and temporal precedence. However, these engage independent sensorimotor vs. nociceptive pathways, with variable duration and thresholds. Unlike pain, auras are not triggered by nitroglycerin, even in migraineurs with aura (Christiansen *et al.*, 1999), nor are they relieved by sumatriptan (Rose, 1994), further evidence that the aura is not a primarily vascular event. In experimentally naïve animals, a single SD produces a biphasic sequence suggesting multiple vascular reflex waves following depressed cortical excitation (Chang *et al.*, 2010).

13.4.4   Gender, estrogen, and interictal excitability phenotype in migraine aura and epilepsy

A key issue is whether migraines and seizures arise from a normal or elevated baseline excitability state, and whether gender or hormones affect this baseline and, hence, co-incidence. Migraine has a clear gender difference, with higher female prevalence (Chai *et al.*, 2014). In contrast, there is little similar evidence in epilepsy, except for X-linked forms (Veliskova, 2006), and little difference in peri-ictal migraine prevalence.

Both migraine frequency (Victor *et al.*, 2010) and juvenile onset epilepsies increase after puberty in both sexes, and may be associated with the menstrual cycle (Herzog, 2015). Direct modulation by estrogen and progesterone contribute to the excitability shift (Borsook *et al.*, 2014), although the biological complexity of fast (membrane) versus slow (genomic) estrogen receptor effects on neurons (Arevalo *et al.*, 2015), glia (Acaz-Fonseca *et al.*, 2014), and the neurovascular unit limit our understanding of this modulation. For example, β-estradiol facilitates experimentally triggered SD within 60 minutes, and is fully reversible in rodent neocortical brain slices, suggesting a direct membrane pathway (Sachs *et al.*, 2007; Chauvel *et al.*, 2013), but slower genomic effects have not been systematically explored.

Despite an excitatory role for estrogen in the adult brain, the contribution to seizure incidence is not always clear, and studies reveal both pro-convulsive (NMDA receptor-mediated) and anti-convulsive (GABA receptor-related) effects in human and animal studies (Veliskova, 2006; Tauboll *et al.*, 2015). Age is also important, since early estradiol exposure in the neonatal period prevents gene-linked epilepsy, but aggravates seizures in adults (Olivetti *et al.*, 2014).

In contrast to simple migraine, the brain in migraine with aura shows interictal hyperexcitability. Human transcranial magnetic stimulation (TMS) studies reveal decreased stimulus thresholds (van der Kamp *et al.*, 1996; Aurora *et al.*, 1999). Visual evoked potential studies also show elevated amplitudes to interictal photic stimuli (Demarquay and Mauguiere, 2015), while FHM1 mouse models show interictal hyperexcitability (Vecchia *et al.*, 2015). In epilepsy, due to its vast monogenic heterogeneity, the presence of interictal brain excitability is too variable to characterize, beyond commenting that, while interictal EEG spikes are a diagnostic hallmark of all epilepsy, they are not uniformly present at all times.

By convention, mouse channelopathy models of epilepsy all show variable degrees of interictal spiking. Interestingly, some epilepsy and migraine human cases show interictal and ictal autonomic (QT interval) disturbances (Duru *et al.*, 2006; Anderson *et al.*, 2014). The basis for the eponymic lateralization of migraine aura in a bilaterally expressed channelopathy or ion pump deficiency is not understood. SD in visual auras can be lateralized (Hougaard *et al.*, 2014), as is the hyperemia of hemiplegia auras in FHM2 (Blicher *et al.*, 2015; Iizuka *et al.*, 2012). Nevertheless it is unclear why mutation of a ubiquitously-expressed P/Q calcium channel or ATPase subunit would selectively lower SD threshold in a single hemisphere beyond the passive constraint that, once triggered, SD is unable to cross the midline via white matter tracts.

13.4.5 Pharmacological overlap

Antiepileptic (AED) pharmacology is a mainstay of migraine prophylaxis, implying that the balance of cortical network excitability is essential in both conditions (Oakley and Kossoff, 2014; Schiefecker *et al.*, 2014). Clinically effective AEDs span various nominal categories, namely sodium channel blockers, histone deacetylase inhibitors, and AMPA receptor blockers. However, each drug has its own off target effects, and there is substantial individual variation and pharmacoresistance in both disorders (Parisi *et al.*, 2007; Bogdanov *et al.*, 2011). In addition to AEDs, some studies report anti-migraine efficacy of non-pharmacological antiepileptic interventions that target interictal excitability, including the ketogenic diet (Stafstrom and Rho, 2012; Di Lorenzo *et al.*, 2015) and vagal nerve stimulation (Cecchini *et al.*, 2009; Goadsby *et al.*, 2014; Chen *et al.*, 2015).

13.5 Acquired and genetic etiologies of migraine with aura and epilepsies

13.5.1 Epilepsy

Acquired epilepsies comprise about one-third of all seizure disorder etiologies, and the large remainder, until recently labeled 'idiopathic', are now considered genetic (Figure 13.1). Heredity is a major cause of epilepsy, and the epilepsy genome is rapidly expanding (Noebels, 2015a). The Online Catalog of Mendelian Inheritance in Man (OMIM, NIH) now lists over 175 human genes in dbSNP monogenically linked to epilepsy and, of these, ion channelopathy, both voltage- and ligand-gated, remains the largest category, although a rich biological diversity of other genes is also recognized (Lerche *et al.*, 2013; Noebels, 2003). Sporadic *de novo* mutations found in clinical exomes account for a majority of new gene discovery in epilepsy, while the remainder arises from family studies and reverse genetic approaches in animal models. The "missing inheritance" is likely due to complex non-Mendelian patterns of pathogenic alleles, with a significant influence of modifier genes, particularly within the ion channel subunit gene family itself (Klassen *et al.*, 2011).

While many epilepsy genes show allegiance to a particular seizure type, channelopathies significantly depart from this rule. Most channels display allelic heterogeneity, giving rise to more than one seizure type, depending on the relative gain or loss of function in the channel protein. Pleiotrophy of *CACNA1A* is clearly seen in patients and mouse models of FHM1, where a gain of P/Q-type calcium current enhances glutamate transmitter release, producing convulsive seizures, hemiplegic migraine, and a low threshold for cortical SD (Tottene *et al.*, 2009), while reduced P/Q

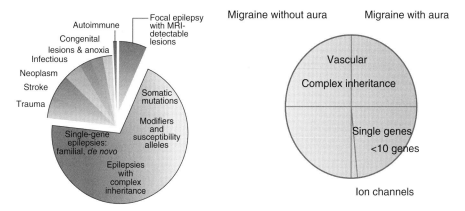

Figure 13.1 Estimated proportion of clinically discoverable and genetically driven etiologies of epilepsy and migraine with aura. Left: In epilepsy, about on-third of cases are secondary to demonstrable brain injury. The remainder are due to genetic mutations, either monogenic or in complex patterns of inheritance. Monogenic causes of seizures exceed 150; each is still considered individually rare forms of epilepsy. Many epilepsy syndromes are exclusively genetic, and show extensive locus heterogeneity (modified from Thomas *et al.*, 2014). Right: In migraine with aura, a similar architecture of acquired causes is plausible, although the overall contributions of both acquired and genetic syndromes are unknown. A likely difference will be in the proportion of vascular etiologies.

current in the tottering mouse and other loss of function alleles (Noebels, 1979, 2012) produce thalamocortical spike-wave absence epilepsy, and a high threshold for cortical SD (Ayata *et al.*, 2000). A second feature of channelopathies is their locus heterogeneity, where several genes for distinct channel subunits all contribute to clinically similar syndromes, and this pattern is emerging in migraine with aura.

13.5.2 Migraine

In migraine with aura, there is less information on the range of acquired etiologies and their cellular neuropathology. Using epileptogenesis as a model, a secondary pathogenic cascade leading to migraine with aura is likely to resemble that in brain injuries causing epilepsy, albeit in altered proportions. OMIM currently shows 118 entries for migraine loci (34 linked to known genes in dbSNP). In migraine with aura, familial pedigrees have led to the isolation of three genes so far. Many cases of FHM are reported without mutation of these genes, indicating that further simple and complex gene discovery can be expected.

Migraine with aura is highly heritable ($\approx$60%) (Russell *et al.*, 2002) and the underlying genetics are under active exploration (Tolner *et al.*, this book). Genomic association studies (Chasman *et al.*, 2011; Anttila *et al.*, 2013) revealed 12 SNPs in genes associated with migraine, including PRDM16, MEF2D, TRPM8, PHACTR1, ASTN2, LRP1, AJAP1, TSPAN2, FHL5, C7orf10 and MMP16. Later studies have validated some of these genes (i.e., LRP1, PRDM16, MMP16 and TRPM8) in different ethnic groups (An *et al.*, 2013; Esserlind *et al.*, 2013; Ghosh *et al.*, 2013, 2014; Fan *et al.*, 2014; Ran *et al.*, 2014; Sintas *et al.*, 2014), but polymorphisms in TRPM8 and LRP1 are also associated with migraine without aura (Freilinger *et al.*, 2012) (see Chapter 14).

A large number of genes for migraine are linked to vascular biology and inflammation (Malik *et al.*, 2015). Systematic and cell type specific analysis may help refine candidate gene sets (de Vries *et al.*, 2015; Eising *et al.*, 2015), but the biological overlap of these genes and their prevalence in epilepsy patients is not yet established. The PRRT2 gene was initially isolated in cases of infantile convulsions, and also paroxysmal dyskinesia with migraine (Ebrahimi-Fakhari *et al.*, 2015). This gene encodes a membrane protein with proline transporter properties that may interact with SNAP25 (Nobile and Striano, 2014), a presynaptic protein linked to epilepsy (Zhang *et al.*, 2004). PRRT2, like others listed above, awaits further biological and functional characterization in a genetic model system.

13.6   Migraine aura is linked to specific genes with locus and allelic heterogeneity

Three genes – FHM1 (*CACNA1A*), FHM2 (*ATP1A2*), and FHM3 (*SCN1A*) – are now securely linked to genetic migraine with aura (Figure 13.2). They are rare causes, not typically detected in GWAS studies. Dominant allele-specific mutations in these genes favor cellular depolarization, with gain of function in P/Q-type calcium current, loss of ATPase activity, and altered sodium channel kinetics. Like all channel subunits, the genes contain multiple functional domains giving rise to significant allelic heterogeneity, and various loss of function and dominant negative gain of function mutations are responsible for multiple phenotypes.

CACNA1A shows multiple allele-specific phenotypes, ranging from convulsions, hemiplegic migraine, aphasia, ataxia, and coma to absence epilepsy and episodic dyskinesias in the loss of function alleles (Noebels, 2012). Not much information exists on *de novo* variants, but a sporadic loss of function *CACNA1A* allele with epilepsy has been reported (Zangaladze *et al.*, 2010). There is a low genetic contribution of P/Q channel mutation to most migraine (Ferrari *et al.*, 2015), and the penetrance of variants in migraine with aura is still poorly understood. In a study of genetically identical but not genotyped twin pairs, 12 monozygotic twins were discordant for an aura, while the headache phase was similar, if not identical (Kallela *et al.*, 1999).

FHM3 shows similar genetic complexity. A very large dataset for genotype-phenotype correlation has been assembled for *SCN1A*, the predominant gene linked to the epilepsy of pediatric Dravet Syndrome (DS), where over 1200 mutations are known (Meng *et al.*, 2015). Interestingly, this correlation shows that severity is dependent on the mode of mutation inheritance, as well as the mutant allele. Most *de novo* mutations produce severe DS epileptic encephalopathy cases, while inherited variants show weaker "generalized epilepsy with febrile seizures ("GEFS+") phenotypes. Mutations in the orthologous gene *SCN8A* are a recent and less frequent cause of DS (Wagnon and Meisler, 2015).

Functional analysis of SCN1A in migraine cases reveals a mixed spectrum of decreased current, trafficking, and inactivation defects that may produce net excitatory or inhibitory effects, depending on the cell type and circuit (Kahlig *et al.*, 2008), similar to the variation in DS. Functional analysis of DS mutations in heterologous systems and mice on different genetic backgrounds (Rubinstein *et al.*, 2015b) show that answers may differ from those obtained in induced pluripotent stem cells containing the patient's own genomic variant profile (Liu *et al.*, 2013).

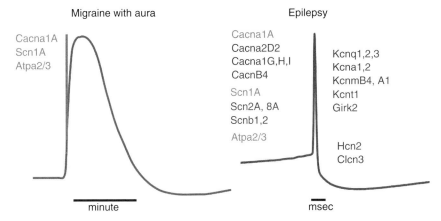

Figure 13.2 Monogenic voltage-gated ion channel genes of migraine with aura and epilepsy, plotted along the voltage trace of their excitability defect; the slow, minutes-long depolarizing trajectory of the spreading cortical wave (Left), or the millisecond kinetics of action potential electrogenesis. Shared genes are in grey; all confirmed ion channel genes for migraine with aura lower the threshold for spreading depolarization, yet also produce robust epilepsy phenotypes with abnormal neuronal burst firing.

13.7   Correspondence of regional brain susceptibility for migraine in genetic epilepsy syndromes

Classic migraine auras include nausea, vomiting, photophobia, photopsia, visual scotomata, hemiparesis, hemisensory deficit, aphasia, and vertigo. Auditory aura has been described as a rare migraine aura variant (Whitman and Lipton, 1995). The aura in a single patient may vary even in a monogenic syndrome such as FHM, which can be occasionally mistaken for basilar artery territory migraine (Haan *et al.*, 1995).

Auras in epilepsy are related to seizure type and location. While *occipital lobe epilepsy* is relatively uncommon (≈1%), occipital seizures are frequently associated with migraine-like visual auras (photophobia, fortification spectra, micropsia) (Ito *et al.*, 2004), and both migraine and seizures can be triggered by visual stimulation. In *Lennox-Gastaut Syndrome* (LGS), a genetic childhood epilepsy, visually evoked occipital seizure activity is common (Caraballo *et al.*, 2009), and about 50% of LGS patients experience peri-ictal migraine headache (Wakamoto *et al.*, 2011), likely due to local seizure or spike activity (Andermann and Zifkin, 1998; Shu *et al.*, 2013).

The GABA receptor *β*3 subunit GABABR3 is one of several candidate genes for LGS (Papandreou *et al.*, 2015). Similarly, migraine and occipital seizures are a common (≈2/3) comorbidity of *Panayiotopoulos* syndrome (PS), a genetically-undefined epilepsy (Andermann and Zifkin, 1998; Clarke *et al.*, 2009). *POLG* mutations impair polymerase gamma, a mitochondrial DNA that maintains the mitochondrial genome, and are also associated with occipital epilepsy and migraine (Janssen *et al.*, 2015).

In frontocentral cortical regions, *Juvenile Myoclonic Epilepsy* (JME) is a common (≈4–10%) generalized spike-wave epilepsy syndrome, with myoclonic and absence seizures arising in the second decade. Most patients are photosensitive and have migraine (Schankin *et al.*, 2011). JME has a strong genetic contribution, and at least

40% of cases show a positive family history (Welty, 2006). Four genes are linked to JME, including *EFHC1, GABRD, GABRA1, and CACNB4.*

Rolandic Epilepsy, also known as benign partial epilepsy of childhood with centrotemporal spikes (BECTS), is a juvenile seizure syndrome with frequent migraine. Candidate genes have been identified (Lal *et al.*, 2015; Reinthaler *et al.*, 2015), and one is near, but not within, the *ATP1A2* gene in the FHM locus (Addis *et al.*, 2014).

In *temporal lobe epilepsies* (TLE*)*, olfactory perceptions often precede seizures, activating the amygdala and the uncus in the parahippocampal gyrus ("uncinate fits"). These auras feature autonomic, abdominal/visceral, and nausea, likely through central autonomic projections from forebrain to medullary brainstem centers, such as vagal nerve nuclei and area postrema. In a study of 876 auras in 400 patients with mesial TLE, 12 categories were assigned (Dupont *et al.*, 2015). Most common were autonomic, abdominal, experiential (déjà vu, confusion), followed by non-specific somatosensory, visual and auditory perceptual, gustatory, olfactory, and vestibular. A majority ($\approx$65%) of these cases reported complex aura profiles with more than one type. While human TLEs have only a few solid monogenic links (*LGI1, RELN*), a larger number of causative genes for TLE have been identified in mouse mutant models, including *Glyt1, Kcna1,* and *Kcnmb4.*

These human comorbid epilepsy/migraine syndromes lend support for gene-directed regional control of excitability and SD threshold. Understanding how specific regions are selectively vulnerable to mutations in a particular gene will require considering how distributions of gene expression, heteroplasmy of mitochondrial DNA, and vasoreactivity combine with local cortical synaptic neurochemistry and connectivity.

13.8   Are SD thresholds plastic?

A hallmark of experimental epileptogenesis is the kindling phenomenon, where chronic stimulation progressively lowers seizure threshold, although there is less evidence for this phenomenon in humans than in rodent models (Bertram, 2007). An important aspect of comorbidity is to understand whether migraine episodes might lower the threshold for seizures, or vice versa. Current evidence provides no support for this relationship and, in fact, shows that chronically epileptic brain is more resistant to SD. In a study of convulsant kindling in rats, seizures initially triggered SD although, with repeated stimulation, the cortical SD threshold increased (Koroleva *et al.*, 1993). Similarly, rats with pilocarpine-induced epilepsy showed a higher SD threshold than naïve animals (Guedes and Cavalheiro, 1997).

In the first study of spreading depression threshold in genetic mouse models, *Tottering* mutant mice with a *Cacna1a* loss of function mutation showed an elevated threshold for SD, despite frequent spontaneous spike-wave seizures, and the SD threshold in *stargazer* mice with similar seizures arising from mutation of a separate gene was unaffected (Ayata *et al.*, 2000). The SD threshold is therefore independent of this seizure type. An elevated SD threshold in chronic epileptic brain has also been reported in human cortical slices *in vitro* using K^+ bath-evoked SD (Maslarova *et al.*, 2011). Acute seizure foci prevent invasion of SD (Bures *et al.*, 1975), and vice versa (McIntyre and Gilby, 2008). Finally, daily repetitive SD generation raises, rather than lowers, the threshold for subsequent SD in rat cortex (Sukhotinsky *et al.*, 2011). These studies suggest that neither an acute nor a prolonged history of seizures or SD is likely to promote its counterpart in patients.

13.9 Spreading depolarization in cardiorespiratory brainstem regions, a candidate mechanism of SUDEP

Migraine aura and seizures share postictal autonomic instability, and may modulate headache pain by activating central autonomic pathways that reach pontine trigeminal and medullary cardiorespiratory brainstem centers. A more tragic outcome of a seizure is Sudden Unexpected Death in Epilepsy (SUDEP), a forensic diagnosis affecting about 10–15% of those with epilepsy (Thurman *et al.*, 2014; Massey *et al.*, 2014). Monitored cases show severe autonomic deregulation, and die within hours after a seizure during a period of apneas, bradycardia, and cardiac asystoles (Ryvlin *et al.*, 2013).

SUDEP has been linked to cardiac LQT gene mutations responsible for sudden death, including the potassium channels KCNQ1 (Goldman *et al.*, 2009) and Kv1.1 (Glasscock *et al.*, 2010), as well as SCN1A1 in Dravet Syndrome (Sakauchi *et al.*, 2011).

Migraine and autonomic deregulation are a common comorbidity of Panayiotopoulos Syndrome (Parisi *et al.*, 2005), and life-threatening cases have been reported (Dirani *et al.*, 2015). Autonomic imbalance, arrhythmias and sudden cardiac death have been reported in migraineurs (May *et al.*, 2015; Monroe *et al.*, 2015). Alternating hemiplegia of childhood (AHC), an infantile form of hemiplegic migraine with seizures due to ATP1A2/3 (Swoboda *et al.*, 2004; Clapcote *et al.*, 2009), is a further addition to the epilepsy/migraine/autonomic borderland. Mutations in the *ATP1A3* gene, expressed in heart and brain, lead to episodic hemiplegia and cardiac repolarization defects, seizures (Jaffer *et al.*, 2015), and prolonged SD (Hunanyan *et al.*, 2015). Migraine also increases the risk of vagal mediated autonomic deregulation, producing vagal syncope (Thijs *et al.*, 2006; Vallejo *et al.*, 2014) and cardiac arrhythmias (Aygun *et al.*, 2003; Melek *et al.*, 2007). These genes, and other channel-interacting genes linked to SUDEP (Qi *et al.*, 2014), alter excitability within central and peripheral parasympathetic pathways and the heart, promoting cardiorespiratory dysfunction.

Since the risk of monogenic SUDEP is congenital, yet SUDEP events occur throughout the lifespan (Thurman *et al.*, 2014), an unexplained feature of gene-linked SUDEP is why younger individuals are not preferentially affected, and even why the first seizure is not lethal. Genetic mouse models of SUDEP with sodium and potassium channelopathy display vagally mediated peri-ictal cardiac arrhythmias and apneas and, in the Kv1 model of SUDEP, about 50% die by one month of age, while those that survive young adulthood live a normal lifespan (Glasscock *et al.*, 2010; Kalume *et al.*, 2013). If hyperexcitability in autonomic pathways were a simple direct mechanism of mortality, early seizures would be fatal events. Therefore both human and animal data imply the participation of a second, independent threshold for a life-threatening seizure.

13.10   Brainstem SD is a "second hit" leading to SUDEP

To test whether SD might be the critical event terminating a lethal seizure, two genetic SUDEP mouse models were studied (Aiba and Noebels, 2015). Evoked cortical seizures in urethane-anesthetized Kv1 KO mice produced SD in dorsal medulla accompanied by apneas, arrhythmias, and cardiorespiratory arrest in over half of the experiments, while cortical seizures never produced brainstem SD or death in wild type adult mice (Figure 13.3). Interestingly, brainstem SD has a low threshold in immature wild type brain that increases during adolescence (Richter, Rupprecht *et al.*, 2003; Funke, Kron *et al.*, 2009).

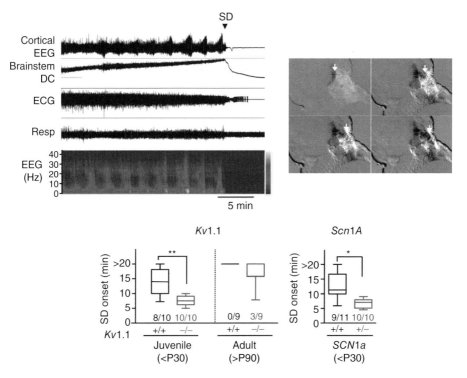

Figure 13.3 Brainstem SD is related to sudden death in SUDEP mouse models. Left: terminal SD recorded from medullary cardiorespiratory nuclei in a Kv1 KO mouse model of SUDEP. After repeated seizures following cortical application of 4aminopyridine, severe irreversible apnea and cardiac arrhythmia only commenced with the onset of brainstem SD. Right: serial photos of IOS signal showing SD-induced transparency change (dark) in brainstem slice of Kv1 mouse, following oxygen and glucose deprivation (OGD). In coronal slices of medulla, a depolarizing wave reliably initiated at the rim of the solitary tract nucleus (NTS) (upper left frame), and invaded adjacent vagal nerve nuclei (lower right frame). Lower: *in vitro* brainstem slices from both Kv1$^{-/-}$ and Nav1$^{-/-}$ mutants showed a strikingly reduced SD threshold compared to wild type slices induced by OGD. Aiba *et al.* (2015). Reproduced from Science Translational Medicine.

13.11   Tau ablation prevents seizures, SUDEP and brainstem SD threshold in models of SUDEP

Deletion of the gene for the microtubule-associated protein tau (*MAPT*) prevents inherited epilepsy, and prolongs survival in mouse and fly models of Kv1 and Scn1a hyperexcitability (Holth *et al.*, 2013; Gheyara *et al.*, 2014). *In vitro* analysis of brainstem SD threshold in Kv1 KO/tau KO double mutants showed that loss of tau rescues the lowered SD threshold phenotype (Aiba and Noebels, 2015). This is the second gene (along with *CACNA1A* loss of function) (Glasscock *et al.*, 2007) that is known to correct the hyperexcitability phenotype of Kv1 SUDEP, and predicts an interesting array of SD modifier genes.

13.12   Conclusion

Genes for a small subset of voltage-gated ion channels and regulators of cellular depolarization identify shared molecular pathways for seizures and migraine auras, and confirm that the "borderland" designation of these comorbid disorders is well founded. Future research can define the edges of this genetic borderland and, ultimately explain why some epilepsy genes possess or lack a migraine aura-like component, and what developmental features tilt the brain toward either phenotype. By providing a broad spectrum of models for individual electroclinical syndromes, regional brain thresholds, and pharmacological selectivity, the experimental study of these genes can reveal critical insights into the molecular and network complexity of both conditions, and strategies to lower the risk for premature death.

13.13   Acknowledgements

The authors acknowledge support from the American Heart Association (IA, Postdoctoral Fellowship 14POST20130031) and NIH (JLN, NS2907, NS090340 and Center for SUDEP Research, and the Blue Bird Circle Foundation.

References

Acaz-Fonseca, E., R. Sanchez-Gonzalez, *et al.* (2014). Role of astrocytes in the neuroprotective actions of 17beta-estradiol and selective estrogen receptor modulators. *Molecular and Cellular Endocrinology* **389**(1–2): 48–57.

Addis, L., T. Chiang, *et al.* (2014). Evidence for linkage of migraine in Rolandic epilepsy to known 1q23 FHM2 and novel 17q22 genetic loci. *Genes, Brain and Behavior* **13**(3): 333–340.

Aiba, I. and J. L. Noebels (2015). Spreading depolarization in the brainstem mediates sudden cardiorespiratory arrest in mouse SUDEP models. *Science Translational Medicine* **7**(282): 282ra246.

An, X. K., Q. L. Ma, *et al.* (2013). PRDM16 rs2651899 variant is a risk factor for Chinese common migraine patients. *Headache* **53**(10): 1595–1601.

Andermann, F. and B. Zifkin (1998). The benign occipital epilepsies of childhood: an overview of the idiopathic syndromes and of the relationship to migraine. *Epilepsia* **39**(Suppl 4): S9–23.

Anderson, J. H., J. M. Bos, *et al.* (2014). Prevalence and spectrum of electroencephalogram-identified epileptiform activity among patients with long QT syndrome. *Heart Rhythm* **11**(1): 53–57.

Anttila, V., B. S. Winsvold, *et al.* (2013). Genome-wide meta-analysis identifies new susceptibility loci for migraine. *Nature Genetics* **45**(8): 912–917.

Appel, S., A. D. Sharan, *et al.* (2015). A comparison of occipital and temporal lobe epilepsies. *Acta Neurologica Scandinavica* **132**(4): 284–290.

Arevalo, M. A., I. Azcoitia, *et al.* (2015). The neuroprotective actions of oestradiol and oestrogen receptors. *Nature Reviews Neuroscience* **16**(1): 17–29.

Aurora, S. K., F. al-Sayeed, *et al.* (1999). The cortical silent period is shortened in migraine with aura. *Cephalalgia* **19**(8): 708–712.

Ayata, C., M. Shimizu-Sasamata, *et al.* (2000). Impaired neurotransmitter release and elevated threshold for cortical spreading depression in mice with mutations in the alpha1A subunit of P/Q type calcium channels. *Neuroscience* **95**(3): 639–645.

Aygun, D., L. Altintop, *et al.* (2003). Electrocardiographic changes during migraine attacks. *Headache* **43**(8): 861–866.

Berg, A. T., S. F. Berkovic, *et al.* (2010). Revised terminology and concepts for organization of seizures and epilepsies: report of the ILAE Commission on Classification and Terminology, 2005–2009. *Epilepsia* **51**(4): 676–685.

Bertram, E. (2007). The relevance of kindling for human epilepsy. *Epilepsia* **48**(Suppl 2): 65–74.

Blicher, J. U., A. Tietze, *et al.* (2015). Perfusion and pH MRI in familial hemiplegic migraine with prolonged aura. *Cephalalgia* **36**(3): 279–83.

Bogdanov, V. B., S. Multon, *et al.* (2011). Migraine preventive drugs differentially affect cortical spreading depression in rat. *Neurobiology of Disease* **41**(2): 430–435.

Borsook, D., N. Erpelding, *et al.* (2014). Sex and the migraine brain. *Neurobiology of Disease* **68**: 200–214.

Bures, J., I. von Schwarzenfeld, *et al.* (1975). Blockage of cortical spreading depression by picrotoxin foci of paroxysmal activity. *Epilepsia* **16**(1): 111–118.

Cai, S., L. D. Hamiwka, *et al.* (2008). Peri-ictal headache in children: prevalence and character. *Pediatric Neurology* **39**(2): 91–96.

Caraballo, R., M. Koutroumanidis, *et al.* (2009). Idiopathic childhood occipital epilepsy of Gastaut: a review and differentiation from migraine and other epilepsies. *Journal of Child Neurology* **24**(12): 1536–1542.

Cecchini, A. P., E. Mea, *et al.* (2009). Vagus nerve stimulation in drug-resistant daily chronic migraine with depression: preliminary data. *Neurological Sciences* **30**(Suppl 1): S101–104.

Chai, N. C., B. L. Peterlin, *et al.* (2014). Migraine and estrogen. *Current Opinion in Neurology* **27**(3): 315–324.

Chang, J. C., L. L. Shook, *et al.* (2010). Biphasic direct current shift, haemoglobin desaturation and neurovascular uncoupling in cortical spreading depression. *Brain* **133**(Pt 4): 996–1012.

Chasman, D. I., M. Schurks, *et al.* (2011). Genome-wide association study reveals three susceptibility loci for common migraine in the general population. *Nature Genetics* **43**(7): 695–698.

Chauvel, V., J. Schoenen, *et al.* (2013). Influence of ovarian hormones on cortical spreading depression and its suppression by L-kynurenine in rat. *PLoS One* **8**(12): e82279.

Chen, S. P., I. Ay, *et al.* (2015). Vagus Nerve Stimulation Inhibits Cortical Spreading Depression. *Pain* **157**(4): 797–805.

Christiansen, I., L. L. Thomsen, *et al.* (1999). Glyceryl trinitrate induces attacks of migraine without aura in sufferers of migraine with aura. *Cephalalgia* **19**(7): 660–667; discussion 626.

Clapcote, S. J., S. Duffy, *et al.* (2009). Mutation I810N in the alpha3 isoform of Na^+,K^+-ATPase causes impairments in the sodium pump and hyperexcitability in the CNS. *Proceedings of the National Academy of Sciences of the United States of America* **106**(33): 14085–14090.

Clarke, T., Z. Baskurt, *et al.* (2009). Evidence of shared genetic risk factors for migraine and rolandic epilepsy. *Epilepsia* **50**(11): 2428–2433.

de Vries, B., V. Anttila, *et al.* (2015). Systematic re-evaluation of genes from candidate gene association studies in migraine using a large genome-wide association data set. *Cephalalgia* **36**(7): 604–14.

Demarquay, G. and F. Mauguiere (2015). Central Nervous System Underpinnings of Sensory Hypersensitivity in Migraine: Insights from Neuroimaging and Electrophysiological Studies. *Headache* **56**(9): 1418–1438.

Di Lorenzo, C., G. Coppola, *et al.* (2015). Migraine improvement during short lasting ketogenesis: a proof-of-concept study. *European Journal of Neurology* **22**(1): 170–177.

Dirani, M., W. Yamak, *et al.* (2015). Panayiotopoulos syndrome presenting with respiratory arrest: A case report and literature review. *Epilepsy & Behavior Case Reports* **3**: 12–14.

Dreier, J. P. and C. Reiffurth (2015). The stroke-migraine depolarization continuum. *Neuron* **86**(4): 902–922.

Dupont, S., Y. Samson, *et al.* (2015). Are auras a reliable clinical indicator in medial temporal lobe epilepsy with hippocampal sclerosis? *European Journal of Neurology* **22**(9): 1310–1316.

Duru, M., I. Melek, *et al.* (2006). QTc dispersion and P-wave dispersion during migraine attacks. *Cephalalgia* **26**(6): 672–677.

Ebrahimi-Fakhari, D., A. Saffari, *et al.* (2015). The evolving spectrum of PRRT2-associated paroxysmal diseases. *Brain* **138**(Pt 12): 3476–3495.

Eising, E., C. de Leeuw, *et al.* (2015). Involvement of astrocyte and oligodendrocyte gene sets in migraine. *Cephalalgia* **36**(7): 640–7.

Esserlind, A. L., A. F. Christensen, *et al.* (2013). Replication and meta-analysis of common variants identifies a genome-wide significant locus in migraine. *European Journal of Neurology* **20**(5): 765–772.

Fan, X., J. Wang, *et al.* (2014). Replication of migraine GWAS susceptibility loci in Chinese Han population. *Headache* **54**(4): 709–715.

Ferrari, M. D., R. R. Klever, *et al.* (2015). Migraine pathophysiology: lessons from mouse models and human genetics. *Lancet Neurology* **14**(1): 65–80.

Freilinger, T., V. Anttila, *et al.* (2012). Genome-wide association analysis identifies susceptibility loci for migraine without aura. *Nature Genetics* **44**(7): 777–782.

Funke, F., M. Kron, *et al.* (2009). Infant brain stem is prone to the generation of spreading depression during severe hypoxia. *Journal of Neurophysiology* **101**(5): 2395–2410.

Gheyara, A. L., R. Ponnusamy, *et al.* (2014). Tau reduction prevents disease in a mouse model of Dravet syndrome. *Annals of Neurology* **76**(3): 443–456.

Ghosh, J., S. Pradhan, *et al.* (2013). Genome-wide-associated variants in migraine susceptibility: a replication study from North India. *Headache* **53**(10): 1583–1594.

Ghosh, J., S. Pradhan, *et al.* (2014). Multilocus analysis of hormonal, neurotransmitter, inflammatory pathways and genome-wide associated variants in migraine susceptibility. *European Journal of Neurology* **21**(7): 1011–1020.

Glasscock, E., J. Qian, *et al.* (2007). Masking epilepsy by combining two epilepsy genes. *Nature Neuroscience* **10**(12): 1554–1558.

Glasscock, E., J. W. Yoo, *et al.* (2010). Kv1.1 potassium channel deficiency reveals brain-driven cardiac dysfunction as a candidate mechanism for sudden unexplained death in epilepsy. *Journal of Neuroscience* **30**(15): 5167–5175.

Gniel, H. M. and R. L. Martin (2010). Changes in membrane potential and the intracellular calcium concentration during CSD and OGD in layer V and layer II/III mouse cortical neurons. *Journal of Neurophysiology* **104**(6): 3203–3212.

Goadsby, P. J., B. M. Grosberg, *et al.* (2014). Effect of noninvasive vagus nerve stimulation on acute migraine: an open-label pilot study. *Cephalalgia* **34**(12): 986–993.

Goldman, A. M., E. Glasscock, *et al.* (2009). Arrhythmia in heart and brain: KCNQ1 mutations link epilepsy and sudden unexplained death. *Science Translational Medicine* **1**(2): 2ra6.

Gowers, W. R. (1906). Clinical Lectures on the borderland of epilepsy. III – Migraine. *British Medical Journal* **2**(2397): 1617–1622.

Guedes, R. C. and E. A. Cavalheiro (1997). Blockade of spreading depression in chronic epileptic rats: reversion by diazepam. *Epilepsy Res* **27**(1): 33–40.

Haan, J., G. M. Terwindt, *et al.* (1995). Is familial hemiplegic migraine a hereditary form of basilar migraine? *Cephalalgia* **15**(6): 477–481.

Hadjikhani, N., M. Sanchez Del Rio, *et al.* (2001). Mechanisms of migraine aura revealed by functional MRI in human visual cortex. *Proceedings of the National Academy of Sciences of the United States of America* **98**(8): 4687–4692.

Hartl, E., J. Remi, *et al.* (2015). Two Patients With Visual Aura – Migraine, Epilepsy, or Migralepsy? *Headache* **55**(8): 1148–1151.

Headache Classification Committee of the International Headache, S. (2013). The International Classification of Headache Disorders, 3rd edition (beta version). *Cephalalgia* **33**(9): 629–808.

Herzog, A. G. (2015). Catamenial epilepsy: Update on prevalence, pathophysiology and treatment from the findings of the NIH Progesterone Treatment Trial. *Seizure* **28**: 18–25.

Holth, J. K., V. C. Bomben, *et al.* (2013). Tau loss attenuates neuronal network hyperexcitability in mouse and Drosophila genetic models of epilepsy. *Journal of Neuroscience* **33**(4): 1651–1659.

Hougaard, A., F. M. Amin, *et al.* (2014). Interhemispheric differences of fMRI responses to visual stimuli in patients with side-fixed migraine aura. *Human Brain Mapping* **35**(6): 2714–2723.

Hunanyan, A. S., N. A. Fainberg, *et al.* (2015). Knock-in mouse model of alternating hemiplegia of childhood: behavioral and electrophysiologic characterization. *Epilepsia* **56**(1): 82–93.

Iizuka, T., Y. Takahashi, *et al.* (2012). Neurovascular changes in prolonged migraine aura in FHM with a novel ATP1A2 gene mutation. *Journal of Neurology, Neurosurgery & Psychiatry* **83**(2): 205–212.

Ito, M., N. Adachi, *et al.* (2004). Characteristics of postictal headache in patients with partial epilepsy. *Cephalalgia* **24**(1): 23–28.

Jaffer, F., A. Avbersek, *et al.* (2015). Faulty cardiac repolarization reserve in alternating hemiplegia of childhood broadens the phenotype. *Brain* **138**(Pt 10): 2859–2874.

Janssen, W., A. Quaegebeur, *et al.* (2015). The spectrum of epilepsy caused by POLG mutations. *Acta Neurologica Belgica* **116**: 17

Kahlig, K. M., T. H. Rhodes, *et al.* (2008). Divergent sodium channel defects in familial hemiplegic migraine. *Proceedings of the National Academy of Sciences of the United States of America* **105**(28): 9799–9804.

Kalachikov, S., O. Evgrafov, *et al.* (2002). Mutations in LGI1 cause autosomal-dominant partial epilepsy with auditory features. *Nature Genetics* **30**(3): 335–341.

Kallela, M., M. Wessman, *et al.* (1999). Clinical characteristics of migraine concordant monozygotic twin pairs. *Acta Neurologica Scandinavica* **100**(4): 254–259.

Kalume, F., R. E. Westenbroek, *et al.* (2013). Sudden unexpected death in a mouse model of Dravet syndrome. *Journal of Clinical Investigation* **123**(4): 1798–1808.

Kanemura, H., Sano, F., Ishii, S., Ohyama, T., Sugita, K., Aihara, M. (2013). Characteristics of headache in children with epilepsy. *Seizure* **22**(8): 647–50.

Kelley, S. A., A. L. Hartman, *et al.* (2012). Comorbidity of migraine in children presenting with epilepsy to a tertiary care center. *Neurology* **79**(5): 468–473.

Klassen, T., C. Davis, *et al.* (2011). Exome sequencing of ion channel genes reveals complex profiles confounding personal risk assessment in epilepsy. *Cell* **145**(7): 1036–1048.

Koroleva, V. I. and J. Bures (1979). Circulation of cortical spreading depression around electrically stimulated areas and epileptic foci in the neocortex of rats. *Brain Research* **173**(2): 209–215.

Koroleva, V. I. and J. Bures (1980). Blockade of cortical spreading depression in electrically and chemically stimulated areas of cerebral cortex in rats. *Electroencephalography and Clinical Neurophysiology* **48**(1): 1–15.

Koroleva, V. I. and J. Bures (1983). Cortical penicillin focus as a generator of repetitive spike-triggered waves of spreading depression in rats. *Experimental Brain Research* **51**(2): 291–297.

Koroleva, V. I., L. V. Vinogradova, *et al.* (1993). Reduced incidence of cortical spreading depression in the course of pentylenetetrazol kindling in rats. *Brain Research* **608**(1): 107–114.

Lal, D., K. Pernhorst, *et al.* (2015). Extending the phenotypic spectrum of RBFOX1 deletions: Sporadic focal epilepsy. *Epilepsia* **56**(9): e129–133.

Leao, A.A. (1947). Further observations on the spreading depression of activity in the cerebral cortex. *Journal of Neurophysiology* **10**(6): 409–14.

Lerche, H., M. Shah, *et al.* (2013). Ion channels in genetic and acquired forms of epilepsy. *Journal of Physiology* **591**(Pt 4): 753–764.

Liu, Y., L. F. Lopez-Santiago, *et al.* (2013). Dravet syndrome patient-derived neurons suggest a novel epilepsy mechanism. *Annals of Neurology* **74**(1): 128–139.

Ludvigsson, P., D. Hesdorffer, *et al.* (2006). Migraine with aura is a risk factor for unprovoked seizures in children. *Annals of Neurology* **59**(1): 210–213.

Malik, R., T. Freilinger, *et al.* (2015). Shared genetic basis for migraine and ischemic stroke: A genome-wide analysis of common variants. *Neurology* **84**(21): 2132–2145.

Martens, D., I. Oster, *et al.* (2012). Cerebral MRI and EEG studies in the initial management of pediatric headaches. *Swiss Medical Weekly* **142**: w13625.

Martinet, L. E., O. J. Ahmed, *et al.* (2015). Slow Spatial Recruitment of Neocortex during Secondarily Generalized Seizures and Its Relation to Surgical Outcome. *Journal of Neuroscience* **35**(25): 9477–9490.

Maslarova, A., M. Alam, *et al.* (2011). Chronically epileptic human and rat neocortex display a similar resistance against spreading depolarization in vitro. *Stroke* **42**(10): 2917–2922.

Massey, C. A., L. P. Sowers, *et al.* (2014). Mechanisms of sudden unexpected death in epilepsy: the pathway to prevention. *Nature Reviews Neurology* **10**(5): 271–282.

May, L. J., K. Millar, *et al.* (2015). QTc Prolongation in Acute Pediatric Migraine. *Pediatric Emergency Care* **31**(6): 409–411.

McIntyre, D. C. and K. L. Gilby (2008). Mapping seizure pathways in the temporal lobe. *Epilepsia* **49**(Suppl 3): 23–30.

Melek, I. M., E. Seyfeli, *et al.* (2007). Autonomic dysfunction and cardiac repolarization abnormalities in patients with migraine attacks. *Medical Science Monitor* **13**(3): RA47–49.

Meng, H., H. Q. Xu, *et al.* (2015). The SCN1A mutation database: updating information and analysis of the relationships among genotype, functional alteration, and phenotype. *Human Mutation* **36**(6): 573–580.

Milner, P. M. (1958). Note on a possible correspondence between the scotomas of migraine and spreading depression of Leao. *Electroencephalography and Clinical Neurophysiology* **10**(4): 705.

Monroe, D. J., J. T. T. Meehan, *et al.* (2015). Sudden Cardiac Death in a Young Man with Migraine-associated Arrhythmia. *Journal of Forensic Sciences* **60**(6): 1633–6.

Nobile, C. and P. Striano (2014). PRRT2: a major cause of infantile epilepsy and other paroxysmal disorders of childhood. *Progress in Brain Research* **213**: 141–158.

Noebels, J. (2015a). Pathway-driven discovery of epilepsy genes. *Nature Neuroscience* **18**(3): 344–350.

Noebels, J.L. (2012). The Voltage-Gated Calcium Channel and Absence Epilepsy. In: J. L. Noebels, M. Avoli, M. A. Rogawski, R. W. Olsen and A. V. Delgado-Escueta (eds). *Jasper's Basic Mechanisms of the Epilepsies*. Bethesda (MD).

Noebels, J.L. (2015b). Single-Gene Determinants of Epilepsy Comorbidity. *Cold Spring Harbor Perspectives in Medicine* **5**(11).

Noebels, J.L. and Sidman, R.L. (1979). Inherited epilepsy: spike-wave and focal motor seizures in the mutant mouse tottering. *Science* **204**(4399): 1334–6.

Noebels, J.L. (2003). The biology of epilepsy genes. *Annual Review of Neuroscience* **26**: 599–625.

Nye, B. L. and V. M. Thadani (2015). Migraine and epilepsy: review of the literature. *Headache* **55**(3): 359–380.

Oakley, C. B. and E. H. Kossoff (2014). Migraine and epilepsy in the pediatric population. *Current Pain and Headache Reports* **18**(3): 402.

Olivetti, P. R., A. Maheshwari, *et al.* (2014). Neonatal estradiol stimulation prevents epilepsy in Arx model of X-linked infantile spasms syndrome *Science Translational Medicine* **6**(220): 220ra212.

Ophoff, R. A., G. M. Terwindt, *et al.* (1996). Familial hemiplegic migraine and episodic ataxia type-2 are caused by mutations in the Ca^{2+} channel gene CACNL1A4. *Cell* **87**(3): 543–552.

Papandreou, A., A. McTague, *et al.* (2015). GABRB3 mutations: a new and emerging cause of early infantile epileptic encephalopathy. *Developmental Medicine & Child Neurology* **58**(4): 416–20.

Parisi, P., R. Ferri, *et al.* (2005). Ictal video-polysomnography and EEG spectral analysis in a child with severe Panayiotopoulos syndrome. *Epileptic Disorders* **7**(4): 333–339.

Parisi, P., D. G. Kasteleijn-Nolst Trenite, *et al.* (2007). A case with atypical childhood occipital epilepsy Gastaut type: an ictal migraine manifestation with a good response to intravenous diazepam. *Epilepsia* **48**(11): 2181–2186.

Parisi, P., Matricardi, S., Tozzi, E., Sechi, E., Martini, C., Verrotti, A. (2012). Benign epilepsy of childhood with centro-temporal spikes (BECTS) versus migraine: a neuropsychological assessment. *Child's Nervous System* **28**(12): 2129–35.

Parisi, P., A. Verrotti, *et al.* (2015). Diagnostic criteria currently proposed for ictal epileptic headache: Perspectives on strengths, weaknesses and pitfalls. *Seizure* **31**: 56–63.

Pietrobon, D. and M. A. Moskowitz (2013). Pathophysiology of migraine. *Annual Review of Physiology* **75**: 365–391.

Punia, V., P. Farooque, *et al.* (2015). Epileptic auras and their role in driving safety in people with epilepsy. *Epilepsia* **56**(11): e182–185.

Qi, Y., J. Wang, *et al.* (2014). Hyper-SUMOylation of the Kv7 potassium channel diminishes the M-current leading to seizures and sudden death. *Neuron* **83**(5): 1159–1171.

Ran, C., L. Graae, *et al.* (2014). A replication study of GWAS findings in migraine identifies association in a Swedish case-control sample. *BMC Medical Genetics* **15**: 38.

Reinthaler, E. M., B. Dejanovic, *et al.* (2015). Rare variants in gamma-aminobutyric acid type A receptor genes in rolandic epilepsy and related syndromes. *Annals of Neurology* **77**(6): 972–986.

Richter, F., S. Rupprecht, *et al.* (2003). Spreading depression can be elicited in brain stem of immature but not adult rats. *Journal of Neurophysiology* **90**(4): 2163–2170.

Rogawski, M. A. (2012). Migraine and Epilepsy-Shared Mechanisms within the Family of Episodic Disorders. In: J. L. Noebels, M. Avoli, M. A. Rogawski, R. W. Olsen and A. V. Delgado-Escueta (eds). *Jasper's Basic Mechanisms of the Epilepsies*. Bethesda (MD).

Rose, F. C. (1994). Sumatriptan does not arrest migraine aura. *Headache* **34**(7): 446.

Rossignol, E., I. Kruglikov, *et al.* (2013). CaV 2.1 ablation in cortical interneurons selectively impairs fast-spiking basket cells and causes generalized seizures. *Annals of Neurology* **74**(2): 209–222.

Rubinstein, M., S. Han, *et al.* (2015a). Dissecting the phenotypes of Dravet syndrome by gene deletion. *Brain* **138**(Pt 8): 2219–2233.

Rubinstein, M., R. E. Westenbroek, *et al.* (2015b). Genetic background modulates impaired excitability of inhibitory neurons in a mouse model of Dravet syndrome. *Neurobiology of Disease* **73**: 106–117.

Russell, M. B., V. Ulrich, *et al.* (2002). Migraine without aura and migraine with aura are distinct disorders. A population-based twin survey. *Headache* **42**(5): 332–336.

Ryvlin, P., L. Nashef, *et al.* (2013). Incidence and mechanisms of cardiorespiratory arrests in epilepsy monitoring units (MORTEMUS): a retrospective study. *Lancet Neurology* **12**(10): 966–977.

Sachs, M., H. C. Pape, *et al.* (2007). The effect of estrogen and progesterone on spreading depression in rat neocortical tissues. *Neurobiology of Disease* **25**(1): 27–34.

Sakauchi, M., H. Oguni, *et al.* (2011). Retrospective multiinstitutional study of the prevalence of early death in Dravet syndrome. *Epilepsia* **52**(6): 1144–1149.

Schankin, C. J., J. Remi, *et al.* (2011). Headache in juvenile myoclonic epilepsy. *Journal of Headache and Pain* **12**(2): 227–233.

Schiefecker, A. J., R. Beer, *et al.* (2014). Clusters of Cortical Spreading Depolarizations in a Patient with Intracerebral Hemorrhage: A Multimodal Neuromonitoring Study. *Neurocritical Care* **22**(2): 293–298.

Schulte, U., J. O. Thumfart, *et al.* (2006). The epilepsy-linked Lgi1 protein assembles into presynaptic Kv1 channels and inhibits inactivation by Kvbeta1. *Neuron* **49**(5): 697–706.

Shoffner, J. M., M. T. Lott, *et al.* (1990). Myoclonic epilepsy and ragged-red fiber disease (MERRF) is associated with a mitochondrial DNA tRNA(Lys) mutation. *Cell* **61**(6): 931–937.

Shu, X. M., G. P. Zhang, *et al.* (2013). The characterization of childhood occipital epilepsy of Gastaut: a study of seven patients. *Cell Biochemistry and Biophysics* **67**(3): 991–995.

Sintas, C., J. Fernandez-Morales, *et al.* (2014). Replication study of previous migraine genome-wide association study findings in a Spanish sample of migraine with aura. *Cephalalgia* **35**(9): 776–82.

Somjen, G. G. (2002). Ion regulation in the brain: implications for pathophysiology. *Neuroscientist* **8**(3): 254–267.

Sperling, M. R. and M. J. O'Connor (1990). Auras and subclinical seizures: characteristics and prognostic significance. *Annals of Neurology* **28**(3): 320–328.

Stafstrom, C. E. and J. M. Rho (2012). The ketogenic diet as a treatment paradigm for diverse neurological disorders. *Frontiers in Pharmacology* **3**: 59.

Sukhotinsky, I., E. Dilekoz, *et al.* (2011). Chronic daily cortical spreading depressions suppress spreading depression susceptibility. *Cephalalgia* **31**(16): 1601–1608.

Swoboda, K. J., E. Kanavakis, *et al.* (2004). Alternating hemiplegia of childhood or familial hemiplegic migraine? A novel ATP1A2 mutation. *Annals of Neurology* **55**(6): 884–887.

Tauboll, E., L. Sveberg, *et al.* (2015). Interactions between hormones and epilepsy. *Seizure* **28**: 3–11.

Thijs, R. D., M. C. Kruit, *et al.* (2006). Syncope in migraine: the population-based CAMERA study. *Neurology* **66**(7): 1034–1037.

Thomas, R.H. and S.F. Berkovic (2014). The hidden genetics of epilepsy – a clinically important new paradigm. *Nature Reviews Neurology* **10**(5): 283–92.

Thurman, D. J., D. C. Hesdorffer, *et al.* (2014). Sudden unexpected death in epilepsy: assessing the public health burden. *Epilepsia* **55**(10): 1479–1485.

Toldo, I., E. Perissinotto, *et al.* (2010). Comorbidity between headache and epilepsy in a pediatric headache center. *Journal of Headache and Pain* **11**(3): 235–240.

Tottene, A., R. Conti, *et al.* (2009). Enhanced excitatory transmission at cortical synapses as the basis for facilitated spreading depression in Ca(v)2.1 knockin migraine mice. *Neuron* **61**(5): 762–773.

Vallejo, M., L. A. Martinez-Martinez, *et al.* (2014). Frequency of migraine in patients with vasovagal syncope. *International Journal of Cardiology* **171**(2): e14–15.

van der Kamp, W., A. Maassen VanDenBrink, *et al.* (1996). Interictal cortical hyperexcitability in migraine patients demonstrated with transcranial magnetic stimulation. *Journal of the Neurological Sciences* **139**(1): 106–110.

Vecchia, D., A. Tottene, *et al.* (2015). Abnormal cortical synaptic transmission in CaV2.1 knockin mice with the S218L missense mutation which causes a severe familial hemiplegic migraine syndrome in humans. *Frontiers in Cellular Neuroscience* **9**: 8.

Veliskova, J. (2006). The role of estrogens in seizures and epilepsy: the bad guys or the good guys? *Neuroscience* **138**(3): 837–844.

Verrotti, A., P. Striano, *et al.* (2011). Migralepsy and related conditions: advances in pathophysiology and classification. *Seizure* **20**(4): 271–275.

Victor, T. W., X. Hu, *et al.* (2010). Migraine prevalence by age and sex in the United States: a life-span study. *Cephalalgia* **30**(9): 1065–1072.

Wagnon, J. L. and M. H. Meisler (2015). Recurrent and Non-Recurrent Mutations of SCN8A in Epileptic Encephalopathy. *Frontiers in Neurology* **6**: 104.

Wakamoto, H., H. Nagao, *et al.* (2011). Idiopathic childhood occipital epilepsy of Gastaut: report of 12 patients. *Pediatric Neurology* **44**(3): 183–186.

Wei, Y., G. Ullah, *et al.* (2014). Unification of neuronal spikes, seizures, and spreading depression. *Journal of Neuroscience* **34**(35): 11733–11743.

Welty, T. E. (2006). Juvenile myoclonic epilepsy: epidemiology, pathophysiology, and management. *Pediatric Drugs* **8**(5): 303–310.

Whitman, B. W. and R. B. Lipton (1995). Oscillocusis: an unusual auditory aura in migraine. *Headache* **35**(7): 428–429.

Whitty, C. W. (1953). Familial hemiplegic migraine. *Journal of Neurology, Neurosurgery & Psychiatry* **16**(3): 172–177.

Yankovsky, A.E., F. Andermann, *et al.* (2005). Preictal headache in partial epilepsy. *Neurology* **65**(12): 1979–81.

Zangaladze, A., A. A. Asadi-Pooya, *et al.* (2010). Sporadic hemiplegic migraine and epilepsy associated with CACNA1A gene mutation. *Epilepsy & Behavior* **17**(2): 293–295.

Zeviani, M., F. Muntoni, *et al.* (1993). A MERRF/MELAS overlap syndrome associated with a new point mutation in the mitochondrial DNA tRNA(Lys) gene. *European Journal of Human Genetics* **1**(1): 80–87.

Zhang, Y., A. P. Vilaythong, *et al.* (2004). Elevated thalamic low-voltage-activated currents precede the onset of absence epilepsy in the SNAP25-deficient mouse mutant coloboma. *Journal of Neuroscience* **24**(22): 5239–5248.

14

Genetics of monogenic and complex migraine

Else A. Tolner[1], Else Eising[2], Gisela M. Terwindt[1], Michel D. Ferrari[1] and Arn M.J.M. van den Maagdenberg[2]

[1] Department of Neurology, Leiden University Medical Center, Leiden, the Netherlands
[2] Department of Human Genetics, Leiden University Medical Center, Leiden, the Netherlands

Migraine is a common, debilitating brain disorder that affects over 15% of the general population – women three times more often than men (Goadsby *et al.*, 2002; Headache Classification Committee of the IHS, 2013). In 30% of patients, attacks may be preceded by neurological aura symptoms (i.e., transient visual, sensory, motor or speech disturbances), the likely consequence of a wave of neuronal and glial depolarization called cortical spreading depression (CSD) (Lauritzen, 1994). The presence of an aura defines the two main migraine types: migraine with aura (MA), and migraine without aura (MO). Activation of the trigeminovascular system is likely responsible for migraine headaches (Goadsby *et al.*, 2002).

The aim of this chapter is to discuss the status of molecular genetic findings in migraine, both in rare monogenic forms of migraine, such as familial hemiplegic migraine (FHM), and in the common complex polygenic forms (i.e., MA and MO).

14.1   Migraine is a genetic disease

Migraine shows strong familial aggregation and is a multifactorial (i.e., complex) genetic disorder (Russell and Olesen, 1995; Stewart *et al.*, 1997, 2006), in which genetic and environmental factors seem to play an equally important role (Mulder *et al.*, 2003). There is debate whether MA and MO should be considered separate disease entities, or different expressions of one disease. Several epidemiological studies have suggested that MA and MO are distinct disorders (Russell *et al.*, 1996, 2002), whereas other studies suggested the existence of a migraine continuum with pure MA and pure MO on both ends of the clinical spectrum (Kallela *et al.*, 2001; Nyholt *et al.*, 2004; Ligthart *et al.*, 2006). The latter view seems more in line with clinical observations that headache characteristics are identical in MA and MO, and that many patients experience both types of attacks during their lifetime. Genetic studies may shed light on the debate as they may reveal migraine susceptibility genes that may be shared by both migraine types.

Neurobiological Basis of Migraine, First Edition. Edited by Turgay Dalkara and Michael A. Moskowitz.
© 2017 John Wiley & Sons, Inc. Published 2017 by John Wiley & Sons, Inc.

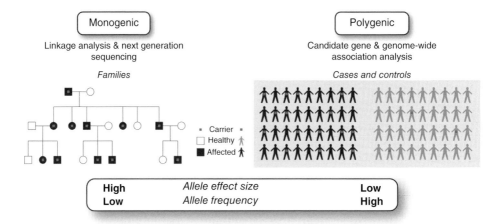

Figure 14.1 Different categories of genetic variation exist, based on the frequency and effect size of the allele. Mendelian monogenic disorders are caused by rare alleles with high effect sizes. A classical linkage approach (combined with Sanger sequencing of candidate genes to identify the causal mutation) was used to identify migraine genes, but has been replaced by next generation sequencing. For polygenic common forms of migraine typically common variants with a low effect size are identified. Hypothesis-free genome-wide association studies (GWAS) have been successful in identifying such variants, and have replaced the candidate gene association approach. Adapted from Tolner *et al.* (2015) and reproduced by permission of Wolters Kluwer Health, Inc.

14.2 How to identify genes for migraine?

For many disorders, including migraine, there are two main categories of diseases when considering their genetic architecture: rare monogenic forms; and common genetically complex, oligogenic or polygenic forms. With respect to monogenic forms of migraine, most prominent is Familial Hemiplegic Migraine (FHM), an autosomal dominant sub-type of MA, characterized by a transient hemiparesis during the aura and headache characteristics that are identical to those found with the common forms of migraine (Thomsen *et al.*, 2002). Other rare monogenic disorders exist in which migraine is a prominent clinical feature, such as, for example, Cerebral Autosomal Dominant Arteriopathy with Subcortical Infarcts and Leukoencephalopathy (CADASIL), characterized by mid-adult onset of vascular dementia and stroke (Joutel *et al.*, 1996), and Familial Advanced Sleep Phase Syndrome (FASPS), characterized by abnormal sleep-wake cycles (Brennan *et al.*, 2013). As the approaches to identify genes for the various categories differ (Figure 14.1), they are discussed separately in the next paragraphs.

14.3 Gene identification in monogenic Familial Hemiplegic Migraine

The classical linkage approach in migraine research was applied to large families in which the disorder showed a clear monogenic pattern of inheritance. Several hundreds of polymorphic genetic markers, evenly spread over the genome, with alleles that allow tracking of them from one generation to the next, were tested for co-segregation with disease in a family-based setting. The causal gene mutation was then identified in the genomic region shared by affected individuals, often after tedious sequencing of protein-coding regions of individual genes.

More recent technical developments, referred to as next generation sequencing (NGS), allow parallel sequencing of all protein coding regions ("exome sequencing") or the whole genome ("whole genome sequencing") in a single experiment, which has given an enormous boost to gene identification for monogenic disorders (Kuhlen-baumer *et al.*, 2011). Knowledge of mutations in genes of monogenic disorders can be directly applied for clinical diagnosis, because these mutations have a high effect size. In other words, the presence of a mutation in an individual has a very high probability of revealing the molecular cause of the disorder that may or may not yet be present.

The traditional approach has been very successful for familial hemiplegic migraine (FHM), with currently three undisputed genes identified – *CACNA1A* (FHM1) (Ophoff *et al.*, 1996), *ATP1A2* (FHM2) (De Fusco *et al.*, 2003), and *SCN1A* (FHM3) (Dichgans *et al.*, 2005) – that encode subunits of voltage-gated calcium channels, sodium-potassium ATPases, and voltage-gated sodium channels, respectively. Combined knowledge on these FHM gene products reveals the importance of the tripartite synapse and, therefore, neurotransmission in the pathophysiology of the disease (Figure 14.2; Ferrari *et al.*, 2015; Tolner *et al.*, 2015).

Genotype-phenotype correlations of mutation carriers have shown a spectrum of associated symptoms, in addition to hemiplegic migraine, ranging from cerebellar ataxia, seizures, to mild head trauma induced cerebral edema that can be fatal (De Vries *et al.*, 2009). Genetic studies have also been performed in isolated cases of sporadic hemiplegic migraine (SHM) (i.e., patients with no first- or second-degree family members suffering from hemiplegic migraine). A study in 105 SHM patients and their first-degree family members (Thomsen *et al.*, 2003) indicated that:

i)   more than half of the patients also had non-hemiplegic MA attacks;
ii)   one-third had additional MO attacks; and
iii) first-degree relatives had an increased risk of MA.

Genetic analyses in SHM patients revealed only very few mutations in one of the FHM genes (De Vries *et al.*, 2007; Gallanti *et al.*, 2011; Thomsen *et al.*, 2008), indicating that most patients have the disease because of:

i)   a yet unidentified hemiplegic migraine gene;
ii)   an interplay of multiple genetic variants with a small effect size, similar to what is the case for the common migraine forms; or
iii) a non-genetic cause.

Still, patients with an early age of onset, and who exhibit additional neurological symptoms such as ataxia, epilepsy or intellectual inabilities, carry, in approximately 75% of cases, an (in most cases) *de novo* mutation in *CACNA1A* or *ATP1A2* (Riant *et al.*, 2010).

Recently, truncating deletions in the *PRRT2* gene, which encodes a proline-rich transmembrane protein, were identified in a few patients with (hemiplegic) migraine, as a result of which *PRRT2* was put forward as the fourth hemiplegic migraine gene (Riant *et al.*, 2012). However, as the same (or very similar) *PRRT2* deletions were also found in several hundred patients with paroxysmal kinesigenic dyskinesia (PKD), benign familial infantile convulsions (BFIC) and infantile convulsion choreoathetosis (ICCA), without signs of migraine, the relation of *PRRT2* and migraine seems far from straightforward (Pelzer *et al.*, 2014).

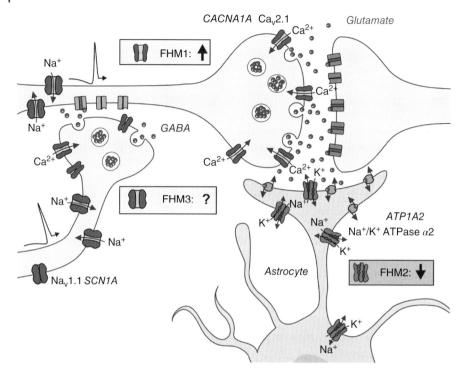

Figure 14.2 Products of the Familial Hemiplegic Migraine (FHM) genes FHM1 (*CACNA1A*), FHM2 (*ATP1A2*), and FHM3 (*SCN1A*) genes play important roles in the tripartite synapse. FHM1 mutations cause a gain-of-function of Ca$_V$2.1 calcium channels that are located at presynaptic terminals of glutamatergic and GABAergic neurons. When an action potential reaches the presynaptic terminal, Ca$_V$2.1 channels open, allowing Ca^{2+} to enter, trigger vesicle fusion and glutamate release into the synaptic cleft, which causes subsequent activation of post-synaptic receptors and action potential generation. FHM2 mutations cause loss-of-function of α2-isoform containing Na$^+$/K$^+$-ATPases that are located in astrocytic membranes, where they assist in removing extracellular K$^+$ and generating a Na$^+$ gradient required for the uptake of glutamate from the synaptic cleft. FHM3 mutations cause loss-of-function of Na$_V$1.1 voltage-gated sodium channels that are located on inhibitory interneurons. Na$_V$1.1 channels serve to initiate and propagate action potentials. Gain-of-function mutations in Ca$_V$2.1 (FHM1) and loss-of-function mutations in the Na$^+$/K$^+$-ATPase (FHM2) and Na$_V$1.1 (FHM3) will each generate a net increase of general neuronal excitability. Tolner *et al.* (2015), with permission from Wolters Kluwer Health, Inc).

14.4 Functional studies of gene mutations in monogenic Familial Hemiplegic Migraine

The large effect sizes of gene mutations in monogenic FHM allow their functional characterization in cellular and transgenic animal models. Most cellular studies have shown that FHM1 mutations exert gain-of-function effects by shifting neuronal Ca$_V$2.1 channels' voltage-dependence towards more negative membrane potentials, while enhancing channel open probability (Pietrobon, 2010), although loss-of-function effects have also been reported (Cao *et al.*, 2004; Tao *et al.*, 2012). Loss of glial Na^+/K^+ ATPase function seems the most likely mechanism for FHM2 mutations (Tavraz *et al.*, 2008) (see Chapter 15).

Most FHM3 mutations seem to exert loss-of-function effects of $Na_V 1.1$ sodium channels, which appear primarily to affect inhibitory neurons, but gain-of-function effects have also been proposed (Kahlig *et al.*, 2008; Cestèle *et al.*, 2008). Even more astounding, when expressed in neurons, partial rescue from abnormal protein folding can transform mutant protein from a loss-of-function to a gain-of-function mutation (Cestèle *et al.*, 2013). Whether, and to what extent, this transition also occurs *in vivo* remains to be established, as no FHM3 knock-in (KI) mouse model is currently available to test this. Taken together, the cellular studies of FHM mutations predict increased neurotransmitter and potassium ion levels at the synaptic cleft (Figure 14.2), especially after high intensity neuronal firing, which would facilitate CSD (Somjen, 2001).

Effects of FHM1 and FHM2 mutations have also been investigated at the organismal level, by introducing pathogenic human FHM mutations in the endogenous *Cacna1a* or *Atp1a2* gene, respectively. Two transgenic FHM1 KI mouse models have been generated, expressing the gain-of-function missense mutations R192Q or S218L in the *Cacna1a* gene (van den Maagdenberg, 2004; van den Maagdenberg *et al.*, 2010). Mutant mice homozygous for the S218L mutation exhibit the complex phenotype of cerebellar ataxia and spontaneous seizures that is also part of the clinical phenotype in S218L patients (Stam *et al.*, 2009), whereas mutant R192Q mice, like patients with this mutation (Ophoff *et al.*, 1996), do not exhibit these additional clinical features.

A migraine-relevant feature is the susceptibility to CSD that, at least in animals, has been shown to activate brainstem and other centers of the brain relevant for the activation of headache mechanisms (Bolay *et al.*, 2002; Zhang *et al.*, 2011b; Karatas *et al.*, 2013). In FHM1 R192Q and S218L mutant mice, the susceptibility to experimentally induced CSD is increased (van den Maagdenberg, 2004; van den Maagdenberg *et al.*, 2010; Eikermann-Haerter *et al.*, 2009). These features were:

i) more prominent in the severer S218L mutant (capturing the difference in clinical severity when compared to R192Q mutants);
ii) more pronounced in homozygous versus heterozygous animals; and
iii) in line with the female preponderance in migraineurs – more pronounced in female than male mutant mice (with no gender difference in wild type animals) (Eikermann-Haerter *et al.*, 2009).

Heterozygous FHM2 KI mice, which express the mutant *Atp1a2* product due to a loss-of-function W887R missense mutation, also display an increased CSD susceptibility (Leo *et al.*, 2011). Similar to homozygous *Atp1a2* knock-out mice (James *et al.*, 1999), homozygous FHM2 KI mice are not viable.

Only the FHM1 mouse models were studied in greater detail, which resulted in considerable insight in pathophysiological mechanisms of hemiplegic migraine and, to a certain extent, also common forms of migraine (for reviews, see Ferrari *et al.* (2015) and Tolner *et al.* (2015)). Neurobiological studies in cortical brain slices of FHM1 R192Q and S218L KI mice demonstrated enhanced neuronal calcium influx as a direct consequence of hyperactivity of $Ca_V 2.1$ channels (Tottene *et al.*, 2009; Vecchia *et al.*, 2015) which, when normalized, resulted in normalization of CSD characteristics in brain slices of R192Q mutants (Tottene *et al.*, 2009). CSD waves in mutant animals were shown to travel to subcortical brain regions and, in S218L mice, could even reach thalamus or re-enter the cortex (Eikermann-Haerter *et al.*, 2011a).

Studies in Calyx of Held brainstem neurons in brain slices and *in vivo* indicated that S218L-mutated $Ca_V2.1$ channels cause an increase of basal intracellular $[Ca^{2+}]$, which is suggested to be the dominant factor causing a gain-of-function at the synaptic level (Di Guilmi *et al.*, 2014). Investigations in cerebellar slices of R192Q and S218L mice indicated that FHM1-mutated channels are already in a facilitated state at rest (Adams *et al.*, 2010). This is underscored by a recent Ca^{2+} imaging study in the somatosensory cortex of heterozygous S218L mice, which revealed an altered synaptic morphology compatible with stronger synapses and a hyperexcitability phenotype (Eikermann-Haerter *et al.*, 2015). These data support the concept that FHM1 mutations cause a $Ca_V2.1$ gain-of-function, leading to cerebral hyperexcitability that could also explain the more severe neurological deficits associated with the S218L mutation in patients.

Given the widespread expression of $Ca_V2.1$ channels throughout the nervous system, it remains quite an enigma why the hyperexcitability phenotype associated with FHM1 mutations causes no severer phenotype than an episodic disease like migraine. Some important light was shed by studies suggesting that functional effects of FHM1 mutations may be neuron type-specific. For example, the absence of an effect of FHM1 mutations on cortical fast-spiking cortical interneurons, in comparison to the clear gain-of-function effect observed for excitatory pyramidal neurons (Inchauspe *et al.*, 2010; Tottene *et al.*, 2009), is likely due to the expression of interneuron-specific Cav2.1 channels, whose gating properties are not modified by the FHM1 mutation (Vecchia *et al.*, 2014). Context-dependency may cause different effects of FHM1 mutations across brain regions, and could result in dynamic disturbances in the balance between excitation and inhibition in neuronal circuits (Vecchia and Pietrobon, 2012), which can be speculated to underlie the observed phenotypes.

Behavioral changes suggestive of spontaneous unilateral head pain have been identified in FHM1 mutant mice, typified as an increased amount of head grooming, with unilateral oculotemporal strokes and increased blink rates with one eye closed (Chanda *et al.*, 2013). These behaviors appeared to be novelty or restraint stress induced, and could be normalized by serotonergic anti-migraine drugs (Goadsby *et al.*, 2002), suggesting involvement of trigeminal pain pathways. Further evidence for spontaneous head pain in FHM1 mice was obtained from using the so-called mouse grimace scale, an objective measure of facial pain expression in mice (Langford *et al.*, 2010); in addition, FHM1 mice displayed signs of photophobia by displaying light-avoidance behavior (Chanda *et al.*, 2013).

Insight into molecular pain-related mechanisms in FHM1 mice came from investigating the functionality of purinergic receptors (Köles *et al.*, 2011) – more specifically, P2X3 receptors that are mostly expressed by nociceptive sensory neurons and participate in transduction of pain signals (Giniatullin and Nistri, 2013), and P2Y receptors, which are proposed as new targets for analgesic and antimigraine drugs (Magni and Ceruti, 2013). Trigeminal (TG) sensory neurons of R192Q mice revealed excessively enhanced ATP-gated purinergic P2X3 receptor activity, due to constitutive activation of P2X3 receptors in TGs of mutant mice (Nair *et al.*, 2010). Notably, TG neurons of

R192Q mice exhibited increased release of various soluble migraine-relevant mediators, such as CGRP, BDNF and TNFα, already at baseline (Hullugundi *et al.*, 2013). The enhanced baseline activity of P2X3 receptors could explain why further potentiation of these receptors by exogenous CGRP or TNFα was not observed.

The combination of enhanced purinergic activity and soluble "migraine mediators" (Giniatullin *et al.*, 2008) may underlie the abnormal cytokine and chemokine profiles and activated macrophages observed for TG neurons of R192Q mice (Franceschini *et al.*, 2013). When FHM1 TG neurons were co-cultured with satellite glial cells, mimicking their native environment, an increased CGRP release at baseline, and upon neuronal activation, resulted in potentiation of glial P2Y receptors and subsequent glial cell activation (Ceruti *et al.*, 2011). The observed neuro-inflammatory state of TGs in FHM1 mice with constitutively activated purinergic receptors in both neurons and glial cells could facilitate pain signal transduction, given the proposed role of inflammatory pain mediators, including TNFα on meningeal nociceptors, for development of head pain (Zhang *et al.*, 2011a). Such a cascade was recently proposed to be triggered by CSD via activation of neuronal Pannexin channels (Karatas *et al.*, 2013).

Given the enhanced susceptibility of FHM1 mice to CSD (van den Maagdenberg *et al.*, 2004, 2010; Eikermann-Haerter *et al.*, 2009), the baseline inflammatory characteristics of TG in FHM1 mice may convert acute activation of trigeminal pathways by CSD into a chronic trigeminal pain state reflecting headaches of long duration. If, indeed, *in vitro* findings from TG neurons would translate to the *in vivo* level, FHM1 mice could serve as a valuable model for investigating effects of existing and novel migraine drugs, which may involve modulation of CGRP and inflammatory pathways (Wrobel Goldberg and Silberstein, 2015; Russo, 2015).

14.5 Genetic studies in monogenic disorders in which migraine is a prominent part of the clinical phenotype

Other rare monogenic disorders in which migraine is prevalent may provide useful additional insight in pathophysiological mechanisms involved in migraine (Figure 14.3). The clearest example is Cerebral Autosomal Dominant Arteriopathy with Subcortical Infarcts and Leukoencephalopathy (CADASIL), which is caused by mutations in the *NOTCH3* gene that plays an important role in vascular smooth muscle cells of small blood vessels of the brain (Joutel *et al.*, 1996). Some one-third of CADASIL patients have migraine with aura (Dichgans *et al.*, 1998), supporting involvement of a vascular component in migraine pathophysiology. Another clear example is Familial Advanced Sleep Phase Syndrome (FASPS), which is causal by missense mutation in the casein kinase 1δ (*CSNK1D*) gene. All eight patients from two FASP families also suffered from migraine with aura (Brennan *et al.*, 2013).

The mutant gene product of CK1D, a known regulator of circadian rhythms, seems to cause vascular dysfunction through abnormal astrocytic signaling. Both CADASIL and FASP are monogenic disorders that link abnormal vascular and, in the case of FASP, are also glial, dysfunction to migraine pathophysiology. Transgenic mice in which CADASIL or FASPS mutations were overexpressed, similar to what was found for mice that express FHM1 mutations, showed a reduced threshold for CSD (Brennan *et al.*, 2013; Eikermann-Haerter *et al.*, 2011b). Exactly how mutations in *NOTCH3* or

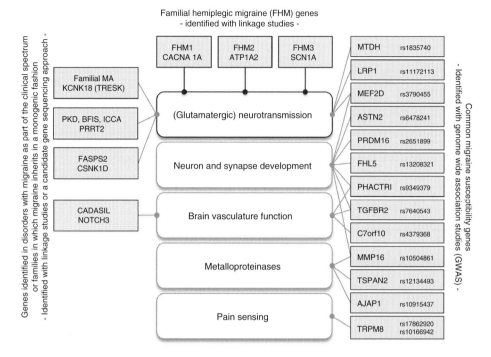

Figure 14.3 Genes and pathways involved in Familial Hemiplegic Migraine (FHM), common forms of migraine, and other disorders in which migraine is prominent. Arrows connect genes to the presumed function of that gene. Adapted from Tolner *et al.* 2015 and reproduced with permission from Wolters Kluwer Health, Inc.

CSNK1D cause vascular phenotypes that might explain the occurrence of migraine in mutation carriers is not yet known.

There is one example of a presumed monogenic gene identification in pure familial common non-hemiplegic migraine (Lafrenière *et al.*, 2010). In *KCNK18*, which encodes the TRESK protein, and was selected as candidate gene for targeted sequencing because of its role in controlling neuronal excitability, a truncating non-functional F139WfsX24 mutation was identified that could explain all migraine cases in a multigenerational family with migraine with aura. As several rare TRESK variants, including a variant that, like the F139WfsX24 mutation, showed complete loss of function, were also observed in control individuals, *KCNK18* is now regarded a genetic modifier of a migraine phenotype, and not the direct cause (Andres-Enguix *et al.*, 2012).

14.6   Genome-wide association studies in common polygenic migraine

For the identification of genetic factors for common polygenic disorders, traditionally a candidate gene approach has been used that tested the distribution of alleles (DNA variants) at one location in a single candidate gene that had been selected on prior knowledge of migraine pathophysiology. Evidence for causality of the DNA variant (and the gene it belongs to) should come from statistical differences in allele frequencies when comparing cases and controls. Most studies used only a few hundred cases, or even fewer, but still many claims for migraine susceptibility genes were made (for review, see De Vries *et al.* (2009)), despite the fact that, in virtually all studies, no efforts were made to replicate findings in independent cohorts.

Since a few years ago, the candidate gene approach has been replaced by the hypothesis-free genome-wide association (GWA) approach. GWA studies (GWAS) test up to several million common variants (single-nucleotide polymorphisms – SNPs), covering the whole genome for association with a trait, in very large cohorts of patients and controls (at least several thousands). The distribution of allele frequencies between cases and controls is compared for each SNP. To correct sufficiently for multiple testing, *P*-values below 5×10^{-8} are considered to be genome-wide significant. Effect sizes of variants identified through GWAS tend to be very low, so GWAS results have no relevance to very little for clinicians and patients, as yet. This may be different when many tens, to perhaps hundreds, of DNA variants associated with migraine have been identified in the future.

Several GWAS have been performed for migraine. Two studies focused on patients that were collected by specialized headache clinics (Anttila *et al.*, 2010; Freilinger *et al.*, 2012). One study focused on patients with MA, and identified a single associated DNA variant that linked to the *MTDH* gene (Anttila *et al.*, 2010). The other study focused on MO, and identified six loci that led to *MEF2D, TGFBR2, PHACTR1, ASTN, TRPM8* and *LRP1* as the likely susceptibility genes (Freilinger *et al.*, 2012). Combining genotyped samples of those studies with those of a large population-based GWAS (Chasman *et al.*, 2011), and several additional cohorts, yielded an enormous data set, with over 23 000 cases and 100 000 controls, which was used for a meta-analysis by the International Headache Genetics Consortium (Anttila *et al.*, 2013).

The meta-analysis yielded 13 migraine susceptibility loci, with genes involved in neuronal pathways (*MTDH, LRP1, PRDM16, MEF2D, ASTN2, PHACTR1, FHL5, MMP16*), metalloproteinases (*MMP16, TSPAN2, AJAP1*) and vascular pathways (*PHACTR1, TGFBR2, C7orf10*) (Figure 14.3). The genetic associations detected by migraine GWAS are statistically very robust (with successful replication in many independent cohorts), though they explain only very little of the genetic variance and, therefore, they hardly have predictive value. The GWAS data set gives a unique opportunity to re-evaluate findings from candidate gene association studies. None of the previously reported associated gene variants could be replicated in a large GWAS data set of over 5000 cases and 13 000 controls (De Vries *et al.*, 2015) which, in retrospect, suggests that candidate gene association studies yielded false-positive results, likely due to the fact that these studies were heavily underpowered.

14.7   Future directions in genetic migraine research

Several novel approaches and methodologies are now available that will further the identification of genetic factors in migraine and the understanding of their functional consequences. The most relevant ones are discussed below.

14.7.1 Future avenues of genetic research

Although an increasing number of genetic migraine susceptibility variants have been identified, considerable efforts are still needed to fully harvest from GWAS. The main obstacle is that GWAS hits at the moment are SNPs that merely "tag" the disease locus, implying that the identified associated SNP is not the disease-causing variant, but in linkage disequilibrium with the real variant. Hence, it is doubtful whether many of the current associated SNP variants are, in fact, the real causal variants and do pinpoint the causal genes. Fine-scale mapping of each GWAS locus would enable the identification of truly functional variant(s) – that is, those variants with the greatest effect sizes and/or lowest *P*-value.

Expensive efforts are needed to perform large-scale targeted sequencing of a locus to first capture all variants and, to a certain extent, this can be overcome by imputation with publically available 1000 Genomes Project data (Abecasis *et al.*, 2012). Subsequent genotyping of rare variants (using custom-made chip arrays), and haplotyping efforts in large cohorts, is expected to prioritize variants, but this is not straightforward at the moment (Edwards *et al.*, 2013).

A second major obstacle is that the majority of GWAS hits will not affect amino acid sequences in encoded proteins. Instead, they are located in intronic or intergenic regions more likely to have subtle influences on gene regulation. A popular approach is to perform pathway-based analyses to examine GWAS signals of a group of genes involved in the same (or similar) biological process(es), to explore pathways affected by multiple GWAS hits (Wang *et al.*, 2010). Mining of gene expression databases (The GTEx Consortium, 2013; http://www.gtexportal.org/), databases of the NIH Roadmap Epigenomics Roadmap project (The NIH Roadmap Epigenomics Mapping Consortium, 2010; http://www.roadmapepigenomics.org), and the Allen Brain Atlas project (Hawrylycz *et al.*, 2012; www.brain-map.org) can be of use to obtain relevant (functional) information from GWAS hits, even when the associated variants are not in a protein-coding region.

A third major obstacle is to investigate the functional consequences of associated SNPs (or linked genes) with respect to disease-relevant pathways. There are several layers of complexity:

i) the initially associated SNP may not be the causal variant in a GWAS locus (so fine mapping is needed to confirm/identify the true causal variant);

ii) there may be multiple SNPs, in multiple combinations (i.e., on multiple haplotypes), in a GWAS locus that confer actual migraine risk (the combination of SNPs on a haplotype may be particularly relevant when specific variants can increase or decrease disease risk);

iii) the associated/causal SNP may be not evolutionary conserved (problems may occur when a model system is used that is non-human).

There are sufficient challenges to functionally study the importance of GWAS hits to understand migraine pathophysiology, as only the combined effect of multiple variants is regarded sufficient to cause the disease (unlike in monogenic forms of migraine, for which a single mutation suffices). Even when all migraine susceptibility genes would have been identified (and there may be many hundreds), the issue remains which *combination* in a given patient will cause disease. For obvious reasons, it will be a *force majeure* to perform such investigation by modulating the genome in cellular or animal (e.g., zebrafish or mouse) models.

14.7.2 Novel sequencing strategy for gene identification

Genetic research in migraine will certainly benefit from recent breakthroughs in massive parallel DNA sequencing, such as next generation sequencing (NGS), which allows cost-efficient sequencing of all protein-coding regions ("exome"), or the complete genome ("whole genome") in a single experiment. Despite successes in many genetic studies (Stranneheim and Wedell, 2016), more sophisticated procedures for data pooling, bioinformatic filtering and variant prioritization methods need to be developed to identify disease-related DNA variants among a huge number of non-related variants, especially when used on larger sets of patients with monogenic or complex polygenic forms of migraine. Novel technologies are emerging, but remain challenging at the moment, to help harvesting from recent GWAS discoveries.

References

Abecasis GR, Auton A, Brooks LD, DePristo MA, Durbin RM, Handsaker RE, Kang HM, Marth GT and McVean GA, 1000 Genomes Project Consortium (2012). An integrated map of genetic variation from 1,092 human genomes. *Nature* **491**: 56–65.

Adams PJ, Rungta RL, Garcia E, van den Maagdenberg AM, MacVicar BA and Snutch TP (2010). Contribution of calcium-dependent facilitation to synaptic plasticity revealed by migraine mutations in the P/Q-type calcium channel. *Proceedings of the National Academy of Sciences of the United States of America* **107**: 18694–18699.

Andres-Enguix I, Shang L, Stansfeld PJ, Morahan JM, Sansom MS, Lafrenière RG, Roy B, Griffiths LR, Rouleau GA, Ebers GC, Cader ZM and Tucker SJ (2012). Functional analysis of missense variants in the TRESK (KCNK18) K channel. *Scientific Reports* **2**: 237.

Anttila V, Stefansson H, Kallela M, Todt U, Terwindt GM, Calafato MS, Nyholt DR, Dimas AS, Freilinger T, Müller-Myhsok B, Artto V, Inouye M, Alakurtti K, Kaunisto MA, Hämäläinen E, de Vries B, Stam AH, Weller CM, Heinze A, Heinze-Kuhn K, Goebel I, Borck G, Göbel H, Steinberg S, Wolf C, Björnsson A, Gudmundsson G, Kirchmann M, Hauge A, Werge T, Schoenen J, Eriksson JG, Hagen K, Stovner L, Wichmann H-E, Meitinger T, Alexander M, Moebus S, Schreiber S, Aulchenko YS, Breteler MMB, Uitterlinden AG, Hofman A, van Duijn CM, Tikka-Kleemola P, Vepsäläinen S, Lucae S, Tozzi F, Muglia P, Barrett J, Kaprio J, Färkkilä M, Peltonen L, Stefansson K, Zwart J-A, Ferrari MD, Olesen J, Daly M, Wessman M, van den Maagdenberg AM, Dichgans M, Kubisch C, Dermitzakis ET, Frants RR, Palotie A and International Headache Genetics Consortium (2010). Genome-wide association study of migraine implicates a common susceptibility variant on 8q22.1. *Nature Genetics* **42**: 869–873.

Anttila V, Winsvold BS, Gormley P, Kurth T, Bettella F, McMahon G, Kallela M, Malik R, de Vries B, Terwindt G, Medland SE, Todt U, McArdle WL, Quaye L, Koiranen M, Ikram MA, Lehtimäki T, Stam AH, Ligthart L, Wedenoja J, Dunham I, Neale BM, Palta P, Hämäläinen E, Schürks M, Rose LM, Buring JE, Ridker PM, Steinberg S, Stefansson H, Jakobsson F, Lawlor DA, Evans DM, Ring SM, Färkkilä M, Artto V, Kaunisto MA, Freilinger T, Schoenen J, Frants RR, Pelzer N, Weller CM, Zielman R, Heath AC,

Madden PAF, Montgomery GW, Martin NG, Borck G, Göbel H, Heinze A, Heinze-Kuhn K, Williams FMK, Hartikainen A-L, Pouta A, van den Ende J, Uitterlinden AG, Hofman A, Amin N, Hottenga J-J, Vink JM, Heikkilä K, Alexander M, Müller-Myhsok B, Schreiber S, Meitinger T, Wichmann HE, Aromaa A, Eriksson JG, Traynor BJ, Trabzuni D, Rossin E, Lage K, Jacobs SBR, Gibbs JR, Birney E, Kaprio J, Penninx BW, Boomsma DI, van Duijn C, Raitakari O, Järvelin M-R, Zwart J-A, Cherkas L, Strachan DP, Kubisch C, Ferrari MD, van den Maagdenberg AMJM, Dichgans M, Wessman M, Smith GD, Stefansson K, Daly MJ, Nyholt DR, Chasman DI, Palotie A, North American Brain Expression Consortium, UK Brain Expression Consortium and International Headache Genetics Consortium (2013). Genome-wide meta-analysis identifies new susceptibility loci for migraine. *Nature Genetics* **45**: 912–917.

Bolay H, Reuter U, Dunn AK, Huang Z, Boas DA and Moskowitz MA (2002). Intrinsic brain activity triggers trigeminal meningeal afferents in a migraine model. *Nature Medicine* **8**: 136–142.

Brennan KC, Bates EA, Shapiro RE, Zyuzin J, Hallows WC, Huang Y, Lee HY, Jones CR, Fu YH, Charles AC and Ptáček LJ. (2013). Casein kinase idelta mutations in familial migraine and advanced sleep phase. *Science Translational Medicine* **5**: 1–11.

Cao YQ, Piedras-Rentería ES, Smith GB, Chen G, Harata NC and Tsien RW (2004). Presynaptic Ca^{2+} channels compete for channel type-preferring slots in altered neurotransmission arising from Ca^{2+} channelopathy. *Neuron* **43**: 387–400.

Ceruti S, Villa G, Fumagalli M, Colombo L, Magni G, Zanardelli M, Fabbretti E, Verderio C, van den Maagdenberg AM, Nistri A and Abbracchio MP (2011). Calcitonin gene-related peptide-mediated enhancement of purinergic neuron/glia communication by the algogenic factor bradykinin in mouse trigeminal ganglia from wild-type and R192Q Cav2.1 Knock-in mice: implications for basic mechanisms of migraine pain. *Journal of Neuroscience* **31**: 3638–3649.

Cestèle S, Scalmani P, Rusconi R, Terragni B, Franceschetti S and Mantegazza M. (2008). Self-limited hyperexcitability: Functional effect of a familial hemiplegic migraine mutation of the Nav1.1 (SCN1A) Na^+ channel. *Journal of Neuroscience* **28**: 7273–7283.

Cestèle S, Schiavon E, Rusconi R, Franceschetti S and Mantegazza M (2013). Nonfunctional NaV1.1 familial hemiplegic migraine mutant transformed into gain of function by partial rescue of folding defects. *Proceedings of the National Academy of Sciences of the United States of America* **110**: 17546–17551.

Chanda ML, Tuttle AH, Baran I, Atlin C, Guindi D, Hathaway G, Israelian N, Levenstadt J, Low D, Macrae L, O'Shea L, Silver A, Zendegui E, Mariette Lenselink A, Spijker S, Ferrari MD, van den Maagdenberg AM and Mogil JS (2013). Behavioral evidence for photophobia and stress-related ipsilateral head pain in transgenic Cacna1a mutant mice. *Pain* **154**: 1254–1262.

Chasman DI, Schürks M, Anttila V, de Vries B, Schminke U, Launer LJ, Terwindt GM, van den Maagdenberg AMJM, Fendrich K, Völzke H, Ernst F, Griffiths LR, Buring JE, Kallela M, Freilinger T, Kubisch C, Ridker PM, Palotie A, Ferrari MD, Hoffmann W, Zee RYL and Kurth T (2011). Genome-wide association study reveals three susceptibility loci for common migraine in the general population. *Nature Genetics* **43**: 695–698.

De Fusco M, Marconi R, Silvestri L, Atorino L, Rampoldi L, Morgante L, Ballabio A, Aridon P and Casari G (2003). Haploinsufficiency of ATP1A2 encoding the Na^+/K^+ pump alpha2 subunit associated with familial hemiplegic migraine type 2. *Nature Genetics* **33**: 192–196.

De Vries B, Freilinger T, Vanmolkot KRJ, Koenderink JB, Stam AH, Terwindt GM, Babini E, van den Boogerd EH, van den Heuvel JJMW, Frants RR, Haan J, Pusch M, van den Maagdenberg AM, Ferrari MD and Dichgans M (2007). Systematic analysis of three FHM genes in 39 sporadic patients with hemiplegic migraine. *Neurology* **69**: 2170–2176.

De Vries B, Frants RR, Ferrari MD and van den Maagdenberg AM (2009). Molecular genetics of migraine. *Human Genetics* **126**: 115–132.

De Vries B, Anttila V, Freilinger T, Wessman M, Kaunisto MA, Kallela M, Artto V, Vijfhuizen LS, Göbel H, Dichgans M, Kubisch C, Ferrari MD, Palotie A, Terwindt GM, van den Maagdenberg AM and on behalf of the International Headache Genetics Consortium (2015). Systematic re-evaluation of genes from candidate gene association studies in migraine using a large genome-wide association data set. *Cephalalgia* **36**(7): 604–14.

Di Guilmi MN, Wang T, Inchauspe CG, Forsythe ID, Ferrari MD, van den Maagdenberg AM, Borst JG and Uchitel OD (2014). Synaptic gain-of-function effects of mutant Cav2.1 channels in a mouse model of familial hemiplegic migraine are due to increased basal [Ca^{2+}]i. *Journal of Neuroscience* **34**: 7047–7058.

Dichgans M, Mayer M, Uttner I, Brüning R, Müller-Höcker J, Rungger G, Ebke M, Klockgether T and Gasser T (1998). The phenotypic spectrum of CADASIL: clinical findings in 102 cases. *Annals of Neurology* **44**: 731–739.

Dichgans M, Freilinger T, Eckstein G, Babini E, Lorenz-Depiereux B, Biskup S, Ferrari MD, Herzog J, van den Maagdenberg AM, Pusch M and Strom TM (2005). Mutation in the neuronal voltage-gated sodium channel SCN1A in familial hemiplegic migraine. *Lancet* **366**: 371–377.

Edwards SL, Beesley J, French JD and Dunning AM (2013). Beyond GWASs: illuminating the dark road from association to function. *American Journal of Human Genetics* **93**: 779–797.

Eikermann-Haerter K, Dileköz E, Kudo C, Savitz SI, Waeber C, Baum MJ, Ferrari MD, van den Maagdenberg AM, Moskowitz MA and Ayata C (2009). Genetic and hormonal factors modulate spreading depression and transient hemiparesis in mouse models of familial hemiplegic migraine type 1. *Journal of Clinical Investigation* **119**: 99–109.

Eikermann-Haerter K, Yuzawa I, Qin T, Wang Y, Baek K, Kim YR, Hoffmann U, Dilekoz E, Waeber C, Ferrari MD, van den Maagdenberg AM, Moskowitz MA and Ayata C (2011a). Enhanced subcortical spreading depression in familial hemiplegic migraine type 1 mutant mice. *Journal of Neuroscience* **31**: 5755–5763.

Eikermann-Haerter K, Yuzawa I, Dilekoz E, Joutel A, Moskowitz MA and Ayata C (2011b). Cerebral autosomal dominant arteriopathy with subcortical infarcts and leukoencephalopathy syndrome mutations increase susceptibility to spreading depression. *Annals of Neurology* **69**: 413–418.

Eikermann-Haerter K, Arbel-Ornath M, Yalcin N, Yu ES, Kuchibhotla KV, Yuzawa I, Hudry E, Willard CR, Climov M, Keles F, Belcher AM, Sengul B, Negro A, Rosen IA, Arreguin A, Ferrari MD, van den Maagdenberg AM, Bacskai BJ and Ayata C (2015). Abnormal synaptic Ca($^{2+}$) homeostasis and morphology in cortical neurons of familial hemiplegic migraine type 1 mutant mice. *Annals of Neurology* **78**: 193–210.

Ferrari MD, Klever RR, Terwindt GM, Ayata C, van den Maagdenberg AM (2015). Migraine pathophysiology: lessons from mouse models and human genetics. *Lancet Neurology* **14**: 65–80.

Franceschini A, Vilotti S, Ferrari MD, van den Maagdenberg AM, Nistri A and Fabbretti E (2013). TNFalpha levels and macrophages expression reflect an inflammatory potential of trigeminal ganglia in a mouse model of familial hemiplegic migraine. *PLoS One* **8**: e52394.

Freilinger T, Anttila V, de Vries B, Malik R, Kallela M, Terwindt GM, Pozo-Rosich P, Winsvold B, Nyholt DR, van Oosterhout WPJ, Artto V, Todt U, Hämäläinen E, Fernández-Morales J, Louter MA, Kaunisto MA, Schoenen J, Raitakari O, Lehtimäki T, Vila-Pueyo M, Göbel H, Wichmann E, Sintas C, Uitterlinden AG, Hofman A, Rivadeneira F, Heinze A, Tronvik E, van Duijn CM, Kaprio J, Cormand B, Wessman M, Frants RR, Meitinger T, Müller-Myhsok B, Zwart J-A, Färkkilä M, Macaya A, Ferrari MD, Kubisch C, Palotie A, Dichgans M, van den Maagdenberg AM and International Headache Genetics Consortium (2012). Genome-wide association analysis identifies susceptibility loci for migraine without aura. *Nature Genetics* **44**: 777–782.

Gallanti A, Cardin V, Tonelli A, Bussone G, Bresolin N, Mariani C and Bassi MT (2011). The genetic features of 24 patients affected by familial and sporadic hemiplegic migraine. *Neurological Sciences* **32**(Suppl 1): S141–142.

Giniatullin R and Nistri A (2013). Desensitization properties of P2X3 receptors shaping pain signaling. *Frontiers in Cellular Neuroscience* **7**: 245.

Giniatullin R, Nistri A and Fabbretti E (2008). Molecular mechanisms of sensitization of pain-transducing P2X3 receptors by the migraine mediators CGRP and NGF. *Molecular Neurobiology* **37**: 83–90.

Goadsby PJ, Lipton RB and Ferrari MD (2002). Migraine--current understanding and treatment. *New England Journal of Medicine* **346**: 257–270.

GTEx Consortium (2013). The Genotype-Tissue Expression (GTEx) project. *Nature Genetics* **45**: 580–585.

Hawrylycz MJ, Lein ES, Guillozet-Bongaarts AL, Shen EH, Ng L, Miller JA, van de Lagemaat LN, Smith KA, Ebbert A, Riley ZL, Abajian C, Beckmann CF, Bernard A, Bertagnolli D, Boe AF, Cartagena PM, Chakravarty MM, Chapin M, Chong J, Dalley RA, Daly BD, Dang C, Datta S, Dee N, Dolbeare TA, Faber V, Feng D, Fowler DR, Goldy J, Gregor BW, Haradon Z, Haynor DR, Hohmann JG, Horvath S, Howard RE, Jeromin A, Jochim JM, Kinnunen M, Lau C, Lazarz ET, Lee C, Lemon TA, Li L, Li Y, Morris JA, Overly CC, Parker PD, Parry SE, Reding M, Royall JJ, Schulkin J, Sequeira PA, Slaughterbeck CR, Smith SC, Sodt AJ, Sunkin SM, Swanson BE, Vawter MP, Williams D, Wohnoutka P, Zielke HR, Geschwind DH, Hof PR, Smith SM, Koch C, Grant SG and Jones AR (2012). An anatomically comprehensive atlas of the adult human brain transcriptome. *Nature* **489**: 391–399.

Headache Classification Committee of the International Headache Society (2013). The International Classification of Headache Disorders, 3rd edition (beta version). *Cephalalgia* **33**: 629–808.

Hullugundi SK, Ferrari MD, van den Maagdenberg AM and Nistri A (2013). The mechanism of functional up-regulation of P2X3 receptors of trigeminal sensory neurons in a genetic mouse model of familial hemiplegic migraine type 1 (FHM-1). *PLoS One* **8**: e60677.

Inchauspe CG, Urbano FJ, Di Guilmi MN, Forsythe ID, Ferrari MD, van den Maagdenberg AM and Uchitel OD (2010). Gain of function in FHM-1 Cav2.1 knock-in mice is related to the shape of the action potential. *Journal of Neurophysiology* **104**: 291–299.

James PF, Grupp IL, Grupp G, Woo AL, Askew GR, Croyle ML, Walsh RA and Lingrel JB (1999). Identification of a specific role for the Na,K-ATPase alpha 2 isoform as a regulator of calcium in the heart. *Molecular Cell* **3**: 555–563.

Joutel A, Corpechot C, Ducros A, Vahedi K, Chabriat H, Mouton P, Alamowitch S, Domenga V, Cécillion M, Marechal E, Maciazek J, Vayssiere C, Cruaud C, Cabanis EA, Ruchoux MM, Weissenbach J, Bach JF, Bousser MG and Tournier-Lasserve E (1996). Notch3 mutations in CADASIL, a hereditary adult-onset condition causing stroke and dementia. *Nature* **383**: 707–710.

Kahlig KM, Rhodes TH, Pusch M, Freilinger T, Pereira-Monteiro JM, Ferrari MD, van den Maagdenberg AM, Dichgans M and George AL Jr, (2008). Divergent sodium channel defects in familial hemiplegic migraine. *Proceedings of the National Academy of Sciences of the United States of America* **105**: 9799–9804.

Kallela M, Wessman M, Havanka H, Palotie A and Färkkila M (2001). Familial migraine with and without aura: clinical characteristics and co-occurence. *European Journal of Neurology* **8**: 441–449.

Karatas H, Erdener SE, Gursoy-Ozdemir Y, Lule S, Eren-Koçak E, Sen ZD and Dalkara T. (2013). Spreading depression triggers headache by activating neuronal Panx1 channels. *Science* **339**: 1092–1095.

Köles L, Leichsenring A, Rubini P and Illes P (2011). P2 receptor signaling in neurons and glial cells of the central nervous system. *Advances in Pharmacology* **61**: 441–493.

Kuhlenbaumer G, Hullmann J and Appenzellerm S (2011). Novel genomic techniques open new avenues in the analysis of monogenic disorders. *Human Mutation* **32**: 144–151.

Lafrenière RG, Cader MZ, Poulin JF, Andres-Enguix I, Simoneau M, Gupta N, Boisvert K, Lafrenière F, McLaughlan S, Dubé MP, Marcinkiewicz MM, Ramagopalan S, Ansorge O, Brais B, Sequeiros J, Pereira-Monteiro JM, Griffiths LR, Tucker SJ, Ebers G and Rouleau GA (2010). A dominant-negative mutation in the TRESK potassium channel is linked to familial migraine with aura. *Nature Medicine* **16**: 1157–1160.

Langford DJ, Bailey AL, Chanda ML, Clarke SE, Drummond TE, Echols S, Glick S, Ingrao J, Klassen-Ross T, Lacroix-Fralish ML, Matsumiya L, Sorge RE, Sotocinal SG, Tabaka JM, Wong D, van den Maagdenberg AM, Ferrari MD, Craig KD and Mogil JS (2010). Coding of facial expressions of pain in the laboratory mouse. *Nature Methods* **7**: 447–459.

Lauritzen M (1994). Pathophysiology of the migraine aura. *The spreading depression theory. Brain* **117**: 199–210.

Leo L, Gherardini L, Barone V, De Fusco M, Pietrobon D, Pizzorusso T and Casari G (2011). Increased susceptibility to cortical spreading depression in the mouse model of familial hemiplegic migraine type 2. *PLoS Genetics* e1002129.

Ligthart L, Boomsma DI, Martin NG, Stubbe JH and Nyholt DR (2006). Migraine with aura and migraine without aura are not distinct entities: further evidence from a large Dutch population study. *Twin Researchearch and Human Genetics* **9**: 54–63.

Magni G and Ceruti S (2013). P2Y purinergic receptors: new targets for analgesic and antimigraine drugs. *Biochemical Pharmacology* **85**: 466–477.

Mulder EJ, van Baal C, Gaist D, Kallela M, Kaprio J, Svensson DA, Nyholt DR, Martin NG, MacGregor AJ, Cherkas LF, Boomsma DI and Palotie A (2003). Genetic and environmental influences on migraine: a twin study across six countries. *Twin Research* **6**: 422–431.

Nair A, Simonetti M, Birsa N, Ferrari MD, van den Maagdenberg AM, Giniatullin R, Nistri A and Fabbretti E (2010). Familial hemiplegic migraine Ca(v)2.1 channel mutation R192Q enhances ATP-gated P2X3 receptor activity of mouse sensory ganglion neurons mediating trigeminal pain. *Molecular Pain* **6**: 48.

Nyholt DR, Gillespie NG, Heath AC, Merikangas KR, Duffy DL and Martin NG (2004). Latent class and genetic analysis does not support migraine with aura and migraine without aura as separate entities. *Genetic Epidemiology* **26**: 231–244.

Ophoff RA, Terwindt GM, Vergouwe MN, van Eijk R, Oefner PJ, Hoffman SM, Lamerdin JE, Mohrenweiser HW, Bulman DE, Ferrari M, Haan J, Lindhout D, van Ommen GJ, Hofker MH, Ferrari MD and Frants RR (1996). Familial hemiplegic migraine and episodic ataxia type-2 are caused by mutations in the Ca^{2+} channel gene CACNL1A4. *Cell* **87**: 543–552.

Pelzer N, de Vries B, Kamphorst JT, Vijfhuizen LS, Ferrari MD, Haan J, van den Maagdenberg AM and Terwindt GM (2014). *PRRT2* and hemiplegic migraine: a complex association. *Neurology* **83**: 288–290.

Pietrobon D (2010). Insights into migraine mechanisms and CaV2.1 calcium channel function from mouse models of familial hemiplegic migraine. *Journal of Physiology* **588**: 1871–1878.

Riant F, Ducros A, Ploton C, Barbance C, Depienne C and Tournier-Lasserve E (2010). De novo mutations in *ATP1A2* and *CACNA1A* are frequent in early-onset sporadic hemiplegic migraine. *Neurology* **75**: 967–972.

Riant F, Roze E, Barbance C, Méneret A, Guyant-Maréchal L, Lucas C, Sabouraud P, Trébuchon A, Depienne C and Tournier-Lasserve E (2012). PRRT2 mutations cause hemiplegic migraine. *Neurology* **79**: 2122–2124.

Russell MB and Olesen J (1995). Increased familial risk and evidence of genetic factor in migraine. *British Medical Journal* **311**: 541–544.

Russell MB, Iselius L and Olesen J (1996). Migraine without aura and migraine with aura are inherited disorders. *Cephalalgia* **16**: 305–309.

Russell MB, Ulrich V, Gervil M and Olesen J (2002). Migraine without aura and migraine with aura are distinct disorders. A population-based twin survey. *Headache* **42**: 332–336.

Russo AF (2015). CGRP as a neuropeptide in migraine: lessons from mice. *British Journal of Clinical Pharmacology* **80**: 403–414.

Somjen GG (2001). Mechanisms of spreading depression and hypoxic spreading depression-like depolarization. *Physiological Reviews* **81**: 1065–1096.

Stam AH, Luijckx GJ, Poll-Thé BT, Ginjaar IB, Frants RR, Haan J, Ferrari MD, Terwindt GM and van den Maagdenberg AM (2009). Early seizures and cerebral oedema after trivial head trauma associated with the CACNA1A S218L mutation. *Journal of Neurology, Neurosurgery & Psychiatry* **80**: 1125–1129.

Stewart WF, Staffa J, Lipton RB and Ottman R (1997). Familial risk of migraine: a population-based study. *Annals of Neurology* **41**: 166–172.

Stewart WF, Bigal ME, Kolodner K, Dowson A, Liberman JN and Lipton RB (2006). Familial risk of migraine: variation by proband age at onset and headache severity. *Neurology* **66**: 344–348.

Stranneheim H and Wedell A (2016). Exome and genome sequencing: a revolution for the discovery and diagnosis of monogenic disorders. *Journal of Internal Medicine* **279**: 3–15.

Tao J, Liu P, Xiao Z, Zhao H, Gerber BR and Cao YQ (2012). Effects of familial hemiplegic migraine type 1 mutation T666M on voltage-gated calcium channel activities in trigeminal ganglion neurons. *Journal of Neurophysiology* **107**: 1666–1680.

Tavraz NN, Friedrich T, Dürr KL, Koenderink JB, Bamberg E, Freilinger T and Dichgans M (2008). Diverse functional consequences of mutations in the Na$^+$/K$^+$-ATPase alpha2-subunit causing familial hemiplegic migraine type 2. *Journal of Biological Chemistry* **283**: 31097–31106.

The NIH Roadmap Epigenomics Mapping Consortium. Bernstein BE, Stamatoyannopoulos JA, Costello JF, Ren B, Milosavljevic A, Meissner A, Kellis M, Marra MA, Beaudet AL, Ecker JR, Farnham PJ, Hirst M, Lander ES, Mikkelsen TS and Thomson JA (2010). *Nature Biotechnology* **28**: 1045–1048.

Thomsen LL, Eriksen MK, Roemer SF, Andersen I, Olesen J and Russell MB (2002) A population-based study of familial hemiplegic migraine suggests revised diagnostic criteria. *Brain* **125**: 1379–1391.

Thomsen LL, Ostergaard E, Romer SF, Andersen I, Eriksen MK, Olesen J and Russell MB (2003). Sporadic hemiplegic migraine is an aetiologically heterogeneous disorder. *Cephalalgia* **23**: 921–928.

Thomsen LL, Oestergaard E, Bjornsson A, Stefansson H, Fasquel AC, Gulcher J, Stefansson K and Olesen J (2008). Screen for *CACNA1A* and *ATP1A2* mutations in sporadic hemiplegic migraine patients. *Cephalalgia* **28**: 914–921.

Tolner EA, Houben T, Terwindt GM, de Vries B, Ferrari MD and van den Maagdenberg AM (2015). From migraine genes to mechanisms. *Pain* **156**(Suppl 1): S64–74.

Tottene A, Conti R, Fabbro A, Vecchia D, Shapovalova M, Santello M, van den Maagdenberg AM, Ferrari MD and Pietrobon D (2009). Enhanced excitatory transmission at cortical synapses as the basis for facilitated spreading depression in Ca(v)2.1 knockin migraine mice. *Neuron* **61**: 762–773.

van den Maagdenberg AM, Pietrobon D, Pizzorusso T, Kaja S, Broos LA, Cesetti T, van de Ven RC, Tottene A, van der Kaa J, Plomp JJ, Frants RR and Ferrari MD. (2004). A *Cacna1a* knockin migraine mouse model with increased susceptibility to cortical spreading depression. *Neuron* **41**: 701–710.

van den Maagdenberg AM, Pizzorusso T, Kaja S, Terpolilli N, Shapovalova M, Hoebeek FE, Barrett CF, Gherardini L, van de Ven RC, Todorov B, Broos LA, Tottene A, Gao Z, Fodor M, De Zeeuw CI, Frants RR, Plesnila N, Plomp JJ, Pietrobon D and Ferrari MD (2010). High CSD susceptibility and migraine-associated symptoms in CaV2.1 S218L mice. *Annals of Neurology* **67**: 85–98.

Vecchia D and Pietrobon D (2012). Migraine: a disorder of brain excitatory-inhibitory balance? *Trends in Neurosciences* **35**: 507–520.

Vecchia D, Tottene A, van den Maagdenberg AM and Pietrobon D (2014). Mechanism underlying unaltered cortical inhibitory synaptic transmission in contrast with enhanced excitatory transmission in cav2.1 knockin migraine mice. *Neurobiology of Disease* **69**: 225–234.

Vecchia D, Tottene A, van den Maagdenberg AM and Pietrobon D (2015). Abnormal cortical synaptic transmission in Ca$_V$2.1 knockin mice with the S218L missense mutation which causes a severe familial hemiplegic migraine syndrome in humans. Frontiers in Cellular *Neuroscience* **9**: 8.

Wang K, Li M and Hakonarson H (2010). Analysing biological pathways in genome-wide association studies. *Nature Reviews Genetics* **11**: 843–854.

Wrobel Goldberg S and Silberstein SD (2015). Targeting CGRP: A New Era for Migraine Treatment. *CNS Drugs* **29**: 443–445.

Zhang XC, Kainz V, Burstein R and Levy D (2011a). Tumor necrosis factor-alpha induces sensitization of meningeal nociceptors mediated via local COX and p38 MAP kinase actions. *Pain* **152**: 140–149.

Zhang X, Levy D, Kainz V, Noseda R, Jakubowski M and Burstein R (2011b). Activation of central trigeminovascular neurons by cortical spreading depression. *Annals of Neurology* **69**: 855–865.

15

Lessons from familial hemiplegic migraine and cortical spreading depression
Daniela Pietrobon

Department of Biomedical Sciences, University of Padova, and CNR Institute of Neuroscience, Padova, Italy

15.1   Introduction

Migraine is a common episodic neurological disorder with complex pathophysiology. It is generally recognized that: i) most migraine attacks start in the brain; ii) migraine headache depends on the activation and sensitization of the trigeminovascular pain pathway; and iii) cortical spreading depression (CSD) is the neurophysiological correlate of migraine aura (Lauritzen, 1994 ; Noseda and Burstein, 2013; Pietrobon and Moskowitz, 2013, 2014).

CSD is a slowly propagating wave of rapid and nearly complete depolarization of brain cells, that lasts about one minute and silences brain electrical activity for several minutes (Pietrobon and Moskowitz, 2014). It is characterized by collapse of ion homeostasis and profound disruption of transmembrane ionic gradients, plus release of neurotransmitters and other molecules from cellular compartments. Experimental induction of CSD in normally metabolizing brain tissue requires intense depolarizing stimuli that increase the extracellular concentration of potassium ions $[K^+]_e$ above a critical threshold.

As inferred from modeling, initiation of the positive feedback cycle that ignites CSD requires the generation of a net inward current, as a consequence of the activation of a sufficient number of voltage-gated and/or $[K^+]_e$-dependent channels. Net inward current leads to membrane depolarization and increase of $[K^+]_e$ which, in turn, leads to further activation of voltage-gated and/or $[K^+]_e$-dependent channels, further depolarization, and an increase in local $[K^+]_e$. This results in complete neuronal depolarization if the removal of K^+ from the interstitium, mainly due to glial reuptake mechanisms, does not keep pace with its release (Somjen, 2001; Pietrobon and Moskowitz, 2014). Although the nature of the ion channels that are crucial to initiate CSD remains incompletely understood, there is strong pharmacological evidence that NMDA receptors play a key role in CSD initiation (Pietrobon and Moskowitz, 2014).

Experiments in rats have shown that a single CSD can lead to a long-lasting increase in ongoing activity of dural nociceptors and central trigeminovascular neurons, regardless of the cortical region it arises from (Bolay *et al.*, 2002; Zhang *et al.*, 2010, 2011; Zhao and Levy, 2015). The activation process possibly involves CSD-induced opening of neuronal pannexin1 megachannels, resulting in a downstream cascade of events that may lead to release of proinflammatory molecules in the meninges via glia limitans (Karatas *et al.*,

Neurobiological Basis of Migraine, First Edition. Edited by Turgay Dalkara and Michael A. Moskowitz.

2013). These findings are consistent with, and support, the idea that CSD not only causes migraine aura but may also trigger the mechanisms underlying migraine headache.

The mechanisms of the primary brain dysfunction(s) underlying the susceptibility to CSD ignition in the human brain and the onset of a migraine attack remain largely unknown, and these are major open issues in the neurobiology of migraine.

Migraine is a complex genetic disorder, with heritability estimates as high as 50% and a likely polygenic multifactorial inheritance (Russell and Ducros, 2011; Ferrari *et al.*, 2015). Three large genome-wide association studies and a subsequent meta-analysis have identified a few risk factors for both migraine with and without aura (Ferrari *et al.*, 2015). However, most of our current molecular understanding of migraine comes from studies of familial hemiplegic migraine (FHM), a rare monogenic autosomal dominant form of MA (Russell and Ducros, 2011; Ferrari *et al.*, 2015). Three FHM causative genes have been identified, all encoding ion channels or transporters (Ophoff *et al.*, 1996; De Fusco *et al.*, 2003; Dichgans *et al.*, 2005). Additional FHM genes certainly exist, and remain to be identified (Thomsen *et al.*, 2007).

Apart from the motor aura and the possible longer duration of the aura, typical FHM attacks resemble MA attacks, and both types of attacks may alternate in patients and co-occur within families. This suggests that FHM and MA may be part of the same spectrum, and may share some pathogenetic mechanisms, despite clinical observations that the response to infusion of CGRP and glyceriltrinitrate seems to differ (Ashina *et al.*, 2013; Ferrari *et al.*, 2015). Some FHM patients can also have atypical severe attacks (with signs of diffuse encephalopathy, confusion or coma, prolonged hemiplegia and in a few cases seizures) and/or permanent cerebellar symptoms (Russell and Ducros, 2011).

This chapter will focus on:

i) the physiological role of the proteins encoded by the three known FHM genes and the functional consequences of FHM mutations; and
ii) the insights into the mechanisms underlying susceptibility to CSD and initiation of migraine attacks obtained from the functional analysis of FHM mouse models.

15.2 FHM genes and functional consequences of FHM mutations

FHM type 1 (FHM1) is caused by missense mutations in CACNA1A, the gene encoding the pore-forming subunit of neuronal $Ca_V2.1$ (P/Q-type) voltage-gated calcium (Ca) channels (Ophoff *et al.*, 1996; Pietrobon, 2013) (Figure 15.1). These calcium channels are widely expressed in the nervous system, including all structures implicated in the pathogenesis of migraine, and play a dominant role in controlling neurotransmitter release; the somatodendritic localization of $Ca_V2.1$ channels points to additional postsynaptic roles, for example, in neural excitability (Pietrobon, 2013). In particular, in different areas of the cerebral cortex, excitatory synaptic transmission at pyramidal cell synapses, and inhibitory synaptic transmission at both fast-spiking (FS) and somatostatin-expressing interneuron synapses, depend predominantly or exclusively on P/Q-type Ca channels (Pietrobon, 2013 and references therein; Rossignol *et al.*, 2013) (see Chapter 14).

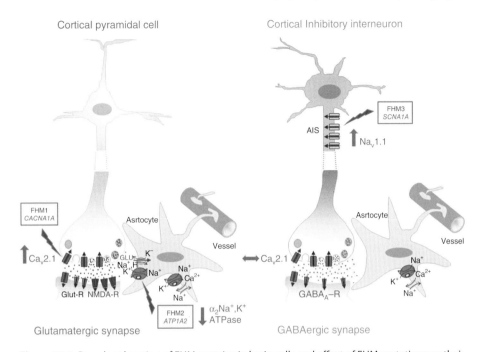

Figure 15.1 Prevalent location of FHM proteins in brain cells and effect of FHM mutations on their function. The Ca$_V$2.1 channels (the mutant proteins in FHM1) are located at the active zones of both excitatory and inhibitory synaptic terminals throughout the brain. FHM1 mutations produce gain-of-function of the Ca$_V$2.1 channels in excitatory cortical pyramidal cells, but do not affect the Ca$_V$2.1 channels in multipolar cortical inhibitory interneurons. In the adult brain, the α2 Na$^+$, K$^+$ ATPases (the mutant proteins in FHM2) are located almost exclusively in astrocytes, where they are colocalized with glutamate transporters in astrocyte processes surrounding excitatory, but not inhibitory, synapses. The Na$_V$1.1 channels (the mutant proteins in FHM3) are located in cortical inhibitory interneurons, especially at the axon initial segment, and play an important role in interneuron (but not pyramidal cell) excitability, particularly in sustaining high-frequency firing. FHM3 mutations produce gain-of-function of Na$_V$1.1 channels in cortical interneurons.

Analysis of the single channel properties of mutant recombinant human Ca$_V$2.1 channels (Tottene *et al.*, 2002; Pietrobon, 2013) and of the P/Q-type calcium current in different neurons of knock-in (KI) mice carrying FHM1 mutations, revealed that the mutations produce gain-of-function of Ca$_V$2.1 channels, mainly due to increased channel open probability and channel activation at lower voltages (van den Maagdenberg *et al.*, 2004, 2010; Tottene *et al.*, 2009; Inchauspe *et al.*, 2010; Fioretti *et al.*, 2011; Gao *et al.*, 2012). FHM1 mutations also reduce the G protein-mediated inhibitory modulation of recombinant Cav2.1 channels, an effect that, if confirmed in neurons, may lead to further gain of function during neuromodulation (Melliti *et al.*, 2003; Weiss *et al.*, 2008; Serra *et al.*, 2009).

The gain-of-function effect of FHM1 mutations may be dependent on the specific Ca$_V$2.1 splice variant and/or auxiliary subunit (Mullner *et al.*, 2004; Adams *et al.*, 2009). The expression of specific Ca$_V$2.1 splice variants and/or auxiliary subunits in different types of neurons may underlie some interesting neuron-specific effects of FHM1 mutations recently uncovered in trigeminal and cortical neurons. In trigeminal ganglion neurons of FHM1 KI mice, the P/Q-type calcium current was increased in small capsaicin-insensitive trigeminal ganglion neurons not innervating the dura, but was unaltered in small capsaicin-sensitive neurons innervating the dura (Fioretti *et al.*, 2011). Congruently, depolarization-evoked CGRP release from the dura was unaltered in FHM1 KI mice, whereas CGRP release from trigeminal ganglia was enhanced (Fioretti *et al*, 2011).

In contrast with the increased current density and left-shifted activation gating of the $Ca_V2.1$ channels in cortical pyramidal cells and other excitatory CNS neurons from FHM1 KI mice (van den Maagdenberg *et al.*, 2004, 2010; Tottene *et al.*, 2009; Inchauspe *et al.*, 2010; Gao *et al.*, 2012), the current density and activation gating of the $Ca_V2.1$ channels expressed in cortical multipolar (mainly FS) inhibitory interneurons were barely affected by the FHM1 mutation (Vecchia *et al.*, 2014). Congruently, cortical excitatory synaptic transmission was enhanced in FHM1 KI mice whereas, in striking contrast, inhibitory neurotransmission at FS (and other multipolar) interneuron synapses was unaltered (Tottene *et al.*, 2009; Vecchia *et al.*, 2014, 2015) (Figure 15.1).

Neuron-specific effects of FHM1 mutations on action potential (AP)-evoked Ca influx may also result from different shape and duration of APs in different neurons. Although in cortical pyramidal cells, the shift to lower voltages of mutant $Ca_V2.1$ channel activation resulted in increased AP-evoked Ca current, a similar activation shift of mutant $Ca_V2.1$ channels at the Calyx of Held synaptic terminals did not alter the AP-evoked Ca current (Inchauspe *et al.*, 2010). The different durations of the AP in pyramidal cells and Calyx (1.8 vs 0.44 ms AP half width) may largely explain the different effects of the FHM1 mutation on the AP-evoked Ca current (Inchauspe *et al.*, 2010). The demonstration of neuron-specific alterations of $Ca_V2.1$ channels and/or AP-evoked Ca influx has an important implication for familial migraine mechanisms, in that it may help to explain why a mutation in a calcium channel that is widely expressed in the nervous system produces the specific neuronal dysfunctions leading to migraine (see next section).

FHM type 2 (FHM2) is caused by (mainly missense) mutations in ATP1A2, the gene encoding the α_2 subunit of the Na^+, K^+ ATPase (NKA) (De Fusco *et al.*, 2003; Bøttger *et al.*, 2012; see Figure 15.1). In the brain, this isoform is expressed primarily in neurons during embryonic development and at time of birth, but almost exclusively in astrocytes in the adult (Pietrobon, 2007 and references therein). While the ubiquitous α1 NKA is thought to fulfill households tasks, the α_2 NKA is thought to have specific important roles in clearance of K^+ and glutamate released during neuronal activity and in astrocyte Ca^{2+} homeostasis (Pietrobon, 2007). Although the lower affinity of the α2 NKA for extracellular K^+ makes it better geared to respond efficiently to activity-dependent increases of $[K^+]_e$, compared with α3 and α1, the relative contribution of the different NKA isoforms in K^+ clearance from the extracellular medium remains unclear, and might vary in different conditions (D'Ambrosio *et al.*, 2002; Ransom *et al.*, 2000; Larsen *et al.*, 2014).

An important role of the α2 NKA in glutamate clearance by astrocytes is suggested by its colocalization with the glial glutamate transporters in astrocytic processes surrounding glutamatergic synapses in the adult somatosensory cortex (Cholet *et al.*, 2002) and the evidence of physical and functional coupling of the α2 NKA with glial glutamate transporters (Pellerin and Magistretti, 1997; Rose *et al.*, 2009; Illarionava *et al.*, 2014). A specific role of α2 NKA in the regulation of intracellular Ca^{2+}, particularly in the endoplasmic reticulum, is suggested by the colocalization of the α2 NKA with the Na^+/Ca^{2+} exchanger, in microdomains that overlie subplasmalemmal endoplasmic reticulum in cultured astrocytes (Pietrobon, 2007 and references therein).

FHM2 mutations cause complete or partial loss-of-function of recombinant α2 NKA, due to loss or reduction of catalytic activity or impairment of plasma membrane delivery and/or protein degradation (Pietrobon, 2007; Boettger *et al*, 2012). The $α_2$ NKA protein is barely detectable in the brain of homozygous FHM2 KI mice, and strongly reduced in the brain of heterozygous mutants (Leo *et al.*, 2011; Figure 15.1).

FHM type 3 (FHM3) is caused by missense mutations in SCNA1A, the gene encoding the pore-forming subunit of neuronal $Na_V1.1$ voltage-gated sodium channels (Dichgans *et al.*, 2005; Figure 15.1). $Na_V.1.1$ channels are highly expressed in cortical inhibitory interneurons, especially at the axon initial segment, and play an important role in interneuron (but not pyramidal cell) excitability, particularly in sustaining interneuron high-frequency firing (Yu *et al.*, 2006; Ogiwara *et al.*, 2007). Indeed loss-of-function mutations in $Na_V.1.1$ channels and consequent selective impairment of firing in inhibitory interneurons cause a spectrum of epilepsy syndromes (Catterall *et al.*, 2010).

Conflicting findings were obtained from the analysis of the functional consequences of FHM3 mutations on recombinant human $Na_V1.1$ channels expressed in non-neuronal cells, pointing to either gain- or loss-of-function effects of FHM3 mutations, depending on the mutation and/or the laboratory (Cestèle *et al.*, 2008; Kahlig *et al.*, 2008). However, recently, it has been shown that the L1649Q mutant Nav1.1 channel, which was non-functional when expressed in a non neuronal cell line because of lack of plasma membrane delivery, shows an overall gain-of-function phenotype, and could sustain high-frequency firing better than the WT channel when expressed in cortical interneurons (Cestèle *et al.*, 2013). This interesting finding suggests that FHM3 is most likely associated with gain-of-function of NaV1.1 channels and consequent selective hyperexcitability of cortical interneurons (Figure 15.1).

15.3 Insights into the mechanisms underlying susceptibility to cortical spreading depression and initiation of migraine attacks from the functional analysis of FHM mouse models

Three different FHM mouse models have been generated by introducing the human FHM1 R192Q or S218L and FHM2 W887R mutations into the orthologous genes (van den Maagdenberg *et al.*, 2004, 2010; Leo *et al.*, 2011). While mutations R192Q and W887R in humans cause typical FHM attacks (Ophoff *et al.*, 1996; De Fusco *et al.*, 2003), mutation S218L causes a particularly dramatic clinical syndrome (Kors *et al.*, 2001). Whereas homozygous R192Q and heterozygous S218L and W887R KI mice do not exhibit an overt phenotype, homozygous S218L mice model the main features of the severe S218L clinical syndrome (van den Maagdenberg *et al.*, 2010).

The investigation of experimental CSD, elicited either by electrical stimulation of the cortex *in vivo* or by focal application of high KCl in cortical slices, revealed a lower threshold for CSD initiation and an increased velocity of CSD propagation in both FHM1 and FHM2 KI mice (van den Maagdenberg *et al.*, 2004, 2010; Tottene *et al.*, 2009;

Leo *et al.*, 2011). Moreover, a single CSD, elicited by brief epidural application of high KCl, more readily propagated into the striatum and produced more severe and prolonged motor deficits (including hemiplegia) in FHM1, compared with WT mice (Eikermann-Haerter *et al.*, 2009b, 2011).

In agreement with the higher female prevalence in migraine, the velocity of propagation and the frequency of CSDs, elicited by continous epidural high KCl application, were larger in female than in male FHM1 mouse mutants. The sex difference was abrogated by ovariectomy and enhanced by orchiectomy, suggesting that female and male gonadal hormones exert reciprocal effects on CSD susceptibility (Eikermann-Haerter *et al.*, 2009a, 2009b). However, no gender differences in the electrical threshold for CSD induction and the velocity of CSD propagation were found in FHM2 KI mice (Leo *et al.*, 2011). The frequency of CSDs was also increased in FHM1 KI mice after administration of the stress hormone corticosterone, but not after acute restrain stress (Shyti *et al.*, 2015).

In homozygous FHM1 KI mice carrying the mild R192Q or the severe S218L mutation, the strength of CSD facilitation, as well as the severity of the post-CSD neurological motor deficits and the propensity of CSD to propagate into subcortical structures, were all in good correlation with the strength of the gain-of-function of the $Ca_V2.1$ channel and the severity of the clinical phenotype produced by the two FHM1 mutations (Kors *et al.*, 2001; van den Maagdenberg *et al.*, 2004, 2010; Tottene *et al.*, 2005; Eikermann-Haerter *et al.*, 2009b, 2011). Propagation of CSD to the hippocampus and thalamus, and repetitive CSD events following a single CSD-inducing stimulus, were observed only in S218L mutants (van den Maagdenberg *et al.*, 2010; Eikermann-Haerter *et al.*, 2011). These unique CSD features might account for the severe attacks, with seizures, coma and cerebral edema, typical of patients with the S218L mutation.

Although FHM3 mouse models are not yet available, the report that FHM3 in two unrelated families co-segregates with a new eye phenotype, with clinical features similar to experimental spreading depression in retina (Vahedi *et al.*, 2009), suggests that the ability to facilitate CSD is likely also shared by FHM3 mutations.

As a whole, the studies of experimental CSD in FHM KI mice strengthen the view of CSD as a key player in the pathogenesis of migraine. Moreover, the investigation of the mechanisms underlying the facilitation of experimental CSD in FHM1 KI mice has provided insights into the mechanisms of initiation of CSD, and into the mechanisms that may make the brain of migraineurs susceptible to "spontaneous" CSDs.

The study of cortical synaptic transmission in FHM1 KI mice revealed enhanced excitatory transmission, due to enhanced action potential-evoked Ca influx through mutant presynaptic $Ca_V2.1$ channels and enhanced probability of glutamate release at cortical pyramidal cell synapses (Tottene *et al.*, 2009; Vecchia *et al.*, 2015). CSD rescue experiments in R192Q KI mice support a causative relationship between increased glutamate release at cortical excitatory synapses and facilitation of (both initiation and propagation of) experimental CSD (Tottene *et al.*, 2009). In fact, the facilitation of CSD in acute cortical slices of homozygous R192Q KI mice was completely eliminated when AP-evoked glutamate release at pyramidal cell synapses was brought back to WT values by partially inhibiting the $Ca_V2.1$ channels (Tottene *et al.*, 2009).

In good correlation with the similar gain-of-function of the neuronal P/Q-type Ca^{2+} current and the similar facilitation of experimental CSD in *heterozygous* S218L and *homozygous* R192Q KI mice (van den Maagdenberg *et al.*, 2010), the gain-of-function of evoked excitatory neurotransmission in cortical pyramidal cells in microculture was quantitatively similar in *heterozygous* S218L and *homozygous* R192Q KI mice (Tottene *et al.*, 2009; Vecchia *et al.*, 2015). This good correlation is consistent with the conclusion that enhanced glutamate release at cortical pyramidal cell synapses may explain the facilitation of experimental CSD in *heterozygous* S218L KI mice, as directly shown in *homozygous* R192Q KI mice.

The data are consistent with, and support, a model of CSD initiation in which a local regenerative $[K^+]_e$ increase, $[K^+]_e$-induced opening of presynaptic $Ca_V2.1$ channels, and consequent glutamate release and activation of NMDA receptors (and possibly activation of postsynaptic $Ca_V2.1$ channels), are key elements in the positive feedback cycle that ignites CSD (Tottene *et al.*, 2009; Pietrobon and Moskowitz, 2014; Figure 15.2). Moreover, the findings are consistent with a model of CSD propagation in which interstitial K^+ diffusion initiates this positive-feedback cycle in contiguous dendritic regions (Tottene *et al.*, 2009; Pietrobon and Moskowitz, 2014).

This model and, in general, the specific requirement of $Ca_V2.1$ channels in the initiation and propagation of CSD (induced by electrical stimulation or brief pulses of high K^+), are further supported by the findings that:

i) in the spontaneous mouse mutants *leaner* and *tottering*, which carry loss-of-function mutations in *cacna1a* (Pietrobon, 2010), the electrical threshold for CSD induction in the cerebral cortex *in vivo* was greatly increased, and the velocity of CSD propagation, as well as K^+-evoked glutamate release (as measured by microdyalisis), were reduced, compared with WT mice (Ayata *et al.*, 2000);

ii) after blockade of either the $Ca_V2.1$ channels or the NMDA receptors, CSD could not be induced in cortical slices of WT mice, even using largely suprathreshold stimuli (Tottene *et al.*, 2011).

In contrast with the larger facilitation of CSD and the larger neuronal P/Q-type Ca^{2+} current in *homozygous* S218L compared with *heterozygous* S218L KI mice (van den Maagdenberg *et al.*, 2010), the strength of excitatory transmission at cortical pyramidal cell synapses is similar in *homozygous* and *heterozygous* S218L KI mice, reflecting a similar AP-evoked presynaptic Ca influx (Vecchia *et al.*, 2015). This suggests the existence of compensatory changes in *homozygous* S218L KI mice that prevent excessive AP-evoked Ca influx and glutamate release. Moreover, these findings suggest that the larger facilitation of experimental CSD in *homozygous*, compared with *heterozygous* S218L KI mice is due to gain-of-function of $Ca_V2.1$-dependent mechanisms different from evoked glutamate release at cortical pyramidal cell synapses (Vecchia *et al.*, 2015). Gain-of-function of $Ca_V2.1$-dependent mechanisms different from evoked-glutamate release should also underlie the unique cortical susceptibility to repetitive CSD events, and the unique propensity of CSD to spread into subcortical structures observed in S218L (both larger in *homozygous* than *heterozygous* mice), but not in R192Q KI mice (van den Maagdenberg *et al.*, 2010; Eikermann-Haerter *et al.*, 2011).

A specific feature of cortical synapses in S218L KI mice not observed in R192Q KI mice is the presence of a fraction of mutant $Ca_V2.1$ channels that is open at resting potential in cortical excitatory synaptic terminals, as revealed by the reduced frequency of spontaneous miniature excitatory postsynaptic currents (mEPSCs) after specific block of $Ca_V2.1$ channels in cortical slices from *heterozygous* and *homozygous* S218L (but not R192Q) KI mice (Vecchia *et al.*, 2015).

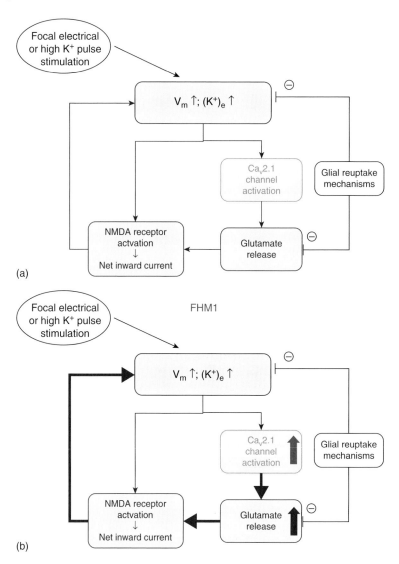

(a)

(b)

Figure 15.2 A model of CSD initiation. (a) A schematic diagram of the initiation mechanisms of experimental CSD induced by a focal electrical or brief K⁺ pulse stimulation. In this model, $Ca_V2.1$-channel dependent release of glutamate from cortical excitatory synapses and activation of NMDA receptors have a key role in the generation of the net inward current necessary to initiate the positive feedback cycle that ignites CSD. The glial reuptake mechanisms play a dampening role, by mediating both K⁺ and glutamate clearance. (b) In FHM1, $Ca_V2.1$ channel activation and glutamate release are larger at any given depolarization and $[K^+]_e$ increase. As a consequence, the positive feedback cycle is amplified, and a smaller depolarizing stimulus is necessary to open a sufficient number of $Ca_V2.1$ channels and release enough glutamate and open enough NMDA receptors to initiate the positive feedback cycle that ignites CSD.

An even larger reduction of mEPSCs frequency after specific block of $Ca_V2.1$ channels as well as an increase in basal $[Ca^{2+}]_i$ in synaptic terminals were measured at Calyx of Held synapses in brainstem slices from *homozygous* S218L KI mice (Di Guilmi *et al.*, 2014). In R192Q KI mice, mEPSCs frequency at both cortical and Calyx synapses was similar to that at WT synapses (Tottene *et al.*, 2009; Inchauspe *et al.*, 2012), indicating that presynaptic $Ca_V2.1$ channels carrying the R192Q mutation are closed at resting potential. Interestingly, an increase of baseline $[Ca^{2+}]_i$ in axonal boutons and shafts in layer 2/3 of cerebral cortex in *heterozygous* S218L KI mice *in vivo* was recently revealed by elegant Ca imaging, using a FRET-based Ca indicator (Eikermann-Haerter *et al*, 2015). Probably as a consequence of the increase in baseline $[Ca^{2+}]_i$, these mice also showed some alterations in axonal and dendritic morphology in the resting state, including slightly larger boutons (Eikermann-Haerter *et al.*, 2015). It would be important to perform similar experiments in R192Q KI mice, to verify whether, as predicted by the work in cortical slices, the increase in baseline $[Ca^{2+}]_i$ is a specific feature of S218L KI mice that might contribute to explain some of the unique features of the *in vivo* CSD in these mice.

A larger facilitation of CSD in *homozygous* compared to *heterozygous* S218L KI mice is expected (even with similar AP-evoked glutamate release in the two genotypes) if a larger fraction of mutant $Ca_V2.1$ channels opens at subthreshold depolarizations induced by local $[K^+]_e$ rise in *homozygous* S218L KI mice. Moreover, in these mice, the increase in basal $[Ca^{2+}]_i$ and Ca^{2+} influx, at negative voltages sub-threshold for AP generation through presynaptic and postsynaptic mutant $Ca_V2.1$ channel, may contribute to lower the threshold for CSD induction through additional mechanisms that remain to be elucidated. For example, in addition to NMDA receptors, $[Ca^{2+}]_i$-activated cationic channels could contribute to the net self-sustaining inward current necessary to initiate the positive feedback cycle that ignites CSD (Somjen *et al.*, 2009; Pietrobon and Moskowitz, 2014).

Moreover, the unique metabolic burden put on cortical neurons by the constant basal Ca^{2+} influx that is specifically produced by the S218L mutation may contribute to the unique features of CSD in S218L KI mice, by, for example, prolonging the transient hypoxia and slowing the recovery of cerebral flow after CSD (Pietrobon and Moskowitz, 2014). Since another peculiarity of mutant S218L Ca^{2+} channels, besides the particularly low threshold of activation, is the incomplete inactivation during prolonged depolarizations (Tottene *et al.*, 2005), a larger increase of $[Ca^{2+}]_i$ during CSD in cortical neurons may also contribute to a slower recovery from CSD in S218L KI mice.

The mechanisms underlying the facilitation of CSD in FHM2 and FHM3 have not yet been experimentally investigated. One may predict that a reduced rate of K^+ clearance and/or a reduced rate of glutamate clearance due to loss-of-function of the α2 NKA pump would lower the threshold for CSD induction and increase the velocity of CSD propagation. It is not straightforward to envisage how gain-of-function of $Na_V1.1$ channels in interneurons and consequent selective hyperexcitability of cortical interneurons may facilitate CSD in FHM3.

In migraineurs, CSD is not induced by experimental depolarizing stimuli, but arises "spontaneously", probably in response to specific triggers that somehow create, in the cortex, the conditions for initiation of the positive feedback cycle that overwhelms the regulatory mechanisms controlling cortical $[K^+]_e$ and ignites CSD. Insights into how this might occur have been provided by the differential effect of FHM1 mutations on synaptic transmission and short-term synaptic plasticity at cortical excitatory and inhibitory synapses (Tottene *et al.*, 2009; Vecchia *et al.*, 2014, 2015). This finding suggests that, very likely, the neuronal circuits that dynamically maintain a tight balance between excitation and inhibition during cortical activity are altered in FHM1. Functional alterations in these circuits are expected to lead to dysfunctional regulation of the cortical excitatory-inhibitory balance and, hence, to abnormal processing of sensory information (Vecchia and Pietrobon, 2012).

A plausible working hypothesis is that dysregulation of the cortical excitatory-inhibitory balance may, under certain conditions (e.g., in response to migraine triggers such as intense, prolonged sensory stimulation), lead to hyperactivity of cortical circuits, that may create the conditions for the initiation of "spontaneous" CSDs (e.g., by increasing $[K^+]_e$ above a critical value). Similar mechanisms might underlie the susceptibility to CSD in FHM2, given that in the cerebral cortex the α2 NKA is localized in glial processes surrounding glutamatergic, but not GABAergic synapses (Cholet *et al.*, 2002).

It is certainly possible that FHM mutations produce parallel dysfunctions in subcortical areas that might also contribute to the altered regulation of cortical function and in general to the disease in a way that remains to be established (e.g., by altering cortical neuromodulation by monoaminergic projections and/or by favoring hyperexcitability of trigeminovascular pathways).

Similar mechanisms may underlie the abnormal regulation of cortical (and possibly subcortical) function in some common migraine subtypes, for which there is indirect evidence consistent with enhanced cortical glutamatergic neurotransmission and enhanced cortico-cortical or recurrent excitatory neurotransmission (Pietrobon and Moskowitz, 2013, and references therein). Some of the susceptibility loci for MA and MO recently identified in genome-wide association studies appear also consistent with the idea of migraine as a disorder of glutamatergic neurotransmission and/or dysregulated brain excitatory-inhibitory balance (Ferrari *et al.*, 2015). Given the wide clinical and genetic heterogeneity of migraine, different molecular and cellular mechanisms that remain largely unknown may well underlie the impaired regulation of brain function and the susceptibility to CSD in different migraineurs.

15.4 Acknowledgements

I gratefully thank Dr. Angelita Tottene for making the figures, and the support of grants from Telethon Italy (GGP14234), from the Italian Ministry of University and Research (PRIN2010) and from the University of Padova (CPDA120811/12).

References

Adams, P.J., Garcia, E., David, L.S., Mulatz, K.J., Spacey, S.D., and Snutch, T.P. (2009). Ca(V)2.1 P/Q-type calcium channel alternative splicing affects the functional impact of familial hemiplegic migraine mutations: implications for calcium channelopathies. *Channels (Austin)* **3**: 110–121.

Ashina, M., Hansen, J.M., and Olesen, J. (2013). Pearls and pitfalls in human pharmacological models of migraine: 30 years' experience. *Cephalalgia* **33**: 540–553.

Ayata, C., Shimizu-Sasamata, M., Lo, E.H., Noebels, J.L., and Moskowitz (2000). Impaired neurotransmitter release and elevated threshold for cortical spreading depression in mice with mutations in the a_{1A} subunit of P/Q type calcium channels. *Neuroscience* **95**: 639–645.

Bolay, H., Reuter, U., Dunn, A.K., Huang, Z., Boas, D.A., and Moskowitz, M.A. (2002). Intrinsic brain activity triggers trigeminal meningeal afferents in a migraine model. *Nature Medicine* **8**: 136–142.

Bøttger, P., Doğanlı, C., and Lykke-Hartmann, K. (2012). Migraine- and dystonia-related disease-mutations of Na^+/K^+-ATPases: Relevance of behavioral studies in mice to disease symptoms and neurological manifestations in humans. *Neuroscience & Biobehavioral Reviews* **36**: 855–871.

Catterall, W.A., Kalume, F., and Oakley, J.C. (2010). NaV1.1 channels and epilepsy. *Journal of Physiology* **588**: 1849–1859.

Cestèle, S., Scalmani, P., Rusconi, R., Terragni, B., Franceschetti, S., and Mantegazza, M. (2008). Self-limited hyperexcitability: Functional effect of a familial hemiplegic migraine mutation of the Na(v)1.1 (SCN1A) Na^+ channel. *Journal of Neuroscience* **28**: 7273–7283.

Cestèle, S., Schiavon, E., Rusconi, R., Franceschetti, S., and Mantegazza, M. (2013). Nonfunctional NaV1.1 familial hemiplegic migraine mutant transformed into gain of function by partial rescue of folding defects. *Proceedings of the National Academy of Sciences* **110**: 17546–17551.

Cholet, N., Pellerin, L., Magistretti, P.J., and Hamel, E. (2002). Similar perisynaptic glial localization for the Na^+,K^+-ATPase alpha 2 subunit and the glutamate transporters GLAST and GLT-1 in the rat somatosensory cortex. *Cerebral Cortex* **12**: 515–525.

D'Ambrosio, R., Gordon, D.S., and Winn, H.R. (2002). Differential role of KIR channel and $Na(^+)/K(^+)$-pump in the regulation of extracellular $K(^+)$ in rat hippocampus. *Journal of Neurophysiology* **87**: 87–102.

De Fusco, M., Marconi, R., Silvestri, L., Atorino, L., Rampoldi, L., Morgante, L., *et al.* (2003). Haploinsufficiency of ATP1A2 encoding the Na^+/K^+ pump alpha2 subunit associated with familial hemiplegic migraine type 2. *Nature Genetics* **33**: 192–196.

Di Guilmi, M.N., Wang, T., Inchauspe, C.G., Forsythe, I.D., Ferrari, M.D., van den Maagdenberg, A.M., *et al.* (2014). Synaptic gain-of-function effects of mutant Cav2.1 channels in a mouse model of familial hemiplegic migraine are due to increased basal $[Ca^{2+}]$i. *Journal of Neuroscience* **34**: 7047–7058.

Dichgans, M., Freilinger, T., Eckstein, G., Babini, E., Lorenz-Depiereux, B., Biskup, S., *et al.* (2005). Mutation in the neuronal voltage-gated sodium channel SCN1A in familial hemiplegic migraine. *Lancet* **366**: 371–377.

Eikermann-Haerter, K., Baum, M.J., Ferrari, M.D., van den Maagdenberg, A.M., Moskowitz, M.A., and Ayata, C. (2009a). Androgenic suppression of spreading depression in familial hemiplegic migraine type 1 mutant mice. *Annals of Neurology* **66**: 564–568.

Eikermann-Haerter, K., Dilekoz, E., Kudo, C., Savitz, S.I., Waeber, C., Baum, M.J., *et al.* (2009b). Genetic and hormonal factors modulate spreading depression and transient hemiparesis in mouse models of familial hemiplegic migraine type 1. *Journal of Clinical Investigation* **119**: 99–109.

Eikermann-Haerter, K., Yuzawa, I., Qin, T., Wang, Y., Baek, K., Kim, Y.R., *et al.* (2011). Enhanced subcortical spreading depression in familial hemiplegic migraine type 1 mutant mice. *Journal of Neuroscience* **31**: 5755–5763.

Eikermann-Haerter, K., Arbel-Ornath, M., Yalcin, N., Yu, E.S., Kuchibhotla, K.V., Yuzawa, I., *et al*. (2015). Abnormal synaptic Ca^{2+} homeostasis and morphology in cortical neurons of familial hemiplegic migraine type 1 mutant mice. *Annals of Neurology* **78**: 193–210.

Ferrari, M.D., Klever, R.R., Terwindt, G.M., Ayata, C., and van den Maagdenberg, A.M.J.M. (2015). Migraine pathophysiology: lessons from mouse models and human genetics. *The Lancet Neurologyogy* **14**: 65–80.

Fioretti, B., Catacuzzeno, L., Sforna, L., Gerke-Duncan, M.B., van den Maagdenberg, A.M., Franciolini, F., *et al*. (2011). Trigeminal ganglion neuron subtype-specific alterations of Ca(V)2.1 calcium current and excitability in a Cacna1a mouse model of migraine. *Journal of Physiology* **589**: 5879–5895.

Gao, Z., Todorov, B., Barrett, C.F., van Dorp, S., Ferrari, M.D., van den Maagdenberg, A.M., *et al*. (2012). Cerebellar ataxia by enhanced Ca(V)2.1 currents is alleviated by Ca^{2+}-dependent K^{+}-channel activators in Cacna1a(S218L) mutant mice. *Journal of Neuroscience* **32**: 15533–15546.

Illarionava, N.B., Brismar, H., Aperia, A., and Gunnarson, E. (2014). Role of Na,K-ATPase α1 and α2 Isoforms in the Support of Astrocyte Glutamate Uptake. *PLoS One* **9**: e98469.

Inchauspe, C.G., Urbano, F.J., Di Guilmi, M.N., Forsythe, I.D., Ferrari, M.D., van den Maagdenberg, A.M., *et al*. (2010). Gain of function in FHM-1 Ca(V)2.1 knock-in mice is related to the shape of the action potential. *Journal of Neurophysiology* **104**: 291–299.

Inchauspe, C.G., Urbano, F.J., Di Guilmi, M.N., Ferrari, M.D., van den Maagdenberg, A.M., Forsythe, I.D., *et al*. (2012). Presynaptic CaV2.1 calcium channels carrying familial hemiplegic migraine mutation R192Q allow faster recovery from synaptic depression in mouse calyx of Held. *Journal of Neurophysiology* **108**: 2967–2976.

Kahlig, K.M., Rhodes, T.H., Pusch, M., Freilinger, T., Pereira-Monteiro, J.M., Ferrari, M.D., *et al*. (2008). Divergent sodium channel defects in familial hemiplegic migraine. *Proceedings of the National Academy of Sciences of the United States of America* **105**: 9799–9804.

Karatas, H., Erdener, S.E., Gursoy-Ozdemir, Y., Lule, S., Eren-Kocak, E., Sen, Z.D., *et al*. (2013). Spreading depression triggers headache by activating neuronal Panx1 channels. *Science* **339**: 1092–1095.

Kors, E.E., Terwindt, G.M., Vermeulen, F.L., Fitzsimons, R.B., Jardine, P.E., Heywood, P., *et al*. (2001). Delayed cerebral edema and fatal coma after minor head trauma: role of the CACNA1A calcium channel subunit gene and relationship with familial hemiplegic migraine. *Annals of Neurology* **49**: 753–760.

Larsen, B.R., Assentoft, M., Cotrina, M.L., Hua, S.Z., Nedergaard, M., Kaila, K., *et al*. (2014). Contributions of the Na^{+}/K^{+}-ATPase, NKCC1, and Kir4.1 to hippocampal K^{+} clearance and volume responses. *Glia* **62**: 608–622.

Lauritzen, M. (1994). Pathophysiology of the migraine aura. The spreading depression theory. *Brain* **117**(Pt 1), 199–210.

Leo, L., Gherardini, L., Barone, V., De Fusco, M., Pietrobon, D., Pizzorusso, T., *et al*. (2011). Increased susceptibility to cortical spreading depression in the mouse model of familial hemiplegic migraine type 2. *PLoS Genetics* **7**: e1002129.

Melliti, K., Grabner, M., and Seabrook, G.R. (2003). The familial hemiplegic migraine mutation R192Q reduces G-protein-mediated inhibition of P/Q-type (Ca(V)2.1) calcium channels expressed in human embryonic kidney cells. *Journal of Physiology* **546**: 337–347.

Mullner, C., Broos, L.A., van den Maagdenberg, A.M., and Striessnig, J. (2004). Familial Hemiplegic Migraine Type 1 Mutations K1336E, W1684R, and V1696I Alter Cav2.1 Ca^{2+} Channel Gating: evidence for beta-subunit isoform-specific effects. *Journal of Biological Chemistry* **279**: 51844–51850.

Noseda, R., and Burstein, R. (2013). Migraine pathophysiology: anatomy of the trigeminovascular pathway and associated neurological symptoms, cortical spreading depression, sensitization, and modulation of pain. *Pain* **154**(Suppl 1): S44–53.

Ogiwara, I., Miyamoto, H., Morita, N., Atapour, N., Mazaki, E., Inoue, I., *et al.* (2007). Nav1.1 Localizes to Axons of Parvalbumin-Positive Inhibitory Interneurons: A Circuit Basis for Epileptic Seizures in Mice Carrying an Scn1a Gene Mutation. *The Journal of Neuroscience* **27**: 5903–5914.

Ophoff, R.A., Terwindt, G.M., Vergouwe, M.N., van Eijk, R., Oefner, P.J., Hoffman, S.M.G., *et al.* (1996). Familial hemiplegic migraine and episodic ataxia type-2 are caused by mutations in the Ca^{2+} channel gene CACNL1A4. *Cell* **87**: 543–552.

Pellerin, L., and Magistretti, P.J. (1997). Glutamate uptake stimulates Na^+,K^+-ATPase activity in astrocytes via activation of a distinct subunit highly sensitive to ouabain. *Journal of Neurochemistry* **69**: 2132–2137.

Pietrobon, D. (2007). Familial hemiplegic migraine. *Neurotherapeutics* **4**: 274–284.

Pietrobon, D. (2010). CaV2.1 channelopathies. *Pflügers Archiv* **460**: 375–393.

Pietrobon, D. (2013). Calcium channels and migraine. *Biochimica et Biophysica Acta* **1828**: 1655–1665.

Pietrobon, D., and Moskowitz, M.A. (2013). Pathophysiology of migraine. *Annual Review of Physiology* **75**: 365–391.

Pietrobon, D., and Moskowitz, M.A. (2014). Chaos and commotion in the wake of cortical spreading depression and spreading depolarizations. *Nature Reviews Neuroscience* **15**: 379–393.

Ransom, C.B., Ransom, B.R., and Sontheimer, H. (2000). Activity-dependent extracellular K^+ accumulation in rat optic nerve: the role of glial and axonal Na^+ pumps. *Journal of Physiology* **522** Pt 3: 427–442.

Rose, E.M., Koo, J.C., Antflick, J.E., Ahmed, S.M., Angers, S., and Hampson, D.R. (2009). Glutamate transporter coupling to Na,K-ATPase. *Journal of Neuroscience* **29**: 8143–8155.

Rossignol, E., Kruglikov, I., van den Maagdenberg, A.M.J.M., Rudy, B., and Fishell, G. (2013). CaV2.1 ablation in cortical interneurons selectively impairs fast-spiking basket cells and causes generalized seizures. *Annals of Neurology* **74**: 209–222.

Russell, M.B., and Ducros, A. (2011). Sporadic and familial hemiplegic migraine: pathophysiological mechanisms, clinical characteristics, diagnosis, and management. *Lancet Neurology* **10**: 457–470.

Serra, S.A., Fernandez-Castillo, N., Macaya, A., Cormand, B., Valverde, M.A., and Fernandez-Fernandez, J.M. (2009). The hemiplegic migraine-associated Y1245C mutation in CACNA1A results in a gain of channel function due to its effect on the voltage sensor and G-protein-mediated inhibition. *Pflügers Archiv* **458**: 489–502.

Shyti, R., Eikermann-Haerter, K., van Heiningen, S.H., Meijer, O.C., Ayata, C., Joëls, M., *et al.* (2015). Stress hormone corticosterone enhances susceptibility to cortical spreading depression in familial hemiplegic migraine type 1 mutant mice. *Experimental Neurology* **263**: 214–220.

Somjen, G.G. (2001). Mechanisms of spreading depression and hypoxic spreading depression-like depolarization. *Physiological Reviews* **81**: 1065–1096.

Somjen, G.G., Kager, H., and Wadman, W.J. (2009). Calcium sensitive non-selective cation current promotes seizure-like discharges and spreading depression in a model neuron. *Journal of Computational Neuroscience* 26: 139–147.

Thomsen, L.L., Kirchmann, M., Bjornsson, A., Stefansson, H., Jensen, R.M., Fasquel, A.C., *et al.* (2007). The genetic spectrum of a population-based sample of familial hemiplegic migraine. *Brain* 130: 346–356.

Tottene, A., Fellin, T., Pagnutti, S., Luvisetto, S., Striessnig, J., Fletcher, C., *et al.* (2002). Familial hemiplegic migraine mutations increase Ca($2+$) influx through single human CaV2.1 channels and decrease maximal CaV2.1 current density in neurons. *Proceedings of the National Academy of Sciences of the United States of America* 99: 13284–13289.

Tottene, A., Pivotto, F., Fellin, T., Cesetti, T., van den Maagdenberg, A.M., and Pietrobon, D. (2005). Specific kinetic alterations of human CaV2.1 calcium channels produced by mutation S218L causing familial hemiplegic migraine and delayed cerebral edema and coma after minor head trauma. *Journal of Biological Chemistry* 280: 17678–17686.

Tottene, A., Conti, R., Fabbro, A., Vecchia, D., Shapovalova, M., Santello, M., *et al.* (2009). Enhanced Excitatory Transmission at Cortical Synapses as the Basis for Facilitated Spreading Depression in Ca(v)2.1 Knockin Migraine Mice. *Neuron* 61: 762–773.

Tottene, A., Urbani, A., and Pietrobon, D. (2011). Role of different voltage-gated Ca^{2+} channels in cortical spreading depression: specific requirement of P/Q-type Ca^{2+} channels. *Channels (Austin)* 5: 110–114.

Vahedi, K., Depienne, C., Le Fort, D., Riant, F., Chaine, P., Trouillard, O., *et al.* (2009). Elicited repetitive daily blindness: a new phenotype associated with hemiplegic migraine and SCN1A mutations. *Neurology* 72: 1178–1183.

van den Maagdenberg, A.M., Pietrobon, D., Pizzorusso, T., Kaja, S., Broos, L.A., Cesetti, T., *et al.* (2004). A Cacna1a knockin migraine mouse model with increased susceptibility to cortical spreading depression. *Neuron* 41: 701–710.

van den Maagdenberg, A.M., Pizzorusso, T., Kaja, S., Terpolilli, N., Shapovalova, M., Hoebeek, F.E., *et al.* (2010). High cortical spreading depression susceptibility and migraine-associated symptoms in Ca(v)2.1 S218L mice. *Annals of Neurology* 67: 85–98.

Vecchia, D., and Pietrobon, D. (2012). Migraine: a disorder of brain excitatory-inhibitory balance? *Trends in Neurosciences* 35: 507–520.

Vecchia, D., Tottene, A., van den Maagdenberg, A.M.J.M., and Pietrobon, D. (2014). Mechanism underlying unaltered cortical inhibitory synaptic transmission in contrast with enhanced excitatory transmission in CaV2.1 knockin migraine mice. *Neurobiology of Disease* 69: 225–234.

Vecchia, D., Tottene, A., van den Maagdenberg, A.M.J.M., and Pietrobon, D. (2015). Abnormal cortical synaptic transmission in CaV2.1 knockin mice with the S218L missense mutation which causes a severe familial hemiplegic migraine syndrome in humans. *Frontiers in Cellular Neuroscience* 9. https://doi.org/10.3389/fncel.2015.00008

Weiss, N., Sandoval, A., Felix, R., Van den Maagdenberg, A., and De Waard, M. (2008). The S218L familial hemiplegic migraine mutation promotes deinhibition of Ca(v)2.1 calcium channels during direct G-protein regulation. *Pflügers Archiv* 457: 315–326.

Yu, F.H., Mantegazza, M., Westenbroek, R.E., Robbins, C.A., Kalume, F., Burton, K.A., *et al.* (2006). Reduced sodium current in GABAergic interneurons in a mouse model of severe myoclonic epilepsy in infancy. *Nature Neuroscience* 9: 1142–1149.

Zhang, X., Levy, D., Noseda, R., Kainz, V., Jakubowski, M., and Burstein, R. (2010). Activation of meningeal nociceptors by cortical spreading depression: implications for migraine with aura. *Journal of Neuroscience* **30**: 8807–8814.

Zhang, X., Levy, D., Kainz, V., Noseda, R., Jakubowski, M., and Burstein, R. (2011). Activation of central trigeminovascular neurons by cortical spreading depression. *Annals of Neurology* **69**: 855–865.

Zhao, J., and Levy, D. (2015). Modulation of intracranial meningeal nociceptor activity by cortical spreading depression: a reassessment. *Journal of Neurophysiology* **113**(7): 2778–2785.

16

From cortical spreading depression to trigeminovascular activation in migraine

Turgay Dalkara[1] and Michael A. Moskowitz[2]

[1] Department of Neurology, Faculty of Medicine and Institute of Neurological Sciences and Psychiatry Hacettepe University, Ankara, Turkey
[2] Departments of Radiology and Neurology, Massachusetts General Hospital, Harvard Medical School, Boston, Massachusetts, USA

16.1 CSD causes the visual aura

Spreading depression (SD) is a transient wave of collective depolarization of neurons and glia which, once initiated, propagates across the gray matter of brain at rate of 2–6 mm/min (Somjen, 2001; Pietrobon and Moskowitz, 2014). This wave is associated with a transient depression of ongoing local electrical activity (e.g., EEG), and with cerebral blood flow (CBF) changes characterized by hyperemia, during the wave and long-lasting oligemia afterwards (Leao, 1944a, 1944b; Lauritzen *et al.*, 1982; and see Chapters 15 and 19).

Lashley, by carefully drawing the progress of his own visual aura, calculated that the physiological correlate must propagate with a speed of 3 mm/min in his own occipital cortex (Lashley, 1941). A few years later, Leao proposed that SD that he discovered in the rabbit cortex might be the cause of slowly propagating visual aura in migraine (Leao and Morrison, 1945). Much later, Milner pointed to the similarity between Lashley's observations and Leao's discovery, in a short communication published in 1958 (Milner, 1958). Unlike experimental animals, DC potential changes and spreading depression of the EEG activity between adjacent channels caused by SD are difficult to detect in humans by scalp recordings. Hence, the hypothesis was met with skepticism, especially on the grounds that human cortex had a much higher threshold for SD induction, compared with the rodent and canine brains commonly used in laboratory studies (Gloor, 1986).

The first convincing evidence in favor of a role of SD in migraine aura came about 40 years later, from SPECT studies registering CBF during induced migraine attacks (Olesen *et al.*, 1981). A wave of oligemia was observed to spread from the occipital lobe to anterior regions of the human brain. This observation was later supported by a PET blood flow study (Woods *et al.*, 1994) and perfusion MR studies (Cutrer *et al.*, 1998; Sanchez del Rio *et al.*, 1999), showing the presence of oligemia within the occipital lobe concordant with the side of visual symptoms, as well as by recording of the magnetic field induced by focal DC potential shifts propagating across the cortex with magnetoencephalography (Bowyer *et al.*, 2001).

Neurobiological Basis of Migraine, First Edition. Edited by Turgay Dalkara and Michael A. Moskowitz.
© 2017 John Wiley & Sons, Inc. Published 2017 by John Wiley & Sons, Inc.

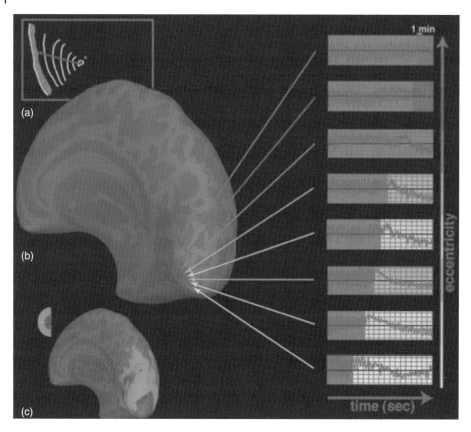

Figure 16.1 Spreading suppression of cortical activation during migraine aura. (a) A drawing showing the progression over 20 minutes of the scintillations and the visual field defect affecting the left hemifield, as described by the patient. The fixation point appears as a small white cross. Shows the overall direction of progression of the visual percept. The front of the scintillation at different times within the aura is indicated by a white line. (b) A reconstruction of the same patient's brain, based on anatomical MR data. The posterior medial aspect of occipital lobe is shown in an inflated cortex format. In this format, the cortical sulci and gyri appear in darker and lighter gray, respectively, on a computationally inflated surface. MR signal changes over time are shown to the right. (c) The MR maps of retinotopic eccentricity from this same subject, acquired during interictal scans. As shown in the logo in the upper left, voxels that show retinotopically specific activation in the fovea are coded dark grey (centered at 1.5° eccentricity). Parafoveal eccentricities are shown, and more peripheral eccentricities are shown in light gray (centered at 3.8° and 10.3°, respectively). The figure and legend were reproduced from Hadjikani *et al.*, (2001). *Proceedings of the National Academy of Sciences of the USA* **98**: 4687–92, with permission.

Compelling evidence was provided by blood oxygenation level-dependent (BOLD) MR, showing characteristics of SD in synchrony with onset and progress of the retinal aura percept that was recorded by the patient while inside the magnet (Hadjikani *et al.*, 2001) (Figure 16.1). MR of this patient suffering a visual aura demonstrated an initial focal increase in BOLD signal within extrastriate cortex, possibly reflecting the SD-induced vasodilation. This BOLD change progressed with a speed of 3.5 ± 1.1 mm/min through the occipital cortex, in close correspondence to the retinotopic march of the visual percept. The BOLD signal then decreased, possibly due to the oligemia following the initial vasodilation.

Not only the baseline BOLD signal but also phasic BOLD increases in response to flickering visual stimuli (checkerboard image) were suppressed during the oligemic phase, possibly due to ongoing cortical SD (CSD)-induced microcirculatory dysfunction (Ostergaard *et al.*, 2015). Like SD, this spreading phenomenon did not cross the prominent sulci, and stopped at the parieto-occipital sulcus. Interestingly, the time course of CBF changes associated with CSDs in the rat and with the migraine aura was strikingly similar, strongly suggesting an association between the two phenomena. Hence, the best current approach to study CSD in humans appears to record the SD-associated CBF changes, given that other techniques, such as magnetoencephalography, have limitations (for example, when detecting deep and penetrating occipital cortical activity (Lauritzen *et al.*, 2011)).

A good correlation reportedly exists between the surface and epidural recordings obtained from surgically-operated patients suffering from recurrent spreading depolarization waves due to vascular or trauma induced brain injury (Drenckhahn *et al.*, 2012; Hartings *et al.*, 2014). However, movement and environmental artifacts frequently complicate detection of surface EEG or DC potential changes. An indirect but highly supportive line of evidence invoking CSD (as the biological substrate of migraine aura) comes from results in transgenic animals. Mutated mice that express human FHM mutations in *CACNA1A* and *ATP1A2* genes exhibit low CSD induction thresholds (Eikermann-Haerter *et al.*, 2009; Leo *et al.*, 2011; and see Chapters 14 and 15). Interestingly, as in FHM patients, the CSD threshold is even lower in females than in males, and in mice bearing the S218L mutation that leads to a more severe clinical phenotype (Eikermann-Haerter *et al.*, 2009).

16.2 SD may underlie transient neurological dysfunctions preceding attacks

SD can be evoked in almost all gray matter regions of the central nervous system in experimental animals. The CA1 sector of the hippocampal formation, followed by the neocortex has the lowest SD induction threshold (Somjen, 2001). Although there is substantial evidence about the putative role of occipital SDs in migraine visual aura, the role of SD in other regions of the human brain remains largely speculative. SDs originating from, or propagating to, other parts of the cortex may underlie unilateral paresthesias over the lips, face or hand, as well as difficulty in finding words (Vincent and Hadjikhani, 2007; and see Chapters 11 and 17). It is also likely that hippocampal SDs might account for transient amnesia preceding headache attacks (Paolino and Levy, 1971; Calandre *et al.*, 2002; Vincent and Hadjikhani, 2007).

Subcortical spread of SD might account for hypothalamic and other limbic symptoms (e.g., food cravings or mood changes) seen just before the headache (Krivanek and Fifkova, 1965; Huston and Bures, 1970; Eikermann-Haerter *et al.*, 2011). Studies in rodents show that propagation of SD to subcortical brain regions is better observed with anesthetics that do not profoundly suppress neuronal excitability, suggesting that the subcortical spread might be a prevalent phenomenon in unanesthetized human brain

(Eikermann-Haerter *et al.*, 2011). Further research is needed to investigate these interesting possibilities in migraine patients.

Another area requiring study is the potential differences between CSD associated with migraine aura and CSD induced in experimental animals (Dahlem *et al.*, 2015). For example, SD induction and propagation should be impacted by the presence of a highly convoluted human cortex with prominent gyri and deep sulci, and a high astrocyte-to-neuron ratio. As noted above, it is generally accepted that the human brain is relatively more resistant to CSD induction, whereas the propagation speed seems to be unaltered, as inferred from spread of CBF changes across the cortex in imaging studies, and from estimates of propagation speed of the visual percept (Hadjikhani *et al.*, 2001; Somjen, 2001).

Recent studies on the convoluted swine brain have demonstrated that the SD propagation could assume several irregular forms other than the radial spread, including the reverberating SDs, which re-enter to the gyrus of origin by circulating around a sulcus (Santos *et al.*, 2014). However, their presence and significance (e.g., in prolonged aura) in migraine remains to be determined. Relatively mild neurological dysfunctions observed during aura also requires a better understanding, and suggest that CSDs in humans might involve only part of the cortical layers and/or spread in a narrow gyral path, rather than engulfing a whole lobe (Richter and Lehmenkuhler, 1993; Dahlem *et al.*, 2015).

16.3   Does SD cause headache?

SD was first posited as a trigger for migraine headache on the basis of clinical and experimental observations (Moskowitz, 1984). For example, the visual aura (experienced as a contralateral visual hallucination) and hemi-cranial pain (experienced most often ipsilateral to the dysfunctional hemisphere, and a source for ipsilateral trigeminovascular activation) suggests that the occipital perturbation underlying the aura could also cause headache (Olesen *et al.*, 1990). The first experimental support for this long-known relationship between aura and headache was provided by detection of c-fos immunostaining (an indirect but histologically detectable marker of intense neuronal activation) in the trigeminal nucleus caudalis after CSD (Moskowitz *et al.*, 1993; Figure 16.2g). Later, hippocampal SDs were also shown to cause c-fos expression in trigeminal nucleus caudalis (Kunkler and Kraig, 2003). Demonstration of the dilation of MMA and dural mast cell degranulation ipsilateral to CSD provided further support for activation of the trigeminovascular system by CSD (Bolay *et al.*, 2002; Karatas *et al.*, 2013; Figure 16.2a-f).

Direct evidence was obtained by electrophysiological recording of discharging nociceptive neurons following CSD in the trigeminal ganglion (first order neuron) and spinal trigeminal nucleus (second order neuron) (Zhang *et al.*, 2010, 2011; Zhao and Levy, 2015; and see Figures in Chapter 7). Consistent with these findings, ultra-high resolution PET imaging reportedly showed increased 2-deoxyglucose uptake in brain regions associated with processing and transmitting nociceptive input many hours after evoking CSD (Cui *et al.*, 2015).

CSDs have also been shown to induce pain-like behavior, as assessed by grimace scale in the mouse (Langford *et al.*, 2010; Karatas *et al.*, 2013; Figure 16.2h, i). This behavioral model has been an important step in demonstrating the algesic potential of the CSD in unanesthetized animals, contrary to the previous reports, which concluded that the

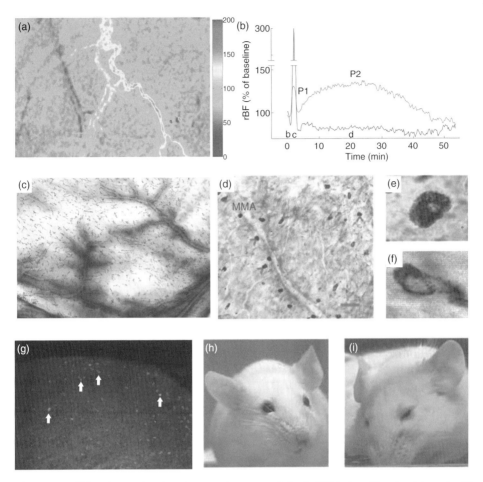

Figure 16.2 CSD activates the trigeminovascular system. A single CSD induced by pinprick can lead to dilatation of the middle meningeal artery (MMA). (a) Laser speckle images of the cortex illustrate the blood flow changes in cortical blood vessels and MMA in a rat under anesthesia. Bright tones show an increase in blood flow compared with baseline. Twenty minutes after induction of a single CSD with a pinprick, the cortex is hypoperfused (darker tone), whereas blood flow in the MMA is increased (bright tone). (b) The MMA flow increase (upper line) peaks around 15–20 min after CSD and lasts about one hour, during which the cortical blood (lower line) remains oligemic. (c) Plasma protein extravasation: leakage of IV-administered HRP in a rat whole-mount dura preparation illustrates plasma protein extravasation from dural vessels after CSD. (d–f) Mast cell degranulation: incubation of dura with methylene blue reveals mast cells (arrowheads) along the course of MMA in a mouse; scale bar = 100 μm (d). Degranulated mast cells (f) can easily be distinguished from resting cells (e) with loss of cytoplasmic granules. (g) c-fos immunoreactivity appears in the trigeminal nucleus caudalis one hour after KCl-induced CSDs. The majority of the labeled cells (arrows) are located in the superficial layers (laminae I and II). (h, i) Pain-related behavior: (h) normal mouse facial appearance; (i) facial expression of a mouse suffering from pain. a, b, c were reproduced from Bolay *et al.* (2002); d, e, f, from Karatas *et al.* (2013); h, i, from Langford *et al.* (2010) and a-i from Erdener and Dalkara (2014), with permission.

CSD might not cause aversive behavior, based on observation of the relatively indirect pain-related behaviors in rodents (Koroleva and Bures, 1993).

The mouse and rat grimace scales demonstrated that rodents surprisingly, have facial expressions displaying their discomfort during pain (Langford *et al.*, 2010; Sotocinal *et al.*, 2011). The model was first developed by monitoring the severe pain induced by intraperitoneal acetic acid administration, and then it was shown to be sensitive enough to detect the CSD-induced headache and its reversal by rizatriptan (Langford *et al.*, 2010). The scoring of CSD-induced facial expressions seems to have the potential to screen analgesic as well as anti-migraine medications such as triptans.

Interestingly, dilatation of the MMA, firing of the first and second order trigeminal neurons and the distressful facial expressions emerged about 15–20 minutes after CSD, in line with the typical time lag between the migraine aura and headache, further supporting the view of a causal relationship between the CSD and headache (Bolay *et al.*, 2002; Zhang *et al.*, 2010, 2011; Karatas *et al.*, 2013; Zhao and Levy, 2015).

This time lag between the aura and headache also provides some clues about the mechanisms of CSD-induced migraine headache. The transient (a few minutes) elevation of potassium, protons, NO, ATP and arachidonic acid in the extracellular environment during CSD can activate the perivascular nociceptive nerves by diffusing to the CSF, as suggested by very brief discharges observed in some nociceptors during CSD before the appearance of delayed persistent activation (Zhang *et al.*, 2010; Zhao and Levy, 2015). However, such activation is expected to lead to a transient headache during the aura, not 15–20 minutes later. This brief elevation may contribute to the headache seen simultaneously with the beginning of aura (Russell and Olesen, 1996; Hansen *et al.*, 2012), and participate in sensitizing trigeminovascular afferents to subsequent more intense and sustained stimulation (Bernstein and Burstein, 2012).

Unfortunately, clinical studies investigating the relationship between the aura and headache onset did not consider changes in the intensity and characteristics of the headache, which are known to vary over time (see Chapter 11). Indeed, electrophysiological recordings in the rat show that C-fiber activation emerges with a longer latency than A∂-fiber activation after CSD (Zhao and Levy, 2015), and mechanosensitivity appears after development of nociceptor sensitization (Bernstein and Burstein, 2012), which better conforms with the progress of headache characteristics after the aura, rather than its presence or absence.

CSD propagating down to subcortical regions might also directly modulate ascending inputs from the second or third order nociceptive neurons (Noseda *et al.*, 2010), but this would not be limited to inputs from trigeminal nociceptive fibers. Direct electrophysiological recordings from the rat brain stem trigeminocervical complex neurons showed that CSD could modulate meningeal nociceptive activity by inhibiting or enhancing their firing, depending on the cortical origin of the descending projections (e.g., occipital V1, sensory S1, S2 or insula) (Noseda *et al.*, 2010; see Chapter 4).

Recently, CSD induced either by a single pinprick or epidural KCl application was found to initiate a parenchymal inflammatory signaling cascade, triggering the release of inflammatory mediators into the subarachnoid space, and stimulating the perivascular trigeminal nociceptors (Karatas *et al.*, 2013; Figure 16.3).

Activation of the trigeminovascular system (monitored by the MMA dilatation) peaked about 15–20 minutes after CSD, and was blocked by inhibiting the cascade at several steps with pharmacological or molecular means. The signaling cascade began

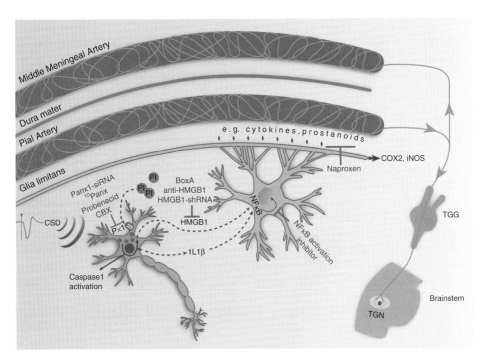

Figure 16.3 Stressed neurons may induce headache by activating the trigeminovascular system via a complex parenchymal signaling cascade. The schema illustrates the cascade of events that take place within 30 minutes after CSD induction. CSD leads to transient opening of pannexin1 (Panx1) channels on neurons, as evidenced by propidium iodide (PI) influx (circles), with subsequent activation of caspase-1 and release of pro-inflammatory mediators (e.g., HMGB1, IL-1β). This causes NF-κB translocation to nucleus, and induces COX2 and iNOS expression in astrocytes. Cytokines, prostanoids and NO are then continuously released to subarachnoid space, via astrocytes forming the glia limitans and, hence, promote sustained activation of the trigeminal nerve fibers around pial vessels. Trigeminal fiber collaterals innervating the middle meningeal artery initiate a sterile dural inflammation, accompanied by mast cell degranulation, whereas the trigeminoparasympathetic reflex causes the late and sustained MMA dilation. T-bars indicate the steps where the cascade was interrupted with inhibitors. It is likely that, over the course of the inflammation, several other cytokines as well as microglia are activated, and the cells illustrated above may assume other roles (for example, NF-κB may also be activated in neurons). The figure and legend were reproduced from supplementary Figure S6 (Karatas *et al.*, 2013). Reproduced with the permission of The American Association for the Advancement of Science.

with opening of the neuronally expressed pannexin-1 large-pore channels, which led to caspase-1 activation, possibly by formation of the inflammasome complex and release of IL-1β and high mobility group box-1 protein (HMGB1) (see also Eising *et al.* (2016) and Takizawa *et al.* (2016)). These pro-inflammatory mediators then activate the NF-κB pathway in astrocytes, which induces expression of the inflammatory enzymes and causes release of their products to the subarachnoid space by way of glia limitans (Figure 16.3).

These findings are in line with numerous independent *in vivo* rat studies, showing robust increases in expression of TNF-alpha, NF-κB, Cox-2 and several interleukins, including IL-1β, in the cortex within hours following KCl-induced repeated CSDs (Caggiano *et al.*, 1996; Jander *et al.*, 2001; Yokota *et al.*, 2003; Horiguchi *et al.*, 2005;

Thompson and Hakim, 2005; Viggiano *et al.*, 2008; Ghaemi *et al.*, 2016). Pannexin-1 channels have been proposed to open at high concentrations of extracellular potassium and glutamate, and of intracellular calcium, as well as by cellular swelling, low pO_2 and activation of P2X7 channels with extracellular ATP (Ma *et al.*, 2009; Chiu *et al.*, 2014; Jackson *et al.*, 2014).

However, there are still controversies about the generalizability of each of these factors detected under specific *in vitro* conditions to neurons *in situ*. Under resting conditions, the opening probability of pannexin-1 channels is low (or opens in a low conductance state), possibly because their unusually large conductance, if opened, may jeopardize the physiological transmembrane ion gradients. Therefore, their activation by the above non-resting physiological conditions (all of which are present during CSD) and their close association with inflammasome formation may serve to detect neuronal stress and then alarm, by activating the parenchymal inflammatory cascade. Unlike the brief release of vasoactive mediators to extracellular space coincident with CSD, the above-summarized inflammatory signaling is more compatible with the appearance and development of sustained headache 15–60 min after the aura.

16.4 Human data supporting the parenchymal inflammatory signaling

Supporting a role for parenchymal inflammatory signaling in migraine headache, the levels of IL-1β, IL-6, TNF-alpha, PGE2 and nitrite in internal jugular blood were reportedly elevated within the first hour of migraine attack (Sarchielli *et al.*, 2000, 2004, 2006). The increase was maximal at the first-hour blood sampling point, and then declined. Since the internal jugular vein in humans drains mainly the brain parenchyma (unlike the internal jugular vein in the rat, which is a rather thin vessel compared to the external jugular vein, which mainly provides the cerebral venous drainage (Szabo, 1995)), these observations suggest production of cytokines in brain parenchyma during a migraine attack as the above outlined hypothesis proposed (Karatas *et al.*, 2013).

It should be noted that the patients in the above reports were studied in the absence of typical visual auras during migraine without aura (MO) attacks, but they clearly document a parenchymal source of cytokines coincident with the beginning of migraine headache. Activation of the parenchymal inflammatory signaling during MO headache suggests that migraine with aura (MA) and MO may use a common signaling pathway to induce headache, even if the initiating mechanisms exhibit dissimilarities (Purdy, 2008). These are not surprising, as both migraine subtypes share very similar headache features, and are treated with the same drugs, including NSAIDs. By contrast, cytokine measurements in peripheral blood during migraine attacks, despite several positive reports, have generally led to inconclusive results, possibly due to plasma volume dilution of relatively small absolute increases in cytokine levels, even in jugular blood, plus the timing of blood sampling (Durham and Papapetropoulos, 2013).

Migraine attacks are also a complaint of patients with cyropyrin-associated periodic syndrome (CAPS), in which IL-1β is overproduced due to mutations in NLRP3, a component protein of the inflammasome (Kitley *et al.*, 2010; Miyamae, 2012). These patients also experience rash, fever, malaise, arthralgia, myalgia, conjunctivitis and non-migrainous headache usually induced by cold. Anti-IL-1β treatment provides relief for headaches in CAPS (Kitley *et al*., 2010; Miyamae, 2012). However, caution is needed in interpreting these observations in favor of activation of the parenchymal pathway. This is because the headache may also be caused by overactivation of inflammasome in dural mast cells, as suggested by dysregulated IL-1β production in skin mast cells in neonatal mice with the CAPS-associated Nlrp3 mutation (Nakamura *et al*., 2012), or by aseptic meningitis seen in the most severe form of this disease (Kitley *et al*., 2010; Miyamae, 2012).

16.5 Meningeal neurogenic inflammation amplifies the parenchymal signal

Clinical observations suggest that some migraine headache attacks may be initiated directly from meninges; for example, on activation of mast cells in allergic diseases or direct activation of TRPA1 channels by umbellulone, a volatile oil from the "headache tree" (*U. californica*) (Monro *et al*., 1984; Nassini *et al*., 2012). Further supporting this view, headaches directly starting from meninges, such as during subarachnoid hemorrhage or meningitis, show several characteristic features of migraine headache, including its throbbing nature and photo/phonophobia, and sometimes they are alleviated by sumatriptan (Lamonte *et al*., 1995; Rosenberg and Silberstein, 2005).

Recent success obtained with antibodies modifying the CGRP pathway clearly demonstrate the important role of meningeal neurogenic inflammation mediated by CGRP in producing migraine headache, since these large macromolecules do not have significant CNS penetration and, hence, act mainly on peripheral targets (see Chapter 9). Prompt alleviation of migraine headache, as well as photo/phonophobia by sumatriptan that is also poorly BBB permeable, is in line with the anti-migraine effect of CGRP antibodies, and underscores the putative role of neurogenic inflammation in the headache phase of migraine (Moskowitz *et al*., 1979; Figure 16.4).

Experimental data have not only established the presence of large networks of neuropeptide-containing meningeal afferents in most vertebrates, including man (See Chapter 1), but calcium-dependent neuropeptide release from these meningeal fibers (Moskowitz *et al*., 1983), as well as evidence for modulation of neurogenic inflammation by ergot alkaloids (Saito *et al*., 1988), the triptans (Buzzi and Moskowitz, 1990), and non-steroidal anti-inflammatory drugs (Buzzi *et al*., 1989). Although, to date, these meningeal networks have received most attention for their role in migraine, in other tissues, neurogenic inflammation is part of an integrative protective response between the peripheral nervous system and the adaptive and innate immune systems, in response to tissue danger signals (Chiu *et al*., 2012).

The parenchymal and meningeal inflammatory signaling cascades seem to be tightly regulated, as they do not lead to overt inflammation characterized by infiltration of leukocytes. The rapid decline in the elevated level of inflammatory mediators in the internal jugular vein of migraine patients supports this idea (Sarchielli *et al*., 2006). It is likely that the algesic signals arise from the parenchymal inflammatory cascade, and are amplified by the meningeal neurogenic inflammation, which may sustain the activation of the nociceptors for development of the sensitization and a lasting headache (see Chapters 6 and 7). Microglia may also take part in the parenchymal inflammatory signaling, although present experimental evidence suggests that this is a relatively delayed

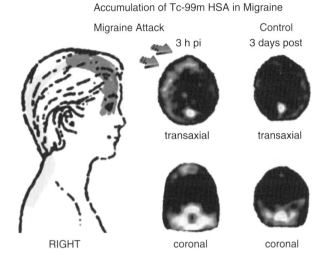

Accumulation of Tc-99m HSA in Migraine

Migraine Attack

3 h pi

transaxial

coronal

RIGHT

Control

3 days post

transaxial

coronal

Figure 16.4 Left: diagram used by the patient to mark the location of the headache epicenter. Right: accumulation of Tc-99m HSA in migraine attack three hours after the intravenous application of 10 mCi of Tc-99m human serum albumin, and three days after the attack (control). The region of increased uptake three hours after the injection corresponded to the diagram where the subject localized her migraine pain epicenter. pi = post-intravenous application. Reproduced from Knotkova and Pappagallo (2007), with permission.

event, perhaps contributing to the prolonged headache. For instance, it has been shown that microglia are activated 7–13 hours after repeated SDs in hippocampal slice cultures prepared from P8-10 rat pups (Grinberg *et al.*, 2011), as well as starting three days after repeated KCl-induced CSDs in the rat cortex *in vivo* (Cui *et al.*, 2009).

Aura attacks without headache suggest that parenchymal signaling initiated by a single CSD may not always be strong enough to activate the nociceptors innervating the meninges. Although there is direct experimental evidence showing activation of the trigeminovascular system with a single or multiple CSDs in rodents (Bolay *et al.*, 2002; Zhang *et al.*, 2010, 2011; Karatas *et al.*, 2013; Zhao and Levy, 2015), some experimental evidence, based on c-fos expression in the brain stem or on pain-related behaviors, suggests that a single CSD may also not always be noxious in rodents (Koroleva and Bures, 1993; Akcali *et al.*, 2010). This conforms with the idea that there may be a threshold to translate the parenchymal stress to neurogenic inflammation and lasting headache.

16.6   Understanding human CSD and migraine without aura

Migraine triggers in general do not reliably "trigger" migraine attacks and the attacks, for example, of visual aura, may not be accompanied by headache in a minority of patients (Aiba *et al.*, 2010; Hoffmann and Recober, 2013). Furthermore, there is a small group of patients who experience only aura without headache (Headache Classification Committee of the International Headache Society, 2013). This suggests that CSD-induced algesic signals have to reach a threshold intensity (concentration) to induce pain.

According to Dahlem's modeling, some CSDs may loose their wave front and spread within a narrow strip of cortex after the initial radial propagation (Dahlem, 2013). A reduced volume of depolarized tissue may, therefore, decrease its algesic potential by reducing the concentrations of cytokines reaching the subarachnoid space, although they may still cause a spreading sensory percept (see also Chapter 17). Moreover, some people may have a higher headache threshold for a number of reasons, as the presence of people who never suffer from headache suggests. For example, their parenchymal inflammatory response may not be strong enough to initiate the meningeal neurogenic inflammation, or the neurogenic inflammation may have a higher threshold. These thresholds may also be modulated by several factors (e.g. hormonal) (Levy, 2009; see Chapter 6). Not infrequently, migraineurs describe transient neurological dysfunctions other than visual aura, such as paresthesias, which are not always followed by headache (Russell and Olesen, 1996; Vincent and Hadjikhani, 2007; DeLange and Cutrer, 2014), and might represent these "subthreshold, non-painful" CSDs as restricted to a small strip of gray matter.

Experimental studies monitoring CSD with CBF changes over the whole surface of the cortex have disclosed that CBF changes do not always propagate radially along a predictable pathway, even in lissencephalic animals – a feature that was not well appreciated, with previous electrophysiological studies recording the CSD propagation with two electrodes (Brennan *et al.*, 2007). The recent observations on the gyrencephalic swine brain are interesting in this regard, and point to a necessity to understand the likely unique features of human CSD (Santos *et al.*, 2014). These approaches may also help explore the possibility that MO and MA share a comparable electrophysiological substrate, as suggested by the therapeutic success of a similar spectrum of migraine prophylactic drugs in both conditions.

The neuronal stress sensed by pannexin-1 large-pore channels, and conveyed by the inflammatory signaling to be reported as headache, may also be experienced during intense neuronal activity under suboptimal homeostatic conditions (e.g., caused by sleep deprivation), as has recently been demonstrated in the mouse by combining prolonged whisker stimulation with inhibition of glycogen use (Karatas *et al.*, 2015). In other words, this alarming pathway initiated during CSD could potentially be activated by other conditions that may trigger MO attacks.

Studies on FHM mutations suggest that increased potassium levels at the synaptic cleft during high-intensity neuronal firing could initiate CSD if the potassium concentration exceeds an estimated threshold of 12 mM (Lothman *et al.*, 1975; Heinemann and Lux, 1977; Pietrobon and Moskowitz, 2014; Tang *et al.*, 2014). Due to the limited extracellular space in the CNS, potassium ions may reach peri-synaptic concentrations sufficiently high to activate pannexin-1 channels during intense synaptic activity, especially in the presence of ATP release that stimulates P2X7 receptors (Jackson *et al.*, 2014). Unlike FHM mutations creating a potential to trigger collective depolarization of a large cohort of neurons (i.e., SD) (Vecchia and Pietrobon, 2012), the more restricted potassium rise around synapses of a smaller neuronal assembly during intense neuronal activity may lead to pannexin-1 activation without SD induction, hence, headache without aura.

The presence of several forms of transient neurological abnormalities preceding attacks of MO, such as the experience of seeing bright colors, or difficulty remembering proper names (Vincent and Hadjikhani, 2007; DeLange and Cutrer, 2014), suggests that an SD-like phenomenon, which causes a milder functional disturbance and does not propagate, may initiate an MO attack (Dahlem, 2013). A PET study, showing a propagating wave of oligemia without focal neurological symptoms (aura) but with headache in a MO patient, suggests that these SD-like phenomena can sometimes propagate without inducing overt neurological dysfunction (aura) (Woods *et al.*, 1994). We should also note that considering a high rate of transient amnesia reported by MO patients (Vincent and Hadjikhani, 2007), it is likely that hippocampal SDs may trigger headaches as well (Paolino and Levy, 1971; Calandre *et al.*, 2002; Kunkler and Kraig, 2003).

16.7 Potential of CSD models to understand migraine and drug development

Despite expected differences in CSDs generated within gyrencephalic and lissencephalic brains, experimental studies in small laboratory animals still hold promise as a tool to understand how a noxious brain event like CSD could cause transient neurological dysfunctions such as aura and headache in migraine patients. In fact, CSDs evoked in rats have been instrumental in exploring a common mechanism of migraine prophylactic drugs (Ayata *et al.*, 2006), and could more realistically model trigeminovascular activation than models using direct chemical or electrical stimulation (Erdener and Dalkara, 2014).

One major goal, then, is to develop genetically engineered mice in which CSDs spontaneously emerge, or can be evoked by minimally invasive triggers (e.g., such as after exposure to blue light) (Houben *et al.*, 2016). The use of such CSD models in awake animals, plus their evaluation by telemetric methods as well as recently developed behavioral tests assessing pain and allodynia, could open a new era in development of acute anti-migraine and prophylactic drugs (Chanda *et al.*, 2013; De Felice *et al.*, 2013; Romero-Reyes and Ye, 2013; Erdener and Dalkara, 2014).

References

Aiba, S., M. Tatsumoto, A. Saisu, H. Iwanami, K. Chiba, T. Senoo, and K. Hirata (2010). Prevalence of typical migraine aura without headache in Japanese ophthalmology clinics. *Cephalalgia* **30**(8): 962–7.

Akcali, D., A. Sayin, Y. Sara, and H. Bolay (2010). Does single cortical spreading depression elicit pain behaviour in freely moving rats? *Cephalalgia* **30**(10): 1195–206.

Ayata, C., H. Jin, C. Kudo, T. Dalkara, and M. A. Moskowitz (2006). Suppression of cortical spreading depression in migraine prophylaxis. *Annals of Neurology* **59**(4): 652–61.

Bernstein, C., and R. Burstein (2012). Sensitization of the trigeminovascular pathway: perspective and implications to migraine pathophysiology. *Journal of Clinical Neurology* **8**(2): 89–99.

Bolay, H., U. Reuter, A. K. Dunn, Z. Huang, D. A. Boas, and M. A. Moskowitz (2002). Intrinsic brain activity triggers trigeminal meningeal afferents in a migraine model. *Nature medicine* **8**(2): 136–42.

Bowyer, S. M., K. S. Aurora, J. E. Moran, N. Tepley, and K. M. Welch (2001). Magnetoencephalographic fields from patients with spontaneous and induced migraine aura. *Annals of Neurology* **50**(5): 582–7.

Brennan, K. C., L. Beltran-Parrazal, H. E. Lopez-Valdes, J. Theriot, A. W. Toga, and A. C. Charles (2007). Distinct vascular conduction with cortical spreading depression. *Journal of Neurophysiology* **97**(6): 4143–51.

Buzzi, M. G., and M. A. Moskowitz (1990). The antimigraine drug, sumatriptan (GR43175), selectively blocks neurogenic plasma extravasation from blood vessels in dura mater. *British Journal of Pharmacology* **99**(1): 202–6.

Buzzi, M. G., D. E. Sakas, and M. A. Moskowitz (1989). Indomethacin and acetylsalicylic acid block neurogenic plasma protein extravasation in rat dura mater. *European Journal of Pharmacology* **165**(2–3): 251–8.

Caggiano, A. O., C. D. Breder, and R. P. Kraig (1996). Long-term elevation of cyclooxygenase-2, but not lipoxygenase, in regions synaptically distant from spreading depression. *Journal of Comparative Neurology* **376**(3): 447–62.

Calandre, E. P., J. Bembibre, M. L. Arnedo, and D. Becerra (2002). Cognitive disturbances and regional cerebral blood flow abnormalities in migraine patients: their relationship with the clinical manifestations of the illness. *Cephalalgia* **22**(4): 291–302.

Chanda, M. L., A. H. Tuttle, I. Baran, C. Atlin, D. Guindi, G. Hathaway, N. Israelian, J. Levenstadt, D. Low, L. Macrae, L. O'Shea, A. Silver, E. Zendegui, A. Mariette Lenselink, S. Spijker, M. D. Ferrari, A. M. van den Maagdenberg, and J. S. Mogil (2013). Behavioral evidence for photophobia and stress-related ipsilateral head pain in transgenic Cacna1a mutant mice. *Pain* **154**(8): 1254–62.

Chiu, I. M., C. A. von Hehn, and C. J. Woolf (2012). Neurogenic inflammation and the peripheral nervous system in host defense and immunopathology. *Nature Neuroscience* **15**(8): 1063–7.

Chiu, Y. H., K. S. Ravichandran, and D. A. Bayliss (2014). Intrinsic properties and regulation of Pannexin 1 channel. *Channels (Austin)* **8**(2): 103–9.

Cui, Y., T. Takashima, M. Takashima-Hirano, Y. Wada, M. Shukuri, Y. Tamura, H. Doi, H. Onoe, Y. Kataoka, and Y. Watanabe (2009). 11C-PK11195 PET for the in vivo evaluation of neuroinflammation in the rat brain after cortical spreading depression. *Journal of Nuclear Medicine* **50**(11): 1904–11.

Cui, Y., H. Toyoda, T. Sako, K. Onoe, E. Hayashinaka, Y. Wada, C. Yokoyama, H. Onoe, Y. Kataoka, and Y. Watanabe (2015). A voxel-based analysis of brain activity in high-order trigeminal pathway in the rat induced by cortical spreading depression. *Neuroimage* **108**: 17–22.

Cutrer, F. M., A. G. Sorensen, R. M. Weisskoff, L. Ostergaard, M. Sanchez del Rio, E. J. Lee, B. R. Rosen, and M. A. Moskowitz (1998). Perfusion-weighted imaging defects during spontaneous migrainous aura. *Annals of Neurology* **43**(1): 25–31.

Dahlem, M. A. (2013). Migraine generator network and spreading depression dynamics as neuromodulation targets in episodic migraine. *Chaos* **23**(4): 046101.

Dahlem, M. A., B. Schmidt, I. Bojak, S. Boie, F. Kneer, N. Hadjikhani, and J. Kurths (2015). Cortical hot spots and labyrinths: why cortical neuromodulation for episodic migraine with aura should be personalized. *Frontiers in Computational Neuroscience* **9**: 29.

De Felice, M., N. Eyde, D. Dodick, G. O. Dussor, M. H. Ossipov, H. L. Fields, and F. Porreca (2013). Capturing the aversive state of cephalic pain preclinically. *Annals of Neurology* **74**(2): 257–65.

DeLange, J. M., and F. M. Cutrer (2014). Our evolving understanding of migraine with aura. *Current Pain and Headache Reports* **18**(10): 453.

Drenckhahn, C., M. K. Winkler, S. Major, M. Scheel, E. J. Kang, A. Pinczolits, C. Grozea, J. A. Hartings, J. Woitzik, J. P. Dreier, and Cosbid study group (2012). Correlates of spreading depolarization in human scalp electroencephalography. *Brain* **135**(Pt 3): 853–68.

Durham, P., and S. Papapetropoulos (2013). Biomarkers associated with migraine and their potential role in migraine management. *Headache* **53**(8): 1262–77.

Eikermann-Haerter, K., E. Dilekoz, C. Kudo, S. I. Savitz, C. Waeber, M. J. Baum, M. D. Ferrari, A. M. van den Maagdenberg, M. A. Moskowitz, and C. Ayata (2009). Genetic and hormonal factors modulate spreading depression and transient hemiparesis in mouse models of familial hemiplegic migraine type 1. *Journal of Clinical Investigation* **119**(1): 99–109.

Eikermann-Haerter, K., I. Yuzawa, T. Qin, Y. Wang, K. Baek, Y. R. Kim, U. Hoffmann, E. Dilekoz, C. Waeber, M. D. Ferrari, A. M. van den Maagdenberg, M. A. Moskowitz, and C. Ayata (2011). Enhanced subcortical spreading depression in familial hemiplegic migraine type 1 mutant mice. *Journal of Neuroscience* **31**(15): 5755–63.

Eising, E., R. Shyti, P. A. t Hoen, L. S. Vijfhuizen, S. M. Huisman, L. A. Broos, A. Mahfouz, M. J. Reinders, M. D. Ferrari, E. A. Tolner, B. de Vries, and A. M. van den Maagdenberg (2016). Cortical Spreading Depression Causes Unique Dysregulation of Inflammatory Pathways in a Transgenic Mouse Model of Migraine. *Molecular Neurobiology*. PMID: 27032388.

Erdener, S. E., and T. Dalkara (2014). Modelling headache and migraine and its pharmacological manipulation. *British Journal of Pharmacology* **171**(20): 4575–94.

Ghaemi, A., A. Sajadian, B. Khodaie, A. A. Lotfinia, M. Lotfinia, A. Aghabarari, M. Khaleghi Ghadiri, S. Meuth, and A. Gorji (2016). Immunomodulatory Effect of Toll-Like Receptor-3 Ligand Poly I: C on Cortical Spreading Depression. *Molecular Neurobiology* **53**(1): 143–54.

Gloor, P. (1986). Migraine and regional cerebral blood flow. *Trends in Neurosciences* **9**: 21.

Grinberg, Y. Y., J. G. Milton, and R. P. Kraig (2011). Spreading depression sends microglia on Levy flights. *PLoS One* **6**(4): e19294.

Hadjikhani, N., M. Sanchez Del Rio, O. Wu, D. Schwartz, D. Bakker, B. Fischl, K. K. Kwong, F. M. Cutrer, B. R. Rosen, R. B. Tootell, A. G. Sorensen, and M. A. Moskowitz (2001). Mechanisms of migraine aura revealed by functional MRI in human visual cortex. *Proceedings of the National Academy of Sciences of the United States of America* **98**(8): 4687–92.

Hansen, J. M., R. B. Lipton, D. W. Dodick, S. D. Silberstein, J. R. Saper, S. K. Aurora, P. J. Goadsby, and A. Charles (2012). Migraine headache is present in the aura phase: a prospective study. *Neurology* **79**(20): 2044–9.

Hartings, J. A., J. A. Wilson, J. M. Hinzman, S. Pollandt, J. P. Dreier, V. DiNapoli, D. M. Ficker, L. A. Shutter, and N. Andaluz (2014). Spreading depression in continuous electroencephalography of brain trauma. *Annals of Neurology* **76**(5): 681–94.

Headache Classification Committee of the International Headache Society (2013). The International Classification of Headache Disorders, 3rd edition (beta version). *Cephalalgia* **33**(9): 629–808.

Heinemann, U., and H. D. Lux (1977). Ceiling of stimulus induced rises in extracellular potassium concentration in the cerebral cortex of cat. *Brain Research* **120**(2): 231–49.

Hoffmann, J., and A. Recober (2013). Migraine and triggers: post hoc ergo propter hoc? *Current Pain and Headache Reports* **17**(10): 370.

Horiguchi, T., J. A. Snipes, B. Kis, K. Shimizu, and D. W. Busija (2005). The role of nitric oxide in the development of cortical spreading depression-induced tolerance to transient focal cerebral ischemia in rats. *Brain Research* **1039**(1–2): 84–9.

Houben, T., I. C. Loonen, S. M. Baca, M. Schenke, J. H. Meijer, M. D. Ferrari, G. M. Terwindt, R. A. Voskuyl, A. Charles, A. M. van den Maagdenberg, and E. A. Tolner (2016). Optogenetic induction of cortical spreading depression in anesthetized and freely behaving mice. *Journal of Cerebral Blood Flow & Metabolism*. PMID: 27107026.

Huston, J. P., and J. Bures (1970). Drinking and eating elicited by cortical spreading depression. *Science* **169**(3946): 702–4.

Jackson, D. G., J. Wang, R. W. Keane, E. Scemes, and G. Dahl (2014). ATP and potassium ions: a deadly combination for astrocytes. *Scientific Reports* **4**: 4576.

Jander, S., M. Schroeter, O. Peters, O. W. Witte, and G. Stoll (2001). Cortical spreading depression induces proinflammatory cytokine gene expression in the rat brain. *Journal of Cerebral Blood Flow & Metabolism* **21**(3): 218–25.

Karatas, H., S. E. Erdener, Y. Gursoy-Ozdemir, S. Lule, E. Eren-Kocak, Z. D. Sen, and T. Dalkara (2013). Spreading depression triggers headache by activating neuronal Panx1 channels. *Science* **339**(6123): 1092–5.

Karatas, H., B. Dönmez-Demir, and T. Dalkara (2015). *Supraphysiological whisker stimulation initiates an inflammatory response in the mouse barrel cortex in vivo.* 9th World Congress International Brain Research Organization, http: //ibro2015.org, Rio de Janerio, Brasil, July 7–11.

Kitley, J. L., H. J. Lachmann, A. Pinto, and L. Ginsberg (2010). Neurologic manifestations of the cryopyrin-associated periodic syndrome. *Neurology* **74**(16): 1267–70.

Knotkova, H., and M. Pappagallo (2007). Imaging intracranial plasma extravasation in a migraine patient: a case report. *Pain Medicine* **8**(4): 383–7.

Koroleva, V. I., and J. Bures (1993). Rats do not experience cortical or hippocampal spreading depression as aversive. *Neuroscience Letters* **149**(2): 153–6.

Krivanek, J., and E. Fifkova (1965). The value of ultramicro-analysis of lactic acid in tracing the penetration of Leao's cortical spreading depression to subcortical areas. *Journal of the Neurological Sciences* **2**(4): 385–92.

Kunkler, P. E., and R. P. Kraig (2003). Hippocampal spreading depression bilaterally activates the caudal trigeminal nucleus in rodents. *Hippocampus* **13**(7): 835–44.

Lamonte, M., S. D. Silberstein, and J. F. Marcelis (1995). Headache associated with aseptic meningitis. *Headache* **35**(9): 520–6.

Langford, D. J., A. L. Bailey, M. L. Chanda, S. E. Clarke, T. E. Drummond, S. Echols, S. Glick, J. Ingrao, T. Klassen-Ross, M. L. Lacroix-Fralish, L. Matsumiya, R. E. Sorge, S. G. Sotocinal, J. M. Tabaka, D. Wong, A. M. van den Maagdenberg, M. D. Ferrari, K. D. Craig, and J. S. Mogil (2010). Coding of facial expressions of pain in the laboratory mouse. *Nature Methods* **7**(6): 447–9.

Lashley, K. S. (1941). Patterns of cerebral integration indicated by the scotomas of migraine. *Archives of Neurology and Psychiatry* **46**: 259–64.

Lauritzen, M., M. B. Jorgensen, N. H. Diemer, A. Gjedde, and A. J. Hansen (1982). Persistent oligemia of rat cerebral cortex in the wake of spreading depression. *Annals of Neurology* **12**(5): 469–74.

Lauritzen, M., J. P. Dreier, M. Fabricius, J. A. Hartings, R. Graf, and A. J. Strong (2011). Clinical relevance of cortical spreading depression in neurological disorders: migraine, malignant stroke, subarachnoid and intracranial hemorrhage, and traumatic brain injury. *Journal of Cerebral Blood Flow & Metabolism* **31**(1): 17–35.

Leao, A. A. P. (1944a). Pial circulation and spreading depression of activity in cerebral cortex. *Journal of Neurophysiology* **7**: 391–6.

Leao, A. A. P. (1944b). Spreading depression of activity in the cerebral cortex. *Journal of Neurophysiology* **7**: 359–90.

Leao, A. A. P., and R. S. Morrison (1945). Propagation of spreading cortical depression. *Journal of Neurophysiology* **8**: 33–45.

Leo, L., L. Gherardini, V. Barone, M. De Fusco, D. Pietrobon, T. Pizzorusso, and G. Casari (2011). Increased susceptibility to cortical spreading depression in the mouse model of familial hemiplegic migraine type 2. *PLoS Genetics* **7**(6): e1002129.

Levy, D. (2009). Migraine pain, meningeal inflammation, and mast cells. *Current Pain and Headache Reports* **13**(3): 237–40.

Lothman, E., J. Lamanna, G. Cordingley, M. Rosenthal, and G. Somjen (1975). Responses of electrical potential, potassium levels, and oxidative metabolic activity of the cerebral neocortex of cats. *Brain Research* **88**(1): 15–36.

Ma, W., H. Hui, P. Pelegrin, and A. Surprenant (2009). Pharmacological characterization of pannexin-1 currents expressed in mammalian cells. *Journal of Pharmacology and Experimental Therapeutics* **328**(2): 409–18.

Milner, P. M. (1958). Note on a possible correspondence between the scotomas of migraine and spreading depression of Leao. *Electroencephalography and Clinical Neurophysiology* **10**(4): 705.

Miyamae, T. (2012). Cryopyrin-associated periodic syndromes: diagnosis and management. *Pediatric Drugs* **14**(2): 109–17.

Monro, J., C. Carini, and J. Brostoff (1984). Migraine is a food-allergic disease. *Lancet* **2**(8405): 719–21.

Moskowitz, M. A. (1984). The neurobiology of vascular head pain. *Annals of Neurology* **16**(2): 157–68.

Moskowitz, M. A., J. F. Reinhard, Jr.,, J. Romero, E. Melamed, and D. J. Pettibone (1979). Neurotransmitters and the fifth cranial nerve: is there a relation to the headache phase of migraine? *Lancet* **2**(8148): 883–5.

Moskowitz, M. A., M. Brody, and L. Y. Liu-Chen (1983). In vitro release of immunoreactive substance P from putative afferent nerve endings in bovine pia arachnoid. *Neuroscience* **9**(4): 809–14.

Moskowitz, M. A., K. Nozaki, and R. P. Kraig (1993). Neocortical spreading depression provokes the expression of c-fos protein-like immunoreactivity within trigeminal nucleus caudalis via trigeminovascular mechanisms. *The Journal of Neuroscience* **13**(3): 1167–77.

Nakamura, Y., L. Franchi, N. Kambe, G. Meng, W. Strober, and G. Nunez (2012). Critical role for mast cells in interleukin-1beta-driven skin inflammation associated with an activating mutation in the nlrp3 protein. *Immunity* **37**(1): 85–95.

Nassini, R., S. Materazzi, J. Vriens, J. Prenen, S. Benemei, G. De Siena, G. la Marca, E. Andre, D. Preti, C. Avonto, L. Sadofsky, V. Di Marzo, L. De Petrocellis, G. Dussor, F. Porreca, O. Taglialatela-Scafati, G. Appendino, B. Nilius, and P. Geppetti (2012). The 'headache tree' via umbellulone and TRPA1 activates the trigeminovascular system. *Brain* **135**(Pt 2): 376–90.

Noseda, R., L. Constandil, L. Bourgeais, M. Chalus, and L. Villanueva (2010). Changes of meningeal excitability mediated by corticotrigeminal networks: a link for the endogenous modulation of migraine pain. *Journal of Neuroscience* **30**(43): 14420–9.

Olesen, J., B. Larsen, and M. Lauritzen (1981). Focal hyperemia followed by spreading oligemia and impaired activation of rCBF in classic migraine. *Annals of Neurology* **9**(4): 344–52.

Olesen, J., L. Friberg, T. S. Olsen, H. K. Iversen, N. A. Lassen, A. R. Andersen, and A. Karle (1990). Timing and topography of cerebral blood flow, aura, and headache during migraine attacks. *Annals of Neurology* **28**(6): 791–8.

Ostergaard, L., J. P. Dreier, N. Hadjikhani, S. N. Jespersen, U. Dirnagl, and T. Dalkara (2015). Neurovascular coupling during cortical spreading depolarization and depression. *Stroke* **46**(5): 1392–401.

Paolino, R. M., and H. M. Levy (1971). Amnesia produced by spreading depression and ECS: evidence for time-dependent memory trace localization. *Science* **172**(3984): 746–9.

Pietrobon, D., and M. A. Moskowitz (2014). Chaos and commotion in the wake of cortical spreading depression and spreading depolarizations. *Nature Reviews Neuroscience* **15**(6): 379–93.

Purdy, R. A. (2008). Migraine with and without aura share the same pathogenic mechanisms. *Neurological Sciences* **29** Suppl 1: S44–6.

Richter, F., and A. Lehmenkuhler (1993). Spreading depression can be restricted to distinct depths of the rat cerebral cortex. *Neuroscience Letters* **152**(1–2): 65–8.

Romero-Reyes, M., and Y. Ye (2013). Pearls and pitfalls in experimental in vivo models of headache: conscious behavioral research. *Cephalalgia* **33**(8): 566–76.

Rosenberg, J. H., and S. D. Silberstein (2005). The headache of SAH responds to sumatriptan. *Headache* **45**(5): 597–8.

Russell, M. B., and J. Olesen (1996). A nosographic analysis of the migraine aura in a general population. *Brain* **119**(Pt 2): 355–61.

Saito, K., S. Markowitz, and M. A. Moskowitz (1988). Ergot alkaloids block neurogenic extravasation in dura mater: proposed action in vascular headaches. *Annals of Neurology* **24**(6): 732–7.

Sanchez del Rio, M., D. Bakker, O. Wu, R. Agosti, D. D. Mitsikostas, L. Ostergaard, W. A. Wells, B. R. Rosen, G. Sorensen, M. A. Moskowitz, and F. M. Cutrer (1999). Perfusion weighted imaging during migraine: spontaneous visual aura and headache. *Cephalalgia* **19**(8): 701–7.

Santos, E., M. Scholl, R. Sanchez-Porras, M. A. Dahlem, H. Silos, A. Unterberg, H. Dickhaus, and O. W. Sakowitz (2014). Radial, spiral and reverberating waves of spreading depolarization occur in the gyrencephalic brain. *Neuroimage* **99**: 244–55.

Sarchielli, P., A. Alberti, M. Codini, A. Floridi, and V. Gallai (2000). Nitric oxide metabolites, prostaglandins and trigeminal vasoactive peptides in internal jugular vein blood during spontaneous migraine attacks. *Cephalalgia* **20**(10): 907–18.

Sarchielli, P., A. Alberti, L. Vaianella, L. Pierguidi, A. Floridi, G. Mazzotta, A. Floridi, and V. Gallai (2004). Chemokine levels in the jugular venous blood of migraine without aura patients during attacks. *Headache* **44**(10): 961–8.

Sarchielli, P., A. Alberti, A. Baldi, F. Coppola, C. Rossi, L. Pierguidi, A. Floridi, and P. Calabresi (2006). Proinflammatory cytokines, adhesion molecules, and lymphocyte integrin expression in the internal jugular blood of migraine patients without aura assessed ictally. *Headache* **46**(2): 200–7.

Somjen, G. G. (2001). Mechanisms of spreading depression and hypoxic spreading depression-like depolarization. *Physiological Reviews* **81**(3): 1065–96.

Sotocinal, S. G., R. E. Sorge, A. Zaloum, A. H. Tuttle, L. J. Martin, J. S. Wieskopf, J. C. Mapplebeck, P. Wei, S. Zhan, S. Zhang, J. J. McDougall, O. D. King, and J. S. Mogil (2011). The Rat Grimace Scale: a partially automated method for quantifying pain in the laboratory rat via facial expressions. *Molecular Pain* **7**: 55.

Szabo, K. (1995). The cranial venous system in the rat: anatomical pattern and ontogenetic development. II. Dorsal drainage. *Annals of Anatomy* **177**(4): 313–22.

Takizawa, T., M. Shibata, Y. Kayama, H. Toriumi, T. Ebine, A. Koh, T. Shimizu, and N. Suzuki (2016). Temporal profiles of high-mobility group box 1 expression levels after cortical spreading depression in mice. *Cephalalgia* **36**(1): 44–52.

Tang, Y. T., J. M. Mendez, J. J. Theriot, P. M. Sawant, H. E. Lopez-Valdes, Y. S. Ju, and K. C. Brennan (2014). Minimum conditions for the induction of cortical spreading depression in brain slices. *Journal of Neurophysiology* **112**(10): 2572–9.

Thompson, C. S., and A. M. Hakim (2005). Cortical spreading depression modifies components of the inflammatory cascade. *Molecular Neurobiology* **32**(1): 51–7.

Vecchia, D., and D. Pietrobon (2012). Migraine: a disorder of brain excitatory-inhibitory balance? *Trends in Neurosciences* **35**(8): 507–20.

Viggiano, E., D. Ferrara, G. Izzo, A. Viggiano, S. Minucci, M. Monda, and B. De Luca (2008). Cortical spreading depression induces the expression of iNOS, HIF-1alpha, and LDH-A. *Neuroscience* **153**(1): 182–8.

Vincent, M. B., and N. Hadjikhani (2007). Migraine aura and related phenomena: beyond scotomata and scintillations. *Cephalalgia* **27**(12): 1368–77.

Woods, R. P., M. Iacoboni, and J. C. Mazziotta (1994). Brief report: bilateral spreading cerebral hypoperfusion during spontaneous migraine headache. *New England Journal of Medicine* **331**(25): 1689–92.

Yokota, C., H. Inoue, Y. Kuge, T. Abumiya, M. Tagaya, Y. Hasegawa, N. Ejima, N. Tamaki, and K. Minematsu (2003). Cyclooxygenase-2 expression associated with spreading depression in a primate model. *Journal of Cerebral Blood Flow & Metabolism* **23**(4): 395–8.

Zhang, X., D. Levy, R. Noseda, V. Kainz, M. Jakubowski, and R. Burstein (2010). Activation of meningeal nociceptors by cortical spreading depression: implications for migraine with aura. *Journal of Neuroscience* **30**(26): 8807–14.

Zhang, X., D. Levy, V. Kainz, R. Noseda, M. Jakubowski, and R. Burstein (2011). Activation of central trigeminovascular neurons by cortical spreading depression. *Annals of Neurology* **69**(5): 855–65.

Zhao, J., and D. Levy (2015). Modulation of intracranial meningeal nociceptor activity by cortical spreading depression: a reassessment. *Journal of Neurophysiology* **113**(7): 2778–85.

Part V

Modeling and imaging in migraine

17

Mathematical modeling of human cortical spreading depression

Markus A. Dahlem

Department of Physics, Humboldt University of Berlin, Berlin, Germany

17.1 Introduction

We are looking back to more than 50 years of mathematical models of cortical spreading depression (CSD). In general, computational neuroscience uses abstract models formulated in mathematical language to interpret data and guide a principled understanding of the nervous systems in health and disease. The complexity of neural systems can make it difficult to assess the value of such models, because they have to abstract from the details and incorporate only the aspects that are considered to be important, yet what is important may only be known in hindsight.

With regard to this difficulty, however, a computational model is often not fundamentally different from animal models. In particular, in animal models of pain, the efficacy of a drug is often first demonstrated in humans and then in the animal model, which is called backward validation [41]. Unlike animal models, a computational model can be deliberately and intentionally changed in any manner – that is, components can be modified or added in any sequence. Therefore, one can feature backward validation by making the computational science process cyclic. In fact, many cycles have been completed in the last 50 years of CSD research. Moreover, experiments on pain using non-human animals, or even human subjects pose great ethical problems. Computer models are an attractive – but limited – remedy for this problem.

Last, but not least, experimental animal models and clinical studies have become increasingly sophisticated, and have given rise to an abundance of biological data across a range of spatial and temporal scales, extending from molecules to whole brain, and from sub-milliseconds of channel gating to several hours of attack duration, and even years in changes in headache history. Accurate biophysical, multi-scale computational models can help to integrate diverse data sets and to unify information.

In this chapter, we will provide various examples of two classes of computer models of CSD, all without trying to parse mathematical details; these can be found in the cited original literature. The common theme that runs through these examples is to elucidate how the respective objective of the model determines the chosen level of abstraction.

First, we introduce microscopic models that include cellular and cytoarchitectonic detail. Such models can address questions related to the electrophysiological

Neurobiological Basis of Migraine, First Edition. Edited by Turgay Dalkara and Michael A. Moskowitz.

characterization of membrane properties during CSD. In the second part, which builds on the first part by further abstraction, we introduce macroscopic models that describe large scale pattern formation in cortical tissue and, with that, we address questions raised by the neurological manifestation of CSD. We end with some predictions from this computational science approach.

17.2   Microscopic models: cellular and cytoarchitectonic detail

A key question addressed by microscopic models concerns which properties of the neuronal membrane contribute to the ignition of CSD. In this case, the computational science process begins by identifying the following physiological observations to be selected for a working model.

17.2.1   Physiological observations: persistent depolarization

Sustained inward currents can drive a persistent depolarization of the neuronal membrane. Such a phenomenon underlies not only spreading depression (CSD), but also tonic-clonic seizure discharges. In both cases, the sustained inward currents add up to a suprathreshold input. The threshold can initially be defined as the minimal current amplitude of, in principle, infinite duration (in practice, several tens of milliseconds suffice), that results in periodic firing – the so-called rheobase current.

When positive electric charge (such as sodium ions) flows into neurons, this defines an inward current. It is unclear whether the inward current during CSD occurs by the same pathways that are involved in normal cellular functioning, such as the generation of action potentials (but this case in some abnormal mode of operation of these known active channels) or, alternatively, if at least some part of the inward current is carried by an ion flow through unknown channels.

17.2.2   Working model: sustained inward currents

How can experimental data on the available electrophysiological measurements [43] be quantitatively interpreted? For this purpose, a computer model was developed [28] to test a hypothesis – namely, that the persistent depolarization is generated by the cooperative action of several known channels, and that blocking any one of the channels can slow down CSD or decrease its intensity, but not prevent it. The step towards a working model is the simplification of the observed cellular system into its quantifiable factors.

Among these quantifiable factors are five active membrane currents, two passive electrical properties (leak currents), and active pumping of sodium ions (Na^+) and potassium ions (K^+). These five active membrane currents are: the transient and persistent Na^+ currents; a delayed rectifier K^+ current; a transient K^+ current; and a NMDA receptor mediated current. Furthermore, the cell morphology of a hippocampal CA1 neuron, in terms of geometrical properties of its soma and apical dendrite, is included as part of this working model of CSD.

17.2.3 Physiological mechanism: excitability

The classical Hodgkin and Huxley (HH) framework of membrane electrophysiology [24] is used to represent the working model as a mechanistic model. This framework formulates membrane electrophysiology, considering the equivalent electrical circuit for a patch of membrane as a fixed capacitance (lipid bilayer) and, in parallel, voltage-gated conductances (ion channels) with, in series, batteries (ion gradients). The voltage-gated ion channel kinetics are described by independent conformational transitions of the channel subunits. The voltage-gating provides the necessary nonlinearity for threshold behavior. Models resulting from the HH framework are also called conductance-based neuron models.

The HH model of action potentials is one of the most successful models in mathematical biology. It is worthwhile to look into this more fully, due to the great significance and relationship between action potentials and spreading depression.

The HH model describes the underlying mechanism of a single spike as a phenomenon of excitability. The reasons for its success can be understood from two connected perspectives. First, cellular transmission of action potentials is one of the most fundamental processes in biology. Second, far beyond the generation of action potentials is the phenomenon of excitability. How this is related to the onset of rhythmic activity, such as bursting, is important to a whole host of other problems outside membrane physiology and even biology, including physics, chemistry, sociology, and engineering. Because the HH model was the first precise biophysical model of excitability, its mathematical structure serves as representative of a whole class of excitable phenomena in various areas, and it set much of the terminology and the way we classify excitable and bursting systems [27].

These two connected perspectives can be irritating when it comes to modeling CSD as an excitable phenomenon, because action potentials set not only the terminology, but also generic forms of mathematical models for excitability, such as the famous FitzHugh-Nagumo model and others [2, 15, 23, 42, 44, 55]. For this reason, we explicitly note that action potentials and spreading depression share many elements that constitute two distinct and separate kinds of excitable phenomena. In particular, they take place on very different space- and timescales. In fact, the very purpose of the computer models developed by Kager, Wadman, and Somjen (KWS), described in the following, was to study how these elements are interlaced, but lead to two distinct excitable phenomena. Excitability means that, while small perturbations return immediately to rest, a stronger – but still brief – stimulus can trigger a large excursion that, eventually, also reverts to the resting state without the need of further input.

An action potential is caused in the neural membrane by a small amplitude depolarization. By definition, the size of the rheobase current can be taken as an inversely proportionate measure of this kind of membrane excitability. In the case of an action potential, the "excursion", as an essential act constituting excitability, is the change of the membrane potential towards a positively polarized state that eventually repolarizes to the negatively polarized resting state. Such a spike lasts 1/1000th of a second. During this period, ions are exchanged across the nerve cell membrane, but only to a negligible degree.

Spreading depression, on the other hand, is caused in the neural membrane by sustained depolarization. Changes in ion concentrations have to become significant to

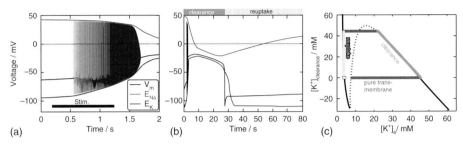

Figure 17.1 Simulated time course of CSD on short and long timescales and the "plane of excitability" of CSD models. (a) The black line is the transmembrane potential V_m simulated in the cell soma; the light and dark gray lines are the Nernst potentials of sodium and potassium, respectively. High-frequency discharges caused by an applied depolarizing stimulation current of 0.15 nA amplitude, lasting one second (black bar), followed by sustained after-discharges (first spiking and then, after a depolarization block at ≈ 1.7 seconds, by non-spiking currents. (b) As in (a), but on a longer timescale; note that even after 80 seconds the Nernst potentials have not completely recovered. The top bar marks time period of the two distinct phases in the "plane of excitability". (c) The "plane of excitability" of CSD models. The plane is spanned by extracellular potassium ion concentration $[K^+]_e$ and potassium ion clearance (measured in mM with virtual reference to the extracellular volume). The resting state is marked by a white square. If a depolarizing stimulation current takes $[K^+]_e$ beyond the dashed line, sustained after-discharges occur and significant potassium ion clearance sets in. At a maximum value of cleared potassium, the membrane potential is driven quickly back by the electrogenic pump to near its resting state. Shortly after this, the neural membrane is functionally no longer significantly impaired, but re-uptake of the lost potassium takes several tens of minutes.

maintain this depolarization. For example, a high-frequency series of action potentials can result from, and cause, persistent depolarization. The hallmarks of the excursion in the case of spreading depression are the energy draining pathological after-discharges that let neurons starve from a transient loss of transmembrane ion gradients.

The original HH framework did not account for changes in ion concentrations, but it can be extended in a rather straightforward manner for this purpose, and then translated into a computational model. Ion currents also determine ion concentration changes by considering the morphology of the cytoarchitecture by only two parameters – the volume fraction between intracellular and interstitial space, and the volume-to-surface-area ratio of the cell. The intra- and extracellular ion concentrations, in turn, determine the Nernst potentials, which are part of the original HH framework.

We shall refrain from presenting mathematical equations of the cellular CSD models. These can be found in the cited literature and, to a certain degree, source code can be found in open source code repositories [25]. Instead, we present the simulations in terms of time series (see Figure 17.1).

Let us first comment on the number of rate equations. In the first KWS model [28], the morphology of the neuron was represented by 201 electrically coupled compartments. For each compartment, a set of extended HH equations is solved with possibly varying parameters. Such a set consists of the following rate equations; one for the transmembrane voltage V_m coming form the Kirchhof law of the equivalent electrical circuit for a patch of membrane; one for each channel's type of subunit with a gated conformational transition; and one for each ion concentration in the neuronal, extracellular, glial, and vascular milieu (to the extent that these are included). Cell volume swelling can add another rate equation.

17.2.4 Results, modeling iterations, and interpretation

17.2.4.1 Increasing physiological detail

The first of a series of KWS models [28] simulated the time course of CSD, similar to the time course shown in Figure 17.1. This simulation has been interpreted in such a way that currents through ion channels that are normally present in neuronal membranes can generate the depolarization state in CSD. Although the onset of CSD can be delayed, in particular if either the persistent sodium or the NMDA mediated current is varied to the extent that it becomes insufficient, the deficit is eventually compensated by the remaining conductance.

Naturally, many factors that also play important roles in CSD have not been included in this first generation. Therefore, further components and features have been added to the working model: more complete representations of ions and channels, and osmotic cell volume changes [29]; calcium ions and calcium currents, calcium membrane transport, an intracellular calcium buffer, and a calcium-dependent potassium current [30]; and voltage-dependent channels in the glial membrane [59, 60]. With each new KWS model generation, more elaborate hypotheses could be tested and compared with experimental evidence. We refer the interested reader to references [28–30, 59, 60].

The objective of the various ever more detailed model generations, including those of other groups [40], was to make a number of differences visible in the time course of CSD, given more physiological detail, but also to highlight common features shared among all models. The most important of these is that all simulations demonstrated the independence of the CSD process from the strength of the triggering stimulus, confirming that it is an excitable phenomenon with all-or-none character, without the need of an unknown channel. However, one should not omit to mention that this does not exclude an unknown conductance, and another model predicts its importance in specific dendritic domains [37].

17.2.4.2 Model reconciliation

The original HH model for action potentials has four dynamical variables. Until recently, extended HH systems which can model CSD ranged between nine and several hundreds of dynamical variables in multi-compartment models, as introduced in the last section.

Various reduction techniques and assumptions have been used to reduce a CSD model to four dynamical variables, while still retaining adequate biophysical realism in modeling action potentials, tonic-clonic seizure discharges, and spreading depression [25]. These reduction techniques help to reconcile various CSD models and to ensure the consistency between them, by reducing the development and propagation of errors. For instance, the so-called "fixed leak" current is naturally eliminated, and will no longer obfuscate the nature of recovery in CSD models.

A reduced CSD model is tractable for a detailed fast-slow analysis and bifurcation analysis using continuation software. These computational analyzing methods reveal fundamental properties of CSD in the "plane of excitability", focusing on principal activator and inhibitor functions (see Figure 17.1c). These analyzing methods also lead to creating a computationally efficient model, needed to study the influence of molecular changes upon cellular and whole-cortex CSD models. For instance, the functional connection between genetic findings in familial hemiplegic migraine and physiological functions on the level of the cell is an area of particular interest for computational studies [13]. They complement studies that experimentally identify and characterize this connection in heterologous cellular systems. Further examples, extending this approach to whole-cortex models, are given in the following sections.

From the reconciled model, two findings stand out, and they guide a principle understanding of CSD. First, although neurons still have access to metabolic energy that, in principle, can be used to re-establish the loss of the transmembrane ion gradients, the neuronal ion pumps alone are insufficient to counterbalance the currents through both leak and open voltage-gated channels [26]. Second, we identified one variable of particular importance to overcome this recovery problem. The potassium ion clearance, and re-uptake by some reservoirs provided by the nerve cell surroundings, play a crucial mechanistic role in recovery (Figure 17.1c). We therefore suggest describing the new type of CSD excitability as a sequence of two fast processes, with constant total ion content in the neural parenchima separated by two slow processes of ion clearance (loss) and re-uptake (gain) by the neurovacular unit [25].

17.3 Macroscopic models: large scale spatiotemporal phenomenology

Macroscopic CSD models are reliant upon the cellular models and reuse the knowledge gained by them. The perspective, however, changes from physiology to neurology. The following is the only fundamental question addressed by macroscopic models, it requires examination of clinical issues that have many ramifications. In which patterns does CSD spread over the cerebral cortex in humans? The working model for that question starts by identifying clinical manifestations of migraine with aura as the expressions of the pattern-forming neural activity during CSD.

17.3.1   Clinical manifestation: march of migraine aura symptoms

Migraine auras are windows on the visual areas in posterior cortex [66]. The march of visual symptoms prompt the key question formulated by Wilkinson, namely whether, in migraine, *"the spreading depression process engulfs all of posterior cortex [...] or alternatively, the activation directly due to spreading depression is much more limited in extent, and the rest of the spreading activation in adjacent cortical areas represents synaptic activation through feed-forward and feedback circuitry."*

An all-engulfing CSD wave illustrates in many migraine textbooks a full-scale attack (cf. Figure 17.2a). This picture originates from the review by Lauritzen [36], and is based on regional cerebral blood flow, as measured by the xenon 133 injection technique [47], but it lacks backing from functional magnetic resonance imaging [19]. The occurrence of an all-engulfing CSD pattern in human cortex has been called into question [8, 10, 12]. It was suggested that instead, in the human cortex, CSD propagates radially outwards

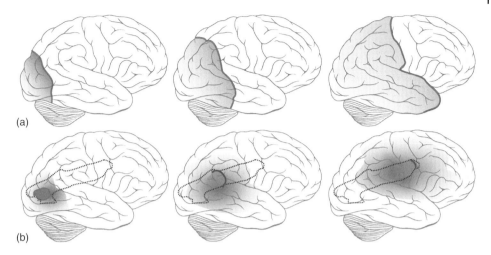

Figure 17.2 Possible patterns of the spread of CSD in a full-scale attack in human cortex (from left to right). (a) All-engulfing CSD wave stopping at the central sulcus. (b) Starting from a "hot spot", a solitary localized CSD breaks away in one direction and is surrounded by activation through synaptic circuitry. The wave segment either propagates along a single continuous path (outlined by dashed line), or is occasionally interrupted, jumps, and reappears in new hot spots at more distant areas, due to the increased non-local synaptic activity (not shown) – see text.

only for a couple of minutes or less and, if longer lasting in a full-scale attack, then CSD propagates only as a localized small wave segment breaking out in one direction [7, 11] (see Figure 17.2b).

Strong evidence for localized CSD wave segments comes from the march of migraine aura symptoms, both within the visual cortex, as a single sensory modality, and across sensory and cognitive modalities. First, the spatio-temporal development of migraine aura symptoms in the visual field is often localized [10, 18, 35, 48, 66] (see Figure 17.3a), and there can be a large variety of localized visual symptoms [20]. Second, aura symptoms follow distinctly variable paths from attack to attack when mapped onto the cortical surface across sensory and cognitive modalities [64] (see Figure 17.2b).

The reformed propagation pattern shown in Figure 17.2, including radially outward-spreading CSD for the first few minutes, and possibly non-local jumps through synaptic circuitry, might consistently explain how such a profound neurophysiological event as CSD could cause such minor neurological symptoms or, in some cases, possibly no symptoms at all [6]. It also suggests that our understanding of how CSD relates to migraine with and without aura is limited in this respect by inappropriate small animal models (but cf. Reference [56]) – hence the need for a complementary computational approach.

17.3.2 Working model: activator inhibitor type description in two spatial dimensions

How can the clinical observations of the march of aura symptoms be interpreted quantitatively? A working model simplifies the observed cortical pattern formation process in terms of activator-inhibitor systems in two spatial dimensions (2D), which provides

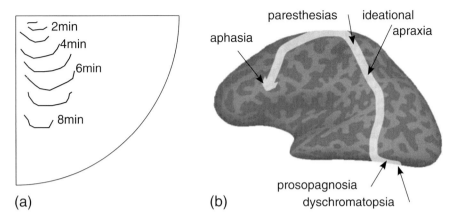

Figure 17.3 Clinical evidence for localized CSD waves. (a) Propagation pattern of self-reported visual field defects during migraine with aura in the lower right visual field quadrant. The time in minutes starts from the first recognition of the migraine aura phase. (b) Human artificially inflated cortical surface, obtained by magnetic resonance imaging (MRI) with add-on aura symptoms (lateral view). The pattern follows contiguous cortical areas successively affected, as indicated by the arrow. Modified from [64]. Reproduced by permission of Sage Publications.

the quantifiable factors to model self-organized activity patterns in the human cortex, on a spatial scale of centimeters and a temporal scale of up to hours.

The quantifiable factors in macroscopic models are lump variables. Such a deliberate simplification gives rise to a high degree of abstraction. Lump variables take the role of an activator and an inhibitor, defined by their respective lump rate functions. Furthermore, other parts of macroscopic working models are cortical functional domains and anatomical landmarks, with an averaged effect of the laminar and cellular tissue heterogeneity and cortical vascularization.

17.3.3 Physiological mechanism: spatiotemporal self-organization

There are various mechanistic ways that activator-inhibitor systems can form cortical activity patterns. Understanding these mechanistic principles of self-organization, and interpreting these patterns in mechanistic terms, remains a key task of computational neuroscience. The important principles for CSD in the human cortex are, broadly speaking, described by reaction-diffusion systems and the neurovascular coupling of neural fields. During normal functioning of the brain, so-called neural fields models describe large-scale dynamics of spatially structured neural networks formed by synaptic connections [1, 4, 67]. The central step from a microscopic cellular description to a macroscopic (continuum) level is conducted in a sequence of approximations. It takes the voltage-based description of spiking neurons and synaptic and dendritic processing to an activity-based description of neural populations.

These concepts of neural field models still apply in some cases of neurological disorders, such as epilepsy. It is unclear, however, how an activity-based description can be rigorously developed under conditions of CSD. During CSD, the energy-draining pathological after-discharges let neurons starve due to a transient loss of transmembrane ion gradients. Neurons can only recover on a rather long timescale, compared to their discharge activity, by metabolizing chemical energy to restore these gradients (see Figure 17.1).

Notwithstanding, our knowledge of the cellular processes during CSD allows a new formulation including, but not limited to, neural field models. The central element is diffusion, due to which the hallmark of CSD emerges – its slow speed.

17.3.4 Results of modeling iterations: from fronts to pulses to solitary localized structures

17.3.4.1 The speed of the front

The first mathematical CSD model, which can be considered the starting-point of a series of macroscopic models introduced below, dates back to the year 1959. Based on mathematical methods developed by Alois Huxley, Alan Hodgkin provided a handwritten manuscript (a transcript and annotated version is in preparation for the *Journal of Neurophysiology*) that gives an order of magnitude calculation of the speed of CSD.

The model supports Grafstein's hypothesis [5, 17], stating that release of K^+ into the cortical extracellular space is the critical self-propagating event in CSD. To be more precise, the model supports that any extracelluar diffusive species that has similar release and removal rates and a similar diffusion coefficient to those of potassium ions can explain the remarkable slow spread of CSD. Whether or not extracellular K^+ is considered a mere coadjuvant on the chain reaction does not affect this essential result, that is, that a reaction-diffusion (RD) process critically determines the speed of CSD – see References [61] and [22] for an up-to-date discussion of this hypothesis.

To sum up, in the context of macroscopic models, "potassium" should be considered a lump variable. In a more detailed microscopic (i.e., cellular) description, the ion homeostasis in general, and potassium homeostasis in particular, is determined by vascular, neuronal, and glial cells and their milieu, as described in the first part. The spatial spread of ions, which determines pattern formation in continuum models and, in particular, the speed of CSD is, in addition to the extracellular diffusion, also critically governed via spatial buffering, achieved by the glial syncytium and by the neurovscular unit. Therefore, at least two relevant potassium ion concentrations need to be considered for the spread of CSD.

Furthermore, charged particles like potassium ions cannot diffuse independently, since they must be accompanied by counter-ions to keep the bulk milieu electroneutral. The lump approach considers all this as an integrated system that works in concert, such that an activator can be called "potassium" because the nonlinear release and removal rate function linked to extracellular K^+ leads to a threshold that triggers a self-activating positive feedback loop, as proposed by Grafstein [16, 17].

The original RD model formulates the potassium rate function by a third-order polynomial describing the nonlinear release with a positive feedback loop in a generic form. The particular values for the three steady states, the roots of the rate function (locations at which the function equals zero), are chosen at resting level concentration, threshold concentration and maximum concentration. The actual values that Hodgkin used were for the extracellular elevation of potassium. The location of the roots should be adjusted, the threshold concentration is sometimes now called ceiling level [21] and lies at around

10 mM, and the maximum concentration is about 55 mM. Together with diffusion, this yields the RD equation:

$$\frac{\partial u}{\partial t} = f(u) + D_u \frac{\partial^2}{\partial x^2} u \qquad (17.1)$$

The potassium ion concentration (i.e., the activator) is called u, the function $f(u)$ is the third order polynomial, and the parameter D_u is the diffusion coefficient of potassium ions in the brain. The space variable is x.

The state of cortical tissue at a maximum concentration of about 55 mM is further away from the 10 mM ceiling level than the resting state value at around 3 mM. The differences to the ceiling level are 45 mM and 7 mM, respectively. These differences are called basins of attraction. In RD systems, the state with the lager basin of attraction wins, and eventually recruits tissue in the state with the smaller one into its state at a fixed speed of millimeters per minute, according to mathematical analysis. While the third order polynomial $f(u)$ in Equation 17.1, suggested by Hodgkin and Huxley, is a generic top-down description, seemingly focusing solely on potassium ion concentration, a similar form is now derived from the bottom-up cellular CSD model within their extended conductance-based HH framework [26].

17.3.4.2 Propagation and zigzag percepts

Reggia and Montgomery have built a hybrid model – a reaction-diffusion (RD) model coupled to neural field dynamics [49, 50]. This was the first computational model that originally aimed at reproducing the typical zigzags of the fortification pattern experienced as visual field defects during migraine with aura (Figure 17.4a). One part of this model is similar to the previous RD model based on potassium dynamics, described in Equation 17.1.

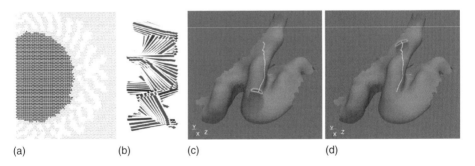

(a)   (b)   (c)   (d)

Figure 17.4 Simulations of zigzag patterns experienced during visual migraine aura and spread of CSD in human cortex. (a) The spread of CSD, with patterns of intense cortical activity in white. The cerebral cortex was modeled as a two-dimensional array of hexagonally tessellated volume elements (figure from [49]) Reproduced by permission of Elsevier. (b) The zigzag percept based on the pinwheel structure of iso-orientation domains in cortical feature map excited by a CSD wave [9]. (c)-(d) Simulation of CSD on an individually shaped cortical surface, obtained by MRI from a migraine sufferer who has drawn his visual field defects, as shown in Figure 17.3a. The surface is the left primary visual cortex, located in the calcarine sulcus (CS). The lower quadrant of the right visual hemifield is mapped onto the dorsal bank of CS and onto the cuneus. (c) Start of simulation with CSD located at the occipital pole about 10 mm into the medial convexity. (d) Near the end of simulation; the line marks the path of the localized CSD takes on the cuneus [50]. Richter and Lehmenkühler (1993). Reproduced by permission of Elsevier. For animated version of (b) please use the link, https://www.youtube.com/watch?v=GFvuC9dxY9I.

The RD system also included an inhibitor to model the wave back in CSD, which recovers the resting state by driving the maximum extracellular potassium ion concentration back to the resting state concentration (note, we call the inhibitor v although, in the original paper, it was called r, for the "resequestration" of ions);

$$\frac{\partial v}{\partial t} = \varepsilon g(u, v) \tag{17.2}$$

with the generic rate function $g(u, v)$ being linear in both its arguments u and v, and introducing the time scale separation $\varepsilon \ll 1$, which renders the dynamics of the inhibitor v slow.[1] This was not the first such model that describes CSD as a pulse (a solitary wave with front and back); see the work by Tuckwell, Miura, and others for a microscopic cellular description [40, 62, 63, 68].

One reason we put emphasis on the macroscopic model by Reggia and Montgomery [49, 50] is that it directly links with later models that also describe the spread of CSD in 2-D on macroscopic scales. For the sake of completeness, the early cellular automata model from Reshodko and Bureš, which modeled reverberating CSD in 2-D, should also be mentioned [52], as well as a paper by Wiener and Rosenbluth [65] that describes a mathematical model for similar re-entry patterns in 2D in cardiac arrhythmia. In the beginning of their article, the authors made the connection to the brain, and possibly to CSD: "*Nervous elements and cardiac and other striate muscle fibers are excitable.* [...] *The laws which apply to the muscle fibers are also applicable to the nerve fibers.*" Arturo Rosenblueth clearly knew about the 2-D phenomenon of CSD, since he was one of the supervisors of Aristides Leão [58].

Another reason to consider the model by Reggia and Montgomery [49, 50] in some detail is that this model focuses on the neurological symptoms caused by CSD in migraine (Figure 17.4a). To this end, the distinguishing and novel feature in the model is that the RD model is coupled to a neural network. This network simulates the lateral long-range connections, a non-local coupling beyond diffusion. The neural network is merely used to predict the visual field defects during migraine with aura. The activity in the neural network dynamics is not fed back to the actual RD equations (Equations 1.1 and 1.2). In this perspective, the neural field is like an epiphenomenon of CSD. More recently, there has been a shift to examine their interaction.

Each network node (cortical cells or populations of cells) has an associated activation level $a(t)$, which is transferred via synaptic connections to other nearby cells. The activation level $a(t)$ represents the mean firing rate of neurons at time t. Within the neural network, lateral coupling is modeled by "Mexican hat" interactions – that is, cortical cells excite nearby cells and inhibit cells more distant. The formulation of the neural network dynamics in terms of the activation level $a(t)$ was not developed specifically to simulate visual field effects in migraine with aura. Rather, it was developed and used to study a variety of issues related to cortical dynamics and reorganization of sensory cortical feature maps [51].

An alternative approach to model the zigzag pattern was suggested later by Dahlem *et al.* [9]. If one merely considers the synaptic activity as an epiphenomenon, one can

---

1 Note that the new variable v is coupled to the potassium dynamics u by simply subtracting v in the rate function – hence, v is called an inhibitor, as it inhibits the release of potassium ions. Due to the occurrence of a second variable, a new rate function, $\tilde{f}(u, v) = f(u) - v$., is introduced, and Equation 17.1, in combination with Equation 17.2, should be adopted accordingly; we drop, however, the tilde in the following.

replace the neural network model, and more easily and precisely consider the effect of an advancing RD wave using a specific sensory cortical feature map that organizes the feature of orientation preferences of neurons in iso-orientation domains around a pinwheel structure [3]. Such a model could realistically simulate visual field effects as zigzag percepts (Figure 17.4b).

This model also makes specific predictions about the zigzags rotation features. Similar suggestions, but without proposing a mathematical model that can simulate zigzag patterns, were made before by Richards [53] and Schwartz [57] – namely, that the zigzags can be explained with reference to the layout of functional domains of orientation preferences in the primary visual cortex and, therefore, keen observations of visual migraine aura actually pre-empted the discovery of a pinwheel structure [3] in human cortex.

17.3.4.3 Propagation of solitary localized patterns

Let us recapitulate the preceding pattern formation principles that build on each other and need to be further expanded to explain the march of symptoms shown in Figure 17.3.

A reaction-diffusion system with a single activator species, which has an activation threshold that triggers a positive feedback loop, provides a mechanistic explanation of front propagation (Section 17.3.4.1, with Equation 17.1). A reaction-diffusion system with one activator, together with its inhibitor, which is usually, but not necessary, immobile, provides a mechanistic explanation of pulse propagation – that is, a solitary single wave with front and back (Section 17.3.4.2, with Equations 17.1 and 17.2). Without further assumptions, the latter system can only explain an all-engulfing CSD wave in the human cortex.

What is the next pattern formation principle? There is one more needed, assuming that the spread of a CSD wave during a full-scale migraine attack is not all-engulfing (as shown in Figure 17.2a) but is, instead, spatially limited to a narrow cortical pathway (as shown in Figure 17.2b), and further assuming that any taken pathway is not determined by territorial conditions, such as cytoarchitecture or vascular. Certainly, we have to take into account the influence of territorial heterogeneity. However, in a computational science process, we must first develop a high level of conceptual coherence, and try to deduce the patterns from a few fundamental principles.

Indeed, it is well known how stable solitary localized structures arise due to mechanisms of self-organization. There is a vast body of literature of activator-inhibitor models describing propagating "spots" in a variety of different systems, such as semiconductor material, gas discharge phenomena, and chemical systems [31, 34, 38, 39, 45, 46]. A plausible hypothesis is that the same generic principles apply to propagation of CSD if it propagates as a localized structure.

Inspired by such a generic model [34], which shows propagation of spots in 2-D by global inhibition, we suggest the following expansion to the reaction-diffusion system of activator inhibitor type described by Equations 17.1 and 17.2 [7, 11]:

$$\frac{\partial u}{\partial t} = \overbrace{\underbrace{f(u,v)}_{\text{front reaction}} + \underbrace{D_u \left(\frac{\partial^2}{\partial x^2} + \frac{\partial^2}{\partial y^2} \right) u}_{\text{diffusion}}}^{\text{activator rate function}} \tag{17.3}$$

$$\frac{\partial v}{\partial t} = \underbrace{\varepsilon}_{\text{slow}} \overbrace{\left(\underbrace{g(uv)}_{\text{back reaction}} + \underbrace{\int k(x,y)a(t)\,\mathrm{d}x\mathrm{d}y}_{\text{non-local coupling}} \right)}^{\text{inhibitor rate function}} \tag{17.4}$$

The activator equation is unchanged (Equation 17.1 → Equation 17.3), except that Fick's diffusion term is now in its 2-D form. The inhibitor equation is expanded by a non-local coupling term reminiscent of a neuronal field.

17.3.5 Interpretation of pattern formation principles

The value of a computational science strategy emerges when we can test predictions obtained from a coherent and efficient explanation for the clinical phenomenology. Therefore, we need to be comprehensible about both the intended purpose and the further consequences of a non-local term that represents, in a CSD model, the activation level of a neural field. Before we can make verifiable clinical predictions in the next section, the physiological interpretation of the fundamental principles in the model is critical.

To put it very clearly, the development of the macroscopic CSD model described by Equations 17.3 and 17.4 is pursued in a targeted manner to produce localized structures. Therefore, the prediction cannot be that CSD exists as a localized structure. Also, the statement that large-scale neural activity is not a mere epiphenomena in itself fails to suffice as a sufficiently clear prediction. Rather, if CSD propagates as a localized solitary wave, then we predict that these patterns are caused by a non-local coupling term with well-defined features. Therefore to tackle the prediction, the interpretation of this term is crucial. However, before we do that, let us mention – to further raise confidence in this approach – that the macroscopic CSD model is able to describe CSD in curved cortical geometry [14, 33] and, in particular, in personalized simulations using individual MRI scanner readings (see Figure 17.4c–d).

We have already encountered non-local neural fields twice before. The model by Reggia and Montgomery [49, 50] introduced a neural field to model the zigzag percept, and Wilkinson raised the question of whether there is spreading activation in the synaptic circuitry, which can be thought of as synonyms for a neural field [66].

In the model described by Equations 17.3 and 17.4 [7, 11], which successfully simulated personalized the aura features shown in Figure 17.3a by the spread shown in Figure 17.4c–d, the long-range coupling did not assume a "Mexican hat" connectivity – that is, nearby excitation and distant inhibition, but the feedback effect of the activation level $a(t)$ spread out by a global inhibition. In mathematical terms, the kernel function $k(x,y)$ in Equation 17.4 was taken as a constant (i.e., $k(x,y) = K$), and not as the difference of two Gaussians.

The interpretation is that, with respect to the tissue susceptibility to CSD, the synaptic footprint does not determine the quality of the feedback to the RD model. Any activity transferred to both synaptic populations (excitatory and inhibitory) will drive the neurovascular unit (NVU) equally. It is the feedback of the NVU, as a lump concept, that preconditions the tissue at risk to be recruit into the CSD state. In other words, we propose that the NVU, in turn, has a neuroprotective effect on the CSD surrounding tissue once the blood flow rises (hyperemia – see the work by Olesen [47]), due to increased activity levels in either population. A generic version of such a physiological mechanism describes the activity level $a(t)$ in a vastly simplified form, namely by the Heaviside function $H(u)$ that assumes one, if the activator is over a threshold, and otherwise zero.

It still remains to be tested how the fast-spreading activity in the neural field influences the CSD dynamics. If, for example, the localized solitary CSD wave propagates with occasional non-local jumps, the fast-spreading activity cannot exclusively be neuroprotective. This may yield an inverted "Mexican hat" coupling effect – that is, nearby inhibition (mandate for localization), and distant excitation or additional cortico-thalamic excitatory interactions.

17.3.6 Clinical predictions

The clinically relevant supplement to the fundamental question addressed by macroscopic CSD models is: are the characteristics of different forms of propagating CSD waves related to the major sub-forms migraine without aura (MO) and migraine with aura (MA) and, if so, how? If CSD is localized, its noxious signature [32] could significantly vary with both the size of affected cortical surface area at any one time, and the location of this area with respect to gyral, sulcal, and laminar position (see Figure 17.5).

In addition to the personalized simulations (Figure 17.4c–d), we performed statistical analysis of the spatio-temporal development in a flat area of the cortex. These simulations of Equations 17.3 and 17.4 were initiated by 8000 different initial conditions, representing homeostatic perturbations, caused by local hyperactivity in pinwheel maps

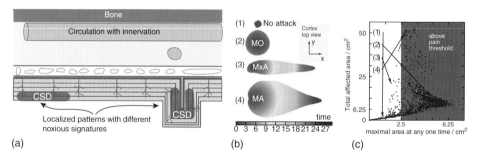

(a) (b) (c)

Figure 17.5 (a) Schematic representation of a cortical cross-section with meninges and skull; not to scale. The effect of CSD and its noxious signature could significantly vary with overall size of affected area and CSD's gyral, sulcal, and laminar location. (b) Spatiotemporal signatures of CSD. The model parameters are chosen such that only transient waves exist; note that we have scaled the dimensionless model such that the units of time are roughly corresponding to minutes, surface area to cm^2, and the speed of CSD to about 3 mm/min. Four stereotypical courses are depicted: (1) Subthreshold – CSD dies out quickly without initial spread. (2) Suprathreshold – CSD dies out after a few minutes, because the front does not break open. This form putatively corresponds to migraine without aura (MO). (3) Suprathreshold – CSD propagates for more than 20 min as a localized wave. The maximal affected area at any one time is below a pain threshold. This form putatively corresponds to typical aura without headache (MxA). (4) As before, but maximal affected area at any one time is above a pain threshold, corresponding to migraine with aura (MA). (c) Statistical analysis of 8000 events following a local random perturbation of the homogeneous steady state – see text (figure from [7]).

[3], triggering CSD [11] (see Figure 17.5b–c). Based on this, we predict that certain features related to shape, size, and duration of CSD determine the aura phase, while others determine the pain phase in migraine. We firstly divide the subtype MA into its two sub-forms, "typical aura with migraine headache" and "typical aura without headache", with the latter being referred to as MxA. Together with MO, we consider three forms and predict that each has a specific signature of CSD. Characteristic for these signatures are the spatio-temporal patterns, as shown by prototypical simulations in Figure 17.5b(1)–(4) and, furthermore, its course in the gyrified human cortex and laminar location [54], as illustrated in Figure 17.5a.

In particular, we predict that a sufficiently large surface area must be instantaneously affected by CSD. Only then can CSD lead into the pain phase in migraine. If the maximal instantaneously affected area is too small, the cascade of subsequent events causing sustained activation of trigeminal afferents [32] is not initiated. The rational behind this suggestion is that the flow of substances in the direction perpendicular to the cortical surface into the pain-sensitive meninges should be significantly convergent in order to reach noxious threshold concentration and initiate central sensitization of second order neurons. The flow driven by a small affected area is sufficiently diluted and, therefore, is tolerated. This makes a prediction that can be tested by noninvasive imaging.

Furthermore, only if CSD assumes a spatio-temporal form that is long-lasting enough (>5 minutes) and, therefore, also propagating further (>1.5 cm beyond the initial large hot spot), will CSD cause noticeable aura symptoms. In fact, this is not a prediction. It merely reflects the diagnostic criteria of migraine aura given by the International Classification of Headache Disorders: "focal neurological symptoms that usually develop gradually over 5–20 minutes". Thus, any neurological events that last less than five minutes are not usually diagnosed as migraine aura.

To summarize, the modeling approach suggest that the primary objective in research relating CSD to migraine pain should be directed to obtain a measure of the different noxious signatures that are transmitted into the meninges and drive the migraine-generator network into the pain state – that is, central sensitization.

References

1 S. Amari (1977). Dynamics of pattern formation in lateral-inhibition type neural fields. *Biological Cybernetics* **27**: 77–87.
2 K.F. Bonhoeffer (1948). Activation of passive iron as a model for the excitation of nerve. *Journal of General Physiology* **32**(1): 69–91.
3 T. Bonhoeffer and A. Grinvald (1991). Iso-orientation domains in cat visual cortex are arranged in pinwheel-like patterns. *Nature* **353**: 429–431.
4 P.C. Bressloff (2012). Spatiotemporal dynamics of continuum neural fields. *Journal of Physics A: Mathematical and Theoretical* **45**(3): 033001.
5 J. Bureš, O. Burešová, and J. Křivánek (1974). *The mechanism and applications of Leão's Spreading Depression*. Academia, New York.
6 A.C. Charles and S.M. Baca (2013). Cortical spreading depression and migraine. *Nature Reviews Neurology* **9**, 637–644.
7 M.A. Dahlem (2013). Migraine generator network and spreading depression dynamics as neuromodulation targets in episodic migraine. *Chaos* **23**: 046101.

8 M.A. Dahlem and E.P. Chronicle (2004). A computational perspective on migraine aura. *Progress in Neurobiology* **74**(6): 351–361.

9 M.A. Dahlem, R. Engelmann, S. Löwel, and S.C. Müller (2000). Does the migraine aura reflect cortical organization. *European Journal of Neuroscience* **12**: 767–770.

10 M.A. Dahlem and N. Hadjikhani (2009). Migraine aura: retracting particle-like waves in weakly susceptible cortex. *PLoS One* **4**: e5007.

11 M.A. Dahlem and T.M. Isele (2013). Transient localized wave patterns and their application to migraine. *Journal of Mathematical Neuroscience* **3**: 7.

12 M.A. Dahlem and S.C. Müller (2004). Reaction–diffusion waves in neuronal tissue and the window of cortical excitability. *Annals of Physics* **13**(7): 442–449.

13 M.A. Dahlem, J. Schumacher, and N. Hübel (2014). Linking a genetic defect in migraine to spreading depression in a computational model. *PeerJ* **2**: e379.

14 M.A. Dahlem, B. Schmidt, I. Bojak, S. Boie, F. Kneer, N. Hadjikhani, and J. Kurths (2015). Cortical hot spots and labyrinths: Why neuromodulation devices for episodic migraine should be personalized. *Frontiers in Computational Neuroscience* **9**: 29.

15 R. FitzHugh (1955). Mathematical models of threshold phenomena in the nerve membrane. *Bulletin of Mathematical Biology* **17**(4): 257–278.

16 B. Grafstein (1956). Locus of propagation of spreading cortical depression. *Journal of Neurophysiology* **19**(4): 308–316.

17 B. Grafstein (1963). Neural release of potassium during spreading depression. In M. A. B. Brazier (ed). *Brain Function. Cortical Excitability and Steady Potentials*, pp. 87–124. University of California Press, Berkeley, CA.

18 O-J. Grüsser (1995). Migraine phosphenes and the retino-cortical magnification factor. *Vision Research* **35**(8): 1125–1134.

19 N. Hadjikhani, M. Sanchez del Rio, O. Wu, D. Schwartz, D. Bakker, B. Fischl, K.K. Kwong, F.M. Cutrer, B.R. Rosen, R.B. Tootell, A.G. Sorensen, and M.A. Moskowitz (2001). Mechanisms of migraine aura revealed by functional MRI in human visual cortex. *Proceedings of the National Academy of Sciences of the United States of America* **98**: 4687–4692.

20 J. Møller Hansen, S.M. Baca, P. VanValkenburgh, and A. Charles (2013). Distinctive anatomical and physiological features of migraine aura revealed by 18 years of recording. *Brain* **136**(12): 3589–3595.

21 U. Heinemann and H.D. Lux (1977). Ceiling of stimulus induced rises in extracellular potassium concentration in the cerebral cortex of cat. *Brain Research* **120**: 231–249.

22 O. Herreras (2005). Electrical prodromals of spreading depression void Grafstein's potassium hypothesis. *Journal of Neurophysiology* **94**: 3656–3657.

23 J.L. Hindmarsh and R.M. Rose (1982). A model of the nerve impulse using two first-order differential equations. *Nature* **296**: 162.

24 A.L. Hodgkin and A.F. Huxley (1952). A quantitative description of membrane current and its application to conduction and excitation in nerve. *Journal of Physiology* **117**: 500–544.

25 N. Hübel and M.A. Dahlem (2014). Dynamics from seconds to hours in Hodgkin-Huxley model with time–dependent ion concentrations and buffer reservoirs. *PLoS Computational Biology* **10**: e1003941.

26 N. Hübel, E. Schöll, and M.A. Dahlem (2014). Bistable dynamics underlying excitability of ion homeostasis in neuron models. *PLoS Computational Biology* **10**: e1003551.

27 E.M. Izhikevich and J. Moehlis (2008). Dynamical systems in neuroscience: The geometry of excitability and bursting. *SIAM Review* **50**(2): 397.

28 H. Kager, W.J. Wadman, and G.G. Somjen (2000). Simulated seizures and spreading depression in a neuron model incorporating interstitial space and ion concentrations. *Journal of Neurophysiology* **84**: 495–512.

29 H. Kager, W.J. Wadman, and G.G. Somjen (2002). Conditions for the triggering of spreading depression studied with computer simulations. *Journal of Neurophysiology* **88**(5): 2700.

30 H. Kager, W.J. Wadman, and G.G. Somjen (2007). Seizure–like afterdischarges simulated in a model neuron. *Journal of Computational Neuroscience* **22**: 105–128.

31 R. Kapral and K. Showalter (eds, 1995). *Chemical Waves and Patterns*. Kluwer, Dordrecht.

32 H. Karatas, S.E. Erdener, Y. Gursoy-Ozdemir, S. Lule, E. Eren-Kocak, Z.D. Sen, and T. Dalkara (2013). Spreading depression triggers headache by activating neuronal Panx1 channels. *Science* **339**(6123): 1092–1095.

33 F. Kneer, E. Schöll, and M.A. Dahlem (2014). Nucleation of reaction-diffusion waves on curved surfaces. *New Journal of Physics* **16**: 053010.

34 K. Krischer and A.S. Mikhailov (1994). Bifurcation to traveling spots in reaction-diffusion systems. *Physical Review Letters* **73**(23): 3165–3168.

35 K. Lashley (1941). Patterns of cerebral integration indicated by scotomas of migraine. *Archives of Neurology & Psychiatry* **46**: 331–339.

36 M. Lauritzen (1987). Cortical spreading depression as a putative migraine mechanism. *Trends in Neurosciences* **10**(1): 8–13.

37 J. Makarova, J.M. Ibarz, S. Canals, and O. Herreras (2007). A steady-state model of spreading depression predicts the importance of an unknown conductance in specific dendritic domains. *Biophysical Journal* **92**: 4216–4232.

38 E. Mihaliuk, T. Sakurai, F. Chirila, and K. Showalter (2002). Feedback stabilization of unstable propagating waves. *Physical Review E: Statistical, Nonlinear, and Soft Matter Physics* **65**(6): 065602.

39 A.S. Mikhailov and K. Showalter (2006). Control of waves, patterns and turbulence in chemical systems. *Physics Reports* **425**: 79–194.

40 R.M. Miura, H. Huang, and J.J. Wylie (2007). Cortical spreading depression: An enigma. *European Physical Journal – Special Topics* **147**(1): 287–302.

41 J.S. Mogil (2009). Animal models of pain: progress and challenges. *Nature Reviews Neuroscience* **10**(4): 283–294.

42 C. Morris and H. Lecar (1981). Voltage oscillations in the barnacle giant muscle fiber. *Biophysical Journal* **35**: 193.

43 M. Müller and G.G. Somjen (1998). Inhibition of major cationic inward currents prevents spreading depression–like hypoxic depolarization in rat hippocampal tissue slices. *Brain Research* **812**(1–2): 1–13.

44 J. Nagumo, S. Arimoto, and S. Yoshizawa (1962). An active pulse transmission line simulating nerve axon. *Proceedings of the IRE* **50**: 2061–2070.

45 F.J. Niedernostheide, B.S. Kerner, and H.G. Purwins (1992). Spontaneous appearance of rocking localized current filaments in a nonequilibrium distributive system. *Physical Review B: Condensed Matter and Materials Physics* **46**: 7559.

46 F.J. Niedernostheide, M. Or-Guil, M Kleinkes, and H.G. Purwins (1997). Dynamical behavior of spots in a nonequilibrium distributive active medium. *Physical Review E: Statistical, Nonlinear, and Soft Matter Physics* **55**: 4107.

47 J. Olesen, B. Larsen, and M. Lauritzen (1981). Focal hyperemia followed by spreading oligemia and impaired activation of rCBF in classic migraine. *Annals of Neurology* **9**: 344–352.

48 E. Pöppel (1973). Fortification illusion during an attack of ophthalmic migraine. *Implications for the human visual cortex. Naturwissenschaften* **60**: 554–555.

49 J.A. Reggia and D. Montgomery (1994). *Modeling cortical spreading depression.* Proceedings of the Annual Symposium on Computer Applications in Medical Care, pp. 873–877.

50 J.A. Reggia and D. Montgomery (1996). A computational model of visual hallucinations in migraine. *Computers in Biology and Medicine* **26**: 133–141.

51 J.A. Reggia, C Lynne D'Autrechy, Granger G Sutton III, and Michael Weinrich (1992). A competitive distribution theory of neocortical dynamics. *Neural Computation* **4**(3): 287–317.

52 L.V. Reshodko and J. Bures (1975). Computer simulation of reverberating spreading depression in a network of cell automata. *Biological Cybernetics* **18**: 181–189.

53 W. Richards (1971). The fortification illusions of migraines. *Scientific American* **224**: 88–96.

54 F. Richter and A. Lehmenkühler (1993). Spreading depression can be restricted to distinct depths of the rat cerebral cortex. *Neuroscience Letters* **152**(1): 65–68.

55 J. Rinzel and J.B. Keller (1973). Traveling Wave Solutions of a Nerve Conduction Equation. *Biophysical Journal* **13**(12): 1313–1337.

56 E. Santos, M. Schöll, R. Sánchez-Porras, M.A. Dahlem, H. Silos, A. Unterberg, H. Dickhaus, and O.W. Sakowitz (2014). Radial, spiral and reverberating waves of spreading depolarization occur in the gyrencephalic brain. *NeuroImage* **99**: 244–255.

57 E. Schwartz (1980). A quantitative model of the functional architecture of human striate cortex with application to visual illusion and cortical texture analysis. *Biological Cybernetics* **37**: 63–76.

58 G.G. Somjen (2005). Aristides Leao's discovery of cortical spreading depression. *Journal of Neurophysiology* **94**: 2–4.

59 G.G. Somjen, H. Kager, and W.J. Wadman (2008). Computer simulations of neuron-glia interactions mediated by ion flux. *Journal of Computational Neuroscience* **25**(2): 349–365.

60 G.G. Somjen, H. Kager, and W.J. Wadman (2009). Calcium sensitive non-selective cation current promotes seizure-like discharges and spreading depression in a model neuron. *Journal of Computational Neuroscience* **26**(1): 139–147.

61 A.J. Strong (2005). Dr. Bernice Grafstein's paper on the mechanism of spreading depression. *Journal of Neurophysiology* **94**: 5–7.

62 H.C. Tuckwell (1981). Simplified reaction-diffusion equations for potassium and calcium ion concentrations during spreading cortical depression. *International Journal of Neuroscience* **12**: 95–107.

63 H.C. Tuckwell and R.M. Miura (1978). A mathematical model for spreading cortical depression. *Biophysical Journal* **23**: 257–276.

64 M. Vincent and N. Hadjikhani (2007). Migraine aura and related phenomena: beyond scotomata and scintillations. *Cephalalgia* **27**: 1368–1377.

65 N. Wiener and A. Rosenblueth (1946). The mathematical formulation of the problem of conduction of impulses in a network of connected excitable elements, specially in cardiac muscle. *Archivos del Instituto de Cardiologia de Mexico* **16**: 205–243.

66 F. Wilkinson (2004). Auras and other hallucinations: windows on the visual brain. Prog. *Brain Research* **144**: 305–320.

67 H.R. Wilson and J.D. Cowan (1972). Excitatory and inhibitory interactions in localized populations of model neurons. *Biophysical Journal* **12**: 1–24.

68 W. Yao, H. Huang, and R.M. Miura (2011). A continuum neural model for the instigation and propagation of cortical spreading depression. *Bulletin of Mathematical Biology* **73**: 2773–2790.

18

Tools for high-resolution *in vivo* imaging of cellular and molecular mechanisms in cortical spreading depression and spreading depolarization

Kıvılcım Kılıç[1], Hana Uhlirova[2], Peifang Tian[3], Payam A. Saisan[1], Mohammad Abbas Yaseen[4], Jonghwan Lee[4], Sergei A. Vinogradov[5], David A. Boas[4], Sava Sakadžić[4] and Anna Devor[6]

[1] Department of Neurosciences, UCSD, La Jolla, California, USA
[2] Department of Radiology, UCSD, La Jolla, California, USA
[3] Department of Physics, John Carroll University, University Heights, Ohio, USA
[4] Martinos Center for Biomedical Imaging, MGH, Harvard Medical School, Charlestown, Massachusetts, USA
[5] Departments of Biochemistry and Biophysics and Chemistry, University of Pennsylvania, Philadelphia, Pennsylvania, USA
[6] Departments of Neurosciences and Radiology, UCSD, La Jolla, California, USA

18.1 Introduction

Cortical spreading depression (CSD) is a commonly used model for migraine aura in animal studies. CSD is a transient, self-propagating wave of cellular depolarization in the cerebral cortex that causes a massive increase in extracellular K^+ and glutamate, and increase in intracellular Ca^{2+} in neurons and astrocytes [1]. This disturbance of ionic homeostasis is accompanied by a spreading wave of arteriolar diameter changes, commonly featuring vasoconstriction, followed by partial relaxation and further sustained constriction in most species [2, 3]. Results in cortical slices suggest that these vascular changes result from astrocytic Ca^{2+} waves [4, 5] causing release of vasoactive metabolites of arachidonic acid (AA) – specifically, a vasoconstrictive messenger 20-hydroxyeicosatetraeonic acid (20-HETE). In support of this hypothesis, an *in vivo* study using 2-photon Ca^{2+} imaging has demonstrated that vasoconstriction occurs when astrocytic Ca^{2+} wave invades a perivascular endfoot and is inhibited upon pharmacological interference targeted to prevent the refill of intracellular Ca^{2+} stores [6].

An increase in intracellular Ca^{2+} is also known to trigger an increase in mitochondrial oxidative phosphorylation [7] and, therefore, in O_2 demand. In agreement with this expectation, a number of *in vivo* rodent imaging studies have indicated that CSD may induce an increase in O_2 demand exceeding vascular O_2 supply [3, 8]. Notably, combining 2-photon imaging of the reduced nicotinamide adenine dinucleotide (NADH) with point measurements of the partial pressure of O_2 (pO_2) in tissue and vasodilation/perfusion measurements, Takano *et al.* concluded that hypoxia was observed even in the presence of an increase in cerebral blood flow (CBF) [8].

The abovementioned studies underscore the importance of microscopic imaging technology for *in vivo* mechanistic investigation of pathophysiology. Below, we will

Neurobiological Basis of Migraine, First Edition. Edited by Turgay Dalkara and Michael A. Moskowitz.

consider a number of microscopic methods for neurovascular and neurometabolic imaging in the context of open questions in the study of CSD.

18.2 Large-scale imaging of vascular dynamics with microscopic resolution

Even in the absence of spreading fronts of neuronal activity, cerebral arteries and arterioles can propagate dilation and constriction along the vessel, and this holds true for both pial and parenchymal vessels. Two-photon imaging in anesthetized rats and mice has revealed that, during normal neurovascular coupling, the initial dilation occurs below layer IV, suggesting that at least some of the underlying mechanisms can be specific to the infragranular layers [9, 10]. In CSD, however, a number of documented mechanisms specifically localize to the brain surface, including activation of pial nociceptors and local neurogenic inflammation [11–13].

Therefore, spatiotemporally resolved microscopic measurements of concrete physiological parameters on the brain surface are of interest in CSD. Among these are measurements of blood oxygenation, diameter and blood flow velocity in pial vessels. These types of measurements can be performed with a relatively simple optical setup, using a CCD camera as a detector. In contrast to scanning optical methods, such as confocal and 2-photon microscopy, a CCD camera captures a 2-D image "at once", leading to higher affordable frame rate. The disadvantage, however, is the lack of true depth resolution: the signal at every pixel represents a weighted sum of the response through the whole depth of light penetration, with the highest sensitivity to the cortical surface [9, 14].

Blood oxygenation can be quantified by measuring the hemoglobin absorption at multiple wavelengths of light, using Optical Intrinsic Signal Imaging (OISI) [15, 16]. Recently, the laboratory of Elizabeth Hillman refined CCD-based technology to determine total hemoglobin, indicative of vasodilation, in the surface vasculature [17–19]. Using high resolution (256×256) and high-speed CCD imaging (30 frames per second), they were able to measure an increase in the total hemoglobin within individual surface vessels across a large field of view (3×3 mm). With this setup, they demonstrated that the same pial artery can propagate the response both upstream and downstream, depending upon the location of the neuronal response. Applied to CSD, this technology would allow a detailed study of propagated dilation and constriction along surface arterioles, and may provide an effective test bed for experimental (e.g., pharmacological or optogenetic) interventions in cases where cellular resolution or sampling of deep tissue is not required.

Relative blood flow changes can be measured with Laser Speckle Contrast Imaging (LSCI) [2, 20, 21] by exploiting the dynamic fluctuations that moving red blood cells (RBC) impose on the random interference pattern of the reflected laser light. Due to its simplicity, imaging speed, and large field of view (FOV), LSCI has been invaluable for investigating CBF changes during spreading depolarizations (SDs). For example, LSCI was utilized to characterize the tri-phasic CBF response during SD [22], and to investigate the vasoconstrictive neurovascular coupling during ischemic depolarizations, which contributes to hemodynamic progression in acute focal cerebral ischemia [23]. In combination with OISI, LSCI was utilized to assess the impact of SDs under different

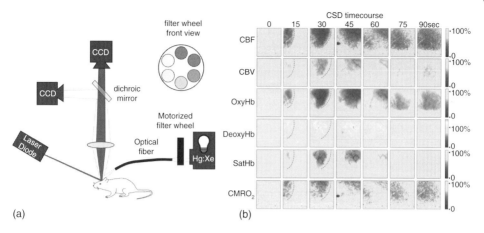

Figure 18.1 Combined OISI and LSCI in CSD. (a) Schematic of instrument used for combined OISI and LSCI. (b) Time-lapse images of hemodynamic and metabolic changes during CSD. For more details see [3]. Reproduced by permission of SAGE.

physiological and pharmacological manipulations [3, 24–26], as well as to investigate mechanisms of triggering SD [27] (Figure 18.1).

In spite of its significant utility, LSCI does not resolve the microvasculature, and does not quantify absolute blood flow. Recent studies suggest that baseline flow is important to understand some aspects of SD, such as tissue susceptibility to SD triggering, SD duration, and polymorphic appearance of CBF transients during SD [27–29]. Furthermore, knowledge about the relation between SD and capillary flow patterns may be essential, both for understanding the impact of SD on tissue viability and for developing novel treatments [6, 30, 31].

This gap in imaging technology can be overcome by Optical Coherence Tomography (OCT), which can provide rapid, depth-resolved imaging of absolute blood flow in individual cortical arterioles and venules over a large FOV, as well as imaging of RBC flux in capillaries [32, 33]. In addition, OCT can assess both tissue scattering, a hallmark of cellular changes associated with depolarizations [34], and tissue motility. These measurements may have an important role in investigating SD impact on tissue viability. Compared to 2-photon microscopy, the advantages of OCT include:

1) increased penetration depth through the thinned skull of mice;
2) >1 mm penetration depth through a cranial window;
3) reliance on endogenous contrast (i.e. optical scattering) instead of exogenous contrast agents; and
4) improved volumetric image acquisition speed.

18.3 Combining measurements of single-vessel diameter with imaging and quantification of intracellular Ca²⁺ in neurons and astrocytes

In vivo measurements of parenchymal vessel diameter typically requires 2-photon microscopy and an intravascular fluorescent agent (e.g., fluorescein isothiocyanate

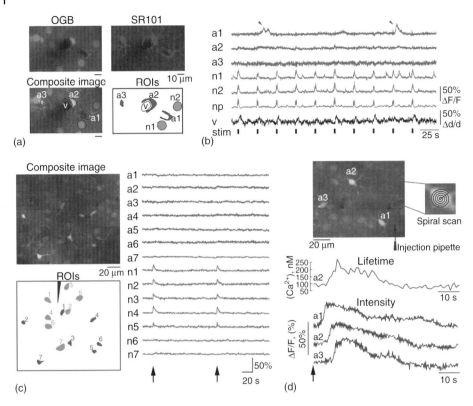

Figure 18.2 Calcium imaging and quantification. (a) Field of view (FOV) 200 μm below the surface, with perivascular astrocytes labeled by OGB (top left frame) and sulforhodamine 101 (SR101, top right frame). Neurons are labeled with OGB only. (b) Time-courses extracted from regions of interest (ROIs) in (a). Arrowheads point to a spontaneous calcium increase in ROI labeled a1. Dilation time-course is labeled with v. (c) Left: Response to puffs of 1 mM glutamate in layer II/III. The injection micropipette contained glutamate. Right: calcium signal time-courses. (d) Quantification of astrocytic calcium *in vivo* with 2-photon FLIM. Top: A composite image of OGB and SR101. A "spiral" sampling trajectory within a single astrocytic cell body is shown on the right. Bottom: FLIM and fluorescence intensity time-courses in response to puff of 1 mM ATP.

(FITC)-labeled dextran [9, 35]). When used with synthetic or genetically encoded Ca^{2+} indicators [48], 2-photon vascular measurements can be combined with imaging of intracellular Ca^{2+} in neurons and astrocytes [36]. Dilation can also be estimated from the expansion of unlabelled vascular cross-section, outlined by the astrocytic endfoot stained with sulforhodamine-101 (Figure 18.2a).

The role of astrocytic Ca^{2+} activity deserves a special note in the context of CSD. Astrocytic Ca^{2+} waves appear secondary to neuronal depolarization (for a recent review see [37]), although it may be required for the CSD-associated vasoconstriction [6]. Interestingly, the same study showed that, in the absence of CSD, spontaneous increases in astrocytic Ca^{2+} did not impact vessel diameter. This finding was recently corroborated by Bonder and McCarthy, who produced Ca^{2+} surges using selective stimulation of astrocytic Gq-GPCR cascades with a designer receptors exclusively activated by designer drugs system (DREADD) [38].

It remains unclear why astrocytic Ca^{2+} increases produce vasoconstriction in the presence of CSD, while spontaneous astrocytic Ca^{2+} activity has no vasoactive effect. It is possible that CSD produces a much larger increase in the absolute intracellular Ca^{2+} concentration necessary to trigger the synthesis and release of the gliotransmitters driving vasoconstriction (e.g., arachidonic acid metabolite 20-HETE). Evaluation of this possibility requires quantitative Ca^{2+} measurements with sufficient temporal resolution to reconstruct dynamic Ca^{2+} signaling events.

Under 2-photon excitation, quantification of Ca^{2+} can be provided by genetically-encoded Ca^{2+}-sensitive Fluorescence Resonance Energy Transfer (FRET) probes [39], or Fluorescence Lifetime Imaging Microscopy (FLIM) [40]. Notably, a commonly used synthetic Ca^{2+} indicator, Oregon Green 488 BAPTA-1 AM (OGB), displays an increase in fluorescent decay lifetime when bound to Ca^{2+} [41], and can be used for 2-photon FLIM *in vivo* [42]. Using optimal laser scanning trajectories, this technology can be successfully employed to obtain the absolute level of Ca^{2+} with cellular resolution in a dynamic regime (Figure 18.2d).

Combined with pharmacological and genetic tools, quantitative imaging of Ca^{2+} in astrocytes may help to unravel the complexity of astrocytic Ca^{2+} activity. In CSD, potentially, the role of Ca^{2+} may be harmful rather than helpful, limiting blood supply and ATP availability for neuronal activity. Suppression of this excitability in turn may prevent the CSD-induced vasoconstriction while not interfering with other vital astrocytic functions such as K^+ uptake [43, 44].

18.4 NADH autofluorescence: an endogenous marker of energy metabolism

NADH is the principal electron carrier in glycolysis, the tricarboxylic acid (TCA) cycle, and the mitochondrial respiratory chain. NADH is generated both during glycolysis in the cytosol and the TCA cycle in the mitochondria, and it is oxidized to NAD^+ in the electron transport chain during oxidative phosphorylation (respiration). The rates of NADH production and its oxidation to NAD^+ accelerate with an increase in the demand for metabolic energy that accompanies an increase in neuronal activity. However, during a transient metabolic response to neuronal perturbation, the rates are mismatched, leading to transient increases or decreases in the $NADH/NAD^+$ ratio. Importantly, the NADH molecule is fluorescent, while NAD^+ is not. Therefore, a change in the ratio of $NADH/NAD^+$ can be observed as a change in NADH fluorescence.

Early cortical surface imaging studies have indicated that, under normal physiological conditions in anesthetized animals, NADH fluorescence decreases in response to an increase in neuronal activity, and increases during a respiratory arrest [45, 46]. Two-photon imaging of NADH is consistent with these observations [47, 48]. Interpretation of NADH fluorescence observations, however, has remained ambiguous, due to its role in both glycolysis (within the cytosol) and respiration (within the mitochondria). Recently, the first genetically encoded NADH probes have been developed, providing a possibility of specific targeting to the cytosol or mitochondria [49, 50]. While 2-photon imaging of these probes has not been attempted yet, studies in cell cultures have estimated a difference of over two orders of magnitude between the mitochondrial and cytosolic NADH ($\approx 30 \, \mu M$ and $\approx 0.15 \, \mu M$, respectively), supporting the notion that intrinsic NADH signals are largely of mitochondrial origin [51]. Thus, glycolysis may be largely invisible to intrinsic NADH imaging.

Another two probes that may provide new insights into the role of glycolysis and oxidative phosphorylation in meeting the energy needs are genetically encoded FRET sensors for lactate and pyruvate, developed by the laboratory of Felipe Barros [52–54]. *In vivo* 2-photon imaging of the lactate probe, targeted to cortical astrocytes, revealed a rapid decrease in the intracellular lactate upon direct cortical stimulation, followed by an overshoot [54]. This result is consistent with previously hypothesized astrocytic lactate release upon an increase in neuronal activity [55]. However, whether this lactate serves a metabolic fuel for neurons or messenger/neuroprotective agent remains unclear [56].

In CSD, *in vivo* 2-photon NADH imaging revealed an increase in NADH fluorescence in between capillaries, even in the presence of blood flow increase. Assuming that the signal reflected an increase in cytosolic glycolysis, the authors concluded that "tissue hypoxia associated with CSD is caused by a transient increase in O_2 demand exceeding vascular O_2 supply." This conclusion, however, may also hold in the case that all the detected fluorescence originates from mitochondria, because an increase in the mitochondrial $NADH/NAD^+$ ratio can serve as an indication of O_2 deficit.

18.5 Direct imaging of molecular O_2 in blood and tissue

Numerous questions important for understanding CSD are related to tissue oxygenation:

- Does CSD cause tissue hypoxia, and what is the level of hypoxia during different phases of CSD?
- How large is the mismatch between oxygen supply and demand during CSD?
- How does CSD influence the cerebral metabolic rate of O_2 ($CMRO_2$), and are the effects of CSD on tissue detrimental?
- What is the relation between tissue oxygen supply and triggering of CSD and the resultant impact on tissue?
- What are the effective strategies for manipulating CSD?

Addressing these questions requires direct measurements of molecular O_2 within capillary domains. Recently, these types of measurements became possible, due to development of a new microscopic imaging technology, termed "2-photon phosphorescence lifetime microscopy" (2PLM), which combines O_2-sensitive two-photon-enhanced phosphorescent nanoprobes with 2-photon microscopy [57]. This method uses phosphorescence quenching to quantify absolute O_2 concentration [58, 59], and is uniquely capable of measuring the partial pressure of O_2 (pO_2) in intact cerebral cortex, because 2-photon excitation is confined to the focal spot, reducing out-of-focus signals, minimizing photodamage, and allowing measurements deeper in the brain's interstitial space and vasculature with high resolution [60–66].

2PLM measurements have revealed that cortical arterioles are responsible for up to 50% of oxygen extraction at rest [64], and that the tissue pO_2 landscape is largely

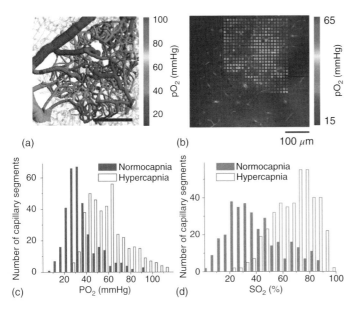

Figure 18.3 Two-photon imaging of O_2 concentration in the brain. (a) Mouse cortical microvascular pO_2 measurements, using 2PLM overlaid with microvascular structures [64]. pO_2 measurements in anesthetized mice were performed down to 450 µm below the cortical surface. Scale bar = 200 µm. (b) A grid of intravascular and tissue pO_2 values measured by 2PLM in a rat somatosensory cortex, superimposed on the vascular reference image [67]. pO_2 in cortical tissue exhibits significant heterogeneity, while the pO_2 landscape is dominated by the oxygen diffusion from the penetrating arterioles. (c–d) Capillary pO_2 and oxygen saturation (SO_2) histograms. (c) Histograms of mouse capillary pO_2 measured by 2PLM during normoxic normocapnia (solid bars) and normoxic hypercapnia (empty bars). (d) Mouse capillary SO_2 histograms, calculated based on data from (c), using Hill's equation [64]. Reproduced by permission of Nature Publishing Group.

dominated by oxygen diffusion from arterioles (Figure 18.3) [60, 67]. In addition, both pO_2 in tissue distant from arterioles, and pO_2 in the capillary network, are very heterogeneous (Figure 18.3). Such heterogeneity suggests that, in spite of the relatively small oxygen extraction fraction from capillaries in the brain cortex, some capillary segments and tissue in their proximity may always have low oxygenation. These tissue regions may be particularly vulnerable to decreases in CBF and/or increases in $CMRO_2$. Since CSD may be associated with simultaneous transient CBF decrease and $CMRO_2$ increase [3, 68], this double perfusion and metabolic impact on tissue may lead to formation of transiently hypoxic tissue regions.

2PLM monitoring of tissue PO_2 in capillary domains may help unravel critical questions about the mismatch between O_2 supply and demand during CSD. In addition, pO_2 measurements enable estimation of $CMRO_2$, which is another key physiological parameter for understanding CSD impact on tissue [69]. Finally, pO_2 and CBF measurements, in combination with the assessment of additional functional markers such as NADH and Ca^{2+} concentration, will help us gain a more complete understanding of this complex phenomenon.

18.6 Employing optogenetics to study inter-cellular communication

Optogenetics is a tool of indisputable significance to neuroscience, from the subcellular to systems level [70–72]. Optogenetics is only starting to make inroads into the study of CSD, and holds great potential in multiple aspects of this complex disorder, including novel ways of triggering the CSD wave [73], as well as dissecting its electrophysiological and neurovascular mechanisms. For example, an overwhelming majority of studies on astrocytic Ca^{2+} surges [74–76] have focused on the effects downstream from activation of metabotropic glutamate receptors (mGluRs) [77]. However, astrocytes express a large repertoire of G-protein coupled receptors (GCPRs), not only for glutamate but also for acetylcholine (ACh), noradrenaline (NA), somatostatin (SST) and vasoactive intestinal peptide (VIP), which can, potentially contribute to the astrocytic Ca^{2+} wave in CSD. Addressing these non-glutamatergic signaling pathways with respect to astrocytic Ca^{2+} activity is challenging, because different neuronal cell types are wired together and are co-activated during circuit activity. Optogenetics, however, allows selective stimulation of a particular cell type (e.g., ACh-positive interneurons [78]). To ensure the specificity, one would have to prevent propagation of activation to other neuronal cell types – for example, using pharmacological means. Optogenetics has already been applied by a number of laboratories, including our own, to study neurovascular/hemodynamic effects [10, 79–84].

18.7 Conclusions and outlook

Above, we emphasized a number of "ready for primetime" technologies for microscopic imaging of vascular, metabolic, and neuroglial parameters, and specific manipulation of brain activity of relevance to CSD research. This list is less than comprehensive. Moreover, both optical instrumentation and optical probes continue to develop rapidly. This growth is likely to experience acceleration in the near future, in light of the BRAIN initiative focused on providing new tools for neuroscience [85, 86]. One of the key goals of the initiative is large-scale imaging with microscopic resolution. In this respect, one "method to watch" is photoacoustic microscopy [87]; another is lightsheet microscopy [88, 89]. Extending the field of view of 2-photon microscopy is also being explored [90].

The efforts to engineer novel optical instrumentation are paralleled by development of novel optical probes/reporters of specific physiological processes. We already mentioned, above, reporters of Ca^{2+}, NADH, lactate, pyruvate, and O_2. Significant progress has also been made towards detecting other metal ions, neurotransmitters (glutamate, NO), H^+, reactive O_2 species, and other biomolecules, such as matrix metalloproteinases (for a recent review, see [91]).

To conclude, a substantial arsenal of already available tools for both imaging and manipulation of the relevant physiological processes provides exciting opportunities for exploring the CSD *in vivo*. We hope that this chapter will find its way into the hands of CSD investigators, and will serve as a motivation to utilize these new methods and form interdisciplinary collaborations. On our side, we deeply believe that a breakthrough in the mechanistic understanding of this physiological phenomenon, as well as many others, will emerge at this interface of biology/medicine and technology/engineering.

References

1 Moskowitz MA, Bolay H, and Dalkara T (2004). Deciphering migraine mechanisms: clues from familial hemiplegic migraine genotypes. *Annals of Neurology* **55**(2): 276–280.

2 Ayata C, *et al.* (2004). Laser speckle flowmetry for the study of cerebrovascular physiology in normal and ischemic mouse cortex. *Journal of Cerebral Blood Flow and Metabolism* **24**(7): 744–755.

3 Yuzawa I, *et al.* (2012). Cortical spreading depression impairs oxygen delivery and metabolism in mice. *Journal of Cerebral Blood Flow and Metabolism* **32**(2): 376–386.

4 Peters O, Schipke CG, Hashimoto Y, and Kettenmann H (2003). Different mechanisms promote astrocyte Ca^{2+} waves and spreading depression in the mouse neocortex. *Journal of Neuroscience* **23**(30): 9888–9896.

5 Basarsky TA, Duffy SN, Andrew RD, and MacVicar BA (1998). Imaging spreading depression and associated intr acellular calcium waves in brain slices. *Journal of Neuroscience* **18**(18): 7189–7199.

6 Chuquet J, Hollender L, and Nimchinsky EA (2007). High-resolution *in vivo* imaging of the neurovascular unit during spreading depression. *Journal of Neuroscience* **27**(15): 4036–4044.

7 Pizzo P, Drago I, Filadi R, and Pozzan T (2012). Mitochondrial Ca(2)(+) homeostasis: mechanism, role, and tissue specificities. *Pflügers Archiv* **464**(1): 3–17.

8 Takano T, *et al.* (2007). Cortical spreading depression causes and coincides with tissue hypoxia. *Nature Neuroscience* **10**(6): 754–762.

9 Tian P, *et al.* (2010). Cortical depth-specific microvascular dilation underlies laminar differences in blood oxygenation level-dependent functional MRI signal. *Proceedings of the National Academy of Sciences of the United States of America* **107**(34): 15246–15251.

10 Uhlirova H, Kılıç K, Tian P, Thunemann M, Desjardins M, Saisan PA, Sakadžić S, Ness TV, Mateo C, Cheng Q, Weldy KL, Razoux F, Vandenberghe M, Cremonesi JA, Ferri CG, Nizar K, Sridhar VB, Steed TC, Abashin M, Fainman Y, Masliah E, Djurovic S, Andreassen OA, Silva GA, Boas DA, Kleinfeld D, Buxton RB, Einevoll GT, Dale AM, Devor A, Elife. (2016). May 31;5. pii: e14315. doi: 10.7554/eLife.14315.

11 Karatas H, *et al.* (2013). Spreading depression triggers headache by activating neuronal Panx1 channels. *Science* **339**(6123): 1092–1095.

12 Zhang X, *et al.* (2010). Activation of meningeal nociceptors by cortical spreading depression: implications for migraine with aura. *Journal of Neuroscience* **30**(26): 8807–8814.

13 Bolay H, *et al.* (2002). Intrinsic brain activity triggers trigeminal meningeal afferents in a migraine model. *Nature Medicine* **8**(2): 136–142.

14 Polimeni JR, Granquist-Fraser D, Wood RJ, and Schwartz EL (2005). Physical limits to spatial resolution of optical recording: clarifying the spatial structure of cortical hypercolumns. *Proceedings of the National Academy of Sciences of the United States of America* **102**(11): 4158–4163.

15 Dunn AK, *et al.* (2003). Simultaneous imaging of total cerebral hemoglobin concentration, oxygenation, and blood flow during functional activation. *Optics Letters* **28**(1): 28–30.

16 Kohl M, *et al.* (2000). Physical model for the spectroscopic analysis of cortical intrinsic optical signals. *Physics in Medicine and Biology* **45**(12): 3749–3764.

17 Bouchard MB, Chen BR, Burgess SA, and Hillman EM (2009). Ultra-fast multispectral optical imaging of cortical oxygenation, blood flow, and intracellular calcium dynamics. *Optics Express* **17**(18): 15670–15678.

18 Chen BR, Bouchard MB, McCaslin AF, Burgess SA, and Hillman EM (2011). High-speed vascular dynamics of the hemodynamic response. *Neuroimage* **54**(2): 1021–1030.

19 Chen BR, Kozberg MG, Bouchard MB, Shaik MA, and Hillman EM (2014). A critical role for the vascular endothelium in functional neurovascular coupling in the brain. *Journal of the American Heart Association* **3**(3): e000787.

20 Draijer M, Hondebrink E, van Leeuwen T, and Steenbergen W (2008). Review of laser speckle contrast techniques for visualizing tissue perfusion. *Lasers in Medical Science* **24**(4): 639–651.

21 Dunn AK, Bolay H, Moskowitz MA, and Boas DA (2001). Dynamic imaging of cerebral blood flow using laser speckle. *Journal of Cerebral Blood Flow and Metabolism* **21**(3): 195–201.

22 Ayata C, *et al.* (2004). Pronounced hypoperfusion during spreading depression in mouse cortex. *Journal of Cerebral Blood Flow and Metabolism* **24**(10): 1172–1182.

23 Shin HK, *et al.* (2006). Vasoconstrictive neurovascular coupling during focal ischemic depolarizations. *Journal of Cerebral Blood Flow and Metabolism* **26**(8): 1018–1030.

24 Shin HK, *et al.* (2007). Normobaric hyperoxia improves cerebral blood flow and oxygenation, and inhibits peri-infarct depolarizations in experimental focal ischaemia. *Brain* **130**(Pt 6): 1631–1642.

25 Shin HK, *et al.* (2008). Mild induced hypertension improves blood flow and oxygen metabolism in transient focal cerebral ischemia. *Stroke* **39**(5): 1548–1555.

26 Jones PB, *et al.* (2008). Simultaneous multispectral reflectance imaging and laser speckle flowmetry of cerebral blood flow and oxygen metabolism in focal cerebral ischemia. *Journal of Biomedical Optics* **13**(4): 044007.

27 von Bornstadt D, *et al.* (2015). Supply-Demand Mismatch Transients in Susceptible Peri-infarct Hot Zones Explain the Origins of Spreading Injury Depolarizations. *Neuron* **85**(5): 1117–1131.

28 Sukhotinsky I, *et al.* (2010). Perfusion pressure-dependent recovery of cortical spreading depression is independent of tissue oxygenation over a wide physiologic range. *Journal of Cerebral Blood Flow and Metabolism* **30**(6): 1168–1177.

29 Sukhotinsky I, Dilekoz E, Moskowitz MA, and Ayata C (2008). Hypoxia and hypotension transform the blood flow response to cortical spreading depression from hyperemia into hypoperfusion in the rat. *Journal of Cerebral Blood Flow and Metabolism* **28**(7): 1369–1376.

30 Unekawa M, Tomita M, Tomita Y, Toriumi H, and Suzuki N (2012). Sustained decrease and remarkable increase in red blood cell velocity in intraparenchymal capillaries associated with potassium-induced cortical spreading depression. *Microcirculation* **19**(2): 166–174.

31 Ostergaard L, Dreier JP, Hadjikhani N, Jespersen SN, Dirnagl U, Dalkara T (2015). Neurovascular coupling during cortical spreading depolarization and depression. *Stroke* **46**(5): 1392–401.

32 Lee J, Wu W, Lesage F, and Boas DA (2013). Multiple-capillary measurement of RBC speed, flux, and density with optical coherence tomography. *Journal of Cerebral Blood Flow and Metabolism* **33**(11): 1707–1710.

33 Srinivasan VJ, *et al.* (2011). Optical coherence tomography for the quantitative study of cerebrovascular physiology. *Journal of Cerebral Blood Flow and Metabolism* **31**(6): 1339–1345.

34 Kohl M, Lindauer U, Dirnagl U, and Villringer A (1998). Separation of changes in light scattering and chromophore concentrations during cortical spreading depression in rats. *Optics Letters* **23**(7): 555–557.

35 Nizar K, *et al.* (2013). *In vivo* Stimulus-Induced Vasodilation Occurs without IP3 Receptor Activation and May Precede Astrocytic Calcium Increase. *Journal of Neuroscience* **33**(19): 8411–8422.

36 Grienberger C and Konnerth A (2012). Imaging calcium in neurons. *Neuron* **73**(5): 862–885.

37 Pietrobon D and Moskowitz MA (2014). Chaos and commotion in the wake of cortical spreading depression and spreading depolarizations. *Ature Reviews Neuroscience* **15**(6): 379–393.

38 Bonder DE and McCarthy KD (2014). Astrocytic Gq-GPCR-linked IP3R-dependent Ca^{2+} signaling does not mediate neurovascular coupling in mouse visual cortex *in vivo. Journal of Neuroscience* **34**(39): 13139–13150.

39 Thestrup T, *et al.* (2014). Optimized ratiometric calcium sensors for functional *in vivo* imaging of neurons and T lymphocytes. *Nature Methods* **11**(2): 175–182.

40 Lakowicz JR, Szmacinski H, Nowaczyk K, Berndt KW, and Johnson M (1992). Fluorescence lifetime imaging. *Analytical Biochemistry* **202**(2): 316–330.

41 Wilms CD, Schmidt H, and Eilers J (2006). Quantitative two-photon Ca^{2+} imaging via fluorescence lifetime analysis. *Cell Calcium* **40**(1): 73–79.

42 Kuchibhotla KV, Lattarulo CR, Hyman BT, and Bacskai BJ (2009). Synchronous hyperactivity and intercellular calcium waves in astrocytes in Alzheimer mice. *Science* **323**(5918): 1211–1215.

43 Kuffler SW (1967). Neuroglial cells: physiological properties and a potassium mediated effect of neuronal activity on the glial membrane potential. *Proceedings of the Royal Society of London. Series B, Biological Sciences* **168**(1010): 1–21.

44 Ransom CB, Ransom BR, and Sontheimer H (2000). Activity-dependent extracellular K^+ accumulation in rat optic nerve: the role of glial and axonal Na^+ pumps. *Journal of Physiology* **522** Pt 3: 427–442.

45 Lothman E, Lamanna J, Cordingley G, Rosenthal M, and Somjen G (1975). Responses of electrical potential, potassium levels, and oxidative metabolic activity of the cerebral neocortex of cats. *Brain Research* **88**(1): 15–36.

46 Mayevsky A (1984). Brain NADH redox state monitored *in vivo* by fiber optic surface fluorometry. *Brain Research* **319**(1): 49–68.

47 Baraghis E, *et al.* (2011). Two-photon microscopy of cortical NADH fluorescence intensity changes: correcting contamination from the hemodynamic response. *Journal of Biomedical Optics* **16**(10): 106003.

48 Yaseen MA, *et al.* (2013). *In vivo* imaging of cerebral energy metabolism with two-photon fluorescence lifetime microscopy of NADH. *Biomedical Optics Express* **4**(2): 307–321.

49 Zhao Y, *et al.* (2011). Genetically encoded fluorescent sensors for intracellular NADH detection. *Cell Metabolism* **14**(4): 555–566.

50 Hung YP, Albeck JG, Tantama M, and Yellen G (2011). Imaging cytosolic NADH-NAD($^+$) redox state with a genetically encoded fluorescent biosensor. *Cell Metabolism* **14**(4): 545–554.

51 Shuttleworth CW (2010). Use of NAD(P)H and flavoprotein autofluorescence transients to probe neuron and astrocyte responses to synaptic activation. *Neurochemistry International* **56**(3): 379–386.

52 San Martin A, *et al.* (2013). A genetically encoded FRET lactate sensor and its use to detect the Warburg effect in single cancer cells. *PLoS One* **8**(2): e57712.

53 San Martin A, *et al.* (2014). Imaging mitochondrial flux in single cells with a FRET sensor for pyruvate. *PLoS One* **9**(1): e85780.

54 Sotelo-Hitschfeld T, *et al.* (2015). Channel-mediated lactate release by K$^+$-stimulated astrocytes. *Journal of Neuroscience* **35**(10): 4168–4178.

55 Pellerin L and Magistretti PJ (2012). Sweet sixteen for ANLS. *Journal of Cerebral Blood Flow and Metabolism* **32**(7): 1152–1166.

56 Barros LF (2013). Metabolic signaling by lactate in the brain. *Trends in Neurosciences* **36**(7): 396–404.

57 Finikova OS, *et al.* (2008). Oxygen microscopy by two-photon-excited phosphorescence. *Chemphyschem* **9**(12): 1673–1679.

58 Rumsey WL, Vanderkooi JM, and Wilson DF (1988). Imaging of phosphorescence: a novel method for measuring oxygen distribution in perfused tissue. *Science* **241**(4873): 1649–1651.

59 Vanderkooi JM, Maniara G, Green TJ, and Wilson DF (1987). An optical method for measurement of dioxygen concentration based upon quenching of phosphorescence. *Journal of Biological Chemistry* **262**(12): 5476–5482.

60 Sakadzic S, *et al.* (2010). Two-photon high-resolution measurement of partial pressure of oxygen in cerebral vasculature and tissue. *Nature Methods* **7**(9): 755–759.

61 Devor A, *et al.* (2011). "Overshoot" of O(2) is required to maintain baseline tissue oxygenation at locations distal to blood vessels. *Journal of Neuroscience* **31**(38): 13676–13681.

62 Devor A, *et al.* (2012). Functional imaging of cerebral oxygenation with intrinsic optical contrast and phosphorescent O$_2$ sensors. *Optical imaging of cortical circuit dynamics* Neuromethods, ed Springer), in press.

63 Lecoq J, *et al.* (2011). Simultaneous two-photon imaging of oxygen and blood flow in deep cerebral vessels. *Nature Medicine* **17**, 893–898.

64 Sakadzic S, *et al.* (2014). Large arteriolar component of oxygen delivery implies a safe margin of oxygen supply to cerebral tissue. *Nature Communications* **5**: 5734.

65 Parpaleix A, Goulam Houssen Y, and Charpak S (2013). Imaging local neuronal activity by monitoring PO(2) transients in capillaries. *Nature Medicine* **19**(2): 241–246.

66 Gagnon L, *et al.* (2015). Quantifying the Microvascular Origin of BOLD-fMRI from First Principles with Two-Photon Microscopy and an Oxygen-Sensitive Nanoprobe. *Journal of Neuroscience* **35**(8): 3663–3675.

67 Devor A, *et al*. (2011). "Overshoot" of O2 is required to maintain baseline tissue oxygenation at locations distal to blood vessels. *Journal of Neuroscience* **31**(38): 13676–13681.

68 Sakadzic S, *et al*. (2009). Simultaneous imaging of cerebral partial pressure of oxygen and blood flow during functional activation and cortical spreading depression. *Applied Optics* **48**(10): D169–177.

69 Sakadžić S, Yaseen MA, Jaswal R, Roussakis E, Dale AM, Buxton RB, Vinogradov SA, Boas DA, Devor A (2016). Two-photon microscopy measurement of cerebral metabolic rate of oxygen using periarteriolar oxygen concentration gradients. *Neurophotonics*. Oct; **3**(4): 045005.

70 Zhang K and Cui B (2015). Optogenetic control of intracellular signaling pathways. *Trends in Biotechnology* **33**(2): 92–100.

71 Yizhar O, Fenno LE, Davidson TJ, Mogri M, and Deisseroth K (2011). Optogenetics in neural systems. *Neuron* **71**(1): 9–34.

72 Miesenbock G (2011). Optogenetic Control of Cells and Circuits. *Annual Review of Cell and Developmental Biology* **27**: 731–758.

73 Baca SM, *et al*. (2013). *Cortical spreading depression triggered by selective activation of astrocytes*. Society for Neuroscience.

74 Petzold GC, Albeanu DF, Sato TF, and Murthy VN (2008). Coupling of neural activity to blood flow in olfactory glomeruli is mediated by astrocytic pathways. *Neuron* **58**(6): 897–910.

75 Schummers J, Yu H, and Sur M (2008). Tuned responses of astrocytes and their influence on hemodynamic signals in the visual cortex. *Science* **320**(5883): 1638–1643.

76 Wang X, *et al*. (2006). Astrocytic Ca^{2+} signaling evoked by sensory stimulation *in vivo*. *Nature Neuroscience* **9**(6): 816–823.

77 Takano T, *et al*. (2006). Astrocyte-mediated control of cerebral blood flow. *Nature Neuroscience* **9**(2): 260–267.

78 Zhao S, *et al*. (2011). Cell type-specific channelrhodopsin-2 transgenic mice for optogenetic dissection of neural circuitry function. *Nature Methods* **8**(9): 745–752.

79 Kahn I, *et al*. (2011). Characterization of the functional MRI response temporal linearity via optical control of neocortical pyramidal neurons. *Journal of Neuroscience* **31**(42): 15086–15091.

80 Scott NA and Murphy TH (2012). Hemodynamic responses evoked by neuronal stimulation via channelrhodopsin-2 can be independent of intracortical glutamatergic synaptic transmission. *PLoS One* **7**(1): e29859.

81 Lim DH, Ledue J, Mohajerani MH, Vanni MP, and Murphy TH (2013). Optogenetic approaches for functional mouse brain mapping. *Frontiers in Neuroscience* **7**: 54.

82 Vazquez AL, Fukuda M, Crowley JC, and Kim SG (2014). Neural and hemodynamic responses elicited by forelimb- and photo-stimulation in channelrhodopsin-2 mice: insights into the hemodynamic point spread function. *Cerebral Cortex* **24**(11): 2908–2919.

83 Kahn I, *et al*. (2013). Optogenetic drive of neocortical pyramidal neurons generates fMRI signals that are correlated with spiking activity. *Brain Research* **1511**: 33–45.

84 Lee JH, *et al*. (2010). Global and local fMRI signals driven by neurons defined optogenetically by type and wiring. *Nature* **465**(7299): 788–792.

85 Devor A, *et al.* (2013). The challenge of connecting the dots in the B.R.A.I.N. *Neuron* **80**(2): 270–274.

86 Insel TR, Landis SC, and Collins FS (2013). Research priorities. The NIH BRAIN Initiative. *Science* **340**(6133): 687–688.

87 Yao J, *et al.* (2015). High-speed label-free functional photoacoustic microscopy of mouse brain in action. *Nature Methods* **12**(5): 407–410.

88 Keller PJ and Ahrens MB (2015). Visualizing whole-brain activity and development at the single-cell level using light-sheet microscopy. *Neuron* **85**(3): 462–483.

89 Bouchard MB, *et al.* (2015). Swept confocally-aligned planar excitation (SCAPE) microscopy for high-speed volumetric imaging of behaving organisms. *Nature Photonics* **9**: 113–119.

90 Tsai PS, Anderson M, Field J, Mateo C, and Kleinfeld D (2013). *Ultrawide-field two photon laser scanning microscope.* Society for Neuroscience.

91 Sakadzic S, Lee J, Boas D, and Ayata C (2015). High-resolution *in vivo* optical imaging of stroke injury and repair. *Brain Research* **1623**: 174–92.

19

Animal models of migraine aura

Shih-Pin Chen[1], Jeremy Theriot[2], Cenk Ayata[3] and KC Brennan[2]

[1] *Department of Neurology, Taipei Veterans General Hospital, Taipei, Taiwan*
[2] *Headache Physiology Laboratory, Department of Neurology, University of Utah, Utah, USA*
[3] *Stroke Service and Neuroscience Intensive Care Unit, Department of Neurology Massachusetts General Hospital, Harvard Medical School, Boston, Massachusetts, USA*

19.1   Introduction: spreading depression and migraine

Spreading depression (SD) is a wave of near-complete neuronal and glial depolarization that slowly propagates in nervous tissue at a speed of $\approx 3\,mm/min$ [1–5]. The loss of transmembrane ion gradients (i.e., K^+ efflux, Na^+ influx), and all spontaneous or evoked synaptic activity and action potentials (i.e., electrocorticogram depression), is accompanied by unregulated release of countless neurotransmitters, neuromodulators and other chemicals [5–7], massive Ca^{2+} influx, cell swelling, and dendritic beading [8, 9], all of which can last up to a minute or more. As a consequence, SD induces severe and long-lasting (minutes to hours) local metabolic and hemodynamic changes [10–12].

Once SD is triggered by a sufficiently intense depolarizing event, extracellular K^+ rapidly rises from $\approx 3\,mM$ to $> 30\,mM$, which then diffuses out to adjacent cells to trigger the same depolarization cycle [5, 13]. In this manner, SD propagates in brain tissue by way of contiguity. The depolarization also depends critically on glutamate release [14–16]. In order for SD to develop and propagate, high neuronal density and low extracellular volume fraction are required. Because of this, SD is limited to the gray matter structures, and never propagates far into the white matter [5, 17]. Indeed, SD propagation can be lamina-specific [18, 19], and inversely correlates with the cortical myelin content [20].

Different regions of the cortex are differentially susceptible to SD [3, 17, 21, 22], suggesting that cytoarchitecture or local receptor expression can modulate this self-propagating regenerative process [23, 24]. SD is an evolutionarily conserved property of central nervous systems of all animals studied to date, from insects to human [25–29]. Among mammals, lissencephalic species appear to be more susceptible to develop and sustain SD than gyrencephalic species [30–35], though little objective comparison has been done.

Spreading depression is thought to be the physiological substrate of the migraine aura. Migraine is classified as being with or without aura, based on the presence of transient

Neurobiological Basis of Migraine, First Edition. Edited by Turgay Dalkara and Michael A. Moskowitz.
© 2017 John Wiley & Sons, Inc. Published 2017 by John Wiley & Sons, Inc.

neurological signs or symptoms (e.g., visual, sensory, motor, or speech disturbances) that develop in up to one-third of patients prior to headache onset, and last 5–60 minutes [36]. Since the discovery of SD by Leão, the similarities between the electrophysiological properties of SD and the symptomatology of aura have suggested that SD is the electrophysiological event underlying migraine aura, implicating a role for SD in migraine pathogenesis [2, 5, 36–38]. Today, an overwhelming amount of evidence supports this notion, including:

- the congruence of cerebrovascular changes during migraine with aura and during SD [39, 40];
- similarities between the direction of modulation of migraine and of SD by the same genetic, hormonal and pharmacological factors; and
- probable common triggers for migraine and SD [37].

A large body of data also indicates that SD can activate inflammatory and nociceptive pathways and trigger headache [41–45]. It remains to be seen whether SD also triggers migraine without a "perceived" aura, at least in a subset of patients [46]. Also, "gold standard" electrophysiological evidence of SD in migraine is still elusive, mainly because of ethical constraints on intracranial recordings. However, it has been conclusively demonstrated, using such recordings, that SD occurs in brain injury states [47].

Over the past decade, SD attracted considerable attention for its translational relevance. Experimental SD models have been used to examine basic migraine mechanisms, test genetic and hormonal modulators, and screen physiological and pharmacological interventions that suppress SD. Here, we provide a critical overview of such models, with their strengths and weaknesses, to better appreciate study quality and interpret the data, and with recommendations to improve intra- and inter-laboratory reproducibility to facilitate future meta-analyses.

19.2   *In vivo* and *in vitro* models of SD susceptibility

The comprehensive investigation of a disease requires both whole-system and reductionist models; the former increase the likelihood of disease-relevance, while the latter are better suited to determining mechanisms. *In vivo* and *in vitro* SD models provide complementary approaches to this basic mechanism of migraine.

CSD was first discovered in an *in vivo* preparation in rabbit [3]. For over 70 years of SD research, work in whole animal preparations has been the predominant technique. *In vivo* models can be challenging and time-consuming, due to microsurgical preparation and maintenance of stable systemic physiological conditions under anesthesia. Nevertheless, they are essential in preclinical therapeutic testing. *In vivo* models have been, for the most part, limited to cerebral cortex, because of ease of access. Most studies have been in rodents, but a wide variety of species, from locust to pigeon, catfish, cat, and monkey have been used [25, 25–27, 29, 48].

There is a fair amount of interspecies variability in SD susceptibility. Although species differences in SD susceptibility and their determinants have not been systematically studied, in general, the larger the brain, the lower the SD susceptibility (e.g., mouse vs. rat), and gyrencephalic species (e.g., cats, swine) are less susceptible to SD than lissencephalic species (e.g., rodents). Gyrencephalic models might simulate SD in human brain better, but studies from lissencephalic species have successfully recapitulated the clinical phenomenology, and have been used to dissect pathophysiology and screen for migraine therapeutics.

The key advantage of *in vivo* models is that they examine SD *in situ*, in a networked, perfused brain. Any brain activity necessarily involves vascular activation, but SD stands out, compared with normal activity and even extreme activity like seizures, in its perturbation of the vasculature. Leão first observed that the vascular concomitants of SD were likely to "condition" the wave [49], and much subsequent experimental evidence has borne this out [10–12, 50–53]. Though perfused whole brain *in vitro* preparations exist [54], and the basic mechanisms of vascular activation have been examined in brain slices [55, 56], it is clear that only whole-animal preparations can capture the whole ensemble of SD-associated neurovascular phenotypes.

In vitro models also have a long history in SD research. Arguably, the first "*in vitro*" model was Bernice Grafstein's use of a disconnected slab of cat cortex for her seminal work on the role of potassium in SD propagation [57]. Though dissimilar to most later techniques, in that it used a whole decerebrate animal, the experiment itself was conducted on a 1.0×0.5 cm piece of tissue that had been disconnected from surrounding tissue (except for vascular connections to preserve viability). The next *in vitro* technique was the isolated retina. Though the retina, unlike the conventional slice, is a complete biological circuit, its characteristics are very similar to those of brain slices. In contrast to the human retina, the chick retina is avascular, and its size and thickness are comparable to brain slices.

In the late 1950s and early 1960s, first toad, and then chick retina, were found to support SD [58, 59]. These were the first SD recording techniques that allowed systematic analysis of the optical changes in tissue generated by the wave; SD in retina generates a concentric series of changes in reflectance as it propagates through the retina. These changes are now typically referred to as optical intrinsic signal (see below). The chick retina was also the first platform on which the pharmacology of CSD could be systematically examined [60].

In the late 1970s and 1980s, tissue slice techniques, which had been in place for other organs since the 1920s, became viable for brain [61]. As mainline neuroscience developed slice preparations, these were adopted as well by CSD researchers. Like retina, brain slice preparations show both optical and electrophysiological changes during CSD, and these have been used to investigate its phenomenology and mechanism with great precision. The first use of modern brain slice recording techniques in SD was a seminal paper by Snow, Taylor, and Dudek in 1983 [62], using both optical imaging and single cell electrophysiology to examine SD.

The key advantages of the brain slice over a whole-animal preparation relate to control. Variables such as anesthesia, temperature, hydration, and blood pressure are eliminated, and near complete control of temperature, oxygenation, pH, ionic, and pharmacological environment can be obtained. Access to cellular resolution imaging and electrophysiology is relatively easy in a slice and, due to environmental control and the limited nature of the network sampled, higher quality electrophysiological recordings can be performed in a slice than *in vivo*.

Another advantage of slice preparations is that they can be used to sample parts of the nervous system inaccessible (at least for now) to *in vivo* techniques, or to examine characteristics that conventional electrode recordings would not allow. For example, slice techniques have been used to examine SD propagation and its effects on synaptic transmission in the amygdala [63]. Slices from brainstem have been used to test hypotheses regarding the possible role of SD in sudden infant death, and sudden death in epilepsy [64–67].

Finally, brain slice techniques can be used to perform basic investigation of human tissue in a manner that would be unethical *in situ*. Human cortical tissue is routinely removed during epilepsy surgery, and survives well *in vitro*, allowing induction of SD and examination of its effects on network excitability [68, 69]. A caveat is that the tissue is from patients with significant baseline disruptions in cortical excitability. Nevertheless, the technique offers access to cellular resolution recording in humans that would otherwise not be available.

Of course, a brain slice is not a networked nervous system; it is literally just a slice of it. Under most circumstances (the thalamocortical slice is an exception), only local circuits (e.g., within cortex, hippocampus, or brainstem, but not between them) can be sampled. For whole-nervous-system diseases like headache, this is a major limitation. However for pursuit of cellular mechanisms, the brain slice has few rivals in its resolving power.

19.3 Experimental preparations

19.3.1 *In vivo* preparations

In vivo SD experiments can take a variety of approaches. Most use anesthesia, although awake preparations have also been used [70–75]. An emphasis on awake techniques in contemporary neuroscience will likely lead to more awake SD preparations in the near future. This makes sense, because migraine aura can only be "perceived" by the awake brain.

For anesthetized technique, a variety of anesthetics can be used, and each has their own considerations (see below). Typically, the animal is restrained in a stereotaxic frame, with comprehensive physiological monitoring (heart rate, respiratory rate, blood pressure, blood gases or capnography), because these physiological variables can affect SD susceptibility. The skull is exposed, and in the simplest preparations, electrodes (active and ground at a minimum) are placed through burr holes (Figure 19.1).

Larger craniotomies can be made to accommodate either more or different electrodes or probes, topical perfusion of drugs, or to allow for imaging [51, 76]. Finally, thin skull preparations give a non-invasive approach to image underlying cortex [50, 51]. Either an additional burr hole or a craniotomy can be used to induce SD, either focally or by exposure of a larger region (e.g., a cortical window made from a craniotomy) to the stimulus (Figure 19.2).

For awake preparations either the animal is woken during surgery, or an initial surgery allows placement of recording equipment – typically either implanted electrodes or closed cortical windows for imaging.

19.3.2 *In vitro* preparations

Brain slice techniques [61] involve the sacrifice of the animal under deep anesthesia, followed by removal of the brain into a cutting solution which is chilled, and whose ionic composition reduces the risk of excitotoxic damage. The slice is glued to a stage,

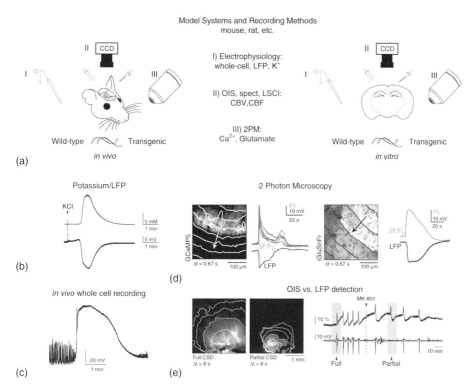

Figure 19.1 Experimental preparations and detection of CSD. (a) *In vivo* and *in vitro* approaches are both available to detect CSD, can take advantage of similar methods, and are complementary. *In vivo* preparations use either burr holes, craniotomies, or thin skull preparations, in wild type or transgenic animals. *In vitro* preparations use brain slices from diverse brain regions. Electrophysiology, wide field optical techniques, or microscopy techniques can all be used to detect CSD. Schematics show detection with electrodes; optical detection with CCD cameras, with light delivery by LED for optical intrinsic signal imaging and by laser for laser speckle contrast imaging; and microscopy. Not shown are magnetic resonance imaging and magnetoencephalographic techniques, which can also be used (see text). (b) Simultaneous detection of CSD, with potassium sensitive electrode and field potential. (c) Detection of a single neuron's depolarization during CSD, with whole cell recording. (d) Imaging and field potential recording of CSD using two photon microscopy. Genetically encoded fluorophores for neuronal calcium (GCaMP5, driven by Synapsin1 promoter) and extracellular glutamate (iGluSnFR) both show propagation of wave *in vivo*. (e) Detection and pharmacological manipulation of CSD, with optical intrinsic signal imaging and field potential. Left panel shows a CSD prior to treatment with the NMDA receptor antagonist MK-801; right panel shows a smaller "partial" CSD after. Traces show OIS and field potential response over the whole experiment. There is a reduction in frequency of CSD with MK-801. However, note that imaging captures a CSD that is not detected by electrode, because it does not propagate far enough to reach the electrode ("Partial CSD"). **Abbreviations:** CCD – charge coupled device camera; LFP – local field potential; K^+ – potassium sensitive electrode; OIS – optical intrinsic signal; LSCI – laser speckle contrast imaging; CBV – cerebral blood volume; CBF – cerebral blood flow; 2PM – two-photon microscopy; Ca^{2+} : calcium imaging.

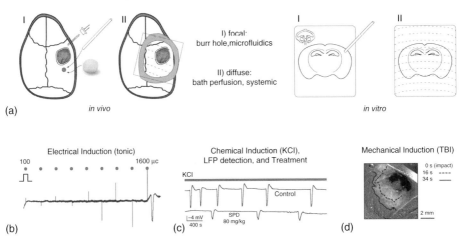

Figure 19.2 Induction of CSD. (a) As with detection of CSD, similar induction techniques can be used *in vivo* and *in vitro*. A variety of induction methods are listed. *In vivo* schematic shows (I) focal induction with optogenetics (laser diode) and with delivery of concentrated KCl, either through tubing or a cotton ball to a burr hole; (II) diffuse delivery of threshold concentrations of KCl (or other inducing substance) over a wider cranial window. *In vitro* schematic shows similarly focal and diffuse approaches, with microfluidics or more conventional tubing for focal induction with KCl, and bath perfusion for a more global approach. (b) CSD thresholding with tonic electrical stimulation. Increasing intensity square current pulses are delivered until CSD is induced (seen on field potential trace). (c) Continuous induction and CSD counting with tonic delivery of KCl through a burr hole. Upper trace shows CSD in control conditions; lower trace shows reduced number (and amplitude) of CSD on treatment with sec-Butylpropylacetamide (SPD), a drug under investigation as a migraine preventive. (d) Mechanical induction of CSD with controlled cortical impact (CCI). Typical mechanical induction of CSD is with pinprick, but this is a stimulus that is difficult to replicate (see text); CCI is a more replicable technique. This experiment also highlights the fact that traumatic brain injury (TBI) causes CSD. TBI is also associated with post-traumatic headache, but little is known about how the effects of TBI (CSD or other) generate these migraine-like headaches.

which is immersed in cutting solution on a vibratome, and the brain is then sliced, most commonly coronally, although horizontal and angulated slices (e.g., thalamocortical slices) are also used. The desired region of brain (e.g., somatosensory cortex, hippocampus) is isolated, either by pre-cutting the brain to expose selected regions, or by the slicing itself. Brain slices range from 150–450 μm in thickness; thin slices are better able to absorb oxygen and nutrients from the bath; thick slices preserve more local connections.

Once the desired slices are cut, they are moved to a recording solution (oxygenated, pH-adjusted, osmolarity adjusted artificial cerebrospinal fluid, including glucose) that is warmed either to room or body temperature, and is allowed to rest prior to experimentation. For the experiment, the slice is placed in a recording chamber – usually under a microscope – on a rig that includes both camera and electrophysiological recording equipment (Figure 19.2). Recording chambers come in many varieties, but are of two types: submerged chambers completely immerse the slice in recording solution [77], while interface chambers immerse the slice up to the top surface, leaving the top surface exposed to humidified oxygen [62, 63, 78–83]. Submerged chambers offer the most control over pharmacology, while interface chambers offer greater exposure to oxygen and can result in "healthier" slices, with behavior more resembling *in vivo* preparations. Induction of SD can either be focal [84–86] or can involve whole-slice exposure to the stimulus [76, 78]. Recording is with electrophysiological techniques (extracellular or intracellular), optical techniques, or both.

19.4   Methods to trigger SD

Experimentally-evoked SD requires intense depolarizing stimuli to ignite (Figure 19.2). This fact highlights one of the greatest remaining mysteries in the study of migraine – that most SD models involve stimuli that are difficult to imagine in an awake behaving human being. An increase of extracellular K^+ above a critical threshold concentration (12 mM) [87, 88] in a minimum critical volume of brain tissue (ranging from 0.03–0.06 mm^3 in mouse cortex *in vitro* to 1 mm^3 in rat cortex *in vivo*) is required [85, 89]. This can be achieved by:

a) direct electrical stimulation;
b) topical application of depolarizing substances, such as high concentrations of K^+, excitatory amino acids, Ca^{2+} channel openers, and Na^+/K^+-ATPase inhibitors;
c) mechanical distortion of tissue, with or without penetrating injury; and
d) hypoxia or ischemia, such as microembolization or topical endothelin-1 application [5, 78, 90–92].

Each approach has its strengths and weaknesses, and different techniques may have different pharmacological profiles [4, 93]. For example, traumatic SD (i.e., needle prick) is reportedly prevented by Na^+ channel blockade, but topical K^+-induced SD is not [94]. Moreover, there is a distinct pharmacological difference between focal and whole-bath induction of SD in brain slices: focally induced SD is readily inhibited by calcium channel and NMDA receptor blockade, while bath-induced SD is not [4]. Therefore, a comprehensive investigation of interventions to suppress SD should, ideally, include more than one form of SD induction to be conclusive.

Electrical stimulation is one of the most direct methods to assess SD susceptibility *in vivo* [88, 93, 95–100], as well as *in vitro* [101]. Stimulation can be delivered as escalating steps of single square wave pulses at an interval of every 4–5min until an SD is evoked (Figure 19.2). The product of stimulus current (mA) and duration (ms) yields the total threshold charge required to trigger SD, expressed in microCoulombs. An alternative to single square wave pulses is high-frequency train stimulation with escalating intensity and/or duration. This mode of SD induction may require action potentials and synaptic transmission to build the depolarization required for SD induction and, therefore, may show a different pharmacological sensitivity profile than single square pulses. On the other hand, large tonic current discharge heats the tissue and electrolyzes water, causing thermal and mechanical effects that need to be taken into account.

It is interesting to note that thresholds obtained with tonic current are approximately an order of magnitude lower than those obtained with tetanic stimulation [95, 97–100]. This may be due to the larger thermal and mechanical effects of tonic stimulation, and the activation of inhibitory networks by tetanic stimulation. Although electrical stimulation threshold is a gold standard in SD susceptibility models, it is also sensitive to many potential confounders, such as stimulus electrode properties (e.g., unipolar or bipolar, size, shape and tip separation, insulation, and duration of use) and the physical conditions of contact with the tissue that determine the stimulus geometry (e.g., presence of dura, bleeding, conductive solutions), increasing the coefficient of variation of the charge threshold [93].

As a corollary to electrical stimulation, intense neuronal activity such as during seizures, or significant afferent pathway stimulation, can also trigger SD. This was first noted by Leão when he induced contralateral SD by electrically stimulating the ipsilateral hemisphere, presumably inducing SD by activation of transcallosal fibers [3]. Blockade of potassium channels with 4-aminopyridine or GABAergic activity with bicuculline is commonly used to generate epileptiform activity; these stimuli also induce SD [102, 103]. In an audiogenic epilepsy model, auditory stimulation evokes *both* seizures and SD; audiogenically driven SD appears to be involved in the subsequent development of seizures [104–107]. Seizure activity also appears to be able to induce SD under certain conditions; seizures provoked by cortical application of 4-aminopyridine in animals with mutations associated with sudden death in epilepsy (SUDEP) lead to a slow, negative DC potential shift, reminiscent of SD in the dorsal medulla [64].

Chemically, topical application of concentrated KCl is most commonly used to evaluate SD susceptibility (Figure 19.2). In one model, a suprathreshold concentration of KCl (e.g., 300 mM for mice and 1 M for rats, or a fixed weight KCl crystal) is applied continuously onto the cortex to trigger repetitive SDs, the frequency of which shows good correlation with the electrical threshold [93]. Alternatively, escalating concentrations of topical or microdialysate KCl can be administered until an SD is triggered at a threshold concentration [76]. Lastly, escalating moles or volumes of a fixed concentration of KCl solution can be administered using iontophoresis or pneumatic injection, via a micropipette, until an SD is triggered [51, 86, 97]. Other depolarizing neurotransmitter receptor agonists have also been used to evoke SD, such as glutamate [15] or N-methyl-D-aspartate [70].

It is also important to consider the size of a stimulus – is it focal, or does it cover a wide area? This is the case for both *in vivo* and *in vitro* preparations. Thresholding can be done with both a focal approach [50, 51, 96–98] or a more diffuse approach, in which a whole craniotomy is bathed in elevated K^+ solution [76]. The same is true in brain slices: both focal [86] and global [78, 83] thresholding can be used (Figure 19.2). Once again, the techniques are not equivalent: in brain slices, the pharmacology of the SD response is different for focal vs. global induction. In particular, SD propagation can be blocked with calcium channel and NMDA receptor blockade for focal induction, but this is not the case for global induction [4]. Given the generally focal onset and concentric propagation of migraine aura, it is likely that focal induction is more relevant, while global induction may be most relevant for ischemic or brain injury models.

Mechanical stimuli have been used to assess susceptibility to CSD [94]. However, especially with needle prick, it is difficult to determine a threshold by escalating mechanical stimulus intensity. The needle size, angle, speed, depth, and strength of insertion are not easily standardized, reproducibility might vary largely between operators and settings, and repeated threshold testing is problematic because of cumulative injury. We do not typically use these methods, because of these factors. The mechanism of mechanical SD induction is unknown, but studies suggest a role for voltage-gated Na^+, AMPA subtype of glutamate receptors, and GABA receptor activity in the perfusion changes accompanying the wave [94, 108].

It is worth noting that mechanical stimulation can be relatively precisely controlled, the best example of this being in controlled cortical impact (CCI) traumatic brain injury. Modern CCI devices [109] can be programmed to deliver very replicable stimuli through the use of voice-coil-controlled pistons. Given the induction of SD with pinprick, it is likely not surprising that CCI reliably generates SD [110] (Figure 19.2). Future attempts at mechanical induction of SD might benefit from either CCI models or techniques based upon them.

Ischemic or hypoxic events can trigger SD. The most obvious example is the generation of peri-infarct depolarizations by various stroke models [111, 112]. However, smaller ischemic injuries – for example, via treatment with the vasoconstrictor endothelin-1, or delivery of microemboli – can also trigger SD [90, 91, 113–115], and may be helpful for our understanding of the pathogenesis of aura and its comorbidity with ischemic stroke.

Persistent ischemia can trigger recurrent SDs via supply-demand mismatch transients [111], which can be suppressed by migraine prophylactic drugs [116]. The primary mechanism of SD onset in the hypoxic/ischemic brain is likely anoxic depolarization, due to failure of Na^+/K^+ ATPase. This can be mimicked by Na^+/K^+ ATPase inhibitors (e.g., ouabain) to trigger SD [78, 117, 118]. Overall, the translational value of hypoxic/ischemic SD induction in migraine is not clear. Speculatively, small reversible areas of ischemia, perhaps occasioned by microemboli, could lead to ignition of CSD in migraine without causing lasting damage [91]. However, thus far, studies in human examining potential causes of microemboli, like patent foramen ovale [119], and trials of patent foramen ovale closure [120], do not support this hypothesis.

19.5 Methods to detect CSD

Because SD is associated with profound ionic, hemodynamic, metabolic and cell volume changes, there are numerous methods to detect SD (Figure 19.1). The gold standard is the detection of a large (15–20 mV when recorded by intracortical glass micropipettes), extracellular direct coupled (DC; frequency < 0.05 Hz) slow potential shift lasting up to a minute, with concurrent and prolonged (several minutes) suppression of the electrocorticographic activity (ECoG). The DC potential shift is observed both *in vivo* and in brain slices [5]. Single unit recordings often detect a brief neuronal spike burst prior to the DC shift [121, 122]. An alternative way to detect the large field potential changes of SD is the use of fluorescent voltage-sensitive dyes, which can be imaged with either cameras or microscopes [113, 123]. The massive extracellular ion shifts of SD (i.e., K^+ increase, Na^+, Ca^{2+} and pH decrease) can also be measured, either *in vivo* or *in vitro*, using ion-selective electrodes [12–14, 25, 118].

SD causes large changes in visible light either reflected or transmitted from the cortex. These changes have been used since Leão to detect the hemodynamic changes associated with CSD [49] and, indeed, the largest change in optical signal for SD *in vivo* is due to changes in perfusion [10]. However, other mechanisms also cause changes in optical signal. SD is associated with significant swelling of neuronal cell bodies and beading of dendritic processes. These changes alter light scattering properties and thus overall reflectance, and are the major component of optical signal in brain slice recordings [124, 125]. Finally, SD causes changes in the intrinsic fluorescence of the brain, which is due to fluorescent components of oxidative metabolism (NADH and flavoproteins) that undergo reduction during the SD wave [9, 126, 127].

For *in vivo* preparations, the reflectance signal is dominated by hemoglobin, which is a major absorber of light at visible wavelengths. Increases in blood volume are observed as a darkening of the tissue, while decreases show brightening [50, 51]. Typically, imaging is done with the reflected light filtered at one of the isosbestic wavelengths of hemoglobin (e.g., green 530 nm light). At these wavelengths, absorption from oxy- and deoxy-hemoglobin is equal, so the signal is an accurate readout of blood volume, uncontaminated by oximetric changes. On the other hand, changes in oxy- and deoxy-hemoglobin can also be measured, by collecting light at wavelengths where the two moieties differ in absorption [12, 128].

Other techniques deployed *in vivo* measure blood flow (as opposed to blood volume and oxygenation, above) during SD. Laser Doppler flowmetry measures the changes in laser light scatter at a point source [129], and laser speckle flowmetry extends the technique to two dimensions, allowing images of blood flow to be generated [50].

To all the above techniques, SD evokes a complex multiphasic hemodynamic response in the tissue. The prototypical response has four distinct phases that vary depending on the species, systemic physiology and detection methods [10, 12, 50, 51, 53, 93, 130, 131]. The hemodynamic response and accompanying changes in tissue oxygenation and metabolic state can be used to detect SD occurrence under normal systemic physiological conditions.

Two-photon microscopy allows the imaging of fluorescence from a very thin plane of tissue, up to hundreds of micrometers deep into tissue, at subcellular spatial resolution. It can be deployed *in vitro* as well as *in vivo*, but its primary advantage is recording cellular level activity in the living (even awake) brain at depth. Two-photon imaging can be used to record calcium and glutamate activity during SD [9, 14, 132], and the current generation of fluorophores are typically delivered in a genetically-encoded manner, allowing specific cell types (e.g., neurons vs. astrocytes) to be imaged [14].

Vessel-impermeant dyes (typically fluorescein or rhodamine dextran) can be used to image vascular diameter and blood flow [132]. The membrane swelling and dendritic beading that occur during the SD wave can be directly imaged from fluorescent cells [9, 133]. Finally, the intrinsic fluorescence of the electron carriers NADH and NADPH can be imaged with two-photon preparations, though these (and other) signals can be contaminated by the very large hemodynamic transients of SD [9, 126].

Diffusion-weighted (DWI) and magnetization transfer MRI have been used to study the spatiotemporal properties of SD *in vivo*, mostly in gyrencephalic brains [30, 134–136], and recently in rodents with the advent of high-field MRI [114, 115]. The transmembrane ion and water shifts during SD are similar to those during anoxic depolarization; therefore, diffusion-weighted MRI changes during SD resemble acute ischemic stroke. However, because SD is a propagating wave of depolarization that lasts only about a minute in any given region, DWI changes are less dramatic than during stroke. Combined with the spatial and temporal averaging of relatively slow image acquisition times, SD can be difficult to detect on MRI. However, MRI has the distinct advantages of being non-invasive and three-dimensional, compared with electrophysiological and optical methods. Moreover, MRI has the potential to be directly translatable between animal and human work.

High-field blood oxygenation level-dependent (BOLD) or spin-lock fMRI have been used to image neurovascular coupling during SD in rodents [137–139]. In humans, fMRI has demonstrated BOLD signal changes consistent with SD, which is time-locked to the onset and propagation of the visual percept of aura [39, 40].

Magnetoencephalography (MEG) can detect magnetic field shifts during SD in lissencephalic rabbit [31], gyrencephalic swine [140], and humans [32, 141, 142]. However, availability and low spatial resolution have thus far restricted its applications.

19.6   SD susceptibility attributes

The term SD susceptibility is defined as the ease with which SD can be initiated and its propagation sustained in a given brain tissue. The stimulus intensity threshold to evoke SD is among the most relevant attributes of SD susceptibility. Depending on the stimulus modality, threshold can be measured in, for example, electrical charge intensity, volume or concentration of a depolarizing agent, or mechanical pressure. Electrical charge intensity to evoke SD correlates well with the threshold concentration of topical KCl [93, 95, 97], and inversely with the frequency of SDs upon continuous topical KCl stimulation [96].

One caveat for determining SD threshold is propagation failure; when the distance between stimulation and recording sites is too long, an SD initiated by threshold stimulus may fail to propagate to the recording site and may be undetected, prompting continued escalation of the stimulus intensity. Hence, longer distance between the stimulation and recording sites might lead to higher perceived SD thresholds, which should be kept in mind when comparing studies. A solution to this problem is to combine optical and electrophysiological approaches [50, 97] (Figure 19.1).

An alternative and complementary SD susceptibility attribute has been the frequency of SDs triggered during continuous topical application of suprathreshold concentrations of depolarizing agents [96, 143]. This attribute is less sensitive to the condition of the underlying tissue and, thus, yields lower coefficients of variation when compared with the threshold [93]. It can, however, be confounded by changes in the refractory period after an SD during which a second SD cannot be triggered, likely determined by neuronal excitability, Na^+/K^+ pump activity, and extracellular K^+ and glutamate clearance by glial cells [4], and it can be affected by genetic and systemic physiological factors.

For example, hypotension prolongs SD duration and thereby the refractory period, thus lowering SD frequency [144–146]. This does not mean reduced SD susceptibility, since the cumulative depolarization duration (i.e., the sum of the durations of all SDs triggered during the test period) may, in fact, stay the same or increase. Hence, when SD frequency is the endpoint, it is mandatory to make sure the physiological conditions of study animals are monitored and maintained. Extending the concept further, a tissue that has a very low threshold for SD, and a long refractory period after the event, might have *fewer* SD induced by continuous stimulation than control tissue.

It is clear that the readouts for continuous stimulation and thresholding are quite different, though they both give an index of susceptibility. It is important to distinguish whether SD number or threshold are being reported, because they are not necessarily equivalent.

SD propagation speed is another commonly measured parameter. SD propagation speed can be calculated using the distance and the latency of SD appearance between two recording sites, and shows good correlation with the SD threshold and frequency [93]. Alternatively, it can be measured using imaging, by generating a kymograph (distance vs. time) plot of the advancing wavefront [51]. The sensitivity, specificity, positive predictive value and negative predictive value are 67%, 76%, 84% and 56%, respectively, for propagation speed in predicting the susceptibility to CSD [93].

However, susceptibility and velocity are certainly not identical parameters, and they do not always correlate. For example, in the casein kinase 1 delta mutant model of migraine, velocity was not significantly increased in mutant mice, though both threshold and number of SD were significantly different [98]. It should be noted that the propagation speed gradually decreases with each successive SD. Hence, it is recommended to measure the propagation speed of only the first SD, taking care not to accidentally induce one or more SDs during experimental preparation. Having two recording sites or imaging also allows the calculation of propagation failure rate, which may also reflect CSD susceptibility, although the predictive value remains to be studied.

The amplitude and duration of the DC shift do not correlate well with the susceptibility to SD [93]. As noted above, systemic physiology can affect SD duration. SD amplitude is less affected by systemic physiology or other confounders, and is the last SD attribute that decreases with SD susceptibility (i.e., least sensitive), and is only rarely used as a primary endpoint [147]. It has been our practice to not include DC potential shifts < 5 mV in amplitude in SD frequency calculations, assuming that small amplitudes are not a result of technical problems, such as poor electrode positioning. However, if imaging is available, such artifacts can be distinguished from real but small SD events (Figure 19.1). If these small amplitude SDs are to be counted, a concomitant ECoG suppression must be sought, to differentiate from electrical noise.

Other properties of SD are less commonly studied, but are worthy of further investigation. The pattern of propagation of SD can be measured if multiple locations are recorded (either with multiple electrodes, or with imaging). It is known that SD does not propagate uniformly [22], and tends to avoid certain regions of cortex (e.g., retrosplenial cortex) [17, 21], but systematic investigation of SD propagation from different cortical regions has not yet been performed. There is also evidence that SD propagates differently in different cortical layers [19, 148], and that different regions of cortex may be differentially susceptible to the event [123, 149]. With the increasing use of 2-D and 3-D techniques, it is likely that more information will emerge on these properties. Meanwhile, it is important, when comparing SD, that induction and recording locations are as identical as possible, to avoid the possible confound of differential susceptibility.

In summary, SD threshold and frequency are recommended susceptibility attributes that can be determined in the same animal, and even in the same hemisphere. Other SD attributes, including propagation speed, duration, and amplitude, are complementary.

19.7   Recommended quality measures for experimental models of migraine aura

19.7.1   Anesthesia

Conventional *in vivo* SD susceptibility models are routinely performed under anesthesia to ensure standard and stable systemic and electrophysiological parameters and reliable stimulus delivery. However, anesthesia can directly suppress SD susceptibility [150–158] and, unfortunately, regimens that are most convenient and best preserve systemic physiology are also the ones that directly suppress SD susceptibility (e.g., inhalational anesthetics, ketamine/xylazine). In addition, it is important to choose an anesthetic regimen that does not interfere with the intervention to be tested. For example, barbiturate anesthesia when testing a GABA agonist, and ketamine when testing an NMDA receptor antagonist, would be less than ideal. Because of potential cardiorespiratory suppressive effects, systemic physiology should be monitored and, if needed, mechanical ventilation should be performed.

19.7.2   Systemic physiology

Arterial blood pressure, blood gas and pH, blood glucose, and body temperature are critical for *in vivo* studies of SD, and should be monitored and controlled carefully during experiments. As mentioned above, hypotension can significantly prolong the SD duration [145, 146]. Interestingly, hypoxia does not appear to affect SD susceptibility unless it is severe [159]. The effect of hypercapnia on SD has not been specifically characterized, but respiratory acidosis may suppress SD susceptibility, as do other causes of acidosis [93, 160]. Hypoglycemia prolongs SD duration [144, 161], whereas hyperglycemia is known to suppress SD susceptibility [144, 162]. Hypothermia has also been shown to inhibit SD susceptibility [163–165].

19.7.3   Surgical preparation and maintenance

Inadvertent tissue injury must be minimized during experimental preparation. Cool saline irrigation during drilling can prevent overheating. Artificial CSF or normal saline, and mineral oil, should be used to prevent cortical drying during preparation and maintenance, respectively. Local anesthesia can minimize activation of trigeminal nociceptive afferents in the scalp or periosteum during cranial surgery, when downstream nociceptive effects of SD are going to be studied. Tissue exposure to blood should be avoided. In rats or larger species, dura should be gently incised, or removed, to standardize stimulation; in mouse, this step is typically omitted, because mouse dura is very thin and is permeable to drugs.

19.7.4   Pharmacokinetic factors

As in any *in vivo* drug testing, therapeutic paradigms must take into account the absorption, bioavailability, distribution, metabolism, and excretion, as well as CNS penetration of the drug candidate. It should be kept in mind that acute efficacy of a single dose may be different than after chronic treatment for many days, weeks or even months. The therapeutic paradigm should also model the intended mode of clinical treatment, such as chronic prophylaxis, preemptive prophylaxis, or acute abortive. Lastly, clinical translation will be greatly facilitated by using a clinically relevant route of administration (e.g., oral, intravenous, or subcutaneous rather than topical or intracerebroventricular). In slice preparations, where drugs are delivered via tubing to the slice chamber, it is important to note whether the drug is soluble in aqueous solutions and, at the other extreme, to what extent it might penetrate or bind to laboratory tubing. For some drugs, a change to more rigid but impermeable tubing (e.g., Teflon) is necessary to allow proper delivery and washout of drugs.

19.7.5 Induction and recording considerations

Differential susceptibility to SD in different brain regions or cortical layers is a real consideration, so both stimulus and recording locations should be maintained as identical as possible; this includes not only the location, but the depth of stimulation or recording devices. In the case of brain slices, it is important that the slices come from the same region (e.g., somatosensory cortex vs. visual or motor cortex), in order that comparisons be valid. For focal KCl stimulation, it is important to make sure that the KCl solution does not spread beyond where it is intended, since this can affect both number of SD elicited, as well as affect electrophysiological readouts (e.g., if KCl solution reaches a ground electrode). For electrical stimulation, electrode parameters must be strictly maintained (impedance, tip separation for bipolar electrodes, active contact area) and, given the currents involved, cleaning biological debris off the electrodes is also important.

19.8   Future directions

Among the next steps in the development and refinement of models of migraine aura should be a focus on methods that allow experimentation on unanesthetized animals, such as electrophysiological recordings in awake freely moving animals using implanted wireless devices, or habituation to an immobilized state on a stereotaxic frame during stimulation studies. Genome-wide association studies and next-generation sequencing may identify novel migraine risk variants [166–169], leading to the development and characterization of novel genetically modified rodent models for pathophysiological investigations, although none of the genetic variants has yet been linked specifically to migraine aura.

As mentioned above, there is little known about the differential susceptibility and propagation of SD in different regions of the brain. There is an unmet need for novel neurobehavioral experimental models (e.g., facial expression, pain and anxiety behavior [170]) to link SD to downstream nociceptive activation and complex behavior patterns related to the postdrome, and to help explain interesting post-SD observations and resolve controversies [44, 74, 171]. Finally, one of the greatest unanswered questions in headache is how SD, a massive depolarization, can arise in uninjured brain. The development of more "naturalistic" models of SD induction is a major priority.

There is also much insight to be gained by the use of tools from other, related fields of neuroscience. The use of *in vivo* cellular resolution techniques (two-photon microscopy [8, 9, 14, 132], *in vivo* whole cell recording [122]) is in its infancy for SD. Brain slice techniques have been incompletely exploited; for example, there is a robust literature on combined vascular and neural recording from brain slices [55, 56] that is highly relevant to SD studies. Brain slice recordings can also help understand the effects of SD on different regions of brain (e.g., brainstem [64] or thalamus and other subcortical regions).

New techniques, such as functional ultrasound, allow both recording [172] and stimulation [173] at depth, and in rodent models the whole brain can be sampled, allowing for the investigation of network effects of SD. Miniaturized microscopes and remote telemetry [174, 175] can now be deployed in awake behaving animals, expanding the possibilities for recording of spontaneous or "naturalistically" induced SD. Finally, the revolution in genetically encoded indicators, optogenetics, chemogenetics, tissue clearing, and other tools for functional circuit mapping, has barely reached the SD field [176–180]. There is much to look forward to.

References

1 Ayata, C. (2009) Spreading depression: from serendipity to targeted therapy in migraine prophylaxis. *Cephalalgia* **29**: 1095–114.

2 Charles, A. and Brennan, K. (2009). Cortical spreading depression-new insights and persistent questions. *Cephalalgia* **29**: 1115–1124.

3 Leao, A. A. P (1944). Spreading depression of activity in the cerebral cortex. *Journal of Neurophysiology* **7**: 359–390.

4 Pietrobon, D. and Moskowitz, M. A. (2014). Chaos and commotion in the wake of cortical spreading depression and spreading depolarizations. *Nature Reviews Neuroscience* **15**: 379–93.

5 Somjen, G. G. (2001). Mechanisms of spreading depression and hypoxic spreading depression-like depolarization. *Physiological Reviews* **81**: 1065–96.

6 Davies, J. A., Annels, S. J., Dickie, B. G., Ellis, Y. and Knott, N. J. (1995). A comparison between the stimulated and paroxysmal release of endogenous amino acids from rat cerebellar, striatal and hippocampal slices: a manifestation of spreading depression? *Journal of the Neurological Sciences* **131**: 8–14.

7 Fabricius, M., Jensen, L. H. and Lauritzen, M. (1993). Microdialysis of interstitial amino acids during spreading depression and anoxic depolarization in rat neocortex. *Brain Research* **612**: 61–9.

8 Eikermann-Haerter, K. *et al.* (2015). Abnormal synaptic Ca(2+) homeostasis and morphology in cortical neurons of familial hemiplegic migraine type 1 mutant mice. *Annals of Neurology* **78**: 193–210.

9 Takano, T. *et al.* (2007). Cortical spreading depression causes and coincides with tissue hypoxia. *Nature Neuroscience* **10**: 754.

10 Ayata, C. and Lauritzen, M. (2015). Spreading Depression, Spreading Depolarizations, and the Cerebral Vasculature. *Physiological Reviews* **95**: 953–993.

11 Brennan, K. C. and Charles, A. (2010). An update on the blood vessel in migraine. *Current Opinion in Neurology* **23**: 266–274.

12 Chang, J. C. *et al.* (2010). Biphasic direct current shift, hemoglobin desaturation, and neurovascular uncoupling in cortical spreading depression. *Brain* **133**: 996–1012.

13 Vyskocil, F., Kritz, N. and Bures, J. (1972). Potassium-selective microelectrodes used for measuring the extracellular brain potassium during spreading depression and anoxic depolarization in rats. *Brain Research* **39**: 255–259.

14 Enger, R. *et al.* (2015). Dynamics of Ionic Shifts in Cortical Spreading Depression. *Cerebral Cortex* **25**(11): 4469–4476.

15 Fifkova, E. and Van Harreveld, A. (1974). Glutamate and spreading depression. *Journal of Neurobiology* **5**: 469–73.

16 Zhou, N. *et al.* (2013). Regenerative glutamate release by presynaptic NMDA receptors contributes to spreading depression. *Journal of Cerebral Blood Flow & Metabolism* **33**: 1582–94.

17 Leao, A. A. P. and Morison, R. S. (1945). Propagation of spreading cortical depression. *Journal of Neurophysiology* **8**: 33–45.

18 Gniel, H. M. and Martin, R. L. (2013). Cortical spreading depression-induced preconditioning in mouse neocortex is lamina specific. *Journal of Neurophysiology* **109**: 2923–36.

19 Herreras, O. and Somjen, G. G. (1993). Propagation of spreading depression among dendrites and somata of the same cell population. *Brain Research* **610**: 276–282.

20 Merkler, D. *et al.* (2009). Propagation of spreading depression inversely correlates with cortical myelin content. *Annals of Neurology* **66**: 355–365.

21 Chen, S. *et al.* (2006). Time-varying spreading depression waves in rat cortex revealed by optical intrinsic signal imaging. *Neuroscience Letters* **396**: 132–6.

22 Eiselt, M. *et al.* (2004). Inhomogeneous propagation of cortical spreading depression-detection by electro- and magnetoencephalography in rats. *Brain Research* **1028**: 83–91.

23 Fujita, S. *et al.* (2015). Cytoarchitecture-Dependent Decrease in Propagation Velocity of Cortical Spreading Depression in the Rat Insular Cortex Revealed by Optical Imaging. *Cerebral Cortex* **26**(4): 1580–9.

24 Ochs, S. (1962). The nature of spreading depression in neural networks. *International Review of Neurobiology* **4**: 1–70.

25 Kraig, R. P. and Nicholson, C. (1978). Extracellular ionic variations during spreading depression. *Neuroscience* **3**: 1045–1059.

26 Marshall, W. (1959). Spreading cortical depression of Leao. *Physiological Reviews* **39**: 239–279.

27 Rodgers, C. I. *et al.* (2007). Stress preconditioning of spreading depression in the locust CNS. *PloS One* **2**: e1366.

28 Rodríguez, E. C. and Robertson, R. M. (2012). Protective effect of hypothermia on brain potassium homeostasis during repetitive anoxia in Drosophila melanogaster. *Journal of Experimental Biology* **215**: 4157–4165.

29 Wise, Y. (1980). Spreading depression in elasmobranch cerebellum. *Brain Research* **199**: 113–126.

30 Bockhorst, K. H. *et al.* (2000). A quantitative analysis of cortical spreading depression events in the feline brain characterized with diffusion-weighted MRI. *Journal of Magnetic Resonance Imaging* **12**: 722–733.

31 Bowyer, S. M. *et al*. (1999). Analysis of MEG signals of spreading cortical depression with propagation constrained to a rectangular cortical strip. I. Lissencephalic rabbit model. *Brain Research* **843**: 71–8.

32 Bowyer, S. M., Aurora, S. K., Moran, J. E., Tepley, J. and Welch, K. M. A. (2001). Magnetoencephalographic fields from patients with spontaneous and induced migraine aura. *Annals of Neurology* **50**: 582–587.

33 Dahlem, M. A. and Hadjikhani, N. (2009).Migraine aura: retracting particle-like waves in weakly susceptible cortex. *PloS One* **4**: e5007.

34 James, M. F. *et al*. (1999). Cortical spreading depression in the gyrencephalic feline brain studied by magnetic resonance imaging. *Journal of Physiology* **519**(Pt 2): 415–25.

35 Santos, E. *et al*. (2014). Radial, spiral and reverberating waves of spreading depolarization occur in the gyrencephalic brain. *Neuroimage* **99**: 244–55.

36 Pietrobon, D. and Moskowitz, M. A. Pathophysiology of migraine. *Annual Review of Physiology***75**: 365–391 (2013).

37 Ayata, C. (2010). Cortical spreading depression triggers migraine attack: pro. *Headache* **50**: 725–30.

38 Lauritzen . (1994). Pathophysiology of the migraine aura. The spreading depression theory. *Brain* **117**(Pt 1): 199–210.

39 Cao, Y., Welch, K. M. A., Aurora, S. and Vikingstad, E. M. (1999). Functional MRI-BOLD of Visually Triggered Headache in Patients With Migraine. *Archives of Neurology* **56**: 548–554.

40 Hadjikhani, N. *et al*. (2001). Mechanisms of migraine aura revealed by functional MRI in human visual cortex. *Proceedings of the National Academy of Sciences of the United States of America* **98**: 4687–92.

41 Bolay, H. *et al*. (2002). Intrinsic brain activity triggers trigeminal meningeal afferents in a migraine model. *Nature Medicine* **8**: 136–42.

42 Zhang, X. *et al* (2010).. Activation of meningeal nociceptors by cortical spreading depression: implications for migraine with aura. *Journal of Neuroscience* **30**: 8807–8814.

43 Zhang, X. *et al*. (2011). Activation of central trigeminovascular neurons by cortical spreading depression. *Annals of Neurology* **69**: 855–865.

44 Karatas, H. *et al*. (2013). Spreading depression triggers headache by activating neuronal Panx1 channels. *Science*. **339**: 1092–5.

45 Zhao, J. and Levy, D. (2015). Modulation of intracranial meningeal nociceptor activity by cortical spreading depression: a reassessment. *Journal of Neurophysiology* **113**: 2778–85.

46 Woods, R., Iacoboni, M. and Mazziotta, J. (1994). Bilateral Spreading Cerebral Hypoperfusion during Spontaneous Migraine Headache. *New England Journal of Medicine* **331**: 1689–1692.

47 Dreier, J. P. (2011). The role of spreading depression, spreading depolarization and spreading ischemia in neurological disease. *Nature Medicine* **17**: 439–447.

48 Santos, E., Schöll, M., Sánchez-Porras, R., Dahlem, M.A., Silos, H., Unterberg, A., Dickhaus, H. and Sakowitz, O.W. (2014). Radial, spiral and reverberating waves of spreading depolarization occur in the gyrencephalic brain. *NeuroImage* **99**: 244–55.

49 Leao, A. A. P. (1944). Pial circulation and spreading depression of activity in cerebral cortex. *Journal of Neurophysiology* **7**: 391–396.

50 Ayata, C. *et al.* (2004). Pronounced hypoperfusion during spreading depression in mouse cortex. *Journal of Cerebral Blood Flow & Metabolism* **24**: 1172–1182.

51 Brennan, K. C. *et al* (2007).. Distinct vascular conduction with cortical spreading depression. *Journal of Neurophysiology* **97**: 4143–4151.

52 Busija, D. W., Bari, F., Domoki, F., Horiguchi, T. and Shimizu, K. (2008). Mechanisms involved in the cerebrovascular dilator effects of cortical spreading depression. *Progress in Neurobiology* **86**: 379–395.

53 Piilgaard, H. and Lauritzen. (2009). Persistent increase in oxygen consumption and impaired neurovascular coupling after spreading depression in rat neocortex. *Journal of Cerebral Blood Flow & Metabolism* **29**: 1517–1527.

54 Dirks, B., Krieglstein, J., Lind, H. H., Rieger, H. and Schutz, H. (1980). Fluorocarbon perfusion medium applied to the isolated rat brain. *Journal of Pharmacological Methods* **4**: 95–108.

55 Filosa, J. A. and Blanco, V. M. (2007).Neurovascular coupling in the mammalian brain. *Experimental Physiology* **92**: 641–646.

56 Gordon, G. R. J., Choi, H. B., Rungta, R. L., Ellis-Davies, G. C. R. and MacVicar, B. A. (2008). Brain metabolism dictates the polarity of astrocyte control over arterioles. *Nature* **456**: 745–749.

57 Grafstein, B. (1956). Mechanism of spreading cortical depression. *Journal of Neurophysiology* **19**: 154–171.

58 Gouras, P. (1958). Spreading Depression of Activity in Amphibian Retina. *American Journal of Physiology* **195**: 28–32.

59 Martins-Ferreira, H. and de Castro, G. O. (1966). Light-scattering changes accompanying spreading depression in isolated retina. *Journal of Neurophysiology* **29**: 715–726.

60 Martins-Ferreira, H., Nedergaard, M. and Nicholson, C. (2000). Perspectives on spreading depression. *Brain Research: Brain Research Reviews* **32**: 215–234.

61 Stricker, C. (1997). *In: Neuroscience methods: a guide for advanced students.* Harwood Academic Publishers,.

62 Snow, R. W., Taylor, C. P. and Dudek, F. E. (1983). Electrophysiological and optical changes in slices of rat hippocampus during spreading depression. *Journal of Neurophysiology* **50**: 561–572.

63 Dehbandi, S., Speckmann, E. J., Pape, H. C. and Gorji, A. (2008). Cortical spreading depression modulates synaptic transmission of the rat lateral amygdala. *European Journal of Neuroscience* **27**: 2057–65.

64 Aiba, I. and Noebels, J. L. (2015). Spreading depolarization in the brainstem mediates sudden cardiorespiratory arrest in mouse SUDEP models. *Science Translational Medicine* **7**: 282ra46.

65 Funke, F., Kron, M., Dutschmann, M. and Müller, M. (2009). Infant brain stem is prone to the generation of spreading depression during severe hypoxia. *Journal of Neurophysiology* **101**: 2395–2410.

66 Richter, F., Rupprecht, S., Lehmenkuhler, A. and Schaible, H.-G. (2003). Spreading Depression Can Be Elicited in Brain Stem of Immature But Not Adult Rats. *Journal of Neurophysiology* **90**: 2163–2170.

67 Richter, F., Bauer, R., Ebersberger, A., Lehmenkühler, A. and Schaible, H.-G. (2012). Enhanced neuronal excitability in adult rat brainstem causes widespread repetitive

brainstem depolarizations with cardiovascular consequences. *Journal of Cerebral Blood Flow & Metabolism* **32**: 1535–1545.

68 Berger, M., Speckmann, E.-J., Pape, H. C. and Gorji, A. (2008). Spreading depression enhances human neocortical excitability in vitro. *Cephalalgia* **28**: 558–562.

69 Gorji and Speckmann. (2004). Spreading depression enhances the spontaneous epileptiform activity in human neocortical tissues. *European Journal of Neuroscience* **19**: 3371–3374.

70 Akcali, D., Sayin, A., Sara, Y. and Bolay, H. (2010). Does single cortical spreading depression elicit pain behaviour in freely moving rats? *Cephalalgia* **30**: 1195–1206.

71 Carew, T. J., Crow, T. J. and Petrinovich, L. F. (1970). Lack of Coincidence between Neural and Behavioral Manifestations of Cortical Spreading Depression. *Science* **169**: 1339–1342.

72 Duckrow, R. B. (1991). Regional cerebral blood flow during spreading cortical depression in conscious rats. *Journal of Cerebral Blood Flow & Metabolism* **11**: 150–154.

73 Faraguna, U., Nelson, A., Vyazovskiy, V. V., Cirelli, C. and Tononi, G. (2010). Unilateral Cortical Spreading Depression Affects Sleep Need and Induces Molecular and Electrophysiological Signs of Synaptic Potentiation In Vivo. *Cerebral Cortex* **20**: 2939–47.

74 Fioravanti, B. *et al.* (2011).Evaluation of cutaneous allodynia following induction of cortical spreading depression in freely moving rats. *Cephalalgia* **31**: 1090–100.

75 Huston, J. P. and Bures, J. (1970). Drinking and eating elicited by cortical spreading depression. *Science* **169**: 702–704.

76 Petzold, G. C. *et al.* (2008). Nitric oxide modulates spreading depolarization threshold in the human and rodent cortex. *Stroke* **39**: 1292–1299.

77 Footitt, D. R. and Newberry, N. R. (1998). Cortical spreading depression induces an LTP-like effect in rat neocortex in vitro. *Brain Research* **781**: 339–342.

78 Basarsky, T. A., Duffy, S. N., Andrew, R. D. and MacVicar, B. A. (1998). Imaging spreading depression and associated intracellular calcium waves in brain slices. *Journal of Neuroscience* **18**: 7189–99.

79 Canals, S. *et al.* (2005). Longitudinal depolarization gradients along the somatodendritic axis of CA1 pyramidal cells: a novel feature of spreading depression. *Journal of Neurophysiology* **94**: 943–951.

80 Canals, S., Larrosa, B., Pintor, J., Mena, M. A. and Herreras, O. (2008). Metabolic challenge to glia activates an adenosine-mediated safety mechanism that promotes neuronal survival by delaying the onset of spreading depression waves. *Journal of Cerebral Blood Flow & Metabolism* **28**: 1835–44.

81 Czeh, G., Aitken, P. G. and Somjen, G. G. (1993). Membrane currents in CA1 pyramidal cells during spreading depression (SD) and SD-like hypoxic depolarization. *Brain Research* **632**: 195–208.

82 Margineanu, D. G. and Klitgaard, H. (2009). Brivaracetam inhibits spreading depression in rat neocortical slices in vitro. *Seizure* **18**: 453–456.

83 Mody, I., Lambert, J. D. and Heinemann, U. (1987). Low extracellular magnesium induces epileptiform activity and spreading depression in rat hippocampal slices. *Journal of Neurophysiology* **57**: 869–888.

84 Tang, Y. T., Kim, J., López-Valdés, H. E., Brennan, K. C. and Ju, Y. S. (2011). Development and characterization of a microfluidic chamber incorporating fluid ports

with active suction for localized chemical stimulation of brain slices. *Lab on a Chip* **11**: 2247–2254.

85 Tang, Y. T. *et al.* (2014). Minimum conditions for the induction of cortical spreading depression in brain slices. *Journal of Neurophysiology* **112**: 2572–2579.

86 Tottene, A. *et al.* (2009). Enhanced excitatory transmission at cortical synapses as the basis for facilitated spreading depression in Ca(v)2.1 knockin migraine mice. *Neuron* **61**: 762–773.

87 Heinemann, U. and Lux, H. D. (1977). Ceiling of stimulus induced rises in extra-cellular potassium concentration in the cerebral cortex of cat. *Brain Research* **120**: 231–249.

88 Reid, K. H., Marrannes, R., De Prins, E. and Wauquier, A. (1987). Potassium translocation and spreading depression induced by electrical stimulation of the brain. *Experimental Neurology* **97**: 345–64.

89 Matsuura, T. and Bures, J. (1971). The minimum volume of depolarized neural tissue required for triggering cortical spreading depression in rat. *Experimental Brain Research* **12**: 238–249.

90 Dreier, J. P. *et al.* (2002). Endothelin-1 potently induces Leao's cortical spreading depression in vivo in the rat: a model for an endothelial trigger of migrainous aura? *Brain* **125**: 102–112.

91 Nozari, A. *et al.* (2010). Microemboli may link spreading depression migraine aura and patent foramen ovale. *Annals of Neurology* **67**(2): 221–229.

92 Smith, J., Bradley, D., James, M. and Huang, C. L. (2006). Physiological studies of cortical spreading depression. *Biological Reviews* **81**: 457–481.

93 Ayata, C. Pearls and pitfalls in experimental models of spreading depression. *Cephalalgia* **33**: 604–13 (2013).

94 Akerman, S., Holland, P. R. and Goadsby, P. J. (2008). Mechanically-induced cortical spreading depression associated regional cerebral blood flow changes are blocked by Na+ ion channel blockade. *Brain Research* **1229**: 27–36.

95 Ayata, C., Shimizu-Sasamata, M., Lo, E. H., Noebels, J. L. and Moskowitz, M. A. (2000). Impaired neurotransmitter release and elevated threshold for cortical spreading depression in mice with mutations in the alpha1A subunit of P/Q type calcium channels. *Neuroscience* **95**: 639–45.

96 Ayata, C., Jin, H., Kudo, C., Dalkara, T. and Moskowitz, M. A. (2006). Suppression of cortical spreading depression in migraine prophylaxis. *Annals of Neurology* **59**: 652–661.

97 Brennan, K. C., Romero Reyes, M., Lopez-Valdes, H. E., Arnold, A. P. and Charles, A. C. (2007). Reduced threshold for cortical spreading depression in female mice. *Annals of Neurology* **61**: 603–6.

98 Brennan, K. C. *et al.* (2013). Casein kinase iδ mutations in familial migraine and advanced sleep phase. *Science Translational Medicine* **5**: 183ra56, 1–11.

99 Leo, L. *et al.* (2011). Increased susceptibility to cortical spreading depression in the mouse model of familial hemiplegic migraine type 2. *PLoS Genetics* **7**: e1002129.

100 Van den Maagdenberg, A. M. *et al.* (2004). A Cacna1a knockin migraine mouse model with increased susceptibility to cortical spreading depression. *Neuron* **41**: 701–10.

101 Kunkler, P. E. and Kraig, R. P. (1998). Calcium waves precede electrophysiological changes of spreading depression in hippocampal organ cultures. *Journal of Neuroscience* **18**: 3416–25.

102 Köhling, R. *et al.* (2003). Differential sensitivity to induction of spreading depression by partial disinhibition in chronically epileptic human and rat as compared to native rat neocortical tissue. *Brain Research* **975**: 129–134.

103 Psarropoulou, C. and Avoli, M. (1993).4-Aminopyridine-induced spreading depression episodes in immature hippocampus: developmental and pharmacological characteristics. *Neuroscience* **55**: 57–68.

104 Guedes, R. C., de Oliveira, J. A., Amancio-Dos-Santos, A. and Garcia-Cairasco, N. (2009). Sexual differentiation of cortical spreading depression propagation after acute and kindled audiogenic seizures in the Wistar audiogenic rat (WAR). *Epilepsy Research* **83**: 207–14.

105 Vinogradova, L. V. (2014). Comparative potency of sensory-induced brainstem activation to trigger spreading depression and seizures in the cortex of awake rats: Implications for the pathophysiology of migraine aura. *Cephalalgia* **35**(11): 979–86.

106 Vinogradova, L. V., Kuznetsova, G. D. and Coenen, A. M. (2005). Audiogenic seizures associated with a cortical spreading depression wave suppress spike-wave discharges in rats. *Physiology & Behavior* **86**: 554–8.

107 Vinogradova, L. V., Kuznetsova, G. D. and Coenen, A. M. (2009). Unilateral cortical spreading depression induced by sound in rats. *Brain Research* **1286**: 201–7.

108 Holland, P. R., Akerman, S. and Goadsby, P. J. (2010). Cortical spreading depression-associated cerebral blood flow changes induced by mechanical stimulation are modulated by AMPA and GABA receptors. *Cephalalgia* **30**: 519–527.

109 Brody, D. L. *et al.* (2007).Electromagnetic controlled cortical impact device for precise, graded experimental traumatic brain injury. *Journal of Neurotrauma* **24**: 657–673.

110 Von Baumgarten, L., Trabold, R., Thal, S., Back, T. and Plesnila, N. (2008). Role of cortical spreading depressions for secondary brain damage after traumatic brain injury in mice. *Journal of Cerebral Blood Flow & Metabolism* **28**: 1353–1360.

111 Von Bornstadt, D. *et al.* (2015). Supply-demand mismatch transients in susceptible peri-infarct hot zones explain the origins of spreading injury depolarizations. *Neuron* **85**: 1117–31.

112 Mies, G., Iijima, T. and Hossmann, K. A. (1993). Correlation between peri-infarct DC shifts and ischaemic neuronal damage in rat. *Neuroreport* **4**: 709–711.

113 Bere, Z., Obrenovitch, T. P., Kozak, G., Bari, F. and Farkas, E. (2014). Imaging reveals the focal area of spreading depolarizations and a variety of hemodynamic responses in a rat microembolic stroke model. *Journal of Cerebral Blood Flow & Metabolism* **34**: 1695–705.

114 Eikermann-Haerter, K. *et al.* (2012). Migraine mutations increase stroke vulnerability by facilitating ischemic depolarizations. *Circulation* **125**: 335–45.

115 Kao, Y. C. *et al.* (2014). Dynamic perfusion and diffusion MRI of cortical spreading depolarization in photothrombotic ischemia. *Neurobiology of Disease* **71**: 131–9.

116 Eikermann-Haerter, K. *et al.* (2015). Migraine prophylaxis, ischemic depolarizations, and stroke outcomes in mice. *Stroke* **46**: 229–36.

117 Balestrino, M., Young, J. and Aitken, P. (1999). Block of (Na+,K+)ATPase with ouabain induces spreading depression-like depolarization in hippocampal slices. *Brain Research* **838**: 37–44.

118 Menna, G., Tong, C. K. and Chesler, M. (2000). Extracellular pH changes and accompanying cation shifts during ouabain-induced spreading depression. *Journal of Neurophysiology* **83**: 1338–45.

119 Rundek, T. *et al.* (2008). Patent foramen ovale and migraine: a cross-sectional study from the Northern Manhattan Study (NOMAS). *Circulation* **118**: 1419–1424.

120 Dowson, A. *et al.* (2008). Migraine Intervention With STARFlex Technology (MIST) Trial: A Prospective, Multicenter, Double-Blind, Sham-Controlled Trial to Evaluate the Effectiveness of Patent Foramen Ovale Closure With STARFlex Septal Repair Implant to Resolve Refractory Migraine Headache. *Circulation* **117**: 1397–1404.

121 Sugaya, E., Takato, M. and Noda, Y. (1975). Neuronal and glial activity during spreading depression in cerebral cortex of cat. *Journal of Neurophysiology* **38**: 822–841.

122 Sawant, P. M., Suryavanshi, P., Mendez, J. M., Dudek, F. E. and Brennan, K. C. (2016). Mechanisms of neuronal silencing after cortical spreading depression. *Cerebral Cortex doi*: 10.1093/cercor/bhv328.

123 Farkas, E., Pratt, R., Sengpiel, F. and Obrenovitch, T. P. (2008).Direct, live imaging of cortical spreading depression and anoxic depolarisation using a fluorescent, voltage-sensitive dye. *Journal of Cerebral Blood Flow & Metabolism* **28**: 251–62.

124 Aitken, P. G., Fayuk, D., Somjen, G. G. and Turner, D. A. (1999). Use of Intrinsic Optical Signals to Monitor Physiological Changes in Brain Tissue Slices. *Methods* **18**: 91–103.

125 Fayuk, D., Aitken, P. G., Somjen, G. G. and Turner, D. A. (2002). Two Different Mechanisms Underlie Reversible, Intrinsic Optical Signals in Rat Hippocampal Slices. *Journal of Neurophysiology* **87**: 1924–1937.

126 Baraghis, E. *et al.* (2011). Two-photon microscopy of cortical NADH fluorescence intensity changes: correcting contamination from the hemodynamic response. *Journal of Biomedical Optics* **16**: 106003.

127 Rex, A., Pfeifer, L., Fink, F. and Fink, H. (1999). Cortical NADH during pharmacological manipulations of the respiratory chain and spreading depression in vivo. *Journal of Neuroscience Research* **57**: 359–370.

128 Shin, H. K. *et al.* (2007). Normobaric hyperoxia improves cerebral blood flow and oxygenation, and inhibits peri-infarct depolarizations in experimental focal ischaemia. *Brain* **130**(Pt 6): 1631–1642.

129 Fabricius, M., Akgoren, N., Dirnagl, U. and Lauritzen, M. (1997). Laminar Analysis of Cerebral Blood Flow in Cortex of Rats by Laser-Doppler Flowmetry: A Pilot Study. *Journal of Cerebral Blood Flow & Metabolism* **17**: 1326–1336.

130 Ostergaard, L. *et al.* (2015). Neurovascular coupling during cortical spreading depolarization and -depression. *Stroke* **46**: 1392–401.

131 Yuzawa, I. *et al.* (2012). Cortical spreading depression impairs oxygen delivery and metabolism in mice. *Journal of Cerebral Blood Flow & Metabolism* **32**: 376–386.

132 Chuquet, J., Hollender, L. and Nimchinsky, E. (2007). High-Resolution In Vivo Imaging of the Neurovascular Unit during Spreading Depression. *Journal of Neuroscience* **27**: 4036–44.

133 Risher, W. C., Ard, D., Yuan, J. and Kirov, S. A. (2010). Recurrent spontaneous spreading depolarizations facilitate acute dendritic injury in the ischemic penumbra. *Journal of Neuroscience* **30**: 9859–9868.

134 Bradley, D. P. *et al.* (2001). Diffusion-weighted MRI used to detect in vivo modulation of cortical spreading depression: comparison of sumatriptan and tonabersat. *Experimental Neurology* **172**: 342–353.

135 Lascola, C. D. *et al.* (2004). Changes in magnetization transfer MRI correlate with spreading depression-induced astroglial reactivity and increased protein expression in mice. *American Journal of Roentgenology* **183**: 1791–7.

136 Smith, M. I. *et al.* (2000). Repetitive cortical spreading depression in a gyrencephalic feline brain: inhibition by the novel benzoylamino-benzopyran SB-220453. *Cephalalgia* **20**: 546–53.

137 Autio, J. A., Shatillo, A., Giniatullin, R. and Grohn, O. H. (2014). Parenchymal spin-lock fMRI signals associated with cortical spreading depression. *Journal of Cerebral Blood Flow & Metabolism* **34**: 768–75.

138 Netsiri, C. *et al.* (2003). A delayed class of BOLD waveforms associated with spreading depression in the feline cerebral cortex can be detected and characterised using independent component analysis (ICA). *Magnetic Resonance Imaging* **21**: 1097–1110.

139 Shatillo, A., Salo, R. A., Giniatullin, R. and Grohn, O. H. (2015). Involvement of NMDA receptor subtypes in cortical spreading depression in rats assessed by fMRI. *Neuropharmacology* **93**: 164–70.

140 Bowyer, S. M. *et al.* (1999). Analysis of MEG signals of spreading cortical depression with propagation constrained to a rectangular cortical strip. II. Gyrencephalic swine model. *Brain Research* **843**: 79–86.

141 Leistner, S. *et al.* (2007). Combined MEG and EEG methodology for non-invasive recording of infraslow activity in the human cortex. *Clinical Neurophysiology* **118**: 2774–80.

142 Leistner, S. *et al.* (2009). Differential infraslow (<0.1 Hz) cortical activations in the affected and unaffected hemispheres from patients with subacute stroke demonstrated by noninvasive DC-magnetoencephalography. *Stroke* **40**: 1683–1686.

143 Kaufmann, D. *et al.* (2015). sec-Butylpropylacetamide (SPD) has antimigraine properties. *Cephalalgia* **36**(10): 924–35.

144 Hoffmann, U., Sukhotinsky, I., Atalay, Y. B., Eikermann-Haerter, K. and Ayata, C. (2012). Increased glucose availability does not restore prolonged spreading depression durations in hypotensive rats without brain injury. *Experimental Neurology* **238**: 130–2.

145 Sukhotinsky, I., Dilekoz, E., Moskowitz, M. . and Ayata, C. (2008). Hypoxia and hypotension transform the blood flow response to cortical spreading depression from hyperemia into hypoperfusion in the rat. *Journal of Cerebral Blood Flow & Metabolism* **28**: 1369.

146 Sukhotinsky, I. *et al.* (2010). Perfusion pressure-dependent recovery of cortical spreading depression is independent of tissue oxygenation over a wide physiologic range. *Journal of Cerebral Blood Flow & Metabolism* **30**: 1168–77.

147 Richter, F. *et al.* (2014). Tumor necrosis factor reduces the amplitude of rat cortical spreading depression *in vivo*. *Annals of Neurology* **76**: 43–53.

148 Gniel, H. M. and Martin, R. L. (2010). Changes in membrane potential and the intracellular calcium concentration during CSD and OGD in layer V and layer II/III mouse cortical neurons. *Journal of Neurophysiology* **104**: 3203–3212.

149 Bere, Z., Obrenovitch, T. P., Bari, F. and Farkas, E. (2014). Ischemia-induced depolarizations and associated hemodynamic responses in incomplete global forebrain ischemia in rats. *Neuroscience* **260**: 217–26.

150 Dhir, A., Lossin, C. and Rogawski, M. A. (2012). Propofol hemisuccinate suppresses cortical spreading depression. *Neuroscience Letters* **514**: 67–70.

151 Guedes, R. C. and Barreto, J. M. (1992). Effect of anesthesia on the propagation of cortical spreading depression in rats. *Brazilian Journal of Medical and Biological Research* **25**: 393–7.

152 Kitahara, Y., Taga, K., Abe, H. and Shimoji, K. (2001). The effects of anesthetics on cortical spreading depression elicitation and c-fos expression in rats. *Journal of Neurosurgical Anesthesiology* **13**: 26–32.

153 Kudo, C., Nozari, A., Moskowitz, M. A. and Ayata, C. (2008). The impact of anesthetics and hyperoxia on cortical spreading depression. *Experimental Neurology* **212**: 201–206.

154 Kudo, C. *et al.* (2013). Anesthetic effects on susceptibility to cortical spreading depression. *Neuropharmacology* **67**: 32–6.

155 Piper, R. and Lambert, G. (1996). Inhalational anesthetics inhibit spreading depression: relevance to migraine. *Cephalalgia* **16**: 87–92.

156 Sonn, J. and Mayevsky, A. (2006). Effects of anesthesia on the responses to cortical spreading depression in the rat brain *in vivo*. *Neurological Research* **28**: 206–219.

157 De Souza, T. K., MB , E. S.-G. , Rodrigues, M. C. and Guedes, R. C. (2015). Anesthetic agents modulate ECoG potentiation after spreading depression, and insulin-induced hypoglycemia does not modify this effect. *Neuroscience Letters* **592**: 6–11.

158 Takagaki, M. *et al.* (2014). Isoflurane suppresses cortical spreading depolarizations compared to propofol – implications for sedation of neurocritical care patients. *Experimental Neurology* **252**: 12–7.

159 Sukhotinsky, I., Dilekoz, E., Moskowitz, M. A. and Ayata, C. (2008). Hypoxia and hypotension transform the blood flow response to cortical spreading depression from hyperemia into hypoperfusion in the rat. *Journal of Cerebral Blood Flow & Metabolism* **28**: 1369–76.

160 Tong, C. K. and Chesler, M. (2000). Modulation of spreading depression by changes in extracellular pH. *Journal of Neurophysiology* **84**: 2449–57.

161 Gido, G., Katsura, K., Kristian, T. and Siesjo, B. K. (1993). Influence of plasma glucose concentration on rat brain extracellular calcium transients during spreading depression. *Journal of Cerebral Blood Flow & Metabolism* **13**: 179–82.

162 Nedergaard, M. and Astrup, J. (1986). Infarct rim: effect of hyperglycemia on direct current potential and [14C]2-deoxyglucose phosphorylation. *Journal of Cerebral Blood Flow & Metabolism* **6**: 607–615.

163 Takaoka, S., Pearlstein, R. D. and Warner, D. S. (1996). Hypothermia reduces the propensity of cortical tissue to propagate direct current depolarizations in the rat. *Neuroscience Letters* **218**: 25–8.

164 Ueda, M. *et al.* (1997). The effect of hypothermia on CSD propagation in rats. *No Shinkei Geka* **25**: 523–8.

165 Yenari, M. A. *et al.* (2000). Diffusion- and perfusion-weighted magnetic resonance imaging of focal cerebral ischemia and cortical spreading depression under
conditions of mild hypothermia. *Brain Research* **885**: 208–19.

166 Anttila, V. *et al.* (2010). Genome-wide association study of migraine implicates a
common susceptibility variant on 8q22.1. *Nature Genetics* **42**: 869–73.

167 Anttila, V. *et al.* (2013). Genome-wide meta-analysis identifies new susceptibility
loci for migraine. *Nature Genetics* **45**: 912–7.

168 Chasman, D. I. *et al.* (2011). Genome-wide association study reveals three susceptibility loci for common migraine in the general population. *Nature Genetics* **43**:
695–8.

169 Freilinger, T. *et al.* (2012). Genome-wide association analysis identifies susceptibility
loci for migraine without aura. *Nature Genetics* **44**: 777–82.

170 Langford, D. J. *et al.* (2010). Coding of facial expressions of pain in the laboratory
mouse. *Nature Methods* **7**: 447–9.

171 Levy, D., Moskowitz, M. A., Noseda, R. and Burstein, R. (2012). Activation of
the migraine pain pathway by cortical spreading depression: do we need more
evidence? *Cephalalgia* **32**: 581–2.

172 Urban, A. *et al.* (2015). Real-time imaging of brain activity in freely moving rats
using functional ultrasound. *Nature Methods* **12**: 873–878.

173 Legon, W. *et al.* (2014). Transcranial focused ultrasound modulates the activity of
primary somatosensory cortex in humans. *Nature Neuroscience* **17**: 322–329.

174 Ghosh, K. K. *et al.* (2011). Miniaturized integration of a fluorescence microscope.
Nature Methods **8**: 871–878.

175 Kadam, S. D., White, A. M., Staley, K. J. and Dudek, F. E. (2010). Continuous elec-
troencephalographic monitoring with radio-telemetry in a rat model of perinatal
hypoxia-ischemia reveals progressive post-stroke epilepsy. *Journal of Neuroscience*
30: 404–415.

176 Chung, K. and Deisseroth, K. (2013). CLARITY for mapping the nervous system.
Nature Methods **10**: 508–513.

177 Knöpfel, T. (2012). Genetically encoded optical indicators for the analysis of neuronal circuits. *Nature Reviews Neuroscience* **13**: 687–700.

178 Rogan, S. C. and Roth, B. L. (2011). Remote control of neuronal signaling. *Pharmacological Reviews* **63**: 291–315.

179 Tye, K. M. and Deisseroth, K. (2012). Optogenetic investigation of neural circuits underlying brain disease in animal models. *Nature Reviews Neuroscience* **13**:
251–66.

180 Yizhar, O., Fenno, L. E., Davidson, T. J., Mogri, M. and Deisseroth, K. (2011). Optogenetics in neural systems. *Neuron* **71**: 9–34.

20

Human models of migraine

Jakob Møller Hansen and Messoud Ashina

Danish Headache Center, Department of Neurology, Rigshospitalet, Glostrup, Faculty of Health and Medical Sciences, University of Copenhagen, Copenhagen, Denmark

20.1   Introduction

Over the past decades, there has been tremendous progress in the understanding of migraine pathophysiology and treatment, but much remains to be learned concerning migraine-initiating mechanisms. Because migraine attacks are fully reversible, and amendable to therapy, the headache- or migraine-provoking property of endogenous signaling molecules can be tested in a human model. If a naturally occurring substance can provoke migraine in humans, then it is possible, although not certain, that blocking specific pathways will be effective in the treatment of migraine. Iversen *et al.* (1989) validated and introduced the experimental model of glyceryl trinitrate (GTN)-induced headache in healthy volunteers. Since then, several studies have demonstrated that human models offer unique possibilities to study migraine pathophysiology and explore the mechanisms of action of existing and future anti-migraine drugs.

The use of the human migraine model has been extensively reviewed (Ashina *et al.*, 2013; Arulmani *et al.*, 2006). This chapter will focus on the most promising molecular targets so far, review and discuss the use of provocation experiments to understand functional consequences of migraine genes, and finally suggest where future studies are needed.

20.2   The first steps: GTN and the NO-hypothesis

Since the middle of the 19th century, when nitrates were introduced for the acute treatment of angina (Murrell, 1879), and factory workers were exposed accidentally to nitrates (McGuinness and Harris, 1961), it has been known that that GTN induces headache (Hering, 1849; Tfelt-Hansen and Tfelt-Hansen, 2009; Hughes and Dake, 1888). GTN is a donor of nitric oxide (NO). The relation between GTN-headache and migraine propensity was explored by Sicuteri and colleagues, who reported a striking difference in the sensitivity to sublingual GTN between healthy controls and migraine patients (Sicuteri *et al.*, 1987).

Neurobiological Basis of Migraine, First Edition. Edited by Turgay Dalkara and Michael A. Moskowitz.
© 2017 John Wiley & Sons, Inc. Published 2017 by John Wiley & Sons, Inc.

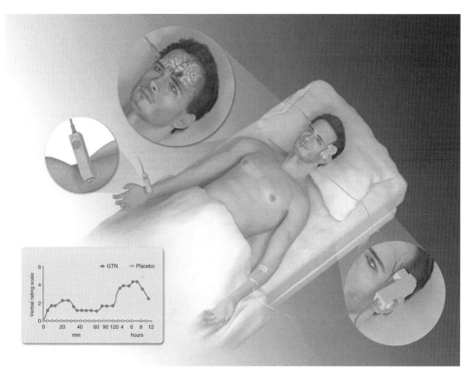

Figure 20.1 The human provocation model. In the main version of this model, patients with migraine are randomly allocated to receive intravenous infusion (25 min) of "target substance" or placebo (isotonic saline) in a double-blind, crossover design. Headache intensity is recorded on a verbal rating scale from 0 to 10 (0 – no headache; 1 – a very mild headache (including a feeling of pressing or throbbing); 5 – moderate headache; 10 – worst imaginable headache). At predefined intervals, hemodynamic variables are recorded (mean velocity of blood flow in the middle cerebral artery by transcranial Doppler with hand-held 2 MHz probes; diameter of the frontal branch of the superficial temporal artery by a high-resolution ultrasonography unit). With the addition of other imaging modalities, such as high-field MRI, even more detailed information can be collected on the vascular response of the cephalic circulation. The subjects are asked to complete a headache diary every hour until 10 hours after discharge. The diary includes headache characteristics and accompanying symptoms necessary to classify the headache according to ICHD-III. Heart rate and blood pressure are measured continuously throughout the study for safety. Olesen *et al.* (2009). Reproduced with permission of SAGE.

Using intravenous GTN, Olesen's migraine research group from Copenhagen investigated and validated the model by providing important details, such as headache time profile, pain characteristics and accompanying symptoms (Ashina *et al.*, 2013). The typical provocation experiment would be set up as a double-blind, crossover study with patients randomly allocated to receive intravenous infusion of the target substance or placebo (isotonic saline) (Figure 20.1).

It was thus demonstrated that patients with migraine were hypersensitive to NO – that is, migraineurs developed significantly stronger headache after GTN infusion than both patients with tension-type headache and healthy subjects (Olesen *et al.*, 1993). When tested in patients with migraine without aura (MO) (Thomsen *et al.*, 1994), most patients reported an immediate headache during GTN infusion but, importantly, 80% of patients developed a delayed headache several hours after the infusion stopped, fulfilling criteria of the International Classification of Headache Disorders for a migraine attack (The International Classification of Headache Disorders, 2013). Other routes of GTN administration (e.g., sublingual) can be used, but results are more variable, and the rate of migraine induction is reduced (Sances *et al.*, 2004) – see also table 20.1.

Collectively, these studies clearly suggest that GTN may trigger a genuine migraine attack in migraine sufferers, and that NO plays a crucial role in migraine pathogenesis.

The success of the model led to increased focus on possible down-stream mediators of the migraine-inducing capabilities of NO. NO activates intracellular soluble guanylate cyclase and, thus, catalyzes the formation of cyclic guanosine monophosphate (cGMP) (Garthwaite *et al.*, 1988). Sildenafil (Viagra®) is a highly selective inhibitor of phosphodiesterase 5 (PDE 5), the major enzyme responsible for the breakdown of cGMP. Inhibition of PDE 5 results in accumulation of cGMP, and the effect of sildenafil could, therefore, mimic the effects of NO, such as activation of soluble guanylate cyclase and increased cGMP formation.

This hypothesis was tested in the human experimental model, where 12 patients with migraine without aura were administered sildenafil 100 mg or placebo in a double-blind, placebo-controlled crossover study (Kruuse *et al.*, 2003). Sildenafil induced delayed migraine-like attack in ten out of 12 patients, compared with two out of 12 after placebo, an effect comparable to that of GTN. Thus, it appears that sildenafil triggered experimental migraine is induced via a cGMP-dependent mechanism – see also table 20.1.

Interestingly, blood flow velocity in the middle cerebral artery (MCA), regional cerebral blood flow in the territory of the middle cerebral artery, and the diameters of radial and temporal artery, were unaffected by sildenafil (Kruuse *et al.*, 2003).

Arterial dilatation may cause headache (Nichols *et al.*, 1990), and GTN infusion does cause a more pronounced dilation of extra- and intracerebral arteries in migraine patients than in controls (Thomsen *et al.*, 1993). The *onset* of the *immediate* GTN-induced headache in healthy volunteers is correlated to dilation of the MCA (Tegeler *et al.*, 1996), but vasodilatation outlasts the headache (Tegeler *et al.*, 1996; Iversen *et al.*, 2008). A *post-hoc* analysis of a series of human experiments found *no* linear relationship between experimental *immediate* headache and dilatation of the intra- and extra cerebral arteries (Ashina *et al.*, 2011). The current understanding, also backed by other studies (Ahn, 2010; Amin *et al.*, 2013; Rahmann *et al.*, 2008), is therefore that vascular changes, though present, are unlikely to be the primary cause for head pain in migraine (Charles, 2013).

Brain imaging research in the last two decades has contributed significantly to advancing our knowledge of the neurobiology of human models of migraine. Using modern brain imaging methods, particularly positron emission tomography (PET) (Ashina *et al.*, 2013), MR angiography (Amin *et al.*, 2013) and functional MRI (Schwedt *et al.*, 2015), researchers have investigated biological markers in migraine (Ashina *et al.*, 2013).

PET studies showed brainstem activation during GTN-induced attacks (Afridi *et al.*, 2005b; Bahra *et al.*, 2001), similar to activation reported during spontaneous migraine attacks (Weiller *et al.*, 1995; Afridi *et al.*, 2005a). Furthermore, GTN induces premonitory symptoms (Afridi *et al.*, 2004) similar to premonitory symptoms reported during spontaneous migraine attacks (Giffin *et al.*, 2003). Using the GTN model, combined with PET, a recent study reported brain activation in hypothalamus during

Table 20.1 Percentages of migraine patient-reported migraine-like attacks in experimental studies.

Compound		Dose	Migraine-like attacks (%)	References
Glyceryl trinitrate (GTN)	Migraine with aura	intravenous 0.5 μg/kg/min	50–67	Afridi *et al.*, 2004; Christiansen *et al.*, 1999
		sublingual 0.9 mg	40.9	Sances *et al.*, 2004
	Migraine without aura	intravenous 0.5 μg/kg/min	80–83	Afridi *et al.*, 2004; Thomsen *et al.*, 1994
		sublingual 0.6 mg / 0.9 mg	66.7 / 82.1	Sicuteri *et al.*, 1987; Sances *et al.*, 2004
	Hemiplegic migraine	intravenous 0.5 μg/kg/min	12.5–30	Hansen *et al.*, 2008a, 2008c, 2010b
Histamine		intravenous 0.5 μg/kg/min intravenous 0.1 mg arterial 0.1 mg (carotid)	70 78 77	Lassen *et al.*, 1995 Northfield, 1938 Northfield, 1938
PDE 5 (Sildenafil)		100 mg per os	83	Kruuse *et al.*, 2003
PDE 3 (Cilostazol)		200 mg per os	86	Guo *et al.*, 2014
Dipyridamole		intravenous 0.142 mg/kg/min	50	Kruuse *et al.*, 2006
Calcitonin gene-related peptide (CGRP)	Migraine with aura	intravenous 1.5 μg/min	57	Hansen *et al.*, 2010a
	Migraine without aura	intravenous 2 μg/min	33–75	Lassen *et al.*, 2002; Asghar *et al.*, 2011
	Hemiplegic migraine	intravenous 1.5 μg/min	9–22	Hansen *et al.*, 2011, 2008b
Vasoactive intestinal peptide (VIP)		intravenous 8 pmol/kg/min	0–18	Amin *et al.*, 2014; Rahmann *et al.*, 2008
Pituitary adenylate cyclase activating polypeptide (PACAP-38)		intravenous 10 pmol/ kg/min	66–73	Schytz *et al.*, 2009; Amin *et al.*, 2014
Prostaglandins	**Prostaglandin E2**	intravenous 0.4 μg/kg/min	58	Antonova *et al.*, 2012
	Prostaglandin I2	intravenous 10 ng/kg/min	50	Wienecke *et al.*, 2009a

the premonitory phase, notably at a time point when the patients were totally pain-free (Maniyar *et al.*, 2014).

Collectively, the experimental studies indicate that NO is involved both in the initiation of, but also throughout, the duration of a migraine attack. Based on the reliable and robust migraine-inducing effects of GTN, the anti-migraine action of non-selective nitric oxide synthase (NOS) inhibitor, N(G)-mono-methyl-L-arginine (L-NMMA) was examined, and it was demonstrated that NOS inhibition was effective in treating spontaneous migraine attacks (Lassen *et al.*, 1997). Clinical trials of selective inhibition of inducible nitric oxide synthase for acute (Van der Schueren *et al.*, 2009) and prophylactic (Hoivik *et al.*, 2010) migraine treatment were negative. This drug class has not yet been developed into available therapy, and NOS inhibitors still have to prove their usefulness in migraine treatment.

In conclusion, the GTN model of migraine has led to a number of important observations, but more studies are still needed to dissect its role in the migraine cascade.

The precise mechanisms of NO-induced migraine are still not fully clarified. Given the ability of NO to penetrate the blood-brain barrier, migraine induction is complex and may include both peripheral and central pain pathways. The imaging studies of NO-provocation do not support the hypothesis of vasodilatation *per se* as the primary source of pain in GTN-induced immediate headache.

20.3 Calcitonin gene-related peptide (CGRP)

CGRP is a 37-amino-acid neuropeptide identified in the early 1980s (Amara *et al.*, 1982; Rosenfeld *et al.*, 1983). Animal models of headache and pain suggest the modulatory role of CGRP in nociceptive transmission (Sun *et al.*, 2003, 2004; Mao *et al.*, 1992; Levy *et al.*, 2005; Oku *et al.*, 1987; Russo, 2014).

Studies in migraine patients have showed elevation of CGRP during (Goadsby *et al.*, 1990) and outside of migraine attacks (Ashina *et al.*, 2000). However, Tvedskov *et al.* challenged these reports, showing no changes in plasma CGRP in the external jugular vein during migraine attacks, compared with outside of attacks (Tvedskov *et al.*, 2005). The strongest human evidence supporting the role of CGRP in migraine has derived from provocation experiments. In a double-blind crossover study, α-CGRP (2 µg/min) or placebo was infused for 20 minutes in 12 patients suffering from migraine without aura (Lassen *et al.*, 2002). During the following 11 hours, all patients experienced headaches after human α-CGRP and only one patient after placebo and, in three patients, the delayed headache fulfilled the IHS criteria for migraine without aura (Lassen *et al.*, 2002). Subsequent studies confirmed that CGRP is, indeed, a trigger of migraine (table 20.1).

The vascular effects of CGRP-infusion in healthy volunteers was investigated with high-resolution 3-Tesla MRI: CGRP causes significant dilation of the extra cerebral middle meningeal artery (MMA), but not of the intra cerebral MCA, compared with placebo (Asghar *et al.*, 2010). Interestingly, the headache-aborting effect of sumatriptan was associated with constriction of the MMA, but not MCA. Furthermore, in contrast to GTN-induced migraine (Schoonman *et al.*, 2008), CGRP-induced migraine without aura was associated with dilatation of extra- and intracerebral arteries, and headache laterality corresponded to the side of vasodilatation (Asghar *et al.*, 2011). This suggests

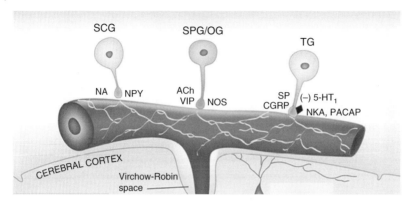

Figure 20.2 Different types of perivascular nerves and their transmitters (modified from Hamel, 2006). Schematic representation of the different types of perivascular nerves and their origin from the superior cervical (SCG), sphenopalatine (SPG), or otic (OG) or trigeminal (TG) ganglion. The most relevant neurotransmitters also discussed in the text are; CGRP, calcitonin gene-related peptide; NOS, nitric oxide synthase; PACAP, pituitary adenylate-cyclase activating polypeptide and VIP, vasoactive intestinal polypeptide. See also Figure 1.1 in chapter 1. Hamel *et al.* (2006). Reproduced by permission of American Physiological Society.

that perivascular release of vasoactive substances, and activation of perivascular sensory afferents, are an integral part of migraine pathophysiology – see Figure 20.2.

The downstream effector of CGRP involves cyclic AMP signaling (Jansen-Olesen *et al.*, 1996). Phosphodiesterase 3 is one of the most important cAMP-degrading enzymes in cerebral arteries, and its activity can be blocked by cilostazol, thus leading to cyclic AMP accumulation. In a provocation study, where 14 migraine patients without aura were examined in a double-blind, placebo-controlled crossover study, cilostazol induced delayed migraine-like attacks in 12 patients (86%), compared with two (14%) patients after placebo. This strongly suggests that intracellular cAMP-accumulation plays a crucial role in migraine induction (Guo *et al.*, 2014) – see also table 20.1.

The importance of CGRP in migraine pathogenesis was underlined after large randomized controlled trials confirmed that CGRP antagonists are effective in a subsets of patients in treating acute migraine attacks (Ho *et al.*, 2008a, 2008b; Olesen *et al.*, 2004; Connor *et al.*, 2009), and also in migraine prophylaxis (Ho *et al.*, 2014).

The exact pathways involved in CGRP-induced migraine attacks and mechanisms of action of CGRP antagonists are not fully clarified, but may involve both peripheral and central site of action (Summ *et al.*, 2010; Sixt *et al.*, 2009). The newest addition to CGRP-based migraine treatment has been the finding that monoclonal antibodies to CGRP are effective in migraine prophylaxis (Sun *et al.*, 2016; Bigal *et al.*, 2015;Dodick *et al.*, 2014a, 2014b). Interestingly, both the anti-migraine action of the CGRP antibodies and their large molecular weight point to a peripheral site of action for CGRP in migraine.

The CGRP studies show that it is possible to go from animal studies, based on anatomy and physiology, into human experimental studies, and on to clinical trials to yield a working drug, based on stringent translational thinking (and, as always, a certain amount of serendipity).

The finding that CGRP causes headache and migraine in MA and MO, and that CGRP antagonism may both abort and prevents migraine attacks is a testament to the validity of the human migraine model. Future human experimental studies with CGRP in conjunction with imaging may help to unravel the site of action of both CGRP and CGRP-based migraine treatment.

20.4 Vasoactive intestinal peptide (VIP) and pituitary adenylate cyclase activating polypeptide (PACAP)

The CGRP studies clearly underlined that neuropeptides are implicated in the pathophysiology of primary headaches. Vasoactive Intestinal Peptide (VIP) and Pituitary Adenylate Cyclase-Activating Polypeptide (PACAP) are both vasoactive peptides belonging to a family of structurally related peptides (Sherwood *et al.*, 2000). They are both found in perivascular parasympathetic nerve fibers (Jansen-Olesen *et al.*, 2004), and PACAP is also found in trigeminal nerve fibers surrounding cerebral blood vessels (Baeres and Moller, 2004). Their release regulates cerebrovascular tone and hemodynamics of the brain (Gulbenkian *et al.*, 2001). Studies of VIP in double-blinded placebo-controlled crossover studies, in both healthy volunteers (Hansen *et al.*, 2006) and migraine patients, (Rahmann *et al.*, 2008; Amin *et al.*, 2014) showed a very modest headache/migraine induction rate (Table 20.1).

In healthy volunteers, PACAP-infusion induced vasodilatation similarly to VIP, but longer-lasting (Birk *et al.*, 2007; Amin *et al.*, 2012), and in migraine patients without aura, PACAP induced both sustained cephalic vasodilatation and migraine attacks (Schytz *et al.*, 2009).

In a randomized head-to-head comparison study of intravenous administration of PACAP and VIP, more patients (73%) reported migraine-like attacks after PACAP38 than after VIP (18%) (Amin *et al.*, 2014; see also table 20.1). PACAP-induced migraine was associated with sustained dilatation of extra cranial arteries and elevated plasma PACAP before the onset of migraine-like attacks. The exact pro-nociceptive mechanisms of PACAP are still not mapped out in details, but central sensitization (Tuka *et al.*, 2012) or mast cell degranulation could be involved (Baun *et al.*, 2012).

Two receptors, $VPAC_1$ (Hosoya *et al.*, 1993) and $VPAC_2$ (Lutz *et al.*, 1993), are activated with equal affinity by PACAP and VIP, but a third receptor, PAC_1, is selectively activated by PACAP (Harmar *et al.*, 1998). The migraine induction by PACAP-38, in contrast to VIP, suggests that the shared VIP/PACAP receptors ($VPAC_1$ and $VPAC_2$) are unlikely to be causal for induction of migraine, but points toward an important role for the PACAP-selective PAC_1 receptor. PACAP has a much higher affinity for the PAC_1 receptor, and it can, therefore, be speculated that the migraine induction by PACAP38 may result from activation of the PAC_1 receptor, which may be an interesting future anti-migraine drug target (Schytz *et al.*, 2010; Amin *et al.*, 2014).

20.4.1 Prostaglandin model

In the last decade, the role of prostaglandins (PGs) in the generation of headache in healthy volunteers and migraine sufferers has been systematically investigated in the human migraine model. The intravenous administration of vasodilating prostaglandins, such as PGI_2 (prostacyclin), PGE_2 and PGD_2, induced headache in healthy volunteers, and PGI_2 triggered migraine-like attacks in migraine patients (Wienecke *et al.*, 2008, 2009a, 2009b, 2011). Interestingly, the infusion of PGE_2 caused *immediate migraine-like attacks*, accompanied by vasodilatation of the middle cerebral artery and insignificant vasodilatation of the superficial temporal artery in migraine patients without aura (Antonova *et al.*, 2012). The fact that PGE_2 selectively triggers *immediate* migraine-like attacks is at odds with all other tested migraine-inducing substances (see table 20.1).

MRI verification of dilatation of cerebral or extra-cerebral arteries in PG-induced headache or migraine is pending. Given that PGs are inflammatory mediators (Hata and Breyer, 2004), capable of activating sensory afferents, it could be speculated that PG-induced vasodilatation does not contribute to provoked headache. To investigate the role of inflammation and vasodilatation in prostaglandin-induced headache, we investigated whether the pro-inflammatory and vaso*constricting* prostanoid prostaglandin F2α (PGF2α) would cause headache in a human model of headache. $PGF_{2\alpha,}$ as opposed to $PGE_2,$ PGI_2 and PGD_2, did not induce headache (Antonova *et al.*, 2011b), but the lack of a dilating effect of $PGF_{2\alpha}$ on cerebral arteries could explain the absence of headache. Based on these data, we suggest that the vasodilating abilities of PGs are important in generating pain in healthy volunteers, and are likely to play a role in the mechanisms of spontaneous migraine attacks.

Drugs were tested in the PGE2 headache model in healthy volunteers. A highly specific and potent EP_4 receptor antagonist, BGC20-1531, did not attenuate PGE_2-induced headache and vasodilatation of intra- or extra-cerebral arteries (Antonova *et al.*, 2011a). The failure of BGC20-1531 to attenuate headache and vasodilatation suggests either that the EP_4 receptor is not involved, or that PGE2 may induce headache via other pathways, and that a single receptor blockade, therefore, may not be enough. It should be emphasized that a lack of efficacy of EP_4 receptor antagonist in PGE_2 model in healthy volunteers does not exclude possible efficacy of EP_4 antagonist as acute or preventive drug in migraine.

20.5   Can we gain from the use of experimental models to study functional consequences of migraine mutations?

Important insights into the genetic and molecular pathophysiology of migraine have come from studies of rare monogenic subtype of migraine, familial hemiplegic migraine (FHM). *In vivo* studies of mice with *knock-ins* of two different FHM genes showed increased susceptibility to cortical spreading depression (CSD) and increased velocity of CSD propagation, compared with wild-type animals (van den Maagdenberg *et al.*, 2004, 2010; Eikermann-Haerter *et al.*, 2009; Leo *et al.*, 2011). The fact that FHM-1 knock-in mice show a relevant pain phenotype (Chanda *et al.*, 2013; Hullugundi *et al.*, 2014) suggests that these transgenic mice are an important model to improve our understanding of migraine pathogenesis, and may be used as a platform for testing novel anti-migraine drugs.

The common types of migraine, MA and MO, are, however, not generally associated with any of the known FHM mutations (Kirchmann *et al.*, 2006; Netzer *et al.*, 2006; Jen *et al.*, 2004; Wieser *et al.*, 2003). In addition, many of the traits found in these monogenic subtypes of migraine (e.g., hemiplegia during aura, progressive ataxia) are not found in common migraine.

The translation from the promising animal studies of the monogenic forms of migraine into a human clinical setting, and the relation between these rare subtypes and MO and MA, may thus not be as straightforward as hoped. A series of experiments using the human experimental model examined whether the FHM mutations were associated with hypersensitivity to the migraine triggers NO and CGRP. Both GTN and CGRP failed to cause more auras or headaches in FHM-patients than healthy controls (Hansen *et al.*, 2008a, 2008b, 2008c). These data indicate that the FHM 1 and 2 genotype does not confer hypersensitivity to migraine triggers such as GTN and CGRP and, thus, suggests different neurobiological mechanisms of migraine initiation in than in the more common migraine types.

20.6   Conclusion

Human models of migraine offer unique possibilities to study mechanisms responsible for migraine and to explore the mechanisms of action of existing and future anti-migraine drugs (Olesen *et al.*, 2009). Results provide insights into the very early migraine symptoms during the premonitory phase (Maniyar *et al.*, 2014), the mechanisms of anti-migraine drugs (Asghar *et al.*, 2011) and the differences between migraine phenotypes (Hansen, 2010a). Human models have played an important role in translational migraine research, leading to the identification and validation of novel targets for the treatment of acute migraine attacks (Olesen *et al.*, 2004; Lassen *et al.*, 1997).

New additions to the model, such as advanced MR, functional MRI (fMRI) using blood-oxygen-level-dependent (BOLD) contrast, and resting state fMRI, positron emission tomography (PET) and multimodal imaging (Schoonman *et al.*, 2008; Amin *et al.*, 2013; Maniyar *et al.*, 2014; Afridi *et al.*, 2005b; Schwedt *et al.*, 2015), may lead to a better understanding of the complex events that constitute a migraine attack, and better and more targeted ways of intervention.

References

Afridi SK, Kaube H, Goadsby PJ (2004). Glyceryl trinitrate triggers premonitory symptoms in migraineurs. *Pain* **110**(3): 675–680.

Afridi SK, Giffin NJ, Kaube H, Friston KJ, Ward NS, Frackowiak RS, Goadsby PJ (2005a). A positron emission tomographic study in spontaneous migraine. *Archives of Neurology* **62**(8): 1270–1275.

Afridi SK, Matharu MS, Lee L, Kaube H, Friston KJ, Frackowiak RS, Goadsby PJ (2005b). A PET study exploring the laterality of brainstem activation in migraine using glyceryl trinitrate. *Brain* **128**(Pt 4): 932–939.

Ahn AH (2010). On the Temporal Relationship Between Throbbing Migraine Pain and Arterial Pulse. *Headache* **50**(9): 1507–1510.

Amara SG, Jonas V, Rosenfeld MG, Ong ES, Evans RM (1982). Alternative RNA processing in calcitonin gene expression generates mRNAs encoding different polypeptide products. *Nature* **298**(5871): 240–244.

Amin FM, Asghar MS, Guo S, Hougaard A, Hansen AE, Schytz HW, van der Geest RJ, de Koning PJ, Larsson HB, Olesen J, Ashina M (2012). Headache and prolonged dilatation of the middle meningeal artery by PACAP38 in healthy volunteers. *Cephalalgia* **32**(2): 140–149.

Amin FM, Asghar MS, Hougaard A, Hansen AE, Larsen VA, de Koning PJ, Larsson HB, Olesen J, Ashina M (2013). Magnetic resonance angiography of intracranial and extracranial arteries in patients with spontaneous migraine without aura: a cross-sectional study. *Lancet Neurology* **12**(5): 454–461.

Amin FM, Hougaard A, Schytz HW, Asghar MS, Lundholm E, Parvaiz AI, de Koning PJ, Andersen MR, Larsson HB, Fahrenkrug J, Olesen J, Ashina M (2014). Investigation of the pathophysiological mechanisms of migraine attacks induced by pituitary adenylate cyclase-activating polypeptide-38. *Brain* **137**(Pt 3): 779–94.

Antonova M, Wienecke T, Maubach K, Thomas E, Olesen J, Ashina M (2011a). The pharmacological effect of BGC20-1531, a novel prostanoid EP4 receptor antagonist, in the prostaglandin E2 human model of headache. *Journal of Headache and Pain* **12**(5): 551–559.

Antonova M, Wienecke T, Olesen J, Ashina M (2011b). Pro-inflammatory and vasoconstricting prostanoid PGF2alpha causes no headache in man. *Cephalalgia* **31**(15): 1532–1541.

Antonova M, Wienecke T, Olesen J, Ashina M (2012). Prostaglandin E2 induces immediate migraine-like attack in migraine patients without aura. *Cephalalgia* **32**(11): 822–33.

Arulmani U, Gupta S, VanDenBrink AM, Centurion D, Villalon CM, Saxena PR (2006). Experimental migraine models and their relevance in migraine therapy. *Cephalalgia* **26**(6): 642–659.

Asghar MS, Hansen AE, Kapijimpanga T, van der Geest RJ, van der Koning P, Larsson HB, Olesen J, Ashina M (2010). Dilation by CGRP of middle meningeal artery and reversal by sumatriptan in normal volunteers. *Neurology* **75**(17): 1520–1526.

Asghar MS, Hansen AE, Amin FM, van der Geest RJ, van der Koning P, Larsson HBW, Olesen J, Ashina M (2011). Evidence for a vascular factor in migraine. *Annals of Neurology* **69**(4): 635–645.

Ashina M, Bendtsen L, Jensen R, Schifter S, Olesen J (2000). Evidence for increased plasma levels of calcitonin gene-related peptide in migraine outside of attacks. *Pain* **86**(1–2): 133–138.

Ashina M, Tfelt-Hansen P, Dalgaard P, Olesen J (2011). Lack of correlation between vasodilatation and pharmacologically induced immediate headache in healthy subjects. *Cephalalgia* **31**(6): 683–690.

Ashina M, Hansen JM, Olesen J (2013). Pearls and pitfalls in human pharmacological models of migraine: 30 years' experience. *Cephalalgia* **33**(8): 540–553.

Baeres FM, Moller M (2004). Origin of PACAP-immunoreactive nerve fibers innervating the subarachnoidal blood vessels of the rat brain. *Journal of Cerebral Blood Flow & Metabolism* **24**(6): 628–635.

Bahra A, Matharu MS, Buchel C, Frackowiak RS, Goadsby PJ (2001). Brainstem activation specific to migraine headache. *Lancet* **357**(9261): 1016–1017.

Baun M, Pedersen MH, Olesen J, Jansen-Olesen I (2012). Dural mast cell degranulation is a putative mechanism for headache induced by PACAP-38. *Cephalalgia* **32**(4): 337–345.

Birk S, Sitarz JT, Petersen KA, Oturai PS, Kruuse C, Fahrenkrug J, Olesen J (2007). The effect of intravenous PACAP38 on cerebral hemodynamics in healthy volunteers. *Regulatory Peptides* **140**(3): 185–191.

Chanda ML, Tuttle AH, Baran I, Atlin C, Guindi D, Hathaway G, Israelian N, Levenstadt J, Low D, Macrae L, O'Shea L, Silver A, Zendegui E, Mariette Lenselink A, Spijker S, Ferrari MD, van den Maagdenberg AM, Mogil JS (2013). Behavioral evidence for photophobia and stress-related ipsilateral head pain in transgenic Cacna1a mutant mice. *Pain* **154**(8): 1254–1262.

Charles A (2013). Vasodilation out of the picture as a cause of migraine headache. *Lancet Neurology* **12**(5): 419–420.

Christiansen I, Thomsen LL, Daugaard D, Ulrich V, Olesen J (1999). Glyceryl trinitrate induces attacks of migraine without aura in sufferers of migraine with aura. *Cephalalgia* **19**(7): 660–667; discussion 626.

Connor KM, Shapiro RE, Diener HC, Lucas S, Kost J, Fan X, Fei K, Assaid C, Lines C, Ho TW (2009). Randomized, controlled trial of telcagepant for the acute treatment of migraine. *Neurology* **73**(12): 970–977.

Dodick DW, Goadsby PJ, Silberstein SD, Lipton RB, Olesen J, Ashina M, Wilks K, Kudrow D, Kroll R, Kohrman B, Bargar R, Hirman J, Smith J (2014a). Safety and efficacy of ALD403, an antibody to calcitonin gene-related peptide, for the prevention of frequent episodic migraine: a randomised, double-blind, placebo-controlled, exploratory phase 2 trial. *Lancet Neurology* **13**(11): 1100–1107.

Dodick DW, Goadsby PJ, Spierings EL, Scherer JC, Sweeney SP, Grayzel DS (2014b). Safety and efficacy of LY2951742, a monoclonal antibody to calcitonin gene-related peptide, for the prevention of migraine: a phase 2, randomised, double-blind, placebo-controlled study. *Lancet Neurology* **13**(9): 885–892.

Eikermann-Haerter K, Dilekoz E, Kudo C, Savitz SI, Waeber C, Baum MJ, Ferrari MD, van den Maagdenberg AM, Moskowitz MA, Ayata C (2009). Genetic and hormonal factors modulate spreading depression and transient hemiparesis in mouse models of familial hemiplegic migraine type 1. *Journal of Clinical Investigation* **119**(1): 99–109.

Garthwaite J, Charles SL, Chess-Williams R (1988). Endothelium-derived relaxing factor release on activation of NMDA receptors suggests role as intercellular messenger in the brain. *Nature* **336**(6197): 385–388.

Giffin NJ, Ruggiero L, Lipton RB, Silberstein SD, Tvedskov JF, Olesen J, Altman J, Goadsby PJ, Macrae A (2003). Premonitory symptoms in migraine: an electronic diary study. *Neurology* **60**(6): 935–940.

Goadsby PJ, Edvinsson L, Ekman R (1990). Vasoactive peptide release in the extracerebral circulation of humans during migraine headache. *Annals of Neurology* **28**(2): 183–187.

Gulbenkian S, Uddman R, Edvinsson L (2001). Neuronal messengers in the human cerebral circulation. *Peptides* **22**(6): 995–1007.

Guo S, Olesen J, Ashina M (2014). Phosphodiesterase 3 inhibitor cilostazol induces migraine-like attacks via cyclic AMP increase. *Brain* **137**(Pt 11): 2951–2959.

Hamel E (2006). Perivascular nerves and the regulation of cerebrovascular tone. *Journal of Applied Physiology (1985)* **100**(3): 1059–1064.

Hansen JM (2010). Familial hemiplegic migraine. *Danish Medical Bulletin* **57**(9): B4183.

Hansen JM, Sitarz J, Birk S, Rahmann AM, Oturai PS, Fahrenkrug J, Olesen J, Ashina M (2006). Vasoactive intestinal polypeptide evokes only a minimal headache in healthy volunteers. *Cephalalgia* **26**(8): 992–1003.

Hansen J, Thomsen L, Marconi R, Casari G, Olesen J, Ashina M (2008a). Familial hemiplegic migraine type 2 does not share hypersensitivity to nitric oxide with common types of migraine. *Cephalalgia* **28**(4): 367–375.

Hansen J, Thomsen L, Olesen J, Ashina M (2008b). Calcitonin gene-related peptide does not cause the familial hemiplegic migraine phenotype. *Neurology* **71**(11): 841–847.

Hansen J, Thomsen L, Olesen J, Ashina M (2008c). Familial hemiplegic migraine type 1 shows no hypersensitivity to nitric oxide. *Cephalalgia* **28**(5): 496–505.

Hansen JM, Thomsen LL, Olesen J, Ashina M (2010). Coexisting typical migraine in familial hemiplegic migraine. *Neurology* **74**(7): 594–600.

Hansen JM, Hauge AW, Olesen J, Ashina M (2010). Calcitonin gene-related peptide triggers migraine-like attacks in patients with migraine with aura. *Cephalalgia* **30**(10): 1179–1186.

Hansen JM, Thomsen LL, Olesen J, Ashina M (2011). Calcitonin gene-related peptide does not cause migraine attacks in patients with familial hemiplegic migraine. *Headache* **51**(4): 544–553.

Harmar AJ, Arimura A, Gozes I, Journot L, Laburthe M, Pisegna JR, Rawlings SR, Robberecht P, Said SI, Sreedharan SP, Wank SA, Waschek JA (1998). International Union of Pharmacology. *XVIII. Nomenclature of receptors for vasoactive intestinal peptide and pituitary adenylate cyclase-activating polypeptide. Pharmacological Reviews* **50**(2): 265–270.

Hata AN, Breyer RM (2004). Pharmacology and signaling of prostaglandin receptors: multiple roles in inflammation and immune modulation. *Pharmacology & Therapeutics* **103**(2): 147–166.

Hering C (1849). Glonoine, a new medicine for headache etc. *American Journal of Homeopathy* (**4**): 3.

Ho TW, Ferrari MD, Dodick DW, Galet V, Kost J, Fan X, Leibensperger H, Froman S, Assaid C, Lines C, Koppen H, Winner PK (2008a). Efficacy and tolerability of MK-0974 (telcagepant), a new oral antagonist of calcitonin gene-related peptide receptor, compared with zolmitriptan for acute migraine: a randomised, placebo-controlled, parallel-treatment trial. *Lancet* **372**(9656): 2115–2123.

Ho TW, Mannix LK, Fan X, Assaid C, Furtek C, Jones CJ, Lines CR, Rapoport AM (2008b). Randomized controlled trial of an oral CGRP receptor antagonist, MK-0974, in acute treatment of migraine. *Neurology* **70**(16): 1304–1312.

Ho TW, Connor KM, Zhang Y, Pearlman E, Koppenhaver J, Fan X, Lines C, Edvinsson L, Goadsby PJ, Michelson D (2014). Randomized controlled trial of the CGRP receptor antagonist telcagepant for migraine prevention. *Neurology* **83**(11): 958–966.

Hoivik HO, Laurijssens BE, Harnisch LO, Twomey CK, Dixon RM, Kirkham AJ, Williams PM, Wentz AL, Lunnon MW (2010). Lack of efficacy of the selective iNOS inhibitor GW274150 in prophylaxis of migraine headache. *Cephalalgia* **30**(12): 1458–1467.

Hosoya M, Onda H, Ogi K, Masuda Y, Miyamoto Y, Ohtaki T, Okazaki H, Arimura A, Fujino M (1993). Molecular cloning and functional expression of rat cDNAs encoding the receptor for pituitary adenylate cyclase activating polypeptide (PACAP). *Biochemical and Biophysical Research Communications* **194**(1): 133–143.

Hughes R, Dake J (1888). *Cyclopedia of drug pathogenesy*. Boerike and Tafel, New York.

Hullugundi SK, Ansuini A, Ferrari MD, van den Maagdenberg AM, Nistri A (2014). A hyperexcitability phenotype in mouse trigeminal sensory neurons expressing the R192Q

Cacna1a missense mutation of familial hemiplegic migraine type-1 (FHM1). *Neuroscience* **266**: 244–54.

International Classification of Headache Disorders (2013). Headache Classification Committee of the International Headache Society (IHS) 3rd edition (beta version). *Cephalalgia*. **33**(9): 629–808.

Iversen HK, Olesen J, Tfelt-Hansen P (1989). Intravenous nitroglycerin as an experimental model of vascular headache. Basic characteristics. *Pain* **38**(1): 17–24.

Iversen HK, Holm S, Friberg L, Tfelt-Hansen P (2008). Intracranial hemodynamics during intravenous infusion of glyceryl trinitrate. *Journal of Headache and Pain* **9**(3): 177–180.

Jansen-Olesen I, Mortensen A, Edvinsson L (1996). Calcitonin gene-related peptide is released from capsaicin-sensitive nerve fibres and induces vasodilatation of human cerebral arteries concomitant with activation of adenylyl cyclase. *Cephalalgia* **16**(5): 310–316.

Jansen-Olesen I, Gulbenkian S, Engel U, Cunha e Sa M, Edvinsson L (2004). Peptidergic and non-peptidergic innervation and vasomotor responses of human lenticulostriate and posterior cerebral arteries. *Peptides* **25**(12): 2105–2114.

Jen JC, Kim GW, Dudding KA, Baloh RW (2004). No mutations in CACNA1A and ATP1A2 in probands with common types of migraine. *Archives of Neurology* **61**(6): 926–928.

Kirchmann M, Thomsen LL, Olesen J (2006). The CACNA1A and ATP1A2 genes are not involved in dominantly inherited migraine with aura. *American Journal of Medical Genetics Part B: Neuropsychiatric Genetics* **141B**: 250–256.

Kruuse C, Thomsen LL, Birk S, Olesen J (2003). Migraine can be induced by sildenafil without changes in middle cerebral artery diameter. *Brain* **126**(Pt 1): 241–247.

Kruuse C, Lassen LH, Iversen HK, Oestergaard S, Olesen J (2006). Dipyridamole may induce migraine in patients with migraine without aura. *Cephalalgia* **26**(8): 925–933.

Lassen LH, Thomsen LL, Olesen J (1995). Histamine induces migraine via the H1-receptor. Support for the NO hypothesis of migraine. *Neuroreport* **6**(11): 1475–1479.

Lassen LH, Ashina M, Christiansen I, Ulrich V, Olesen J (1997). Nitric oxide synthase inhibition in migraine. *Lancet* **349**(9049): 401–402.

Lassen LH, Haderslev PA, Jacobsen VB, Iversen HK, Sperling B, Olesen J (2002). CGRP may play a causative role in migraine. *Cephalalgia* **22**(1): 54–61.

Leo L, Gherardini L, Barone V, De Fusco M, Pietrobon D, Pizzorusso T, Casari G (2011). Increased susceptibility to cortical spreading depression in the mouse model of familial hemiplegic migraine type 2. *PLoS Genetics* **7**(6): e1002129.

Levy D, Burstein R, Strassman AM (2005). Calcitonin gene-related peptide does not excite or sensitize meningeal nociceptors: implications for the pathophysiology of migraine. *Annals of Neurology* **58**(5): 698–705.

Lutz EM, Sheward WJ, West KM, Morrow JA, Fink G, Harmar AJ (1993). The VIP2 receptor: molecular characterisation of a cDNA encoding a novel receptor for vasoactive intestinal peptide. *FEBS Letters* **334**(1): 3–8.

Mainero C, Boshyan J, Hadjikhani N (2011). Altered functional magnetic resonance imaging resting-state connectivity in periaqueductal gray networks in migraine. *Annals of Neurology* **70**(5): 838–845.

Maniyar FH, Sprenger T, Monteith T, Schankin C, Goadsby PJ (2014). Brain activations in the premonitory phase of nitroglycerin-triggered migraine attacks. *Brain* **137**(Pt 1): 232–241.

Mao J, Coghill RC, Kellstein DE, Frenk H, Mayer DJ (1992). Calcitonin gene-related peptide enhances substance P-induced behaviors via metabolic inhibition: *in vivo* evidence for a new mechanism of neuromodulation. *Brain Research* **574**(1–2): 157–163.

McGuinness BW, Harris EL (1961). "Monday head": an interesting occupational disorder. *British Medical Journal (Clinical Research Edition)* **2**(5254): 745–747.

Murrell W (1879). Nitro-glycerine as a remedy for angina pectoris. *Lancet* **113**(2890): 80–81.

Netzer C, Todt U, Heinze A, Freudenberg J, Zumbroich V, Becker T, Goebel I, Ohlraun S, Goebel H, Kubisch C (2006). Haplotype-based systematic association studies of ATP1A2 in migraine with aura. *American Journal of Medical Genetics Part B: Neuropsychiatric Genetics* **141B**: 257–260.

Nichols FT, 3rd, Mawad M, Mohr JP, Stein B, Hilal S, Michelsen WJ (1990). Focal headache during balloon inflation in the internal carotid and middle cerebral arteries. *Stroke* **21**(4): 555–559.

Northfield DWC (1938). Some observations on headache *Brain* **61**(2): 133–162.

Oku R, Satoh M, Fujii N, Otaka A, Yajima H, Takagi H (1987). Calcitonin gene-related peptide promotes mechanical nociception by potentiating release of substance P from the spinal dorsal horn in rats. *Brain Research* **403**(2): 350–354.

Olesen J, Iversen HK, Thomsen LL (1993). Nitric oxide supersensitivity: a possible molecular mechanism of migraine pain. *Neuroreport* **4**(8): 1027–1030.

Olesen J, Diener HC, Husstedt IW, Goadsby PJ, Hall D, Meier U, Pollentier S, Lesko LM (2004). Calcitonin gene-related peptide receptor antagonist BIBN 4096 BS for the acute treatment of migraine. *New England Journal of Medicine* **350**(11): 1104–1110.

Olesen J, Tfelt-Hansen P, Ashina M (2009). Finding new drug targets for the treatment of migraine attacks. *Cephalalgia* **29**(9): 909–920.

Rahmann A, Wienecke T, Hansen JM, Fahrenkrug J, Olesen J, Ashina M (2008). Vasoactive intestinal peptide causes marked cephalic vasodilation, but does not induce migraine. *Cephalalgia* **28**(3): 226–236.

Rosenfeld MG, Mermod JJ, Amara SG, Swanson LW, Sawchenko PE, Rivier J, Vale WW, Evans RM (1983). Production of a novel neuropeptide encoded by the calcitonin gene via tissue-specific RNA processing. *Nature* **304**(5922): 129–135.

Russo AF (2014). Calcitonin Gene-Related Peptide (CGRP): A New Target for Migraine. *Annual Review of Pharmacology and Toxicology* **55**: 533–52.

Sances G, Tassorelli C, Pucci E, Ghiotto N, Sandrini G, Nappi G (2004). Reliability of the nitroglycerin provocative test in the diagnosis of neurovascular headaches. *Cephalalgia* **24**(2): 110–119.

Schoonman GG, van der Grond J, Kortmann C, van der Geest RJ, Terwindt GM, Ferrari MD (2008). Migraine headache is not associated with cerebral or meningeal vasodilatation – a 3T magnetic resonance angiography study. *Brain* **131**(Pt 8): 2192–2200.

Schwedt TJ, Larson-Prior L, Coalson RS, Nolan T, Mar S, Ances BM, Benzinger T, Schlaggar BL (2013). Allodynia and Descending Pain Modulation in Migraine: A Resting State Functional Connectivity Analysis. *Pain Medicine* **15**(1): 154–65.

Schwedt TJ, Chiang CC, Chong CD, Dodick DW (2015). Functional MRI of migraine. *Lancet Neurology* **14**(1): 81–91.

Schytz HW, Birk S, Wienecke T, Kruuse C, Olesen J, Ashina M (2009). PACAP38 induces migraine-like attacks in patients with migraine without aura. *Brain* **132**(Pt 1): 16–25.

Schytz HW, Olesen J, Ashina M (2010). The PACAP receptor: a novel target for migraine treatment. *Neurotherapeutics* **7**(2): 191–196.

Sherwood NM, Krueckl SL, McRory JE (2000). The origin and function of the pituitary adenylate cyclase-activating polypeptide (PACAP)/glucagon superfamily. *Endocrine Reviews* **21**(6): 619–670.

Sicuteri F, Del Bene E, Poggioni M, Bonazzi A (1987). Unmasking latent dysnociception in healthy subjects. *Headache* **27**(4): 180–185.

Sixt ML, Messlinger K, Fischer MJ (2009). Calcitonin gene-related peptide receptor antagonist olcegepant acts in the spinal trigeminal nucleus. *Brain* **132**(11): 3134–3141.

Summ O, Charbit AR, Andreou AP, Goadsby PJ (2010). Modulation of nocioceptive transmission with calcitonin gene-related peptide receptor antagonists in the thalamus. *Brain* **133**(Pt 9): 2540–2548.

Sun RQ, Lawand NB, Willis WD (2003). The role of calcitonin gene-related peptide (CGRP) in the generation and maintenance of mechanical allodynia and hyperalgesia in rats after intradermal injection of capsaicin. *Pain* **104**(1–2): 201–208.

Sun RQ, Lawand NB, Lin Q, Willis WD (2004). Role of calcitonin gene-related peptide in the sensitization of dorsal horn neurons to mechanical stimulation after intradermal injection of capsaicin. *Journal of Neurophysiology* **92**(1): 320–326.

Tegeler CH, Davidai G, Gengo FM, Knappertz VA, Troost BT, Gabriel H, Davis RL (1996). Middle cerebral artery velocity correlates with nitroglycerin-induced headache onset. *Journal of Neuroimaging* **6**(2): 81–86.

Tfelt-Hansen PC, Tfelt-Hansen J (2009). Nitroglycerin headache and nitroglycerin-induced primary headaches from 1846 and onwards: a historical overview and an update. *Headache* **49**(3): 445–456.

Thomsen LL, Iversen HK, Brinck TA, Olesen J (1993). Arterial supersensitivity to nitric oxide (nitroglycerin) in migraine sufferers. *Cephalalgia* **13**(6): 395–399; discussion 376.

Thomsen LL., Kruuse C., Iversen HK., J. O (1994). A nitric oxide donor (nitroglycerin) triggers genuine migraine attacks. *European Journal of Neurology* **1**: 73–80.

Tuka B, Helyes Z, Markovics A, Bagoly T, Nemeth J, Mark L, Brubel R, Reglodi D, Pardutz A, Szolcsanyi J, Vecsei L, Tajti J (2012). Peripheral and central alterations of pituitary adenylate cyclase activating polypeptide-like immunoreactivity in the rat in response to activation of the trigeminovascular system. *Peptides* **33**(2): 307–316.

Tvedskov JF, Lipka K, Ashina M, Iversen HK, Schifter S, Olesen J (2005). No increase of calcitonin gene-related peptide in jugular blood during migraine. *Annals of Neurology* **58**(4): 561–568.

van den Maagdenberg AM, Pietrobon D, Pizzorusso T, Kaja S, Broos LA, Cesetti T, van de Ven RC, Tottene A, van der Kaa J, Plomp JJ, Frants RR, Ferrari MD (2004). A Cacna1a knockin migraine mouse model with increased susceptibility to cortical spreading depression. *Neuron* **41**(5): 701–710.

van den Maagdenberg AM, Pizzorusso T, Kaja S, Terpolilli N, Shapovalova M, Hoebeek FE, Barrett CF, Gherardini L, van de Ven RC, Todorov B, Broos LA, Tottene A, Gao Z, Fodor M, De Zeeuw CI, Frants RR, Plesnila N, Plomp JJ, Pietrobon D, Ferrari MD (2010). High cortical spreading depression susceptibility and migraine-associated symptoms in Ca(v)2.1 S218L mice. *Annals of Neurology* **67**(1): 85–98.

Van der Schueren BJ, Lunnon MW, Laurijssens BE, Guillard F, Palmer J, Van Hecken A, Depre M, Vanmolkot FH, de Hoon JN (2009). Does the unfavorable pharmacokinetic and pharmacodynamic profile of the iNOS inhibitor GW273629 lead to inefficacy in acute migraine? *Journal of Clinical Pharmacology* **49**(3): 281–290.

Weiller C, May A, Limmroth V, Juptner M, Kaube H, Schayck RV, Coenen HH, Diener HC (1995). Brain stem activation in spontaneous human migraine attacks. *Nature Medicine* **1**(7): 658–660.

Wienecke T, Olesen J, Oturai PS, Ashina M (2008). Prostacyclin (epoprostenol) induces headache in healthy subjects. *Pain* **139**(1): 106–116.

Wienecke T, Olesen J, Ashina M (2009a). Prostaglandin I(2) (epoprostenol) triggers migraine-like attacks in migraineurs. *Cephalalgia* **30**(2): 179–90.

Wienecke T, Olesen J, Oturai PS, Ashina M (2009b). Prostaglandin E2(PGE2) induces headache in healthy subjects. *Cephalalgia* **29**(5): 509–519.

Wienecke T, Olesen J, Ashina M (2011). Discrepancy between strong cephalic arterial dilatation and mild headache caused by prostaglandin D (PGD). *Cephalalgia* **31**(1): 65–76.

Wieser T, Mueller C, Evers S, Zierz S, Deufel T (2003). Absence of known familial hemiplegic migraine (FHM) mutations in the CACNA1A gene in patients with common migraine: implications for genetic testing. *Clinical Chemistry and Laboratory Medicine* **41**: 272–275.

21

Imaging pain and headache

Duncan J. Hodkinson, Sophie L. Wilcox and David Borsook

P.A.I.N. Group, Department of Anesthesiology, Perioperative & Pain Medicine, Boston Children's Hospital, Harvard Medical School, Boston, Massachusetts, USA

21.1   Introduction

The trigeminal system is involved in processing nociceptive information from the oral, facial, and cranial territories. Trigeminal mechanisms of nociception have some specific features, compared with the spinal nociceptive system, and many of these will be outlined in this book. In this chapter, we focus on the central processing of trigeminal nociception, described on the basis of human imaging studies, and describe how these studies have provided valuable advances in our understanding of migraine disorders. The following sections will provide an overview of the imaging literature that has helped to uncover the mechanisms underlying the development and evolution of migraine and its specific symptoms. We present evidence that the migraine brain is abnormal outside of attacks, and that repeated attacks may lead to structural alterations in the brain which may, in turn, drive the transformation of migraine to its chronic form. We also highlight some features of other orofacial pain disorders as a way to bring together the CNS mechanisms of trigeminal nociception, and discuss how these relate to the pathophysiology of migraine.

21.2   Functional brain changes in migraine

21.2.1   Headache

From a pain perspective, migraine is unique, in that headache and its associated features are seen in the absence of any obvious cause. Despite many years of investigation, the source of migraine remains elusive. In the past decade, a more "neurocentric" view of the disorder has emerged, based upon findings of human imaging studies, which have shown activations in the brainstem during acute migraine and cluster headache attacks (Weiller *et al.*, 1995; May *et al.*, 1998; Bahra *et al.*, 2001; Afridi *et al.*, 2005). The brainstem activation in almost all these studies appears to be located in the dorsolateral pons, which has led to the hypothesis that dysfunction of this structure is perhaps at the core of the disorder (Akerman *et al.*, 2011). Some authors speculate that this is in fact the

Neurobiological Basis of Migraine, First Edition. Edited by Turgay Dalkara and Michael A. Moskowitz.
© 2017 John Wiley & Sons, Inc. Published 2017 by John Wiley & Sons, Inc.

"generator" of the migraine attack, but this concept has been challenged and remains an area for further investigation (Borsook and Burstein, 2012).

More broadly speaking, there is a large number of imaging and neurophysiological studies which have shown that nociceptive stimuli (trigeminal and somatic) elicit responses in an extensive cortical network, including somatosensory, insular and cingulate areas, as well as frontal and parietal areas. This cortical network may represent a basic mechanism through which significant events for the body's integrity are detected, regardless of the sensory channel through which these events are conveyed (Legrain *et al.*, 2011; Borsook *et al.*, 2013b) (See Figure 21.1).

21.2.2 Aura

It is estimated that approximately one quarter of migraines are preceded by neurological symptoms associated with a transient cortical malfunction, collectively known as *aura* (Lauritzen, 1994). Such cortical disturbances are thought to arise from the phenomenon of cortical spreading depression (CSD), which occurs spontaneously before the onset of the headache. Due to the episodic nature of migraine, it is extremely challenging to perform clinical studies of aura, in particular functional imaging studies of spontaneous migraine events. Nevertheless, Sanchez del Rio and colleagues reported cerebral hypoperfusion (decreased CBF) during aura in the occipital cortex controlaterally to the symptoms (Sanchez del Rio *et al.*, 1999). Also, Hadjikhani and colleagues reported seeing reductions in stimulus-driven BOLD signal fluctuations, in response to checkerboard stimulations, at a rate similar to CSD in the occipital cortex (Hadjikhani *et al.*, 2001). While these findings were preliminary, they strongly supported the idea that CSD may be the cause of migraine aura.

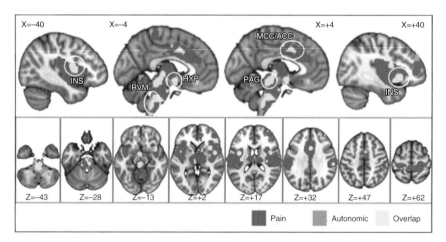

Figure 21.1 Common pathways associated with pain and autonomic function. Brain meta-analytic maps were produced for the terms "pain" (410 studies) and "autonomic" (87 studies), using the NeuroSynth framework (Yarkoni *et al.*, 2011). Automatically generated reverse inference maps show the probability of the term given observed activation (P(term|act.)). Masks for all images are shown only for regions that survived a test of association between term and activation, with a whole-brain correction for multiple comparisons (FDR < 0.05). Abbreviations: INS – insular; RVM – rostral ventral medulla; HYP – hypothalamus; PAG – periaqueductal gray; MCC/ACC – mid cingulate cortex/anterior cingulate cortex.

21.2.3 Allodynia and hyperalgesia

During migraine attacks, approximately 80% of patients exhibit symptomatic or mea-surable cutaneous allodynia (the perception of pain in response to normally innocuous stimuli) and hyperalgesia (hypersensitivity to noxious stimuli) (Burstein *et al.*, 2000). It has been proposed that these symptoms are the consequence of central sensitization of second order neurons at the level of the spinal trigeminal nucleus caudalis and thala-mus (Burstein *et al.*, 1998; Woolf, 2011). One fMRI study, specifically investigating the response to non-trigeminal heat and brush stimuli in migraineurs with extracephalic allodynia, found that thalamic responses were significantly larger when patients were suffering a migraine attack (Burstein *et al.*, 2010). The thalamus is known to be a major site for the processing and modulation of pain (Tracey and Mantyh, 2007), so these find-ings may explain the spread of cutaneous allodynia and hyperalgesia to referred pain areas in the head (localized) or body (extended) (Strassman *et al.*, 1996).

21.2.4 Photophobia, phonophobia, and olfactory discomfort

Sensitivity to light, noise, and/or smells accompanies most attacks of migraine and often persists, to some extent, between attacks. In recent years, a number of neuroimaging studies have been performed to specifically address sensory processing deficits and pho-bic symptoms in migraine patients, with some studies exploring the interrelationship between sensory input and pain processing during the ictal state (Boulloche *et al.*, 2010; Denuelle *et al.*, 2011; Martin *et al.*, 2011; Stankewitz and May, 2011). Common to each of these studies, it appears that sensory processing in migraine is modulated by concomi-tant painful trigeminal stimulation. This finding is supported by recent experimental work in rats, showing that neurons in the thalamus, receiving nociceptive inputs from the dural vasculature, also respond to light (photic) stimuli (Noseda *et al.*, 2010).

Bright light is known to activate nociceptive neurons of the trigeminocervical com-plex (Okamoto *et al.*, 2010) and, thus, sensitivity of the senses may increase during the migraine prodome, and intense sensory stimuli may trigger an attack. Interestingly, the heightened sensitivity in one sensory modality is often associated with heightened sen-sitivity in other modalities, suggesting the involvement of a common mechanism.

21.2.5 Habituation

A hallmark of migraine is the lack of habituation during stimulus repetition. Several studies measuring spontaneous fMRI and EEG responses to evoked sensory stimuli have confirmed the habituation deficits in migraineurs (Wang and Schoenen, 1998; Afra *et al.*, 2000; Coppola *et al.*, 2009; Stankewitz *et al.*, 2013). It has been proposed that this deficit may reflect increased neuronal excitability, decreased inhibition, or decreased preac-tivation levels. The phenomenon is present interictally, not only in adults but also in children, with a significant correlation in deficient habituation between children and their parents (Sandor *et al.*, 1999), indicating a possible heritable character. Migraine type or classification may also be important, as a cohort of familial hemiplegic migraine patients showed increased habituation (Hansen *et al.*, 2011).

21.2.6 Autonomic dysfunction and other non-pain symptoms

Other frequently reported symptoms associated with migraine include altered mood, stress, irritability, fatigue, sleeplessness, exaggerated emotional responses, nausea, and loss of appetite. To elicit such varied symptoms, nociceptive signals that originate in the trigeminovascular pathway during migraine must modulate the activity of hypothalamic, amygdala and basal forebrain structures that integrate sensory, physiological, and cognitive signals that drive behavioral, affective, and autonomic responses (Burstein and Jakubowski, 2005).

The involvement of the hypothalamus in migraine has been the topic of a recent review (Geraud and Donnet, 2013), and activation of hypothalamic regions in spontaneous headache attacks has been demonstrated in two imaging studies (May *et al.*, 1998; Denuelle *et al.*, 2007). Our group recently found that migraine patients in their interictal phase have increased hypothalamic connectivity, with a number of brain regions involved in regulation of autonomic functions, including the locus coeruleus, caudate, parahippocampal gyrus, cerebellum, and the temporal pole (Moulton *et al.*, 2014). In addition, there is strong support for the role of the basal ganglia in pain processing (Borsook *et al.*, 2010), and recent imaging studies suggest a significant role of the basal ganglia in the pathophysiology of episodic migraine (Maleki *et al.*, 2011; Yuan *et al.*, 2013). Altogether, these findings point to an underlying brain dysfunction that causes vulnerability to migraine (Denk *et al.*, 2014), and the susceptibility of an actual attack may be driven by the failure of the brain and body to respond to further stressors (see Figure 21.2).

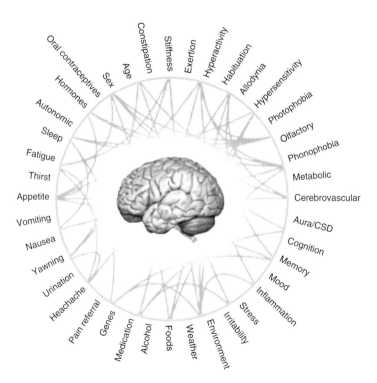

Figure 21.2 Nonlinear network of mediators involved in migraine. There is a central role of the brain in allostasis and the behavioral and physiological response to stressors. Grey lines indicate that each system interacts with the others in a reciprocal manner, creating a nonlinear network.

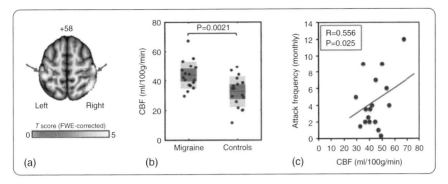

Figure 21.3 Interictal migraine-related increase of regional cerebral blood flow (rCBF) in the primary somatosensory cortices. (a) Quantitative measures of rCBF were acquired using the magnetic resonance imaging (MRI) technique – arterial spin labeling (ASL). Dotted black lines correspond to the boundary of central sulcus (CS) and post-central sulcus (PoCS). Group-wise statistical images (Migraine ($n = 17$) > Controls ($n = 17$)] are displayed with a cluster probability threshold of P < 0.05, corrected for multiple comparisons (FWE). (b) Magnitude of the CBF changes within S1. Plots represent the mean (center line), 95% confidence interval (light-grey region), and one standard deviation (dark-grey region). Individual subjects data are shown as circular markers. (c) Correlations between rCBF and clinical variables. Headache attack frequency was positively correlated with CBF. The underlying dysfunction in S1 and the trigemino-cortical pathway may cause vulnerability to migraine attacks (Figure adapted from Hodkinson *et al.*, 2015b).

21.2.7 Cerebrovascular and metabolic dysfunction

A fundamental role of the autonomic nervous system is regulating cerebral blood flow (CBF) (Goadsby, 2013). Human imaging studies performed during the different phases of attacks, and also in interictal periods, have shown varying effects on CBF (Bartolini *et al.*, 2005). These conflicting results may depend on the different imaging strategies used to measure CBF and the type of migraine disorder; hence, the effects might therefore not be directly comparable.

It is well known that cortical responsivity to sensory stimuli fluctuates over time in relation to the migraine cycle. A recent study suggests that basal CBF expresses both circadian and homeostatic variability (Hodkinson *et al.*, 2014), which may be important in cluster headaches, where the attack patterns show circannual and circadian periodicity. Cerebral metabolic homeostasis may also be disrupted by the increased energy demands caused by the neuronal hyperexcitability during attacks and, to an even greater extent, before attacks (Reyngoudt *et al.*, 2012). This disruption may lead to triggering of the trigeminovascular system and, subsequently, the migraine attack (see Figure 21.3).

21.3 Structural brain changes in migraine

Migraine has been shown not only to involve functional abnormalities over time, but also to be associated with structural changes in the brain. Methods based on high-resolution structural MRI to assess structural changes include: voxel-based morphometry (VBM); surface-based techniques, such as cortical thickness (CT); and diffusion tensor imaging (DTI). These imaging methods have been used extensively to investigate neuroplasticity in grey and white matter in both healthy and patient populations, showing that brain structure may change dynamically.

In chronic pain in general, numerous studies have shown that various chronic pain conditions are associated with changes in brain structure, when compared with healthy controls (Tracey and Bushnell, 2009). These structural alterations, while displaying a degree of pain-type/condition/study specificity, also share some overlap (Smallwood *et al.*, 2013). More specifically in the migraine field, structural imaging studies have also shown evidence that migraine is associated with structural changes in both grey and white matter (Sprenger and Borsook, 2012; Bashir *et al.*, 2013; Hougaard *et al.*, 2014), although interesting studies challenging this conclusion have also arisen. The following section will review the relevant studies of structural changes in migraine, reviewing both grey and white matter alterations.

21.3.1 Grey matter alterations in migraine

Whole-brain VBM is the most frequently used method to assess structural changes in grey matter. It quantifies grey matter volume on a voxel-wise basis, and allows for the detection of volume differences both between groups, and within individuals, over time. Interestingly, the first VBM study by Matharu *et al.* (2003) showed no significant grey matter changes in episodic migraine, compared to healthy controls. A subsequent VBM study by Schmidt-Wilcke *et al.* (2008), with a larger cohort of episodic migraineurs, continued to show no significant grey matter changes at the whole brain level. However, when a region-of-interest approach was employed, "subtle" grey matter reductions in migraineurs were observed in the anterior and posterior cingulate cortex and the insula.

The use of uncorrected statistical thresholds and region of interest approaches in these two pioneering VBM studies may account for the disparity in findings, an issue that has continued in the migraine structural literature (May, 2013). Most recently, Liu *et al.* (2015) reported grey matter increases in the hippocampus, parahippocampal gyrus, amygdala, cerebellum and the occipital cortices, and grey matter reductions in the middle frontal gyrus, superior frontal gyrus, inferior parietal lobule, supramarginal gyrus, temporal cortices and the occipital cortices in female migraineurs with aura, compared with healthy controls. Most interestingly, the authors found evidence that this grey matter increase in the hippocampus of migraineurs may be related to a specific genetic variant, which has been linked to synaptic plasticity and maladaptive stress.

Taken together, these studies present fairly cohesive evidence for grey matter increases and reductions in migraine, particularly in the posterior insula-opercular regions, the prefrontal cortex, and the anterior cingulate cortex (See meta-analyses by Bashir *et al.*, 2013; Dai *et al.*, 2015; Hu *et al.*, 2015). Given the nature of these grey matter changes (namely, being reductions in regions recognized as being involved in pain processing or the response to pain, and having an association with disease duration), several studies have proposed that these structural alterations are a consequence of repeated painful insults during migraine attacks, rather than a causative factor (Maleki *et al.*, 2013; see Figure 21.4). This proposition is supported by evidence from a longitudinal VBM study of newly diagnosed migraineurs by Liu *et al.* (2013), which found grey matter decreases in various brain regions, including the superior frontal

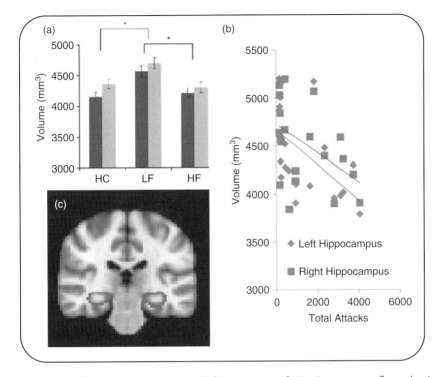

Figure 21.4 Grey matter alterations in the hippocampus of migraineurs may reflect adaptive plasticity in response to repeated migraine attacks and allostatic load. (a) Differences in hippocampal volume. The bar plots show the hippocampus volume comparisons for low frequency (LF), high frequency (HF) and healthy controls (HC). LF migraineurs had a significantly larger hippocampal volume. (b) Migraine attacks and hippocampal volumetric differences. The plots represent the correlation between the left and right hippocampal volumes and estimate of the total number of migraine attacks. (c) The hippocampus represented on the standard MNI152 anatomical template. Figure adapted from Maleki *et al.* (2012).

gyrus, orbitofrontal cortex, hippocampus, precuneus, parietal gyrus and postcentral gyrus at one year follow-up, compared with initial diagnosis.

A more recently developed method to assess structural changes in grey matter, specifically cortical thickness, is surface-based morphometry. The first study to employ this measure in migraine, by Granziera *et al.* (2006), reported increased cortical thickness of motion-processing visual areas MT+ and V3A. Further work also showed increased cortical thickness in the somatosensory cortex (postcentral gyrus) in the region of the somatotopic representation of the head (DaSilva *et al.*, 2007a), a finding replicated by Kim, who also observed a correlation between this increased cortical thickness and disease duration and frequency.

In a manner similar to the VBM literature, there is not complete consensus that migraine is associated with alterations in cortical thickness. Datta *et al.* (2011) reported an absence of changes in cortical thickness in migraineurs, even after specifically investigating specific subregions reported to show differences. As of yet, the lack of structural studies in migraine employing both VBM and surface-based analysis makes it difficult to reconcile the apparent difference in the direction (VBM decreases vs. cortical thickness increases) of grey matter alterations in migraine.

21.3.2   White matter alterations in migraine

The most commonly used method to assess structural changes in white matter is diffusion tenor imaging (DTI), a technique that provides information on the microstructural properties of white matter tracts, based on the diffusion of endogenous water molecules in brain tissue. White matter properties are commonly assessed through several standard diffusion parameters, including fractional anisotropy (FA) and mean diffusivity (MD). White matter connections (fiber pathways) can also be identified and quantified by probabilistic tractography.

The first study that employed DTI to assess white matter in migraineurs identified lower FA values in cortical and sub-cortical regions associated with visual motion perception (V3A, MT+, superior colliculus and lateral geniculate nucleus) in migraineurs both with and without aura (Granziera *et al.*, 2006). Subsequent work by DaSilva *et al.* (2007b) identified reduced FA in aspects of the trigeminal somatosensory pathway (posterior limb of the internal capsule and trigeminothalamic tract), a finding replicated in part by Yu *et al.* (2013), who also found lower FA and MD in the anterior and posterior limb of the internal capsule and throughout the corpus callosum. In turn, lower FA in the corpus callosum was also found by Li *et al.* (2011), who investigated migraineurs both with and without a comorbid emotional (depressive/anxious) disorder.

Both Yu's and Li's studies also found an association between the diffusion parameters in these regions and clinical features, including headache duration and frequency. Taken together, these findings have been interpreted as evidence that repeated migraine attacks may provoke damage in the white matter tracts involved in trigeminal somatosensory processing. However, the interpretation of diffusion findings is highly variable, as changes in FA may be influenced by several factors, such as myelination, axon density, gliosis and inflammation.

In a similar manner, it is still debatable as to whether these white matter alterations are a predisposing factor or a consequence of repeated migraine attacks. While several studies have found a correlation between DTI metrics and clinical features, the aforementioned longitudinal study of newly diagnosed migraineurs by Liu *et al.* (2013) also assessed diffusion changes, and found no differences in white matter structure at one-year follow-up, compared with initial diagnosis. Finally, as with grey matter changes, there is not complete consensus that migraine is associated with structural changes in white matter, with a recent study by Neeb *et al.* (2015) finding no evidence of white matter structural changes in either episodic or chronic migraine.

21.4   Insights from orofacial pain

Certain features of orofacial pain disorders may help bring together CNS mechanisms of trigeminal nociception, and should be considered when discussing the pathophysiology of migraine (Hargreaves, 2011). A recent meta-analysis review of imaging studies found that trigeminal neuropathic pain (TNP) and temporomandibular disorder (TMD) patients show functional and structural changes in the thalamus and the primary somatosensory cortex, suggesting that the thalamocortical pathway is a possible major site of plasticity (Lin, 2014).

Interestingly, direct comparison of these two chronic orofacial pain conditions suggests that some functional and structural changes in the brain may be unique to specific pain types (Gustin *et al.*, 2011). For example, cortical reorganization in the primary somatosensory cortex may be unique to neuropathic pain (TNP), but not to musculoskeletal pain (TMD) (Gustin *et al.*, 2012). In addition, imaging studies frequently report changes in the prefrontal cortex (PFC) and the basal ganglia (Lin, 2014), suggesting the disruption of cognitive (descending) modulation and reward processing in chronic orofacial pain (Navratilova and Porreca, 2014). Other imaging reports of experientially evoked painful and non-painful stimulation have indicated somatotopic representation in the component nociceptive brain regions receiving input from the trigeminal nerve (Jantsch *et al.*, 2005; Upadhyay *et al.*, 2008; Nash *et al.*, 2009; Weigelt *et al.*, 2010).

Further work in patients undergoing trigeminal surgery has demonstrated alterations in regional cerebral blood flow (rCBF) in response to acute ongoing post-surgical pain and recovery with analgesia (Hodkinson *et al.*, 2013, 2015a). Collectively, these trigeminal models of pain, including chronic conditions and post-surgical/prolonged acute pain, represent a unique opportunity to apply neuroimaging techniques to all levels of the ascending (and descending) pain pathway from the level of the primary afferent and synapse (Wilcox *et al.*, 2015a, 2015b) to higher level (cortical) areas (Borsook *et al.*, 2006). The imaging findings and relationship to symptoms are critical in many clinical pain states, and appear to share some similarities with the symptoms reported by patients with migraine. We believe that a better understanding of nociceptive signaling in oral and craniofacial pain may translate into targets for migraine preventative treatments.

21.5 Conclusions

In the last decade, imaging has helped transform our perception that migraine is simply an "event that comes and goes". Those affected by the disorder exhibit clear signs of brain dysfunction in relation to their symptoms, with many changes evolving differently before (pre-ictal), during (ictal), and immediately after (post-ictal) an attack. The imaging literature surrounding brain structural abnormalities is far from clear, but it is generally agreed that the observed changes are not the cause of the disorder but, rather, increase vulnerability to migraine (Denk *et al.*, 2014), thus causing an increased frequency of attacks and the development of chronic daily headache.

A unique feature of migraine that has been overlooked is the fact that attacks are often characterized by passive coping strategies, such as error awareness (Borsook *et al.*, 2013a), which is consistent with sickness behavior. We argue that these deviations from, or interruption of, the normal brain structure or function may be the consequence of allostatic loading (notwithstanding genetic, epigenetic, social or psychological factors), as the repeated migraine attacks start maladaptive mechanisms that may result in a chronic pain of the brain (Borsook *et al.*, 2012).

References

Afra J, Proietti Cecchini A, Sandor PS, Schoenen J (2000). Comparison of visual and auditory evoked cortical potentials in migraine patients between attacks. *Clinical Neurophysiology* **111**: 1124–1129.

Afridi SK, Matharu MS, Lee L, Kaube H, Friston KJ, Frackowiak RS, Goadsby PJ (2005). A PET study exploring the laterality of brainstem activation in migraine using glyceryl trinitrate. *Brain* **128**: 932–939.

Akerman S, Holland PR, Goadsby PJ (2011). Diencephalic and brainstem mechanisms in migraine. *Nature Reviews Neuroscience* **12**: 570–584.

Bahra A, Matharu MS, Buchel C, Frackowiak RS, Goadsby PJ (2001). Brainstem activation specific to migraine headache. *Lancet* **357**: 1016–1017.

Bartolini M, Baruffaldi R, Paolino I, Silvestrini M (2005). Cerebral blood flow changes in the different phases of migraine. *Functional Neurology* **20**: 209–211.

Bashir A, Lipton RB, Ashina S, Ashina M (2013). Migraine and structural changes in the brain: a systematic review and meta-analysis. *Neurology* **81**: 1260–1268.

Borsook D, Burstein R (2012). The enigma of the dorsolateral pons as a migraine generator. *Cephalalgia* **32**: 803–812.

Borsook D, Burstein R, Moulton E, Becerra L (2006). Functional imaging of the trigeminal system: applications to migraine pathophysiology. *Headache* **46**(Suppl 1): S32–38.

Borsook D, Upadhyay J, Chudler EH, Becerra L (2010). A key role of the basal ganglia in pain and analgesia – insights gained through human functional imaging. *Molecular Pain* **6**: 27.

Borsook D, Maleki N, Becerra L, McEwen B (2012). Understanding migraine through the lens of maladaptive stress responses: a model disease of allostatic load. *Neuron* **73**: 219–234.

Borsook D, Aasted CM, Burstein R, Becerra L (2013a). Migraine Mistakes: Error Awareness. *The Neuroscientist* **20**: 291–304.

Borsook D, Edwards R, Elman I, Becerra L, Levine J (2013b). Pain and analgesia: the value of salience circuits. *Progress in Neurobiology* **104**: 93–105.

Boulloche N, Denuelle M, Payoux P, Fabre N, Trotter Y, Geraud G (2010). Photophobia in migraine: an interictal PET study of cortical hyperexcitability and its modulation by pain. *Journal of Neurology, Neurosurgery, and Psychiatry* **81**: 978–984.

Burstein R, Jakubowski M (2005). Unitary hypothesis for multiple triggers of the pain and strain of migraine. *Journal of Comparative Neurology* **493**: 9–14.

Burstein R, Yamamura H, Malick A, Strassman AM (1998). Chemical stimulation of the intracranial dura induces enhanced responses to facial stimulation in brain stem trigeminal neurons. *Journal of Neurophysiology* **79**: 964–982.

Burstein R, Yarnitsky D, Goor-Aryeh I, Ransil BJ, Bajwa ZH (2000). An association between migraine and cutaneous allodynia. *Annals of Neurology* **47**: 614–624.

Burstein R, Jakubowski M, Garcia-Nicas E, Kainz V, Bajwa Z, Hargreaves R, Becerra L, Borsook D (2010). Thalamic sensitization transforms localized pain into widespread allodynia. *Annals of Neurology* **68**: 81–91.

Coppola G, Pierelli F, Schoenen J (2009). Habituation and migraine. *Neurobiology of Learning and Memory* **92**: 249–259.

Dai Z, Zhong J, Xiao P, Zhu Y, Chen F, Pan P, Shi H (2015). Gray matter correlates of migraine and gender effect: A meta-analysis of voxel-based morphometry studies. *Neuroscience* **299**: 88–96.

DaSilva AF, Granziera C, Snyder J, Hadjikhani N (2007a). Thickening in the somatosensory cortex of patients with migraine. *Neurology* **69**: 1990–1995.

DaSilva AF, Granziera C, Tuch DS, Snyder J, Vincent M, Hadjikhani N (2007b). Interictal alterations of the trigeminal somatosensory pathway and periaqueductal gray matter in migraine. *Neuroreport* **18**: 301–305.

Datta R, Detre JA, Aguirre GK, Cucchiara B (2011). Absence of changes in cortical thickness in patients with migraine. *Cephalalgia* **31**: 1452–1458.

Denk F, McMahon SB, Tracey I (2014). Pain vulnerability: a neurobiological perspective. *Nature Neuroscience* **17**: 192–200.

Denuelle M, Fabre N, Payoux P, Chollet F, Geraud G (2007). Hypothalamic activation in spontaneous migraine attacks. *Headache* **47**: 1418–1426.

Denuelle M, Boulloche N, Payoux P, Fabre N, Trotter Y, Geraud G (2011). A PET study of photophobia during spontaneous migraine attacks. *Neurology* **76**: 213–218.

Geraud G, Donnet A (2013). Migraine and hypothalamus. *Revue Neurologique* **169**: 372–379.

Goadsby PJ (2013). Autonomic nervous system control of the cerebral circulation. *Handbook of Clinical Neurology* **117**: 193–201.

Granziera C, DaSilva AF, Snyder J, Tuch DS, Hadjikhani N (2006). Anatomical alterations of the visual motion processing network in migraine with and without aura. *PLoS Medicine* **3**: e402.

Gustin SM, Peck CC, Wilcox SL, Nash PG, Murray GM, Henderson LA (2011). Different pain, different brain: thalamic anatomy in neuropathic and non-neuropathic chronic pain syndromes. *The Journal of Neuroscience* **31**: 5956–5964.

Gustin SM, Peck CC, Cheney LB, Macey PM, Murray GM, Henderson LA (2012). Pain and plasticity: is chronic pain always associated with somatosensory cortex activity and reorganization? *Journal of Neuroscience* **32**: 14874–14884.

Hadjikhani N, Sanchez Del Rio M, Wu O, Schwartz D, Bakker D, Fischl B, Kwong KK, Cutrer FM, Rosen BR, Tootell RB, Sorensen AG, Moskowitz MA (2001). Mechanisms of migraine aura revealed by functional MRI in human visual cortex. *Proceedings of the National Academy of Sciences of the United States of America* **98**: 4687–4692.

Hansen JM, Bolla M, Magis D, de Pasqua V, Ashina M, Thomsen LL, Olesen J, Schoenen J (2011). Habituation of evoked responses is greater in patients with familial hemiplegic migraine than in controls: a contrast with the common forms of migraine. *European Journal of Neurology* **18**: 478–485.

Hargreaves KM (2011). Orofacial pain. *Pain* **152**: S25–32.

Hodkinson DJ, Krause K, Khawaja N, Renton TF, Huggins JP, Vennart W, Thacker MA, Mehta MA, Zelaya FO, Williams SC, Howard MA (2013). Quantifying the test-retest reliability of cerebral blood flow measurements in a clinical model of on-going post-surgical pain: A study using pseudo-continuous arterial spin labelling. *NeuroImage Clinical* **3**: 301–310.

Hodkinson DJ, O'Daly O, Zunszain PA, Pariante CM, Lazurenko V, Zelaya FO, Howard MA, Williams SC (2014). Circadian and homeostatic modulation of functional connectivity and regional cerebral blood flow in humans under normal entrained conditions. *Journal of Cerebral Blood Flow and Metabolism* **34**: 1493–1499.

Hodkinson DJ, Khawaja N, O'Daly O, Thacker MA, Zelaya FO, Wooldridge CL, Renton T, Williams SC, Howard MA (2015a). Cerebral analgesic response to non-steroidal anti-inflammatory drug ibuprofen. *Pain* **156**(7): 1301–10.

Hodkinson DJ, Veggeberg R, Wilcox SL, Scrivani S, Burstein R, Becerra L, Borsook D (2015b). Primary somatosensory cortices contain altered patterns of regional cerebral blood flow in the interictal phase of migraine. *PLoS One* **10**(9): e0137971.

Hougaard A, Amin FM, Ashina M (2014). Migraine and structural abnormalities in the brain. *Current Opinion in Neurology* **27**: 309–314.

Hu W, Guo J, Chen N, Guo J, He L (2015). A meta-analysis of voxel-based morphometric studies on migraine. *International Journal of Clinical and Experimental Medicine* **8**: 4311–4319.

Jantsch HH, Kemppainen P, Ringler R, Handwerker HO, Forster C (2005). Cortical representation of experimental tooth pain in humans. *Pain* **118**: 390–399.

Lauritzen M (1994). Pathophysiology of the migraine aura. The spreading depression theory. *Brain* **117**(Pt 1): 199–210.

Legrain V, Iannetti GD, Plaghki L, Mouraux A (2011). The pain matrix reloaded: a salience detection system for the body. *Progress in Neurobiology* **93**: 111–124.

Li XL, Fang YN, Gao QC, Lin EJ, Hu SH, Ren L, Ding MH, Luo BN (2011). A diffusion tensor magnetic resonance imaging study of corpus callosum from adult patients with migraine complicated with depressive/anxious disorder. *Headache* **51**: 237–245.

Lin CS (2014). Brain signature of chronic orofacial pain: a systematic review and meta-analysis on neuroimaging research of trigeminal neuropathic pain and temporomandibular joint disorders. *PloS One* **9**: e94300.

Liu J, Lan L, Li G, Yan X, Nan J, Xiong S, Yin Q, von Deneen KM, Gong Q, Liang F, Qin W, Tian J (2013). Migraine-related gray matter and white matter changes at a 1-year follow-up evaluation. *Journal of Pain* **14**: 1703–1708.

Liu J, Lan L, Mu J, Zhao L, Yuan K, Zhang Y, Huang L, Liang F, Tian J (2015). Genetic contribution of catechol-O-methyltransferase in hippocampal structural and functional changes of female migraine sufferers. *Human Brain Mapping* **36**(5): 1782–95.

Maleki N, Becerra L, Nutile L, Pendse G, Brawn J, Bigal M, Burstein R, Borsook D (2011). Migraine attacks the Basal Ganglia. *Molecular Pain* **7**: 71.

Maleki N, Becerra L, Upadhyay J, Burstein R, Borsook D (2012). Direct optic nerve pulvinar connections defined by diffusion MR tractography in humans: implications for photophobia. *Human Brain Mapping* **33**(1): 75–88.

Maleki N, Becerra L, Brawn J, McEwen B, Burstein R, Borsook D (2013). Common hippocampal structural and functional changes in migraine. *Brain Structure & Function* **218**: 903–912.

Martin H, Sanchez del Rio M, de Silanes CL, Alvarez-Linera J, Hernandez JA, Pareja JA (2011). Photoreactivity of the occipital cortex measured by functional magnetic resonance imaging-blood oxygenation level dependent in migraine patients and healthy volunteers: pathophysiological implications. *Headache* **51**: 1520–1528.

Matharu MS, Good CD, May A, Bahra A, Goadsby PJ (2003). No change in the structure of the brain in migraine: a voxel-based morphometric study. *European Journal of Neurology* **10**: 53–57

May A, Bahra A, Buchel C, Frackowiak RS, Goadsby PJ (1998). Hypothalamic activation in cluster headache attacks. *Lancet* **352**: 275–278.

May A (2013). Pearls and pitfalls: neuroimaging in headache. *Cephalalgia* **33**: 554–565.

Moulton EA, Becerra L, Johnson A, Burstein R, Borsook D (2014). Altered hypothalamic functional connectivity with autonomic circuits and the locus coeruleus in migraine. *PloS One* **9**: e95508.

Nash PG, Macefield VG, Klineberg IJ, Murray GM, Henderson LA (2009). Differential activation of the human trigeminal nuclear complex by noxious and non-noxious orofacial stimulation. *Human Brain Mapping* **30**: 3772–3782.

Navratilova E, Porreca F (2014). Reward and motivation in pain and pain relief. *Nature Neuroscience* **17**: 1304–1312.

Neeb L, Bastian K, Villringer K, Gits HC, Israel H, Reuter U, Fiebach JB (2015). No microstructural white matter alterations in chronic and episodic migraineurs: a case-control diffusion tensor magnetic resonance imaging study. *Headache* **55**: 241–251.

Noseda R, Kainz V, Jakubowski M, Gooley JJ, Saper CB, Digre K, Burstein R (2010). A neural mechanism for exacerbation of headache by light. *Nature Neuroscience* **13**: 239–245.

Okamoto K, Tashiro A, Chang Z, Bereiter DA (2010). Bright light activates a trigeminal nociceptive pathway. *Pain* **149**: 235–242.

Reyngoudt H, Achten E, Paemeleire K (2012). Magnetic resonance spectroscopy in migraine: what have we learned so far? *Cephalalgia* **32**: 845–859.

Sanchez del Rio M, Bakker D, Wu O, Agosti R, Mitsikostas DD, Ostergaard L, Wells WA, Rosen BR, Sorensen G, Moskowitz MA, Cutrer FM (1999). Perfusion weighted imaging during migraine: spontaneous visual aura and headache. *Cephalalgia* **19**: 701–707.

Sandor PS, Afra J, Proietti-Cecchini A, Albert A, Schoenen J (1999). Familial influences on cortical evoked potentials in migraine. *Neuroreport* **10**: 1235–1238.

Schmidt-Wilcke T, Gansbauer S, Neuner T, Bogdahn U, May A (2008). Subtle grey matter changes between migraine patients and healthy controls. *Cephalalgia* **28**: 1–4.

Smallwood RF, Laird AR, Ramage AE, Parkinson AL, Lewis J, Clauw DJ, Williams DA, Schmidt-Wilcke T, Farrell MJ, Eickhoff SB, Robin DA (2013). Structural brain anomalies and chronic pain: a quantitative meta-analysis of gray matter volume. *Journal of Pain* **14**: 663–675.

Sprenger T, Borsook D (2012). Migraine changes the brain: neuroimaging makes its mark. *Current Opinion in Neurology* **25**: 252–262.

Stankewitz A, May A (2011). Increased limbic and brainstem activity during migraine attacks following olfactory stimulation. *Neurology* **77**: 476–482.

Stankewitz A, Schulz E, May A (2013). Neuronal correlates of impaired habituation in response to repeated trigemino-nociceptive but not to olfactory input in migraineurs: an fMRI study. *Cephalalgia* **33**: 256–265.

Strassman AM, Raymond SA, Burstein R (1996). Sensitization of meningeal sensory neurons and the origin of headaches. *Nature* **384**: 560–564.

Tracey I, Bushnell MC (2009). How neuroimaging studies have challenged us to rethink: is chronic pain a disease? *Journal of Pain* **10**: 1113–1120.

Tracey I, Mantyh PW (2007). The cerebral signature for pain perception and its modulation. *Neuron* **55**: 377–391.

Upadhyay J, Knudsen J, Anderson J, Becerra L, Borsook D (2008). Noninvasive mapping of human trigeminal brainstem pathways. *Magnetic Resonance in Medicine* **60**: 1037–1046.

Wang W, Schoenen J (1998). Interictal potentiation of passive "oddball" auditory event-related potentials in migraine. *Cephalalgia* **18**: 261–265; discussion 241.

Weigelt A, Terekhin P, Kemppainen P, Dorfler A, Forster C (2010). The representation of experimental tooth pain from upper and lower jaws in the human trigeminal pathway. *Pain* **149**: 529–538.

Weiller C, May A, Limmroth V, Juptner M, Kaube H, Schayck RV, Coenen HH, Diener HC (1995). Brain stem activation in spontaneous human migraine attacks. *Nature Medicine* **1**: 658–660.

Wilcox SL, Gustin SM, Macey PM, Peck CC, Murray GM, Henderson LA (2015a). Anatomical changes at the level of the primary synapse in neuropathic pain: evidence from the spinal trigeminal nucleus. *Journal of Neuroscience* **35**: 2508–2515.

Wilcox SL, Gustin SM, Macey PM, Peck CC, Murray GM, Henderson LA (2015b). Anatomical changes within the medullary dorsal horn in chronic temporomandibular disorder pain. *NeuroImage* **117**: 258–266.

Woolf CJ (2011). Central sensitization: implications for the diagnosis and treatment of pain. *Pain* **152**: S2–15.

Yu D, Yuan K, Qin W, Zhao L, Dong M, Liu P, Yang X, Liu J, Sun J, Zhou G, von Deneen KM, Tian J (2013). Axonal loss of white matter in migraine without aura: a tract-based spatial statistics study. *Cephalalgia* **33**: 34–42.

Yuan K, Zhao L, Cheng P, Yu D, Zhao L, Dong T, Xing L, Bi Y, Yang X, von Deneen KM, Liang F, Gong Q, Qin W, Tian J (2013). Altered structure and resting-state functional connectivity of the basal ganglia in migraine patients without aura. *Journal of Pain* **14**: 836–844.

Index

Neurobiological Basis of Migraine, First Edition. Edited by Turgay Dalkara and Michael A. Moskowitz.
© 2017 John Wiley & Sons, Inc. Published 2017 by John Wiley & Sons, Inc.